Technique of the Neurologic Examination

A Programmed Text

TECHNIQUE OF THE NEUROLOGIC EXAMINATION: *A Programmed Text*

234567890WHWH89876543210

This book was set in Alphatype English by John C. Meyer & Son. The editors were Richard S. Laufer and Henry C. De Leo; the production supervisor was Jeanne Skahan. The cover was designed by John Hite. The Whitlock Press, Inc., was printer and binder.

Library of Congress Cataloging in Publication Data

DeMyer, William, date
Technique of the neurologic examination.

Includes bibliographies and index.
1. Neurologic examination. I. Title.
RC348.D44 1980 616.8'04'75 79-26471
ISBN 0-07-016352-9

Technique of the Neurologic Examination

A Programmed Text

Third Edition

William DeMyer, M.D.
Professor of Neurology
Indiana University School of Medicine
Indianapolis

McGRAW-HILL BOOK COMPANY

New York St. Louis San Francisco Auckland Bogotá Hamburg
Johannesburg London Madrid Mexico Montreal New Delhi Panama
Paris São Paulo Singapore Sydney Tokyo Toronto

Contents

Preface to the Third Edition

The major additions to this third edition include a summary of the neurologic examination of the unconscious patient, a discussion of the neuroanatomy of consciousness, and the use of the neurologic examination in the diagnosis of hysteria. The major deletions consist of pruning some of the less successful, mainly verbal, programmed responses. The text comes that much closer to presenting the situations you will actually meet and rehearsing only the real responses you should learn to make. This key principle remains the basis of the text.

I want to thank the many students who have made suggestions for improving the text. Let me hear from you. I am listening.

WILLIAM DeMYER

Preface to the First Edition

The purpose of this textbook is threefold: (1) to teach how to conduct a neurologic examination, (2) to review the anatomy and physiology for interpreting it, and (3) to show which laboratory tests help to clarify the clinical problem. This is not a differential diagnosis text nor a systematic description of diseases.

Anyone who sets out to write a textbook should place his manuscript on one knee and a student on the other. When the student squirms, sighs, or gives a wrong answer, the author has erred. He should correct it right then, before the ink dries. That is the way I have written this text, on the basis of feedback from the students.

The peril of student-on-the-knee teaching is that even though the student moves his lips, the words and voice remain the teacher's. To escape from ventriloquism, my text relies strongly on self-observation and induction. First, you learn to observe yourself, not as Narcissus, but as a sample of every man. Whenever possible you study living flesh, its look, its feel, and its responses. Why study a textbook picture to learn the range of ocular movements if you can hold up a hand mirror? Why memorize the laws of diplopia if you can do a simple experiment on yourself whenever you need to refresh your memory? In the best tradition of science, these techniques supplant the printed word as the source of knowledge. The text becomes a way of extending your own perceptions, of looking at the world through the eyes of experience.

Since programmed instruction is the best way for the learner himself to judge whether learning has taken place most of the text is programmed. He is not abandoned to guess whether he has learned something; the program makes him prove that he has learned. Programming, if abused or overdone, becomes incredibly dull, unmercifully slow. The reader is required to inspect a grain of sand at a time, yet he should have been shown the whole shoreline at a glance. Some programs err by bristling with objectivity, causing one to ask, "Isn't there a human being around here somewhere? Didn't someone think this, decide it, maybe even guess at it a little?" For interludes, I use quotations, anecdotes, and poetry. I even stoop to mnemonics. Sometimes I cajole, not pretending as is customary in textbooks, that the pages have been purified, relieved of an author. I am very much here, poking my head out of a paragraph now and then or peering at you through an asterisk. When I see that you are weary from filling in blanks, I offer some whimsy. When you overflow with something to say, I ask for an essay answer. Sometimes you are invited to anticipate the text, to match wits against the problem without the spoon. At all times as you practice the neurologic examination, I stand at your elbow, guiding your moves and interpretations. You should be able to do a prideful neurologic examination when you finish the book. And lastly, I include references. Only one reader in a hundred uses them? I am interested in him too, in his precious curiosity.

These then are the secrets: a lot of self-observation, a lot of programming, some irony and humor, a few editorials, and occasionally a summarizing paragraph, like this one. And as the leaven, lest they vanish from medical education, reminders of the bittersweet flowers of the mind, of tenderness, of understanding and compassion . . . like this stanza from Yeats, because it is perhaps all that should preface a text like this, into which I have poured the best teaching that I can offer, and yet the wish always exceeds the result, ah me, by far:

Had I the heavens' embroidered cloths,
Enwrought with gold and silver light,
The blue and the dim and the dark cloths
Of night and light and the half light,
I would spread the cloths under your feet;
But I, being poor, have only my dreams;
I have spread my dreams under your feet;
Tread softly because you tread on my dreams.

To the many colleagues who have shared their knowledge with me over the years, I am deeply grateful. I want especially to thank Dr. Alexander T. Ross, my own preceptor in clinical neurology, and many friends in the basic disciplines of neurology, Drs. Ralph Reitan, Charles Ferster, Sidney Ochs, Wolfgang Zeman, and Jans Muller. For their day-to-day help I thank my wife, Dr. Marian DeMyer, Dr. Mark Dyken, and the many medical students, interns, and residents who suffered through the stuttering phases of the programming. And then, Miss Irene Baird, who meticulously, maternally made the drawings; Mrs. Faith Halstead, who typed and retyped the burgeoning manuscript; medical artist James Glore; and photographer Joseph Demma.

WILLIAM DeMYER

Preparation for the Text

I assume that you have finished a year of medical school and have learned the basic concepts of neuroanatomy and neurophysiology (but I review some of them anyway). The text will teach you the vocabulary and intellectual and manual skills needed to do the neurologic examination. Your teachers, then freed from the necessity to transmit this kind of data by lectures, can use precious class hours solely for demonstrating patients who illustrate the material covered in the text. Then if you can go directly to the clinics and wards, you have the ideal situation for learning the neurologic examination.

Since the text requires you to inspect yourself and others, study in your own living quarters, preferably with a partner. You must have some basic examining equipment, which will be listed shortly, and some learning aids. As learning aids get colored pencils, a hand mirror, and a table tennis ball. Don't start until you have all of the items.

Do the text in order. Skipping around invites disaster since each learning sequence locks steps with the one before and presumes mastery of previous material. Allow approximately one hour for each nine pages of material you want to cover.

At the outset, I have found that students want most of all to know: just what is a neurologic examination? Thus I begin my text (and my classes) by outlining a standard complete neurologic examination. Of course you can't do the outline now—that's what the rest of the text is for—but use it in two ways: (1) refer back to it each time you complete a text chapter, to fit what you have learned into the total examination and (2) take it with you to wards and clinics to guide you until you can do it alone.

Abbreviations Used in This Text

ACA Anterior cerebral artery
AComA Anterior communicating artery
AICA Anterior inferior cerebellar artery
AP Anteroposterior
ARAS Ascending reticular activating system
BE Branchial efferent
BP Blood pressure
C Cervical
CAT Computerized axial tomography
cm Centimeter
CNS Central nervous system
cps Cycles per second
CSF Cerebrospinal fluid
EEG Electroencephalogram
EMG Electromyogram
F False
IAA Internal auditory artery
ICA Internal carotid artery
L Lateral, left, or lumbar
LMN Lower motor neuron
MCA Middle cerebral artery
MLF Medial longitudinal fasciculus
mm Millimeters
MSR Muscle stretch reflex
OFC Occipitofrontal circumference
PCA Posterior cerebral artery
PComA Posterior communicating artery
PICA Posterior inferior cerebellar artery
R Right
RBC Red blood cells
S Sacral
SA Somatic afferent
SCA Superior cerebellar artery
SCM Sternocleidomastoid muscle
SE Somatic efferent
SSSS Solely Special Sensory Set (referring to cranial nerves I, II, and VIII)
SVA Special visceral afferent
T True
TNR Tonic neck reflex
UMN Upper motor neuron
V Vertical
VA Visceral afferent
VE Visceral efferent
WBC White blood cells

Summarized Neurological Examination

(The next nine pages summarize the sequence of steps in the neurologic examination. The body of the text, which begins with Chap. 1, explains how to do each step in the sequence.)

I. Introduction

A. How the history guides the examination

1. You can complete much of the neurological examination while you take the history. You appraise the patient's mental status and make several preliminary observations. Inspect his facial features for diagnostic abnormalities; watch his eye movements and eye blinking, and inspect the relation of limbus to lids and the palpebral fissures; look for en- or exophthalmos; note the degree and symmetry of facial movements; listen to his speech pattern, and observe how he swallows saliva; inspect his posture, and look for tremors and involuntary movements.
2. While you will, of course, do a basic routine examination on everyone, the history and preliminary observations tell you how to plan your examination and what areas to emphasize: either central or neuromuscular motor system; sensory system; cranial nerves; or cerebral functions. For example, if the history suggests a spinal cord problem, plan to do a detailed sensory examination of the perianal region for loss or preservation of sacral sensation. But if the history suggests a cerebral lesion, emphasize tests for astereognosis, aphasia, and inattention to simultaneous stimuli.
3. Finally, the history gives clues to or suggests special tests tailored to the particular patient's problems. During the examination, reproduce any conditions which the patient thinks may aggravate or precipitate his complaint. Some common examples are:
   a. Dizziness when standing up: check for orthostatic hypotension.
   b. Episodic complaints of numbness and tingling in extremities, blackout or fainting spells or suspected epilepsy: ask the patient to hyperventilate for a full three minutes.
   c. Weakness in climbing stairs: watch the patient climb stairs.
   d. Trouble swallowing: give the patient something to swallow.
   e. Pathologic fatiguability, particularly of cranial nerve muscles: have patient make 100 repetitive movements and do edrophonium (Tensilon) test for myasthenia gravis.

B. How to remember to do a complete examination

The formal examination must follow an orderly sequence. Neurologists may differ in the order they choose, but they will do essentially the same things. To remember how to follow the order I recommend, you must lay out your instruments in the order of use. As you finish with each one, replace it in your bag. When you have replaced every instrument or laid it aside, you will have done a complete examination, without forgetting anything. Here is the order of use for your instruments:

Instruments	*Use*
1. Flexible steel measuring tape scored in metric system	Measurement of occipitofrontal and other body circumferences, size of skin lesions, length of extremities, etc.
2. Stethoscope	Auscultation of the neck vessels, eyes, and cranium for bruits.
3. Flashlight with rubber adaptor	Pupillary reflexes, inspection of pharynx, and transillumination of the head.
4. Transparent mm ruler	Measurement of pupillary size, diameter of skin lesions, distances on radiographic films.
5. Ophthalmoscope	Funduscopy, examination of ocular media and skin surface for beads of sweat.
6. Tongue blades	Three per patient: one for depressing tongue, one for eliciting gag reflex, one broken for eliciting abdominal and plantar reflexes.
7. Opaque vial of coffee	Testing sense of smell.
8. Opaque vials of salt and sugar	Testing taste.
9. Otoscope	Examination of auditory canal and drum.
10. Tuning fork	Testing vibratory sensation and hearing (256 cps recommended).
11. 10 cc syringe	Caloric irrigation of the ear.
12. Cotton wisp	One end rolled for eliciting corneal reflex, the other loose for testing light touch.
13. Two stoppered plastic tubes	Testing hot and cold discrimination.
14. Disposable straight pins	Testing pain sensation.
15. Reflex hammer	Eliciting muscle stretch reflexes.
16. Penny, nickel, dime, paper clip, and key	Testing stereognosis.
17. Page of figure-stimuli	Screening cerebral and intellectual functions.
18. Blood pressure cuff	Routine BP and orthostatic hypotension.

II. Mental status examination

A. *General behavior and appearance.* Is the patient normal, hyperactive, agitated, quiet, immobile? Is the patient neat or slovenly? Does the patient dress in accordance with age, peers, sex, and background?

B. *Stream of talk.* Does the patient converse normally? Is the speech rapid, incessant, under great pressure, or is it slow and lacking in spontaneity? Is the patient discursive and unable to reach the conversational goal?

C. *Mood and affective responses.* Is the patient euphoric, agitated, inappropriately gay, giggling, or is he silent, weeping, angry? Does his mood swing in a direction appropriate to the subject matter of the conversation? Is he emotionally labile?

D. *Content of thought.* Does the patient have illusions, hallucinations or delusions, and misinterpretations? Is he preoccupied with bodily complaints, fears of cancer or heart disease, or other phobias? Does the patient suffer delusions of persecution and surveillance by malicious persons or forces?

E. *Intellectual capacity.* Is he bright, average, dull, or obviously demented or mentally retarded?

F. *Sensorium*

1. Consciousness
2. Attention span
3. Orientation for time, place, and person
4. Memory, recent and remote, as disclosed during history taking
5. Fund of information
6. Insight, judgement, and planning
7. Calculation

III. Speech. Is it normal or does the patient display

A. *Dysphonia:* difficulty in producing the voice sound.

B. *Dysarthria:* difficulty in articulating the individual sounds or the units (phonemes) of speech: f's, r's, g's, vowels, consonants, the labials (cranial nerve VII), gutturals (X), and linguals (XII).

C. *Dysprosody:* difficulty with the stress of syllables, inflections, pitch of voice, and the rhythm of words.

D. *Dysphasia:* difficulty in expressing or understanding words as the symbols of communication.

IV. Head and face

A. *Inspection*

1. What general impression does the patient's face make? Any unusual features? Is it a diagnostic facial *gestalt?* Does it show normal motility and emotional expression?
2. Inspect the eyes for ptosis, width of palpebral fissures, relation of iris to lids, pupillary size, and interorbital distance.
3. Inspect contours of nose, mouth, chin, and ears.
4. Inspect the hair of scalp, eyebrows, and beard.
5. Inspect the head for abnormalities in shape and symmetry.

B. *Palpate* the skull of a mature patient for lumps, depression or tenderness, and asymmetries and of an infant for fontanelles and sutures. Palpate the carotid and temporal arteries. Measure and record the occipitofrontal circumference in all infants.

C. *Percuss* sinuses and mastoid processes for tenderness if the patient has headaches.

D. *Auscultate* for bruits over the great vessels, eyes, temples, and mastoid processes.

E. *Transilluminate* the sinuses if the patient has headaches. Attempt to transilluminate the skull of every young infant.

V. Cranial nerves

A. Optic group: II, III, IV, and VI

1. Inspect width of palpebral fissures, relation of limbus to lid margins, interorbital distance, and en- or exophthalmos.
2. *Visual functions:* test acuity (central fields) by newsprint (each eye separately), and test peripheral fields by confrontation. Test for inattention to simultaneous stimuli if cerebral lesion suspected.
3. Test pupillary light reflexes, and record size of pupils.
4. Do ophthalmoscopy.
5. *Ocular motility:* test range of ocular movements by having patient's eyes follow your finger through all fields of gaze. During convergence check for miosis. Record nystagmus and any effects of eye movements on it.

B. Branchiomotor group and tongue: V, VII, IX-X, XII, and XI

1. V: inspect masseter and temporalis muscle bulk, and palpate masseter when the patient bites.
2. VII: forehead wrinkling, eyelid closure, mouth retraction, whistle, or puff out cheeks, wrinkle skin over neck (platysma), and labial articulation. Check for Chvostek's sign in selected cases.
3. IX-X: phonation, nasality of articulation, swallowing, gag reflex, palatal elevation.
4. XII: lingual articulations, midline and lateral tongue protrusion, inspect for atrophy, and fasciculations.
5. XI: inspect sternocleidomastoid and trapezius contours, and test strength of head movements and shoulder shrugging.
6. Test for pathologic fatigability by requesting 100 repetitive movements (eye blink, etc) if the history raises this question. Consider edrophonium Cl (Tensilon) test.

C. Special sensory group

1. *Olfaction* (I): use aromatic, nonirritating substance and test each nostril separately.
2. *Taste* (VII): use salt or sugar. (Test if VIIth nerve lesion suspected.)
3. *Hearing* (VIII):
   a. Do otoscopy.
   b. *Threshold and acuity:* adequacy of hearing for conversational speech, ability to hear tuning fork, watch tick or rustling of fingers.
   c. If history or preceding tests suggest a deficit, do air-borne conduction test of Rinné and vertex lateralizing test of Weber.
   d. If the history suggests a cerebral lesion, test for auditory inattention to bilateral simultaneous stimuli, using finger rustling.
   e. In infant or uncooperative patient, use auditopalpebral reflex as crude screening test.
4. *Vestibular function* (VIII): do caloric irrigation in selected patients, and test for positional nystagmus.

D. Somatic sensation of the face (Testing trigeminal area sensation now obviates a return to the face after examining the patient's anogenital area and feet.)

1. Corneal reflex (V-VII arc).
2. Light touch over the three divisions of the Vth nerve.

3. Pain perception over the three divisions of the Vth nerve.
4. Temperature discrimination.
5. Buccal mucosa sensation is tested in selected cases.

VI. Somatic motor system (exclusive of cranial nerves)

A. *Inspection*

1. Initial appraisal of the motor system occurs when you take the history. Inspect the patient for his posture, general activity level, tremors, and involuntary movements.
2. Undress the patient and ponder his somatotype (his build or body *gestalt*).
3. Search his entire skin surface for lesions, particularly neurocutaneous stigmata such as *café au lait* spots.
4. Observe the size and contour of his muscles looking for atrophy, hypertrophy, body asymmetry, joint malalignments, fasciculations, tremors, and involuntary movements.
5. *Gait testing:* free walking, toe and heel walking, tandem walking, deep-knee bend. If a child, have him hop on each foot and run.

B. *Palpation:* palpate muscles if they seem atrophic, hypertrophic, or if the history suggests that they may be tender or in spasm.

C. *Strength testing*

1. *Shoulder girdle:* try to press the patient's arms down after he abducts them to shoulder height. Look for scapular winging.
2. *Upper extremities:* test biceps, triceps, wrist dorsiflexors, and grip. Test strength of finger abduction and extension.
3. *Abdominal muscles:* have patient do a situp. Watch for umbilical migration.
4. *Lower extremities:* test hip flexors, abductors and adductors, knee flexors, foot dorsiflexors, invertors, and evertors. (Knee extensors were tested by the deep knee bend.)
5. Discern whether any weakness follows a distributional pattern such as proximal-distal, right-left, or upper extremity-lower extremity. Grade strength on a scale of 0 to 5 or describe as paralysis, severe, moderate or minimal weakness, or normal.

D. *Percussion:* percuss the thenar eminence for percussion myotonia and test for myotonic grip if patient has generalized muscular weakness.

E. *Muscle tone:* make passive movements of joints to test for spasticity, clonus, or rigidity.

F. *Muscle stretch (deep) reflexes* (Grade 0 to 4+ and designate whether clonic):

1. Jaw jerk (V afferent, V efferent).
2. Biceps reflex (C5-6).
3. Triceps reflex (C7-8).
4. Finger flexion reflex (C7-T1).
5. Quadriceps reflex (L2-4).
6. Hamstrings reflex (L5-S1-2).
7. Triceps surae reflex or ankle jerk (L5-S1-3).
8. Toe flexion reflex (S1-2).

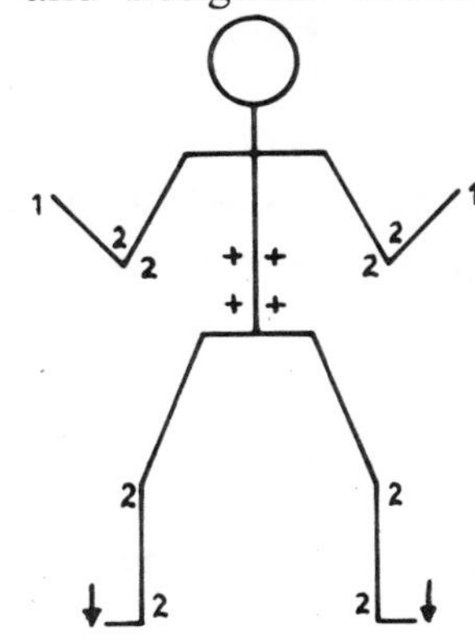

G. Skin-muscle (superficial) reflexes

1. Abdominal skin-muscle reflexes (upper quadrants T 8-9); lower quadrants, (T11-12). Do umbilical migration test (Beevor's sign) in selected cases if a thoracic cord lesion is suspected.
2. Cremasteric reflex (afferent L1—efferent L2).
3. Test anal pucker (S4-5) and bulbocavernosus reflexes in patients suspected of sacral or cauda equina lesions.
4. Extensor toe sign or Babinski sign (afferent S1—efferent L5-S1-2).

H. Cerebellar system: (gait tested previously).

1. Finger-to-nose, rebound, alternating movements.
2. Heel-to-knee.

I. Nerve root stretching tests: done in selected cases:

1. If meningitis is suspected test for nuchal rigidity and concomitant leg flexion (Brudzinski's sign) and do leg raising tests.
2. If disc or low-back disease is suspected, do leg raising tests: straight-knee leg raising test (Laseague's sign) and bent-knee leg raising test (Kernig's sign).

VII. Somatic sensory system

A. Superficial sensory modalities: (include trigeminal area if not previously tested).

1. Light touch over hands, trunk, and feet.
2. Pain perception over hands, trunk, and feet.
3. Temperature discrimination.

B. Deep sensory modalities

1. Vibration perception at knuckles, fingernails, and malleoli of ankles.
2. Position sense of fingers and toes (4th digits).
3. Romberg (swaying) test.
4. Stereognosis.

C. Determine the distributional pattern of any sensory loss: dermatomal, peripheral nerve(s), central pathway, or nonorganic.

D. Summary of dermatomal relations: Trigeminal nerve to interaural line and abuts on C2 (no C1). C3-4 over "cape" area of shoulders, 5-6-7-8-1 are pulled out on arms, C4 abuts on T2, T4 is nipple level, T10 is umbilical level, L5 to big toe, S1 to small toe, S4 and 5 supply perianal zone.

VIII. Cerebral functions

A. When the history or antecedent examination suggests a cerebral lesion, test for agraphognosia, finger agnosia, poor two-point discrimination, right-left disorientation, atopognosia, and tactile, auditory, and visual inattention to bilateral simultaneous stimuli. Test for tactile inattention to simultaneous ipsilateral stimulation of face-hand and foot-hand.

B. Have the patient do the cognitive, constructional, and performance tasks of the Halstead-Reitan cerebral function screening test. See the tables on pages xix and xx and refer to text pages 344–349 for additional instructions.

Table: Halstead-Reitan Cerebral Function Screening Test.

Patient's Task	Examiner's Instructions To the Patient
1. Copy SQUARE (A). (See Figs. A–O, page xxi.)	FIRST, DRAW THIS ON YOUR PAPER. (Point to Square, item A). I WANT YOU TO DO IT WITHOUT LIFTING YOUR PENCIL FROM THE PAPER. MAKE IT ABOUT THIS SAME SIZE.
2. Name SQUARE	WHAT IS THAT SHAPE CALLED?
3. Spell SQUARE	WOULD YOU SPELL THAT WORD FOR ME?
4. Copy CROSS (B)	DRAW THIS ON YOUR PAPER. GO AROUND THE OUTSIDE LIKE THIS UNTIL YOU GET BACK TO WHERE YOU STARTED. MAKE IT ABOUT THIS SAME SIZE.
5. Name CROSS	WHAT IS THAT SHAPE CALLED?
6. Spell CROSS	WOULD YOU SPELL THAT WORD FOR ME?
7. Copy TRIANGLE (C)	Similar to 1 and 4 above.
8. Name TRIANGLE	WHAT IS THAT SHAPE CALLED?
9. Spell TRIANGLE	WOULD YOU SPELL THAT WORD FOR ME?
10. Name BABY (D)	WHAT IS THIS? (Show baby, item D).
11. Write CLOCK (E)	NOW, I AM GOING TO SHOW YOU ANOTHER PICTURE BUT DO *NOT* TELL ME THE NAME OF IT. I DON'T WANT YOU TO SAY ANYTHING OUT LOUD. JUST WRITE THE NAME OF THE PICTURE ON YOUR PAPER. (Show clock, item E).
12. Name FORK (F)	WHAT IS THIS? (Show fork, item F).
13. Read 7 SIX 2 (G)	I WANT YOU TO READ THIS. (Show item G).
14. Read M G W (H)	READ THIS. (Show item H).
15. Reading I (I)	NOW, I WANT YOU TO READ THIS. (Show item I).
16. Reading II (J)	CAN YOU READ THIS? (Show item J).
17. Repeat TRIANGLE	NOW, I AM GOING TO SAY SOME WORDS. I WANT YOU TO LISTEN CAREFULLY AND SAY THEM AFTER ME AS CAREFULLY AS YOU CAN. SAY THIS WORD: TRIANGLE.

Patient's Task	Examiner's Instructions To the Patient
18. Repeat MASSACHUSETTS	THE NEXT ONE IS A LITTLE HARDER BUT DO YOUR BEST. SAY THIS WORD: MASSACHUSETTS.
19. Repeat METHODIST EPISCOPAL	NOW REPEAT THIS ONE: METHODIST EPISCOPAL.
20. Write SQUARE (K)	DON'T SAY THIS WORD OUT LOUD. JUST WRITE IT ON YOUR PAPER. (Point to stimulus word "square," item K).
21. Read SEVEN (L)	CAN YOU READ THIS WORD OUT LOUD. (Show item L.)
22. Repeat SEVEN	NOW, I WANT YOU TO SAY THIS AFTER ME: SEVEN.
23. Repeat-explain. HE SHOUTED THE WARNING	I AM GOING TO SAY SOMETHING THAT I WANT YOU TO SAY AFTER ME. SO LISTEN CAREFULLY: HE SHOUTED THE WARNING. NOW YOU SAY IT. WOULD YOU EXPLAIN WHAT THAT MEANS?
24. Write: HE SHOUTED THE WARNING	NOW, I WANT YOU TO WRITE THAT SENTENCE ON THE PAPER.
25. Compute $85 - 27 =$ (M)	HERE IS AN ARITHMETIC PROBLEM. COPY IT DOWN ON YOUR PAPER ANY WAY YOU LIKE AND TRY TO WORK IT OUT. (Show item M).
26. Compute $17 \times 3 =$	NOW, DO THIS ONE IN YOUR HEAD: 17×3
27. Name KEY (N)	WHAT IS THIS: (Show item N).
28. Demonstrate use of KEY (N)	IF YOU HAD ONE OF THESE IN YOUR HAND, SHOW ME HOW YOU WOULD USE IT. (Show item N).
29. Draw KEY (N)	NOW, I WANT YOU TO DRAW A PICTURE THAT LOOKS JUST LIKE THIS. TRY TO MAKE YOUR KEY LOOK ENOUGH LIKE THIS ONE SO THAT I WOULD KNOW IT WAS THE SAME KEY FROM YOUR DRAWING. (Point to key, item N.)
30. Read (O)	WOULD YOU READ THIS? (Show item O).
31. Place LEFT HAND TO RIGHT EAR	NOW, WOULD YOU DO WHAT IT SAID?
32. Place LEFT HAND TO LEFT ELBOW	NOW, I WANT YOU TO PUT YOUR LEFT HAND TO YOUR LEFT ELBOW.

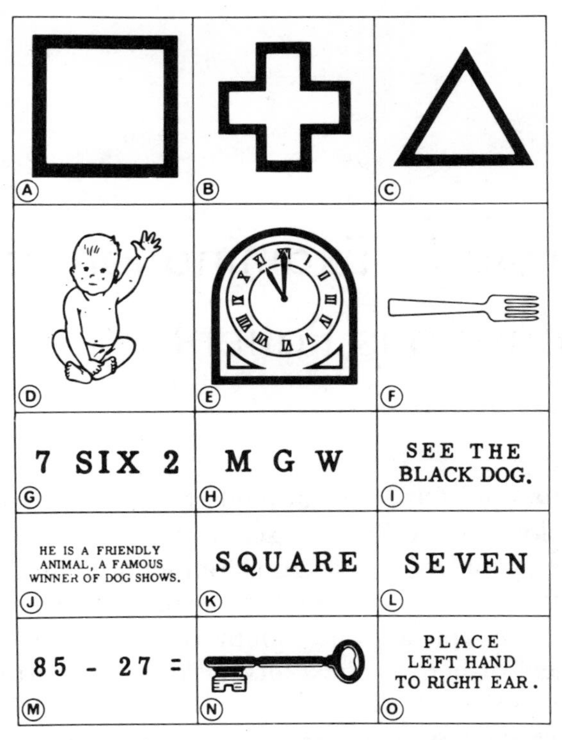

Stimulus figures for testing cerebral functions. This test is the Halstead-Wepman screening test as modified by Dr. Ralph Reitan and currently used in the Neuropsychology Laboratory at Indiana University and many other testing centers.

IX. Case summary

A. Write a three-line summary of the pertinent positive and negative historical and physical findings. (If you can't put it in three lines, you don't understand the problem).

B. Write down a provisional clinical diagnosis and outline the differential diagnosis.

C. Write down a sequential plan of management for:

1. Diagnostic tests to discriminate between the diagnostic possibilities.
2. Therapy: state the therapeutic goals.
3. Management of the emotional, educational, and socioeconomic problems which the illness causes the patient.
4. Identification of and prophylaxis for other persons now known to be "at risk" because of the patient's illness, if his illness is infectious, genetic, or environmentally induced.

Neurologic Examination of the Unconscious Patient

1. *Check respiration.* Observe rate and rhythm of respiration. Note the patient's color and verify air exchange by inspection, palpation, or auscultation. Look for suprasternal retraction and abdominal respiration. For inspiratory stridor, pull the mandible forward and reposition the patient. For apnea, start mouth-to-mouth resuscitation or insert oropharyngeal or endotracheal airway and apply artificial respiration. Assist ventilation with Ambu bag or ventilator as needed. Note any odors such as alcohol. In all maneuvers, stabilize the spine if the patient may have had a neck injury.
2. *Check circulation.* Palpate and auscultate the precordium. Inspect for jugular distension and pedal edema. Palpate the carotid and femoral pulses. Take the blood pressure. If the patient has no heart beat, start cardiac resuscitation.
   a. With hypotension, consider shock or hypovolemia. Restore blood volume with fluids: saline, Ringer's lactate, colloids, or blood.
   b. With hypertension, consider a cardiac or cerebral vascular accident or hypertensive encephalopathy as the cause for the unconsciousness. Consider apresoline, but lower the blood pressure gradually over hours.
3. *Check the blood sugar level.* Prick the patient's finger and do a glucose oxidase tape test (Dextrostix). Give 50 cc of 50% glucose IV stat for demonstrated or suspected hypoglycemia.
4. *Check pupils.* Measure the size of the pupils in millimeters and write it down. Use a ruler, do not guess. Check the pupillary light reflex. With unilaterally or bilaterally dilated pupils that are nonreactive to light, call a neurosurgeon stat. Remove contact lenses to preserve the cornea.
5. *Strip the patient completely.* Empty all of the patient's pockets, purse, wallet, or belongings. Look for Identacards for diabetes or epilepsy, medications, suicide notes, or drug paraphernalia.
6. *Search the entire skin surface* for needle marks indicating subcutaneous injections of insulin or intravenous injections, bruises, petechiae, entry wounds, and turgor. Roll the patient over and check the back. Stabilize the neck to prevent spinal cord injury.
7. *Dispatch an aide, preferably a physician, to obtain a history* from rela-

tives, friends, ambulance drivers, police, the patient's past physicians, or anyone who witnessed the patient's predicament. Ask about the circumstances under which the patient lost consciousness as well as the past medical history.

Inquire about:

a. Possibility of head trauma.
b. A seizure disorder.
c. Insulin/diabetes mellitus.
d. A recent change in mood, behavior, thinking, or neurologic condition.
e. Depression or access to depressant drugs.
f. Other medicines.
g. Allergies, insect bites, and other causes of anaphylactic shock.
h. Cardiac, hepatic, pulmonary, or lung disease.
i. Past hospitalizations for serious health problems. Rule out red herrings. Does the patient have preexisting neurologic or physical anomalies or dysfunctions? (For example, has previous disease altered pupillary size or reactions? Has the patient had prior strabismus?)

8. *Monitor pupillary size, pulse, blood pressure, respiration, and temperature* continuously or at regular, frequent intervals. Consult a neurosurgeon about inserting an intracranial pressure monitor, if the patient may have increased intracranial pressure.
9. *Determine the patient's level of consciousness by responsivity* to voice, startling sound, light, and pain. Check the responses to pain inflicted by compression of the supraorbital ridge and nail beds of all four extremities. Record the extremity response as *none*, *extension*, *flexion*, *appropriate brushing*, or *movement on command*.
10. *Inspect and palpate the patient's head.* Look for localized edema or swelling; look for blood behind the ear (Battle's sign) and around the eyes (raccoon eyes); and for blood or CSF from the nose.
11. *Test for nuchal rigidity.*
12. *Check the patient's eyes for the following signs:*
    a. Blinking and ptosis
    b. Eyelid release test and corneal reflex
    c. Re-measure and record pupillary size
    d. Re-test pupillary light reflex
    e. Test the faciociliary and spinociliary reflexes
    f. Examine ocular alignment, position, and motility
        (1) Record alignment and the position of the eyes
        (2) Record any spontaneous movements of the eyes
        (3) Do doll's eye test
        (4) Do ophthalmoscopic examination
        (5) Otoscopy (look for blood behind the eardrum)
        (6) Do caloric irrigation
13. *Inspect the patient for persistent diagnostic postures and spontaneous patterned or repetitive movements.*
    a. Note whether the patient makes spontaneous and equal movements of face and all four extremities, or lies still, in a flaccid-compliant,

dumped-in-a-heap posture indicating deep coma or flaccid quadriparesis.

b. Look for a predominant posture:
   (1) Persistent deviation of the eyes and head
   (2) Opisthotonus
   (3) Decerebrate or decorticate posturing
   (4) Clenched jaws or immobile neck or extremities indicating tetanus

c. Check specifically for hemiplegia by looking for absence of movement of the face and extremities on one side, with some spontaneous or pain-induced movements of the opposite side. Acute hemiplegia in the unconscious patient is usually flaccid. Do the eyelid release test, look for flaccidity of the cheek manifested by retraction on inspiration and puffing out during expiration, and inflict pain by supraorbital compression to check for unilateral absence of grimacing. Test muscle tone by passive manipulation of all extremities and do the wrist-, arm-, and leg-dropping tests. The intact side of the hemiplegic patient may show the hypertonia known as *paratonia.* Record the result of tonus testing as *normal, flaccid, spastic, rigid, paratonia,* or *flexibilitas cerea* (waxy flexibility), seen in catatonic schizophrenia as well as some organic encephalopathies.

d. Look for cyclic changes in motor activity: shivering, chewing movements, and tremors. Look for overt as well as subtle manifestations of epilepsy: eyelid fluttering, mouth twitching, myoclonic jerks, finger or toe twitching, or frank tonic-clonic generalized seizures.

14. *Elicit the muscle stretch reflexes:* Begin with the glabellar tap to elicit the orbicularis oculi reflexes. Next, do the jaw jerk and work down through the customary stretch reflexes. Directly compare the reflexes on the two sides of the body.
15. *Try to elicit Chvostek's sign.*
16. *Elicit the superficial reflexes.* Corneal, sucking, and lip-pursing reflexes, abdominal, cremasteric, and plantar reflexes.
17. *Attempt to elicit grasp reflexes, forced groping, and traction responses.*
18. *Complete the physical examination,* including abdominal palpation and percussion, rectal and vaginal examinations.
19. *Draw blood sample and anchor IV catheter:*
   a. Blood sugar
   b. Complete blood count (CBC) and hematocrit
   c. Blood-urea nitrogen (BUN)
   d. Gases
   e. Electrolytes (Na, K, Ca, and Cl)
   f. pH
   g. Osmolality
   h. Toxicology
   i. Other ____________________

   ____

Place a sample of the patient's serum in the refrigerator for later chemical or toxicological testing as may be indicated by new information, medicolegal problems, or if the patient dies of unknown causes.

20. *Obtain urine specimen.* Use an external bag or catheterize if the patient is incontinent or has a distended bladder. Freeze a sample of urine for later testing as may be indicated by new information. On the routine testing of the first specimen, order these tests:
    a. Specific gravity
    b. Sugar and ketones
    c. Protein
    d. Toxicology screen
    e. Other ______________________,
    ____
21. *Consider whether to pass a nasogastric tube.* Do it if the patient is likely to have ingested poison, is vomiting, or is not improving and the diagnosis is obscure. Since it may induce vomiting or gagging, and cause extreme increases in intrathoracic and therefore intracranial pressure, pass it with extreme care in a patient who may have had subarachnoid or intracranial hemorrhage, increased intracranial pressure, or is threatening brain herniation. Aspirate as often as needed to avoid fluid accumulation in the stomach and vomiting. Save a sample of any material aspirated for subsequent toxicological analysis.
22. *Make a provisional diagnosis.* At the least, assign the patient to one of the five basic etiologic types of coma: intracranial, toxic-metabolic, anoxic, ischemic, or mental illness. See Figure on page xxvi.
23. *Select the safest and most critical additional test to confirm or reject your provisional diagnosis.* The neurologic tests to consider include skull radiographs, echoencephalography, electroencephalography, lumbar puncture, CAT scan, angiography, pneumoencephalography, and ventriculography. Proper selection of the last four radiographic contrast procedures rests with the neurologist or neurosurgeon.

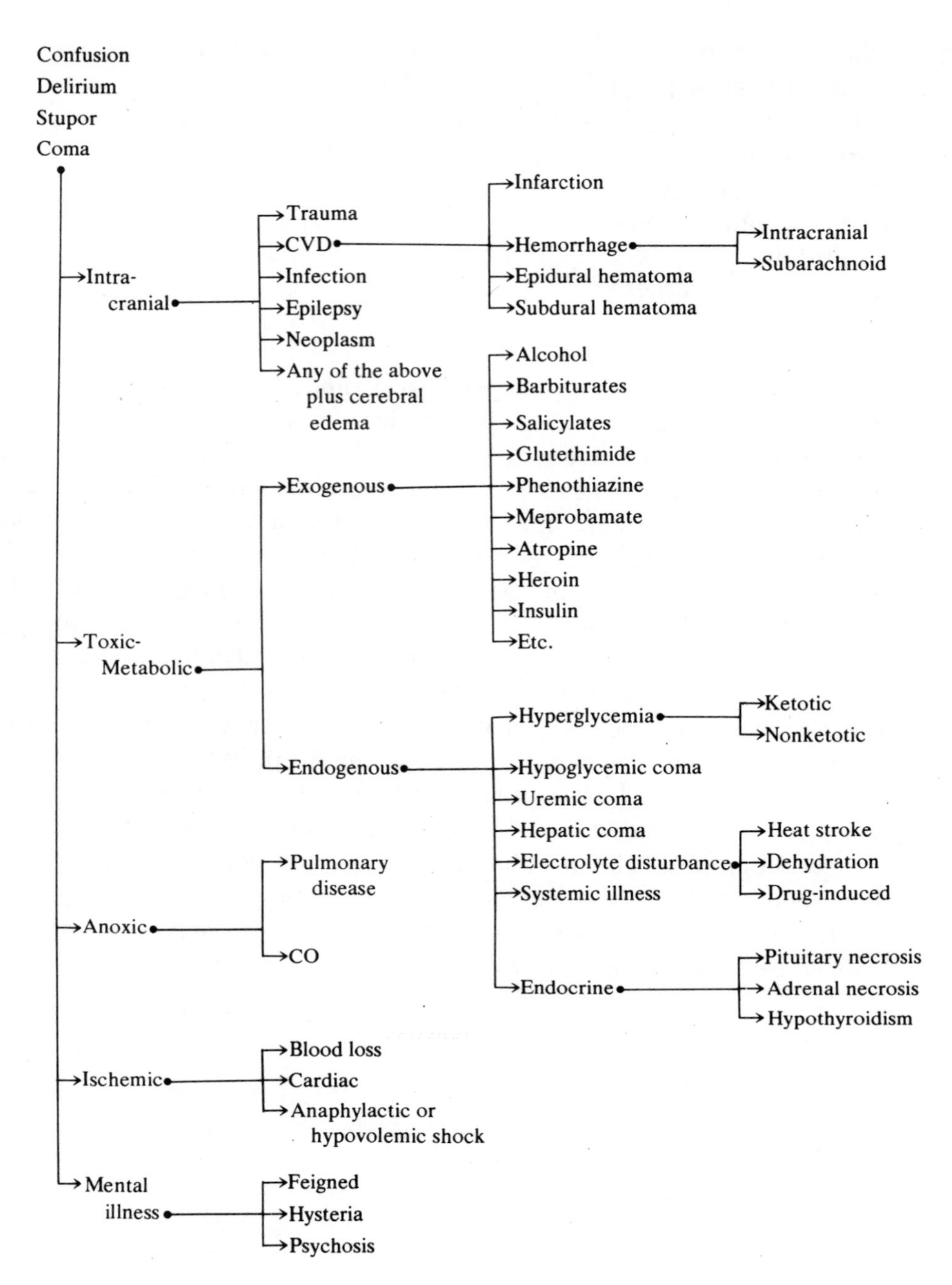

Categories for the differential diagnosis of the unconscious patient.

1

Examination of the Face and Head

Disease is of antiquity and nothing about it changes. It is we who change as we learn to recognize what was formerly imperceptible.

— Jean Martin Charcot

I. Inspection

A. Introduction

If permitted to do only one part of the clinical examination, you should choose to look at the patient. Inspection is the most efficient method of physical diagnosis. It begins the moment you approach your patient and look into his eyes. Suppose he has pinpoint pupils and numerous needle scars over his antecubital veins. In two glances you have recognized a drug addict. This is the diagnostic power of inspection. But hold on a minute. The pupils may be small from eyedrops used to treat glaucoma, and the antecubital veins may be scarred from repeated blood donations. Every sign or combination of signs has a differential diagnosis. The medical significance of a sign emerges only from the background provided by a complete history and physical examination. No single diagnostic technique, by itself, is sufficient.

Because you have had a lifetime of experience in looking, you may think you are already a keen observer. As a test of how well you have observed something, try to draw it. What you have seen well, you can draw well. Complete the requested drawings faithfully. They are tremendous teachers.

B. Inspection of the eyes

1. Using a hand mirror to observe yourself, draw (on a piece of scrap paper) the contours of your eyelid margins. Heed the configuration at the medial and lateral angles. After completing your drawing, compare it with Fig. 1-1 and learn the names in 1*A* and 1*C*.

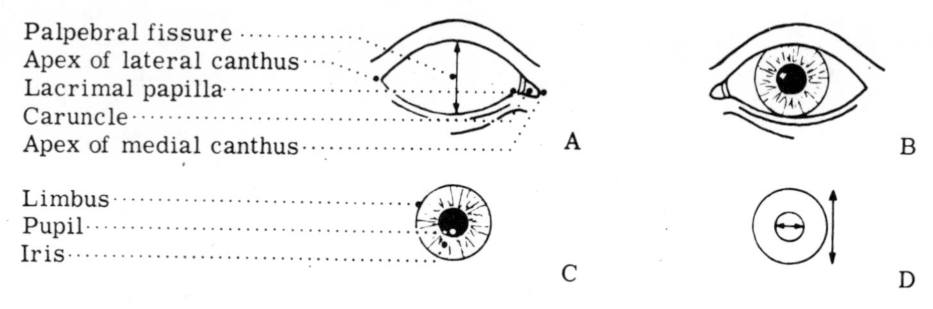

FIG. 1-1. Nomenclature of the eye.

2. Look into your mirror to identify the parts of your eye as listed in Fig. 1-1*A*. (Some students at this point do not yet have a mirror. Are you one? Come on now, be fair. Give these tactics a chance.)
3. In your mirror study your own limbus, iris, and pupil. The limbus, the junction of cornea and sclera, also approximates the external circumference of the iris.
4. The internal circumference of the iris forms the pupil, the opening which admits light into the eye. See the horizontal arrow, Fig. 1-1*D*.
5. Notice the caruncle, the tiny meaty mound of tissue occupying the medial canthus.
6. With your mirror study the relation of the upper and lower lid margins to the limbus when you look straight ahead. Does one lid margin cover more of the iris than the other?

Note: The vertical line on the left side sets off an answer column. Use the card to cover the answers until after you have responded to the text. Then each time you make a response slide the card down to check your answer.

The upper lid partially covers the upper part of the limbus, while the lower lid forms a tangent.

7. Set aside your mirror and from memory draw the iris of the left eye in Fig. 1-2, showing its exact relation to the lid margins.

See Fig. 1-1*B*. If you erred, redraw the iris in the right eye of Fig. 1-2.

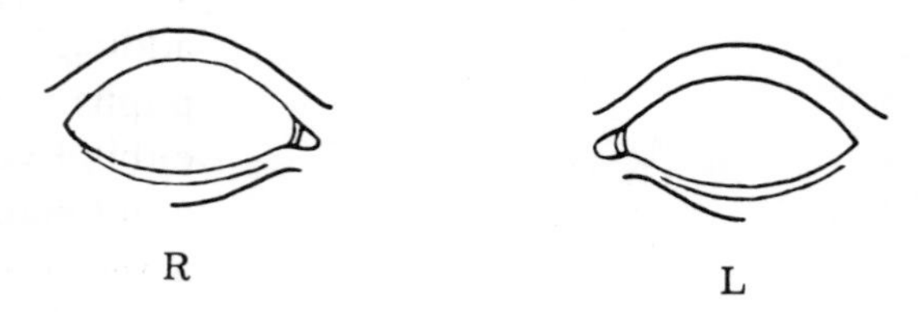

FIG. 1-2. Blank for drawing the relation of the limbus, iris, and pupil to the lid margins when the patient looks straight ahead.

Check your labels against Fig. 1-1.

8. From memory label Fig. 1-2 with the names learned in Fig. 1-1.
9. Look in your mirror and study another person to learn the relationship of the limbus to the canthi and caruncles when the eyes are turned as far as possible to the *right* or *left* sides. If you wear glasses, remove them.
   a. With the eyes turned to one side as far as possible, how much scleral white shows between the limbus and the *apex* of the lateral canthus

None, or virtually none

apex

caruncle

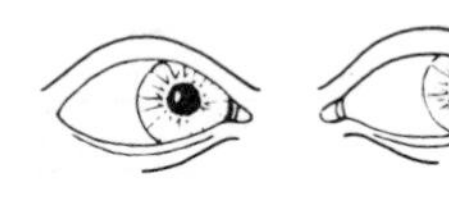

of the *abducted* eye? 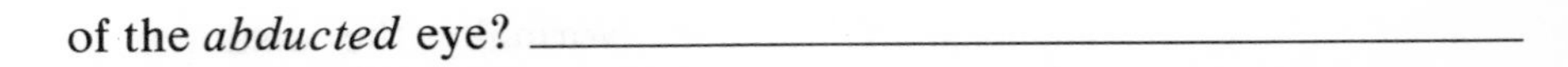

b. Since the caruncle occupies the medial canthus, the limbus cannot reach it. Instead the limbus reaches to, or nearly to, the lateral margin of the caruncle. Thus, with the eyes to one side the limbus of the *abducted* eye reaches to, or nearly to, the ______ of the lateral canthus and the limbus of the *add*ucted eye reaches to, or nearly to, the margin of the ______.

c. In Fig. 1-3 draw the relation of the limbus, iris, and pupils to the lids when the patient looks to his left.

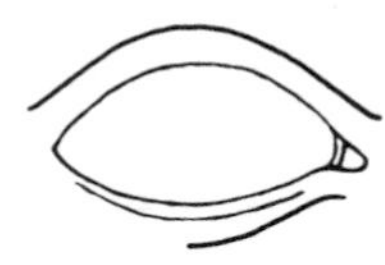 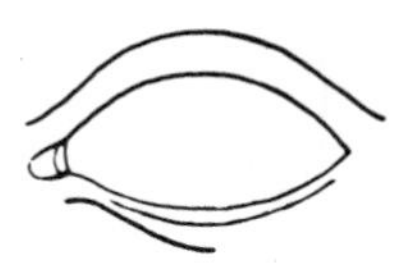

FIG. 1-3. Blank for drawing the relation of the limbus, iris, and pupil to the lid margins when the patient looks to his left as far as possible.

10. A line drawn through the canthi defines the angle of the palpebral fissure, when compared to the horizontal plane. Study Fig. 1-4.

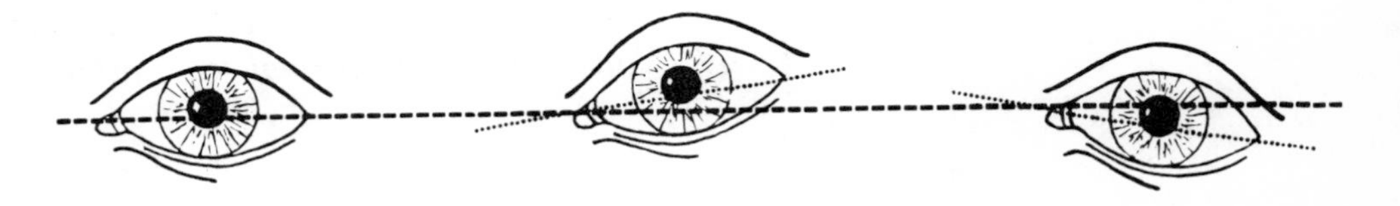

A. Normal B. Mongoloid slant C. Antimongoloid slant

FIG. 1-4. Left eye, showing angulations of the palpebral fissure.

11. Anatomic variations of the medial canthus.
    a. If you have an infant or young child, notice that the medial canthus covers more of the conjunctiva than in adults.
    b. Fig. 1-5 shows anatomic variations in the relation of the medial canthus to the corneal limbus when the eye is looking straight ahead.

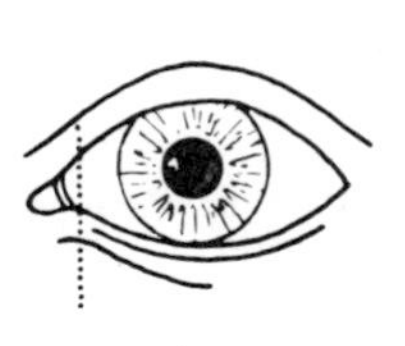 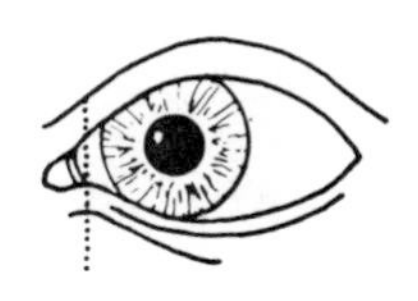 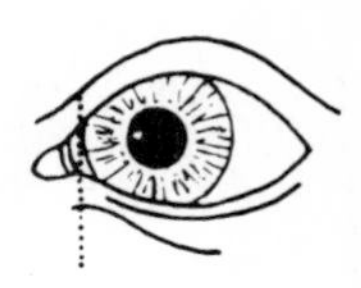

A. Normal adult B. Young child C. Canthus dystopia

FIG. 1-5. Left eye, showing variations in the relation of the medial canthus and lacrimal papilla (vertical line) to the corneal limbus. Notice the decreasing distance between the caruncle and the limbus in A, B, and C.

c. Normally the distance between the iris and medial and lateral margins of the eyelids is about equal. See Fig. 1-5*A*. When the medial canthus is displaced laterally relative to the limbus, as in many young children, the patient *appears* to have inward deviation of the eyes, although the eyes are perfectly straight, as in Fig. 1-5*B*.

d. When the medial canthus is laterally displaced so that the lacrimal papilla falls at the level of the limbus, the anomaly is called *canthus dystopia* (dys = bad; topos = place; hence, badly placed canthus). See Fig. 1-5*C*.

e. State how you would decide whether a patient has canthus dystopia.

____

____

____

____

Ans: With the patient looking straight ahead, compare the distance between the limbus and the lateral and medial canthi (or caruncle medially).

f. Sometimes a fold of skin covers the medial canthus. Since the fold is *upon* the canthus, it is called an *epicanthal* fold. In the spaces beside *A, B,* and *C,* in Fig. 1-6, write down your diagnosis, whether *epicanthal fold, normal,* or *canthus dystopia.*

A. Normal

B. Canthus dystopia

C. Epicanthal fold

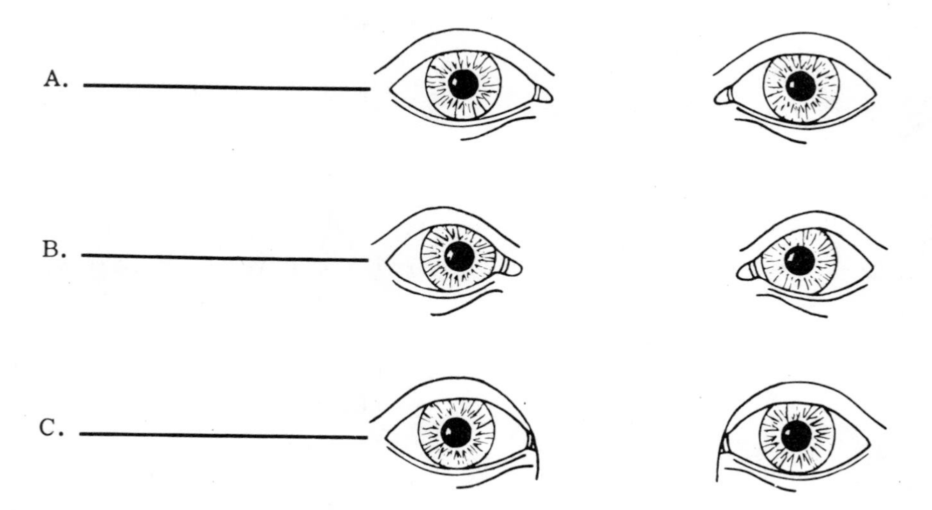

FIG. 1-6. Write your diagnosis in blanks *A, B,* and *C.*

Make the measurements!

12. In Fig. 1-6, measure the distance between the apices of the medial canthi in the normal eyes and in canthus dystopia. The intercanthal distance in the normal eye is ____________ mm and in canthus dystopia it is ____________ mm. Therefore in canthus dystopia, the intercanthal distance is ☐ increased / ☐ decreased / ☐ unchanged.

hypotelorism

epicanthal folds or canthus dystopia

skull radiographs

hypertelorism
hypotelorism

anisocoria

corectasia

cormiosis

corectopia

down

ptosis

enophthalmos

13. The patient with canthus dystopia or epicanthal folds may present the illusion of an increased distance between the eyes. The actual interorbital distance is set by the bone forming the medial walls of the orbits. This distance can be measured only from skull radiographs. If the medial orbital walls and consequently the eyes are too far apart, the patient has *orbital hypertelorism* (hyper = excessive; tele = far, as in *tele*phone). If the medial orbital walls and consequently the eyes are too close together, the patient has orbital *hypo* ______________ ______________.

14. What canthal or lid anomaly could produce the illusion of hypertelorism even with a short interorbital distance? ______________ ______________

15. What diagnostic procedure would you order to decide whether a patient has an abnormal interorbital distance? ______________ ______________.

16. If the interorbital distance is too great, the patient is said to have ______________; if too small, ______________.

17. By holding up your millimeter ruler as you look in the mirror, measure and record the size of one pupil: ______________mm. Is your other pupil the same size? ______________. Are your pupils exactly round? ______________.
    a. Most people have exactly equal pupils, or *isocoria* (iso = equal, cor = pupil — the core is the center of anything). The prefix *a-* or *an-* negates the term that follows. Thus, any congenital or acquired difference in pupillary size is called *an* ______________, which means *not equal pupils.*
    b. An enlarged pupil can be called *pupillodilation,* but since *cor* means pupil, pupillodilation can be called ______________*ectasia.* (Similarly, an enlarged bronchial diameter is called *bronchiectasia*).
    c. An abnormally small pupil is called ______________ *miosis,* or simply *miosis.*
    d. Study the width of your iris and its concentricity with the pupils. An eccentric pupil is called ______________ *ectopia.*
    e. Although the pupils normally are exactly equal, the height of the palpebral fissures may differ slightly in normal subjects, because of slight drooping of an eyelid. Pathologic or excessive drooping of the upper lid is called *ptosis*. Check to see whether one of your lids droops more than the other.
    f. Look into your mirror to observe the surface area of your upper lid as you move your mirror up and down as far as possible. Hold your head still and follow the mirror only with your eyes. In which direction do you see most of the surface area of the lid? ☐ looking up / ☐ straight ahead / ☐ down.
    g. If an eyelid droops too much when the patient looks straight ahead, the condition is called ______________.

18. A palpebral fissure that is too wide may result from protrusion of the eye, *exophthalmos.* If the fissure is too narrow, it may be the result of a sunken eye, called *en* ______________.

ptosis
enophthalmos

anophthalmos

A. Ptosis and cormiosis on L (anisocoria)
B. Exophthalmos on R

C. Normal

D. Canthus dystopia

E. Macrocornea and corectasia

F. Cormiosis on L (anisocoria)

Measure the interorbital distance on skull radiographs

19. Two conditions which might reduce the height of the palpebral fissure are drooping of an eyelid, called ______________ or a sunken eyeball, called ______________.
20. A pathologically small eyeball is called *micro*phthalmos, or if too large *macro*phthalmos. Correspondingly the eyeball may have a *micro*cornea or *macro*cornea. What term would describe complete absence of an eyeball? (What prefix negates?) ______________.
21. Beside the figures of Fig. 1-7, write the correct diagnosis. Be sure to compare the two eyes *systematically*—pupils, iris, and lids.

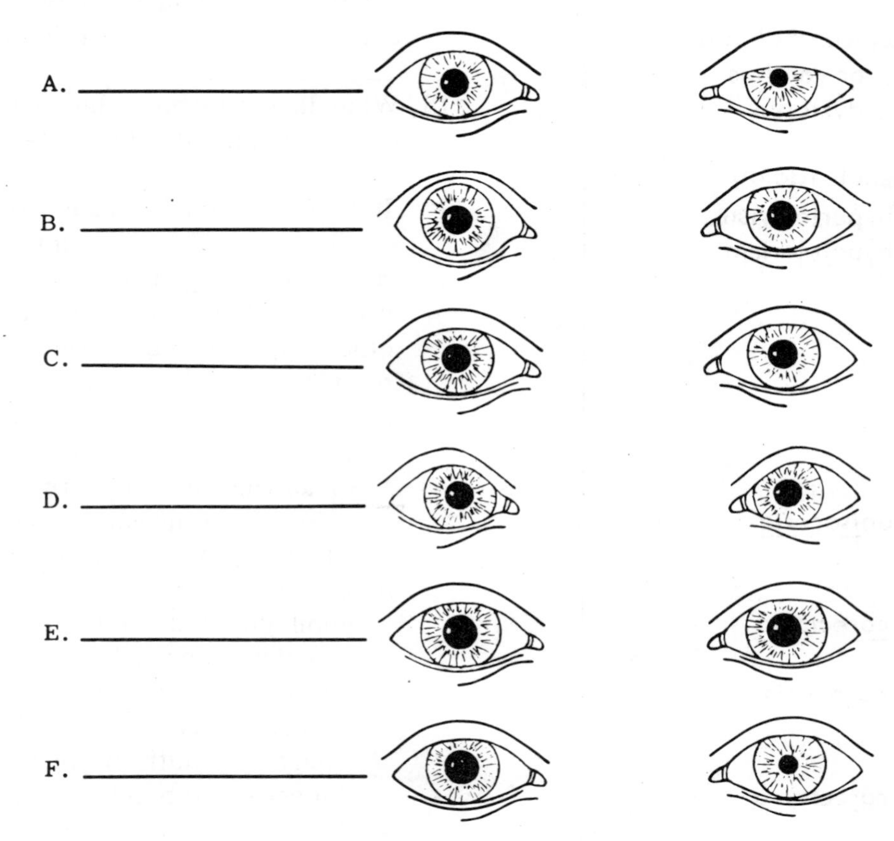

FIG. 1-7. Write your diagnosis in blanks *A* to *F*.

22. By what nonclinical diagnostic procedure do you verify whether a patient has hypo- or hypertelorism? ______________
______________.

Bibliography

DeMyer, W.: The median cleft face syndrome: Differential diagnosis of cranium bifidum, hypertelorism, and median cleft nose, lip, and palate, *Neurology,* 17:961-971, 1967.

Feingold, M., and Bossert, W. H.: Normal values for selected physical parameters: An aid to syndrome delineation. *Birth Defects: Original Article Series,* 10: No. 13, 1-15, 1974.

Laestadius, N., Aase, J. and Smith, D.: Normal inner canthal and outer orbital dimensions, *J. Pediat.,* 74:465-468, 1969.

Pryor, H.: Objective measurement of interpupillary distance, *Pediatrics,* 44:973-977, 1969.

C. Inspection of the nose, mouth, chin, and ears

1. After inspecting the eyes, look systematically at the nose, mouth, chin, and ears.
2. *Nose:* consider the bridge, the nostrils, and the relation of the nose to other facial proportions.
3. *Mouth:* consider the vermillion border of the lips, the median labial tubercle of the upper lip, and the line formed by lip closure. Are the lips closed when the patient's face is at rest? Do they make a horizontal closure line?
4. *Chin:* look for a small chin, *micrognathia,* or a large protuberant chin, *macrognathia* as in pituitary gigantism (acromegaly).
5. *Ears:* check for contour, shape, and asymmetry. Learn to draw a normal ear and label its parts as shown in Fig. 1-8.

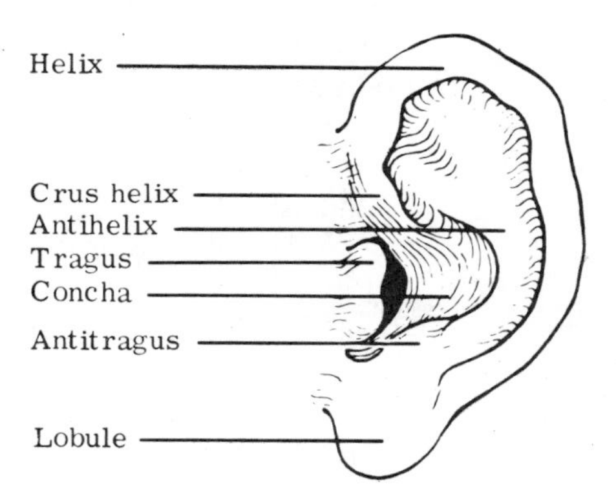

FIG. 1-8. Anatomy of the normal ear, lateral view. Compare your own ear with the drawing and identify the parts.

D. Inspection of the hair of scalp, eyebrows, and beard

1. Notice the border of the hairline of the scalp. How does it relate to the forehead and to the nape of the neck? Is the hairline too high or too low? What is the texture of the scalp hair?
2. Observe whether the eyebrows are full, scanty, absent, or joined in the midline.
3. Inspect the hair of the beard and face for distribution and texture. Inquire of a male patient how often he has to shave. Alterations in the distribution and texture of the hair occur in diverse disorders, in infections, congenital malformations, endocrine, and intersex syndromes.

E. A note on facial diagnosis

When the patient's face looks a little odd, that is to say the *gestalt* or expression seems unusual, pay heed to it. From abnormalities in the face alone, the perceptive physician can diagnose literally hundreds of disorders, ranging from infectious diseases such as leprosy through endocrinopathies, mental and neurologic disorders, and especially malformation syndromes. In many malformation syndromes with abnormal facies, the brain also suffers, causing mental retardation. Knowing the face of such a patient, the physician often can predict with a fair degree of certainty the patient's intellectual potential. Thus, in these instances the face predicts the brain.

Begin by observing the patient's facial *gestalt.* Then dissect the face into parts for individual inspection. Imagine the face as a pair of eyes. Are they too close together or too far apart? Are the pupils equal? Simply ask each question for which your observations will provide an answer. Then visualize him as a nose, a mouth, a chin, a pair of ears. Even if you cannot recite all the possible pathologic deviations of these structures, you can at least know what is normal, and then if you become suspicious of something, consult one of the following sources.

Bibliography

Bergsma, D. (ed.): Morphogenesis and malformation of face and brain. *Birth Defects: Original Article Series,* 10: No. 7, 1975.

DeMyer, W.: Median facial malformations and their implications for brain malformations. *Birth Defects: Original Article Series,* 11: No. 7, 155-181, 1975.

——: "Median Cleft Lip" in W. Grabb (ed.), *Cleft Lip and Palate,* Boston, Little, Brown and Co., 1971.

Goodman, R., and Gorlin, R.: *The Face in Genetic Disorders,* St. Louis, C. V. Mosby, 1970.

Gorlin, R. J., Pindborg, J. J., and Cohen, M. M.: *Syndromes of the Head and Neck,* 2nd ed., New York, McGraw-Hill, 1976.

Greer Walker, D.: *Malformations of the Face,* London, E. & S. Livingstone, Ltd., 1961.

Herzka, H.: *Das Gesicht des Säuglings Ausdruck und Reifung,* Basel, Schwabe & Co., 1965.

Holmes, L., Moser, H., Halldorsson, S., Mack, C., Pant, S., and Matzilevich, B.: *Mental Retardation*—An Atlas of Diseases with Associated Physical Abnormalities, New York, The Macmillan Co., 1972.

Leiber, B., and Olbrich, G.: *Die klinischen Syndrome,* Band I and II, Munchen, Urban & Schwarzenberg, 1972.

Pruzansky, S.: *Congenital Anomalies of the Face and Associated Structures,* Springfield, Charles C. Thomas, 1961.

Smith, D.: *Recognizable Patterns of Human Malformation,* 2nd ed., Philadelphia, W. B. Saunders, 1976.

Warkany, J.: *Congenital Malformations,* Chicago, Year Book Medical Publishers, 1971.

II. Palpation and percussion of the head

A. Palpation

1. *Skull:* It is perfectly natural to touch what you look at. The laying on of hands, an ancient habit of healers, serves at once as a source of information to the physician and of comfort to the patient. Therefore, after extracting all the information by looking, grasp the patient's head between your fingertips (or your own head in lieu of a patient's) and, using fairly firm pressure, search for soft spots, lumps, depressions, and areas of tenderness. Notice your own frontal and parietal eminences. By feel-

ing along the midline and then out laterally, locate the depression between the prominences of the frontal and parietal bones, the depression marking the site of the coronal suture. Feel in the midline posteriorly, where nape of neck meets skull, and find your external occipital protuberance.

2. *Arteries:* Palpate the major accessible arteries, the carotid and temporal. See the carotid arteries in Fig. 1-9*A* and palpate along the anterior edge of your sternocleidomastoid muscles until you find your own. A pulseless carotid artery indicates occlusion. Lay your index finger lightly, just in front of your tragus, and follow the pulsating temporal artery as far distally as you can.

B. Percussion over the sinuses or mastoid processes may help to confirm tenderness in these areas, but the percussion note from the skull itself has little value in adults and can be used only with caution and after great practice in pediatric patients.

III. Auscultation of the head and neck

A. Aneurysms, arteriovenous malformations or fistulae, and occlusive vascular disease may cause bruits over the carotid arteries or head. Loud cardiac sounds transmit along the great vessels. In normal infants and children to five years of age, benign bruits are common. Sometimes you will hear bruits over the carotid arteries of normal adults, but a strong, localized bruit at the carotid bifurcation suggests an obstructive lesion at that point.

B. To survey for cephalic bruits, place a rubber-edged stethoscope bell at various sites over the carotid and vertebral arteries. Then place the bell over the mastoid processes, frontal and parietal regions, and over each eye after the patient gently closes his eyelid. In Fig. 1-9*A*, notice the course of the carotid and vertebral arteries. In 1-9*B*, draw lines showing where the stethoscope bell is placed to listen for carotid or vertebral artery bruits, and then make an X at the other sites where you should place the bell to listen for a bruit.

C. Using your stethoscope, listen to what (I hope) will be silence over your own head. Can you hear heart sounds when you auscultate your carotid arteries?

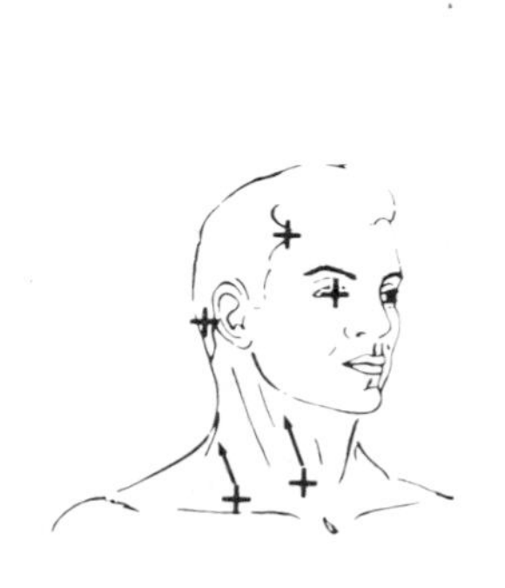

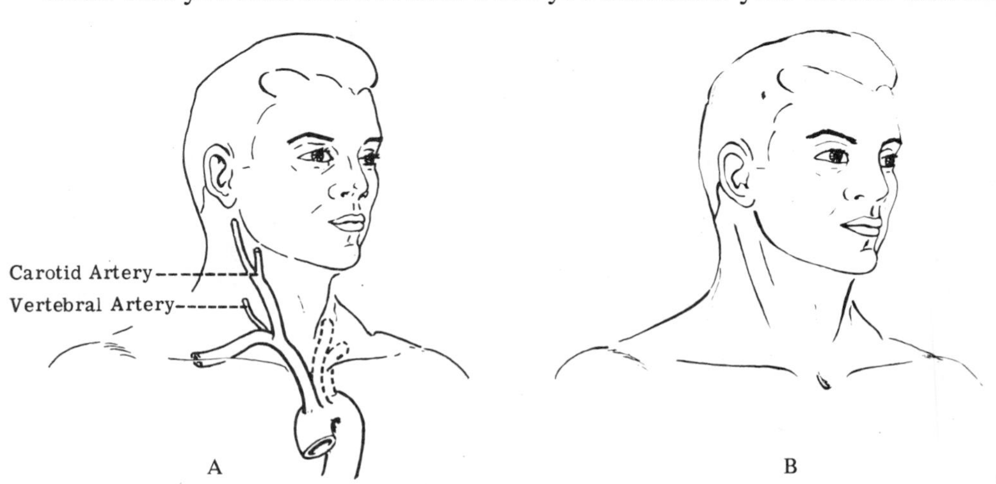

A. Phantom view of carotid and vertebral arteries in the neck.

B. Blank to mark sites of auscultation.

FIG. 1-9. Sites for auscultation of head and neck.

Relax his eyelid

When you place the bell over the eye, what do you have to tell the patient to do to eliminate muscle "noise"? ______________________.

Bibliography

Mace, J., Peters, E., and Matheis, A., Jr.: Cranial bruits in purulent meningitis in childhood, *New Eng. J. Med.,* 278:1420-1422, 1968.

Toole, J. F., and Patel, A. N.: *Cerebrovascular Disorders,* 2nd ed., New York, McGraw-Hill, 1974.

Ziegler, D., Zileli, T., Dick, A., and Sebaugh, J. L.: Correlation of bruits over the carotid artery with angiographically demonstrated lesions, *Neurology,* 21: 860-865, 1971.

IV. Abnormalities in the size and shape of the head

A. *Origin of skull bones and functional arthrology of the skull*

1. The cephalic mesoderm produces skull bones by two different histogenetic sequences. Endochondral bone forms the cranial base. Membranous bone forms the cranial vault and facial skeleton. See Fig. 1-10.

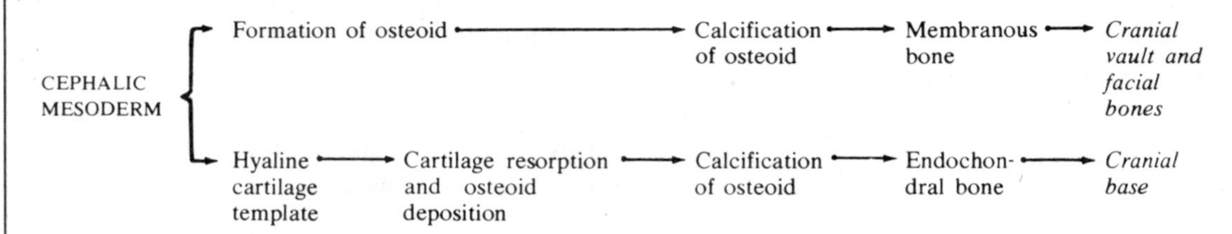

FIG. 1-10. Histogenesis of the two types of cranial bone, *membranous* and *endochondral*. (For reference only. Do not memorize.)

Learn the four endochondral bones of the cranial base in Fig. 1-11. Then you can easily remember the membranous origin of the others.

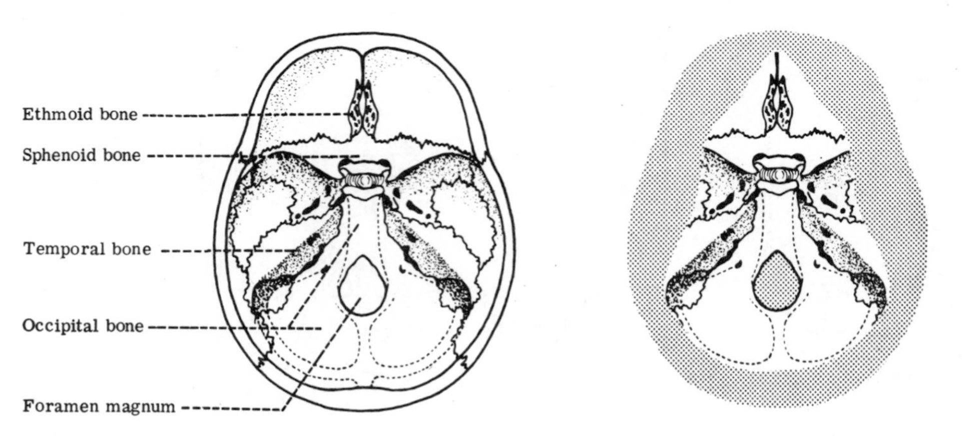

FIG. 1-11. Interior view of skull base on the left. On the right, only the endochondral bone is shown.

Bibliography

Bosma, J. F. (ed.): *Symposium on Development of the Basicranium,* Bethesda, DHEW Publication No. (NIH) 76-989, 1973.

2. *Functional arthrology of the skull*

   a. When a joint cavity separates the two bones at a joint, the joint is called a *diarthrosis.* If connective tissue occupies the space between the bones, leaving no joint cavity, the joint is a *synarthrosis.* In Fig. 1-12, joint A represents the type of joint called a ________________________ .

synarthrosis

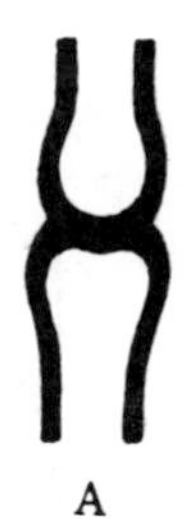

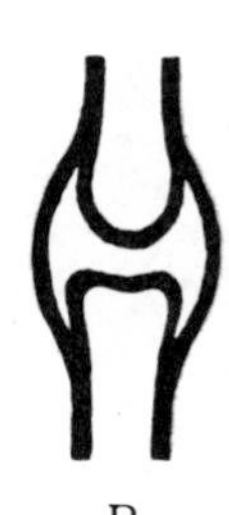

A B

FIG. 1-12. The two types of joints:
Joint A is a ___arthrosis.
Joint B is a ___arthrosis.

synarthrosis
diarthrosis

   b. During morphogenesis, *cartilaginous* connective tissue united the joints of the endochondral bones at the cranial base. Such synarthroses are called *synchrondroses.* During morphogenesis, *fibrous* connective tissue united the membranous bones of cranial vault and face to each other and to endochondral bones. Such synarthroses are called *sutures.* Thus, the two types of skull synarthroses are ________________ and ________________.

synchrondroses, sutures

   c. What is the basis for distinguishing the two types of cranial synarthroses? ____.

type of uniting connective tissue during morphogenesis, fibrous or cartilaginous

   d. Wherever membranous bones contact each other or endochondral bones, the joints are called ________________, but wherever endochondral bones contact other endochondral bones, the joints are called ________________.

sutures

synchondroses

   e. In fetuses, the fibrous connective tissue at the sutures is broad and loose. It forms large, non-ossified membranes between the margins of some skull bones. These sites are called *fontanels.* Review the sutures, fontanels, and bones named in Fig. 1-13*A* and *B.*

   f. The largest fontanel is the ☐ anterior / ☐ posterior fontanel.

   g. It is formed at the junction of four bones, the two ________________ bones and the two ________________ bones.

anterior
frontal
parietal

3. *Pliancy of the synarthroses in the infant's skull*

   a. At the fontanels, the broad sheet of connective tissue allows an up and down, diaphragm-like action, whereas the narrower connective tissue strip at the sutures permits only a limited, hinging action. Thus the infant skull is most pliant at the ☐ sutures / ☐ fontanels.

fontanels

   b. The endochondral bones are united by synchondroses composed of ☐ cartilaginous / ☐ fibrous connective tissue.

cartilaginous

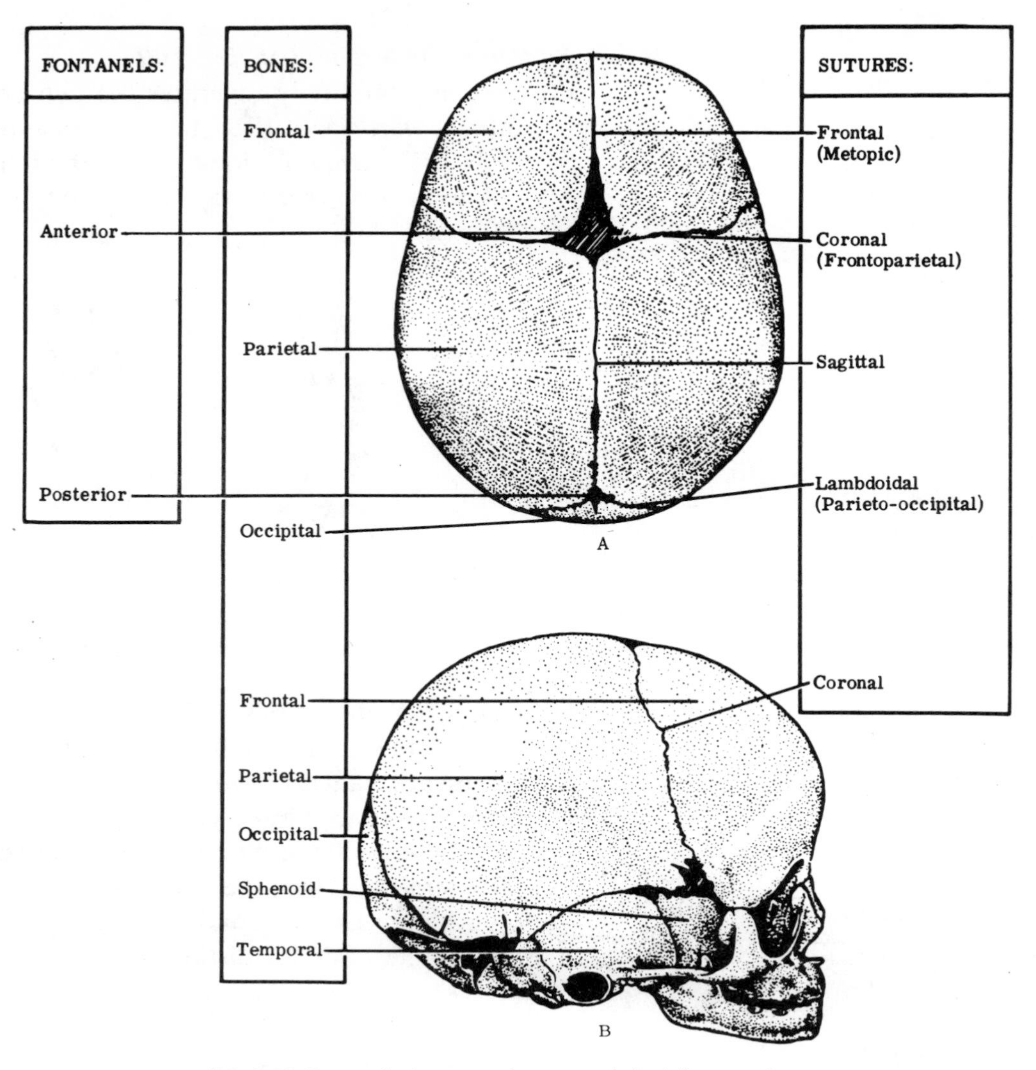

FIG. 1-13. Fontanels, bones, and sutures of the infant cranium.

fontanels
sutures
synchondroses

c. Cartilaginous connective tissue is less pliant than fibrous. Rank the three skull synarthroses, the synchondroses, fontanels, and sutures in order from most to least pliant: ______________, ______________, ______________.

4. *Ossification of skull synarthroses*

a. During morphogenesis, the skull serves the contradictory functions of plasticity and rigidity. The plastic fetal cranium yields to accommodate the expanding brain. It is deformed during passage through the birth canal when the sutures and fontanels permit a hinge-like action and may allow one cranial bone margin to overlap another. The brain may be damaged by compression or by rupture of veins and venous sinuses. The rigidity of the synchondroses prevents buckling of the skull base against the brainstem, which would imperil the passenger even more than deformation of the cranial vault.

b. With maturation, the cranium becomes relatively rigid. The synchondroses, sutures, and fontanels progressively unite and finally ossify completely. Before the synarthroses ossify, we say they are "open." Afterwards, they are "closed." The time of closure varies considerably, as summarized in Table 1-1.

TABLE 1-1. Time of Ossification of Some Cranial Synarthroses. (Reference only, do not memorize.)

Synarthrosis	Ossification (years)
Frontal (metopic) suture	2 years
Coronal suture	30 years
Basilar synchrondroses	2-20 years
Anterior fontanel	1.5 years (range 3-27 months)
Posterior fontanel	Birth to 2 months

5. *Response of the skull to increased intracranial pressure before closure of the synarthroses.*
   a. To the palpating finger, the anterior fontanel is resilient, as every mother knows, for she calls it the "soft spot." When an infant is held upside down, gravity distends the intracranial veins with blood and forces the brain against the roof of the skull. The anterior fontanel, the soft spot, bulges. When the infant is held upright, the opposite shift in intracranial contents occurs and the fontanel ☐ bulges more / ☐ becomes sunken / ☐ is unchanged in contour.

becomes sunken

   b. When an infant cries, he expires against a partially closed glottis. Contraction of the expiratory muscles increases intrathoracic pressure, which is transmitted intracranially by the venous system. The anterior fontanel ☐ becomes sunken / ☐ bulges as the intracranial pressure increases.

bulges

   c. Dehydration reduces the blood and tissue volume, reducing intracranial pressure. The anterior fontanel ☐ becomes sunken / ☐ bulges.

becomes sunken

   d. Write a statement relating the contour of the anterior fontanel to the intracranial pressure. ______________________________

Ans: When the anterior fontanel bulges, the intracranial pressure is increased; when it is sunken, the intracranial pressure is decreased.

   e. Normally the head increases in size as the skull yields to the growth pressure of the brain. A pathologic increase in head size may result from two basic classes of conditions:
      (1) Presence of abnormal substances within the cranium, such as neoplasms, hematomas, hyperplasia, edema, or abnormal accumulation of metabolic substances.
      (2) Presence of increased amounts of cerebrospinal fluid, either from obstruction to its absorption or to its excessive production.

   f. If the intracranial pressure increases, what part of the fetal or infant skull would yield most rapidly and obviously to the increased intracranial pressure? ☐ anterior fontanel / ☐ sutures / ☐ synchrondroses.

Ans: The soft spot! Bulging of the anterior fontanel is the first sign.

g. What position would you place an infant in to inspect whether his fontanel was bulging from a pathologic increase in intracranial pressure? ☐ inverted / ☐ reclining / ☐ upright. Explain:

____

____

Ans: Upright to remove any bulging caused by gravity, which might confuse the evaluation.

☑ No

h. Should you try to estimate pathologic increased pressure from examination of the fontanel if the infant is struggling or crying vigorously? ☐ Yes / ☐ No / ☐ Makes no difference.
Explain: ____

____

____

Ans: When the intrathoracic pressure increases, the intracranial pressure also increases. You may err in considering physiologic bulging as pathologic.

sutures (If you erred, review frame 3c.)

i. The anterior fontanel usually closes by 18 months. Suppose increased intracranial pressure began after that time. Which synarthrosis would yield next to the pressure, the synchondroses of the cranial base, or the sutures of the cranial vault?__________.

increases

j. Wide separation or "splitting" of the sutures can be detected by palpation. Otherwise, skull radiographs are essential. If the sutures split, what happens to the head size? __________.

4 to 6 years

k. Although suture closure by ossification continues into adulthood, *functional* closure occurs earlier. By 10 to 12 years of age the sutures usually adhere so firmly, although nonossified, that they no longer yield to increased intracranial pressure. Suppose you have examined a 16-year-old boy with a big head and spreading of his sutures, as shown by a skull radiograph. What is the *minimum* time the patient could have had increased intracranial pressure? __________

__________.

☑ B

l. In Fig. 1-23, page 27, select the skull radiograph which shows split sutures: ☐ A / ☐ B / ☐ C.

Bulging fontanels
Split sutures
Increased head size

m. List three physical signs of pathologic increased intracranial pressure in a young infant:__________

__________.

6. *The size of the head*

a. Every infant's head circumference must be recorded at every examination. A steel tape measure is placed around the maximum occipitofrontal circumference (OFC), from the external occipital protuberance (inion) to the glabella. Compare with the normal values given in Fig. 1-14. Any OFC value ± 2.5 cm from the mean is suspicious, while any value $\pm$ 3.0 cm is virtually certain to be pathologic, if the body weight, chest circumference, length, and other proportions are normal. However, allowances have to be made for extreme somatotypes.

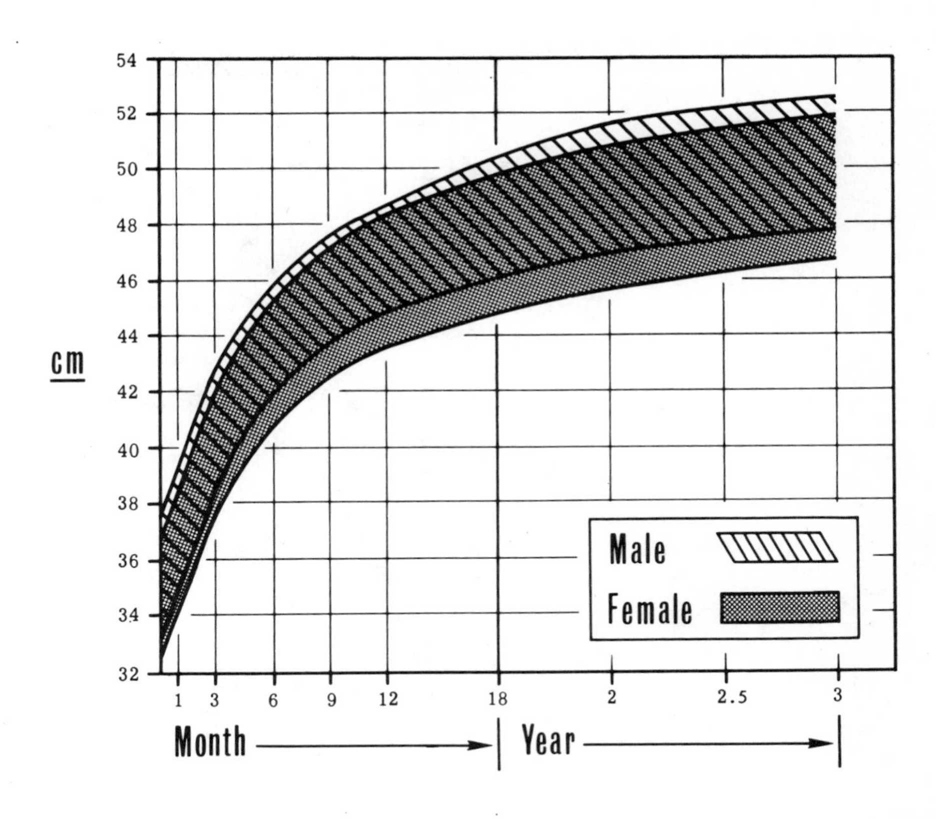

FIG. 1-14. Growth curve for the head circumference of normal infants. The areas shown for males and females include two standard deviations above and below the mean. Ninety-five percent of normal children fall within these areas.

b. To best recognize an abnormal trend in head size, plot successive OFC measurements on a chart. See Fig. 1-15. In Fig. 1-15, trend line *A* displays an abnormally enlarging head (macrocephaly) while trend line *B* shows a lagging head size (microcephaly).

c. If the head is too small, call it *microcephaly*. If too large, ____________cephaly.

*macro*cephaly

d. If the brain or encephalon is too small and weighs too little the condition is called *micrencephaly*. If the brain is too large and heavy, it is called ____________ *encephaly*.

*megal*encephaly or *macr*encephaly

e. Of necessity, a patient with microcephaly has ☐ macrencephaly/ ☐ micrencephaly/ ☐ a normal brain size.

micrencephaly

f. Of necessity, a patient with a big brain must have a big head, but it is not true that a patient with a big head must have a big brain. In macrocephaly, the brain may be normal in weight or too small. In fact, patients with little or no cerebrum may have microcephaly, normocephaly, or macrocephaly. Study Fig. 1-16.

Thus we can conclude that:

☐ (1) The OFC and brain weight have a strict, linear correlation.

☐ (2) While the OFC and brain weight correlate roughly, the OFC predicts the maximum weight the brain may have, but not the minimum.

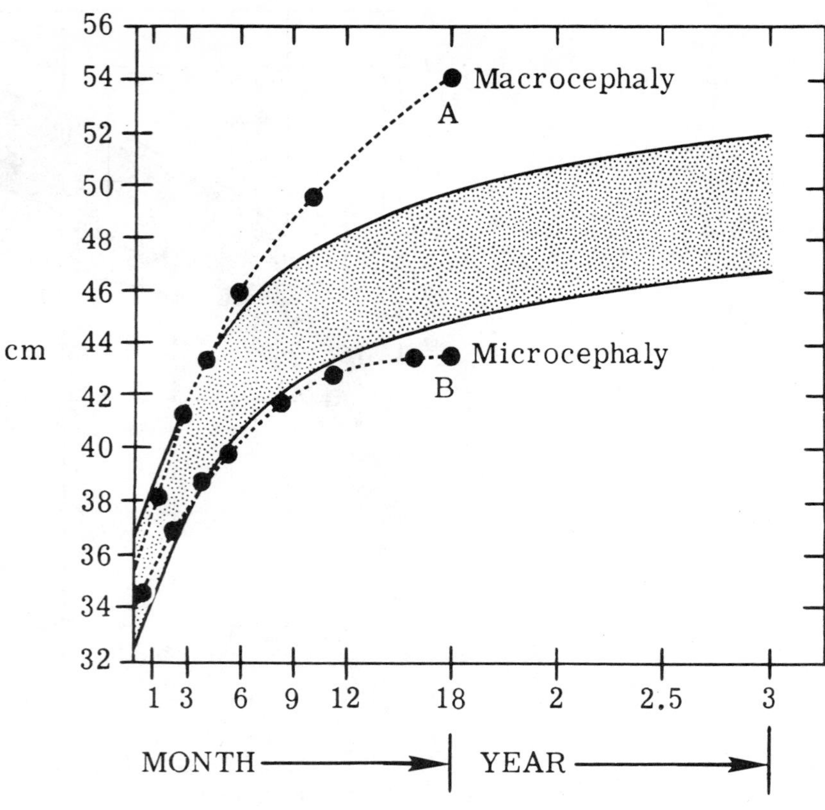

FIG. 1-15. Successive plots of abnormal head sizes.

☐ (3) While the OFC and brain weight correlate roughly, the OFC predicts the minimum weight the brain may have, but not the maximum.

☐ (4) None of the foregoing answers apply.

☒ (2)

g. When the brain volume is small relative to skull volume, as in Fig. 1-16, the space unoccupied by brain contains cerebrospinal fluid (CSF). Whenever the volume of CSF is significantly increased, the condition is called *hydrocephaly,* irrespective of brain size or head size, irrespective of the location of the fluid within the ventricles or subarachnoid space, and irrespective of the intracranial pressure. Thus, the one condition necessary to justify the term *hydrocephaly* is that the ____
____.

volume of CSF is significantly increased

h. It happened that the patient in Fig. 1-16 had *microcephaly* and *micrencephaly.* The disproportionately small brain left a large space to be filled with fluid. Thus, this patient had ☐ macrencephaly/ ☐ anencephaly/ ☐ hydrocephaly as well as microcephaly.

hydrocephaly

i. Thus far the combining terms *micro-*, *macro-*, and *hydro-* have been used in a purely quantitative sense to mean too much or too little of something. Thus, they are descriptive terms like *gigantism* or *dwarfism,* not diagnoses. It is customary to use *hydrocephaly* in a second sense to mean a triad of increased head size, increased CSF, and increased intracranial pressure. If the excessive CSF is

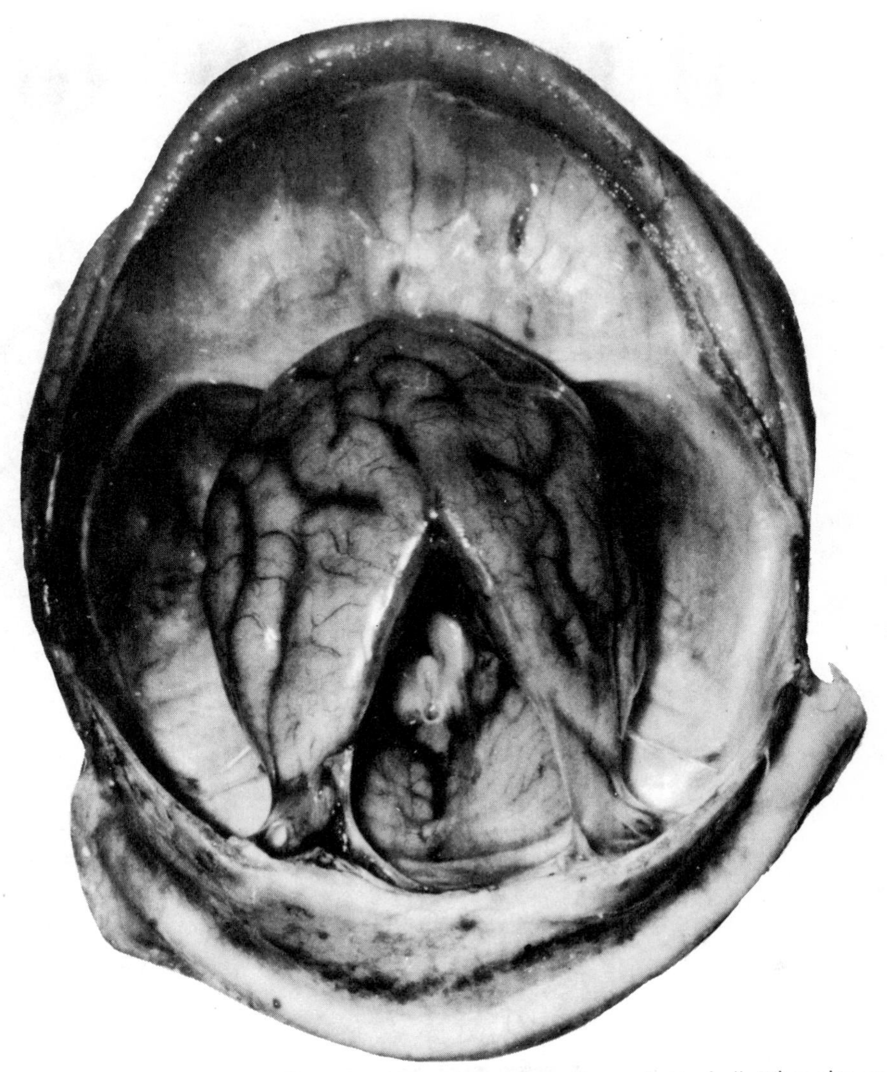

FIG. 1-16. Postmortem photograph of a micrencephalon in a microcephalic skull. When this patient died at the age of 4 months, the OFC was only 32 cm (normal 41 cm). In spite of the tiny head, the disproportionately small brain failed to fill the intracranial space. (*From W. DeMyer and P. White: EEG in holoprosencephaly (arhinencephaly), Arch. Neurol.*, 11: 507-520, 1964.)

under pressure in the ventricles, the cerebral wall thins and the ventricles dilate. See Fig. 1-17.

j. When the brain is too small, as from atrophy, hypoplasia, or destructive lesions, and the excessive CSF merely fills in the unoccupied space, the intracranial pressure may be normal. Is the term *hydrocephaly* admissible in this context? ☐ Yes / ☐ No. Explain: ________
____
____

Ans: Yes, the first definition, the purely quantitative one of frame 6g, applies.

k. If you detect or suspect an abnormal head size, you will want to visualize the size and shape of the brain and the size of the ventricles. You can do this by one of several radiographic methods. *Computerized axial tomography* is the simplest, safest, and most pain-free procedure, as explained in Chapter 13. A second procedure called

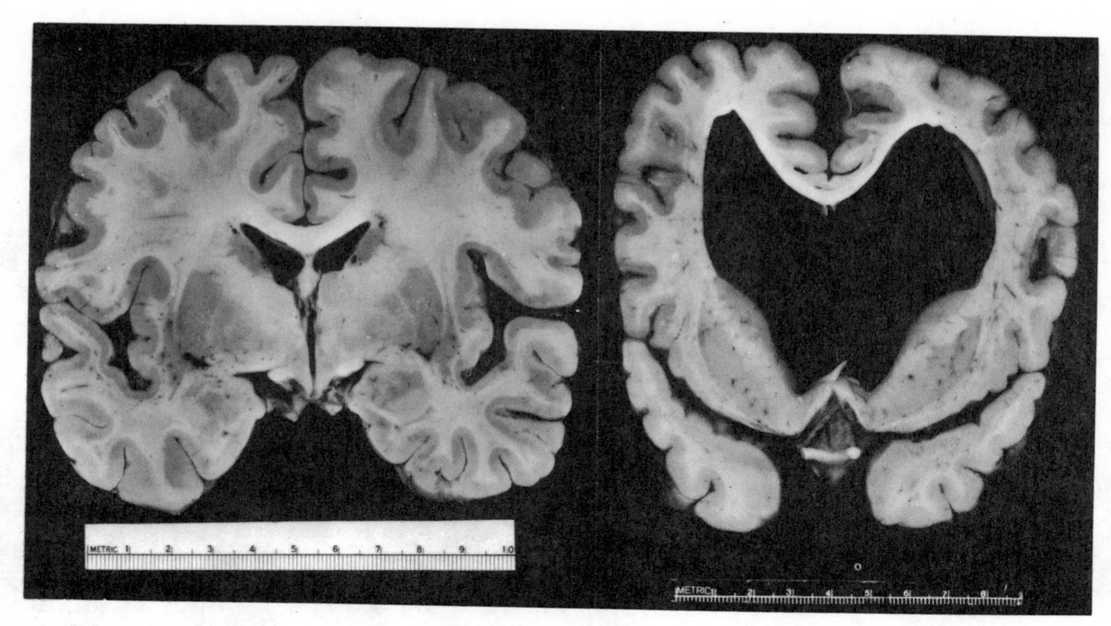

FIG. 1-17. Coronal sections of the brain. *A*. Normal brain to show the configuration of the anterior horns of the lateral ventricles. *B*. Hydrocephalic brain to show the enormous symmetrical dilation of the lateral ventricles. The septum pellucidum, which is shown intact in *A*, is stretched thin and has ruptured.

air encephalography or *pneumoencephalography* requires the insertion of air into the cerebrospinal fluid. The radiolucency of air as compared to brain, fluid, or bone, causes the ventricular cavities and subarachnoid spaces to stand out. Although showing greater detail than computerized axial tomography, air encephalography causes discomfort and carries a slight risk of infection. See Figs. 1-17 and 1-18.

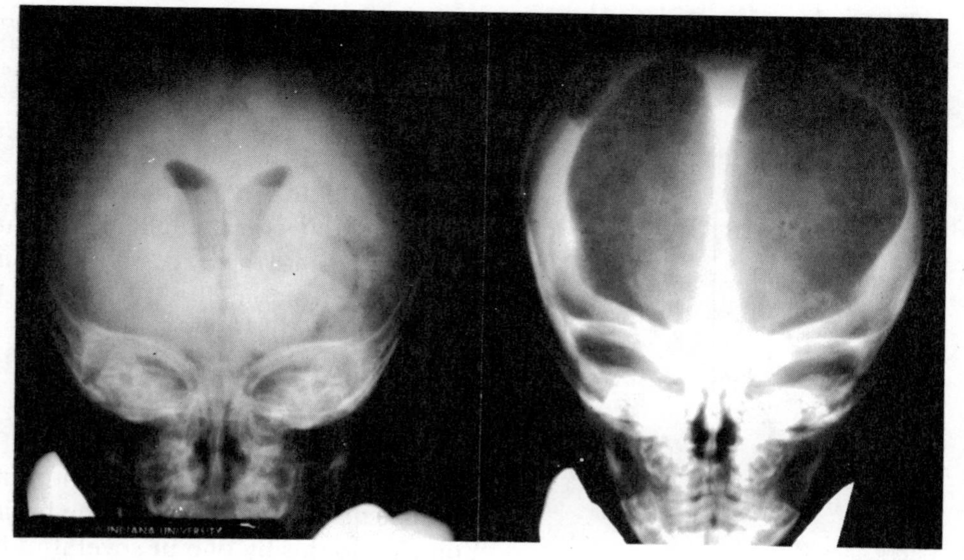

FIG. 1-18. Anteroposterior pneumoencephalograms of young infants. The fluid in the ventricular system has been replaced by air, which is radiolucent. *A*. Normal ventricular configuration. *B*. Hydrocephaly. Compare *A* and *B* of Figs. 1-17 and 1-18.

Bibliography

Baum, J., and Searls, D.: Head shape and size of newborn infants, *Develop. Med. Child Neurol.,* 13:572-575, 1971.

———: Head shape and size of pre-term low-birthweight infants, *Develop. Med. Child Neurol.,* 13:576-581, 1971.

Davies, P., and Davis J.: Very low birthweight and subsequent head growth, *Lancet,* No. 7685, Dec. 12, 1970.

Dekaban, A. S.: Tables of cranial and orbital measurements, cranial volume, and derived indexes in males and females from 7 days to 20 years of age, *Ann. Neurol.,* 2:485-491, 1977.

Finnstrom, O.: Studies on maturity in newborn infants. I: Birth weight, crown-heel length, head circumference, and skull diameters in relation to gestational age. *Acta Paediat. Scand.,* 60:685-694, 1971.

Nellhaus, G.: Head circumference from birth to eighteen years, *Pediatrics,* 41: 106-114, 1968.

Nelson, K., and Deutschberger, J.: Head circumference as a predictor of 4 year I.Q., *Develop. Med. Child Neurol.,* 12:487-495, 1970.

O'Neill, E., Normal head growth and the prediction of head size in infantile hydrocephalus, *Arch. Dis. Child.,* 36:241-252, 1961.

———: Minimal rates of head growth in the first four months of life, *Arch. Dis. Child.,* 37:363-365, 1962.

Sher, P. K., and Brown, S. B.: A longitudinal study of head growth in pre-term infants. II: Differentiation between "catch-up" head growth and early infantile hydrocephalus. *Dev. Med. Child Neurol.,* 17:711-718, 1975.

B. *Transillumination of the head*

1. **Whenever you examine an infant, you must attempt to transilluminate the head. See Fig. 1-19.**

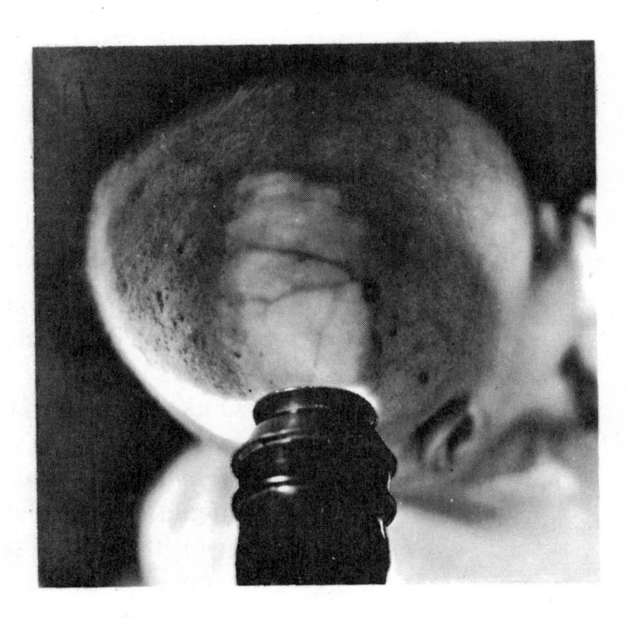

FIG. 1-19. Localized transillumination of the parietal region. A parietal craniotomy was done to relieve an intracerebral and subdural hematoma caused by a head injury. Clear fluid then accumulated between the dura and cerebrum (subdural hygroma) and gradually bulged through the surgical defect in the parietal bone. Scalp vessels can be seen coursing over the bulge.

a. Procedure. Take the infant into a completely dark closet and allow several minutes for dark-adaptation of your eyes. Press an ordinary flashlight fitted with a rubber adaptor against the infant's head, and move it over the various regions of the cranial vault.

b. Results. Normally, a small halo of transillumination, less than a centimeter in diameter, will appear around the adaptor margin. Under four conditions, the halo will be large or even the entire head will light up.

(1) Increased fluid or edema in the scalp or in the subgaleal space between the galea aponeurotica and cranium. See Fig. 1-20*A*.

(2) Increased fluid in the subdural space, between the dura mater and the brain. See Fig. 1-20*B*.

(3) Increased fluid within the brain because of thinning by stretching, destruction, atrophy, or hypoplasia. See Fig. 1-20*C* and *D*.

(4) Premature infants with huge fontanels and very thin cranial bones.

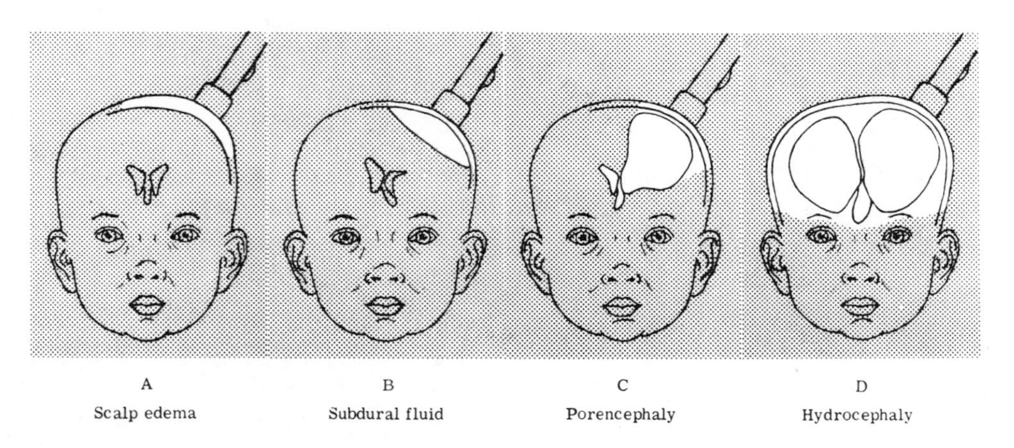

FIG. 1-20. Head transillumination with lesions of different types.

c. Systematic analysis of the cause for transillumination

(1) You will have to decide whether the fluid which causes the transillumination is outside or inside of the skull. Consider first outside fluid.

(a) Outside of the skull, the fluid must be in the scalp or subgaleal space.

Detection of scalp edema: the commonest causes of scalp edema are head injuries and infiltration of intravenous fluid given through a scalp vein. The pitting test discloses scalp edema. Press the ball of your finger firmly against the scalp in the area of transillumination. Hold it firmly and it will sink through the edema fluid, allowing the finger to press the scalp against the bone. After removal of your finger, a pit remains.

(b) *Detection of subgaleal fluid:* subgaleal fluid elevates the scalp from the skull. The skull can be more or less balloted. Finger pressure readily discloses the distance between the scalp and skull, but the scalp does not pit.

(2) Fluid inside of the skull, in the subdural space or intracerebral. (After a head injury, the epidural space may contain blood, but epidural blood never transilluminates.)

(a) To test for subdural fluid, insert a needle through the lateral angle of the anterior fontanel, a subdural tap.

(b) To test for intracerebral fluid, the size and shape of the brain and ventricles have to be visualized. What two radiographic procedures best show the anatomy of the brain in the living patient? ______________________.

computerized axial tomography, air encephalography

d. To prove that you can systematically analyze transillumination, place your hand on top of your head and recite the two extracranial locations and the two intracranial locations of the fluid. Then complete Table 1-2.

TABLE 1-2. Tests for Location of Excess Fluid When the Head Transilluminates

	Location of fluid	Test procedure to verify
Extracranial		
Intracranial		

Scalp/fingertip pressure for pitting edema

Subgaleal space/fingertip pressure for elevation of scalp

Subdural space/subdural taps

Within the brain/air encephalography or computerized axial tomography

e. Rarely, the cerebellum is absent or its region is occupied by a large cyst. The posterior fossa (inferior occipital region) will then transilluminate. This fact demonstrates the principle that you should move the flashlight over the entire cranial vault and inferior occipital region to do a thorough examination.

f. In general, transillumination is useless in patients more than 2 or 3 years of age. The skull is usually too thick and well ossified to transmit light. If you find transillumination in an older patient, almost the only explanation would be that the fluid is located ______________________
____
______________________.

outside the skull in the scalp or subgaleal space

Yes

2 or 3

g. Review Fig. 1-16. Would you expect the head of this young infant to transilluminate? ☐ Yes / ☐ No.

h. Review Fig. 1-17*B*. You would expect this infant's head to transilluminate only if he is less than ________ years old.

i. One of the ironies of a people like ours, who worship technology, is that while many states have passed laws requiring biochemical screening of every infant for phenylketonuria, there is no law requiring a thorough physical examination. By measuring and transilluminating the head of every infant, you will discover countless more lesions, many of them life-threatening yet treatable, such as subdural fluid and hydrocephaly, than by screening for phenylketonuria. Dazzled by laboratory tests, are we demeaned if we have to candle an infants head? Harvey Cushing (1869 - 1939) put it well when he remarked that we have increasing numbers of laboratory tests, ". . . the vast majority of which are but supplementary to, and as *nothing* compared with, the careful study of the patient by a keen observer using his eyes and ears and fingers and a few simple aids."

Bibliography

Rabe, E.: Skull transillumination in infants, *Gen. Practit.,* 36:78-88, 1967.

Sjogren, I., and Engsner, G.: Transillumination of the skull in infants and children, *Acta Paediat. Scand.,* 61:426-428, 1972.

C. *Differential analysis of megalocephaly (macrocephaly)*

1. After you find that a patient has an enlarged head, megalocephaly, you have only made a statistical description of the patient, not a diagnosis. Basically, one of five conditions causes megalocephaly. You should, I think, learn and be able to recite them. The reference on the next page gives a full list of differential diagnoses for megalocephaly.

   Megalocephaly
   - → Hydrocephalus
   - → Brain edema (toxic-metabolic disorders)
   - → Subdural hematoma
   - → Thickened skull
   - → Megalencephaly

2. Two essential steps in the physical examination of a megalocephalic patient are:
   a. Compare the somatotype and OFC of patient, siblings, and parents. Does the patient match or differ from the family pattern?
   b. Attempt to transilluminate the skull.

Bibliography

DeMyer, W.: Megalencephaly in children. Clinical syndromes, genetic patterns and differential diagnosis from other causes of megalocephaly, *Neurology,* 22:634–643, 1972.

D. Mechanism of skull growth

1. Although increased intracranial pressure forces the skull sutures apart, they do not separate in response to the normal pressure of the gently growing brain. Active bone growth along the suture margins keeps them in contact, balancing the intracranial pressure at an optimum level. Clinically, the most important growth occurs along the sagittal and coronal sutures. Study Fig. 1-21.

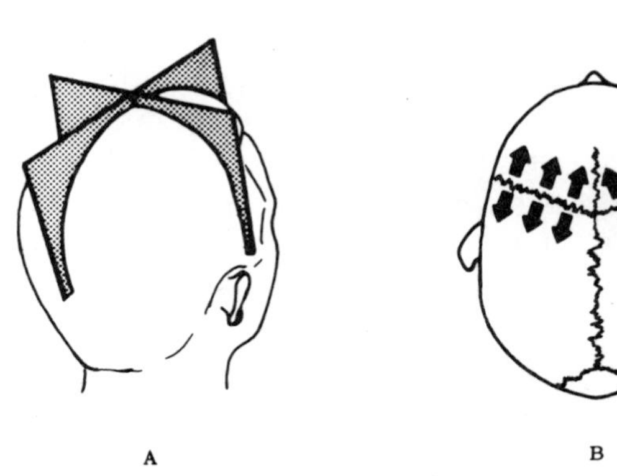

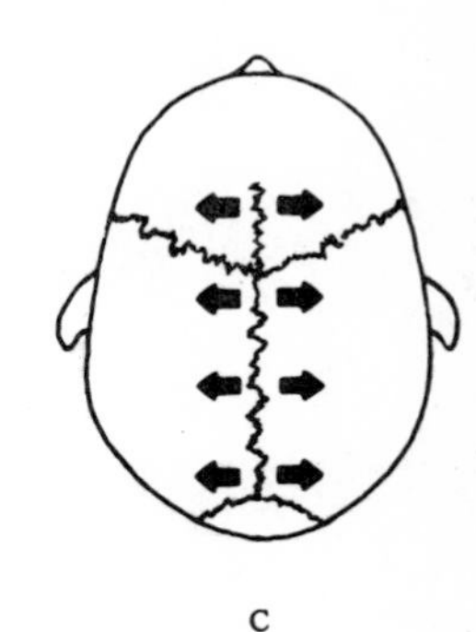

A B C

FIG. 1-21. The sagittal and coronal sutures and the direction of head enlargement from their growth zones. *A.* Schematic projection of the planes of the sagittal and coronal sutures. *B.* Growth along the coronal suture increases the anteroposterior diameter of the head. *C.* Growth along the sagittal suture increases the lateral diameter of the head.

Answers	Frames
☑ A-P	2. Growth along the coronal suture increases the head diameter which is perpendicular to it, the ☐ anteroposterior (A-P) / ☐ lateral diameter.
lateral	3. Growth along the sagittal suture increases the head diameter which is perpendicular to it, the ______________ diameter.
perpendicular	4. As a general law, we can state that growth along a suture margin increases the head diameter which is ______________ to the plane of the suture.
large	5. Look at the heads of your classmates. Some heads will be unusually short and wide and others long and thin. The OFC in the two groups will be approximately the same. Therefore, a head that is relatively small in one diameter will, in compensation, be relatively ______________ in another diameter.

brachycephaly	6. Anthropologists call short-headedness *brachycephaly* (brachy = short) and long-headedness *dolichocephaly* (dolicho = long). Which head type would have the greatest lateral diameter? ______________.
coronal sagittal	7. In brachycephaly, the growth from the ______________ suture proceeds slowly relative to that from the ______________ suture.
dolicho	8. A head that is too long and thin is termed ______________ *cephaly.*
sagittal coronal	9. In dolichocephaly, the growth from the ______________ suture proceeds slowly relative to that from the ______________ suture.

E. Abnormalities in skull shape: the craniosynostoses

1. The terms *dolichocephaly* and *brachycephaly* describe normal variations in the ratio of width and length of the skull. The sutures are basically normal. If a pathologic condition causing bony overgrowth affects the skull, one or more sutures and fontanels do not form or, if formed, close prematurely. Such a condition is called *craniosynostosis* (craniostenosis). You must recognize craniosynostosis in young infants, when surgical treatment is most effective. Removal of strips of bone creates artificial sutures. Early surgery produces the best cosmetic results and prevents later complications: increased intracranial pressure, brain damage, and blindness, which may result from severe craniosynostosis.

	2. *Clinical detection of craniosynostosis*
	a. In craniosynostosis, the overgrowth and fusion of bone at the sutures results in a palpable ridge. The bony overgrowth and absence of the suture can be confirmed by skull radiographs.
☒ C	*b.* From Fig. 1-23, page 27 select the radiograph which shows synostosis of the coronal suture: ☐ A / ☐ B / ☐ C.
coronal	*c.* Suppose you have examined a three-month-old baby whose head looked too short. You would suspect a deficiency of growth from the ______________ suture.
Palpate for a bony ridge and order skull radiographs	3. You would have to decide whether the child's head shape was simple brachycephaly and therefore a normal variant, or whether he had craniosynostosis of the coronal suture. What would you do to determine the state of the sutures? ______________.
	4. *Terminology for craniosynostosis*
	a. Clinicians apply special terms to the abnormal head shapes caused by craniosynostosis. The terms here follow Ford's usage, but there are many synonyms and discrepancies from author to author.
coronal	*b.* The pathologic condition of short-headedness due to craniosynostosis is called *acrobrachycephaly.* See Fig. 1-22*A.* In such a patient, the closed suture is the ______________ suture.

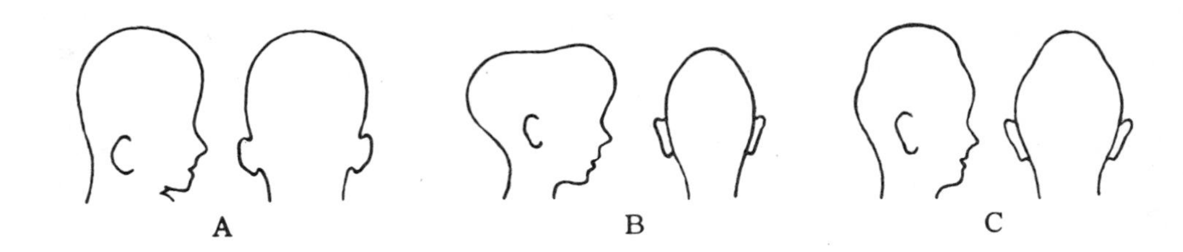

FIG. 1-22. Silhouettes of abnormal head shapes caused by craniosynostosis. *A.* Acrobrachycephaly. *B.* Scaphocephaly. *C.* Oxycephaly.

The sagittal suture permits lateral expansion.

c. In acrobrachycephaly, the head is too short because coronal closure restricts its A-P diameter. Why does the head become too wide? ______ ______________________________.

sagittal

d. The pathologic condition of long-headedness from craniosynostosis is called *scaphocephaly* (scapho = skiff or boat). The head looks like an inverted boat. See Fig. 1-22*B*. The closed suture is the ______ ______ suture.

coronal

e. In scaphocephaly, the head becomes long because it expands perpendicular to the less affected suture, the ______________ suture.

Coronal and sagittal sutures are both synostosed

f. The pathologic head shape in Fig. 1-22*C* is called *oxycephaly* (oxy = keen or sharp). The head is reduced in both the lateral and A-P diameters. What does this head shape imply about the cranial sutures? ______________________________.

g. Complete Table 1-3

brachycephaly/acrobrachycephaly

dolichocephaly/scaphocephaly

oxycephaly

TABLE 1-3. Comparison of Terms for Head Shapes

Skull shape	Term for extreme variation of normal skull	Pathologic term for craniosynostosis
Skull too short and wide		
Skull too long		
Skull too short and narrow	None	

oxycephaly

Neither major suture allows skull growth

h. Would acrobrachycephaly, scaphocephaly, or oxycephaly most likely cause increased intracranial pressure? ______________
Explain: ______________________________.

exopthalmos (proptosis)

i. With increased intracranial pressure in craniosynostosis, the weakest part of the skull yields. The thin orbital plates bulge downwards, protruding the eyes. The general term for eyeball protrusion is ______ ______________.

j. Although usually bilateral, craniosynostosis may obliterate the sutures only on one side of the head. The affected hemicranium is small, and the skull and face are asymmetrical, a condition termed *plagiocephaly* (plagio = oblique). However, the term plagiocephaly crops up indiscriminately for any asymmetrical skull.

k. Craniosynostosis contributes only a share of the misshapen asymmetrical skulls. Intrinsic diseases such as rickets and syphilis deform the skull as does extrinsic pressure. The most striking examples occurred in primitive societies where, in pursuit of beauty, infant's heads were shaped by wrapping them with bandages. (Although artificially shaped heads have gone out of style, the problem of status symbols still prevails.) If an infant has a neurologic deficit which causes him to rest on one part of his head, the head deforms to become flat on the "down" side. If the infant reclines on his back, the occiput becomes flattened. If he reclines on the parieto-occipital region, it flattens and the head becomes skewed. Sometimes no cause for skull asymmetry can be identified. In any event, an abnormal size or shape of the skull warns of an abnormal brain.

l. Complete Table 1-4 to fix the diagnostic terms for head shapes firmly in mind.

Answer	*TABLE 1-4. Terms for Abnormal Head Shapes*	
Acrobrachycephaly	______________ cephaly:	too short a skull because of lack of a coronal suture.
Plagiocephaly	______________ cephaly:	an asymmetrical skull because of lack of sutures on one side.
Scaphocephaly	______________ cephaly:	too long a skull because of lack of a sagittal suture.
Dolichocephaly	______________ cephaly:	too long a skull without craniosynostosis.
Oxycephaly	______________ cephaly:	a short, narrow skull because of craniosynostosis.
Brachycephaly	______________ cephaly:	a short skull without craniosynostosis.

Palpate for suture ridging and premature fontanel closure, and order skull radiographs

m. What do you do to decide whether an infant with an abnormal head shape has craniosynostosis? ____ ______________________.

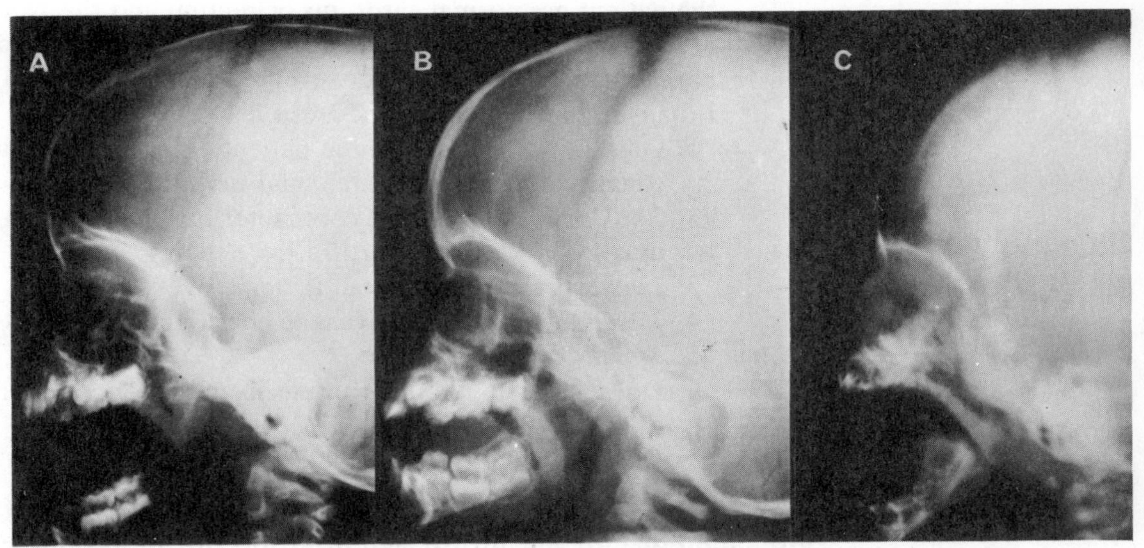

FIG. 1-23. Radiographs of the coronal suture showing various degrees of apposition of frontal and parietal bones.

Bibliography

Bertelsen, T.: The premature synostosis of the cranial sutures, *Acta Ophthal* (Kobenhavn), supp. 51, 1958.

Ford, F.: *Diseases of the Nervous System In Infancy, Childhood and Adolescence,* 5th ed., Springfield, Ill., Charles C Thomas, Publisher, 1966.

Laitinen, L.: Craniosynostosis. Premature fusion of the cranial sutures, *Ann. Paediat. Fenn.,* vol. 2, supp. 6, 1956.

Montaut, J., and Stricker, M.: *Dysmorphies Cranio-faciales. Les Synostoses Prematures (Craniostenoses et Faciostenoses)*, Paris, Masson, 1977.

Shillito, J., Jr. and Matson, D.: Craniosynostosis: a review of 519 surgical patients, *Pediatrics,* 41:829-853, 1968.

V. The philosophy of physical diagnosis

A. *Why examine a patient?* To discover whether the patient's anatomy and physiology deviate significantly from the norm. If he does deviate from the norm, we want to know in what way (qualitatively) and to what degree (quantitatively). In deciding whether a part shows a pathologic deviation, we compare it against three standards:
   1. Compare each part with the theoretical norm for a person of like age and sex.
   2. Compare each part with its mate on the opposite side.
   3. Compare the patient with the other family members. Does he deviate from or repeat the appearances expected from his genetic background?

B. *What attitude do you take in doing the physical examination?* You must assume that everything is abnormal until you examine it. If you start out thinking everything is normal, you will be careless in your examination or even forget part of it.

C. *Why do a complete examination on every patient?* Because you must assume that everything is abnormal until you examine it. You cannot assume that the patient has normal eardrums or rectum and that you don't have to look at them. Suspect everything about the patient to be abnormal. Be absolutely paranoid about it. Thus, do every exam with obsessive-compulsive, yes, ritualistic thoroughness. The steps are:

1. Gather in the *gestalt* of the patient: What is the total impact of his personality, facial appearance, and his somatotype?
2. *Look* over every square centimeter of skin and mucous membrane; look into every orifice, aperture, or opening.
3. *Feel* every part. Poke your finger in every opening.
4. *Listen* to every sound over the chest, abdomen, head, and blood vessels.
5. *Smell* every odor.
6. Do a basic minimum routine examination of every organ system on every patient.
7. Do every additional test indicated by the history.

VIII. Summary of the initial examination of the head and face

How do we insure that you can apply these general principles and the specific data of this chapter to the actual examination of a patient? We do it by instituting a ritual, the ritual of regular rehearsal of just what it is the chapter teaches you to do, until you do it automatically. Although you may prefer to call it rehearsing, the behavioral psychologist would say that he wants you to emit the terminal behavior of the learning sequence. By terminal behavior, he means those recitations and performances which provide evidence to yourself and others that you have learned what you should have. Get a partner and emit the terminal behavior (all right, let's say rehearse) as outlined below. As you do so, notice how the four techniques of inspection, palpation, percussion, and auscultation impose their order on the examination and how the anatomic arrangement of the body parts imposes its order. So turn now to Section IV, A–E of the Summarized Neurologic Examination that precedes Chapter 1 and rehearse it until it becomes yours.

2

The Visual System: Diplopia, Ocular Alignment, and Ocular Muscles

In examining and treating motor anomalies, one never loses an uneasy feeling of incompetence until he has become thoroughly familiar with the physiologic fundamentals from which the signs and symptoms of those anomalies are to be derived. Therefore, a discussion of motor anomalies of the eyes should begin with a synopsis of the physiology of the sensorial and motor apparatus of the eyes.

— Alfred Bielschowsky (1871 - 1940)

I. Diplopia and ocular alignment

A. Visual acuity

1. The concept of visual acuity is basic to understanding ocular alignment. Although the total field of vision when you look straight ahead is nearly 180° wide, you may be surprised at the limited field of visual acuity. Fixate on one book title in a row of books about a meter from you, or place a line of print at that distance. How many book titles or words can you read without shifting fixation?

Do the experiment and find out!

____

2. Visual acuity depends on the light rays striking the central region of the retina, the *fovea centralis* of the macula lutea. Learn Fig. 2-1 — yes, you should be able to draw it.

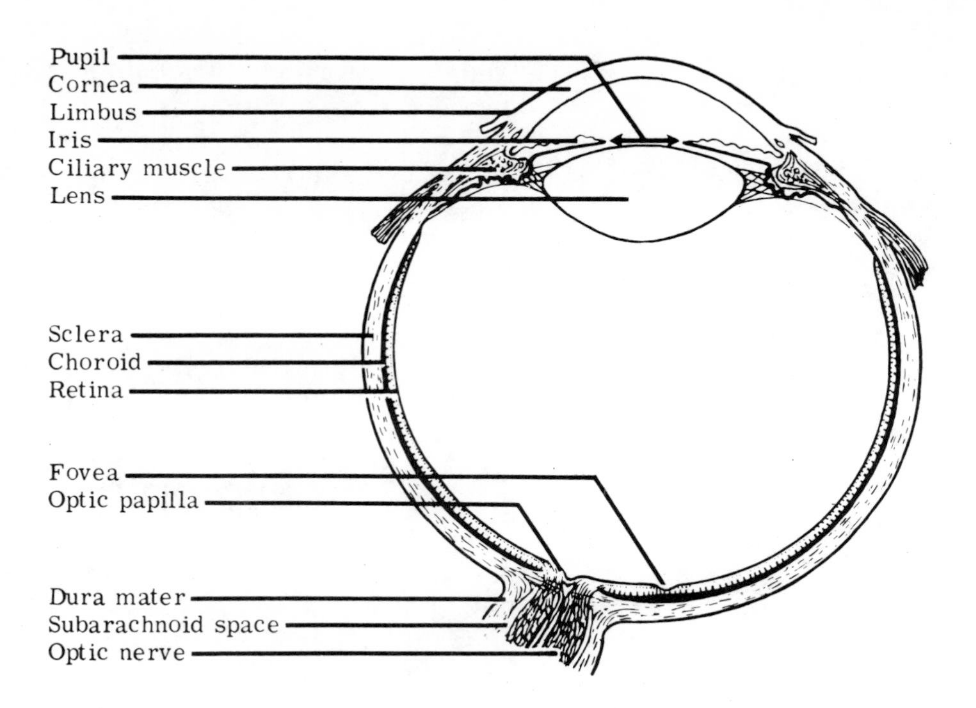

FIG. 2-1. Horizontal section of the right eye.

B. Ocular alignment

1. Ocular alignment is tested by starting with the patient looking straight ahead. The eyes are then said to be in the *primary position*. The point of fixation in the primary position is at infinity distance. See Fig. 2-2.

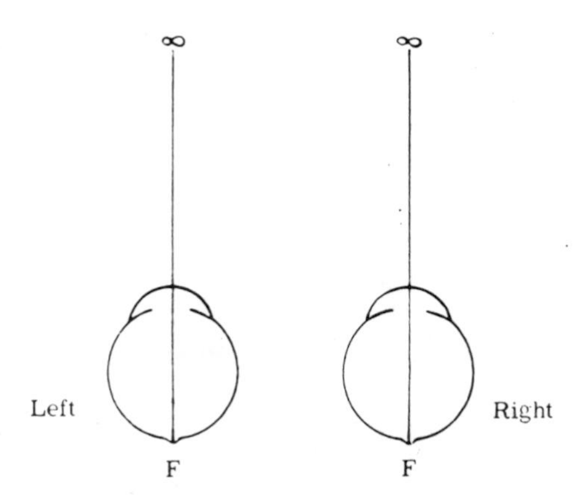

FIG. 2-2. Visual axes when the eyes are in the primary position, fixating on infinity distance. *F* is the fovea.

visual axis

a. A line drawn from the fovea centralis of one eye to the center of the visual field of that eye defines the *visual axis*. Such a line passes through the center of the refractive media of the eye. It is the "line of sight." In Fig. 2-2, the line F-∞ defines the ____________________ ____________________.

essentially parallel

b. When the eyes are in the primary position, fixating on infinity distance, the visual axes are ☐ convergent / ☐ essentially parallel / ☐ divergent.

c. In Fig. 2-3, draw the visual axes when the eyes fixate on a point nearer than infinity. Use a colored pencil.

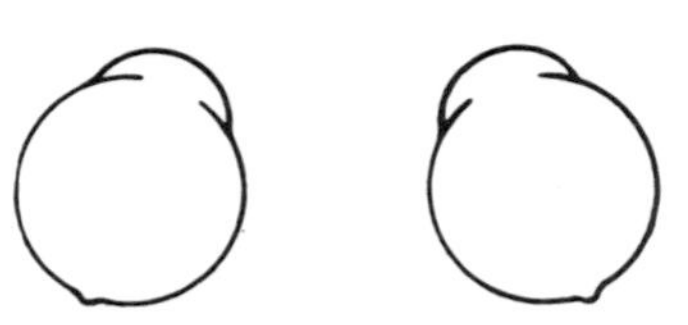

FIG. 2-3. Blank for drawing the visual axes when the eyes fixate on a near point.

fovea centralis

2. When looking at a near point, the eyes converge. With the visual axes properly on target, the central light ray from the fixation point falls on the region of maximum visual acuity. This region is called the ______ ______.

3. *Try this experiment:*
   a. Fixate on some definite point across the room, such as a doorknob.
   b. Hold up the tip of your index finger about 20 cm directly in front of your eyes. Hold the finger so that the doorknob appears to balance on the fingertip.
   c. Fixate *first* on the doorknob, *then* on the very tip of your finger. Keep your gaze firmly on the fingertip and record what happens to the image of the doorknob: ______.
   d. Now fixate *first* on the fingertip and *then* the doorknob. What happens to the appearance of the finger? ______ ______.

becomes double

becomes double

4. In the previous experiment, you found diplopia, *physiologic* diplopia. Fig. 2-4 shows why.
   a. *Explanation of physiologic diplopia.* In Fig. 2-4, rays from only one distance, the fixation point, strike the fovea. All other rays deviate from the fovea in proportion to their distance from the fixation point. Only the rays coming in along the visual axes strike correspondingly on the ______ of each eye.

fovea centralis

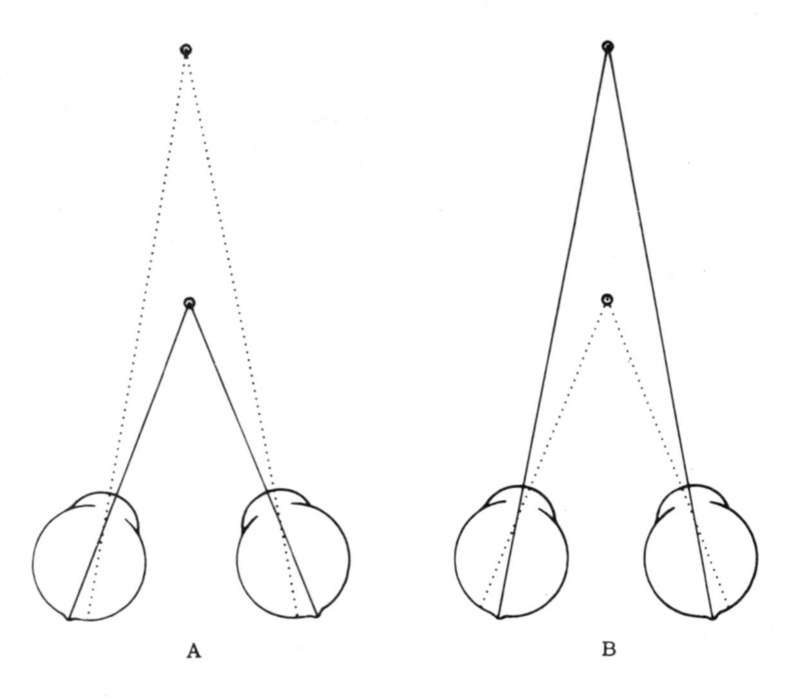

FIG. 2-4. Changes in the angulation of the visual axes when the eyes shift from a near fixation point to a distant one. A. Near fixation. B. Distant fixation.

b. Why don't we have diplopia all the time? Recall that you had to *attend* consciously to the point of *non*fixation to get diplopia. Ordinarily, we have learned to suppress physiologic diplopia. It only appears when we make a determined effort to break through its physiologic suppression. To state it another way, we can say that we only *attend* to the nondiplopic image.

5. *Try this experiment:*
   a. Fixate on the doorknob and place your index fingertip 20 cm away, so that the knob appears to ride on top again.
   b. Alternately wink the right and left eyes as you fix on the doorknob. What happens to the appearance of the finger? __________

   It shifts to one side on closing one eye.

   c. Balance the doorknob on your fingertip again, but this time fixate on your fingertip. Alternately wink the right and left eyes. What happens to the appearance of the doorknob? __________

   It shifts to one side on closing one eye

   d. Explanation. The shift occurs because you *primarily* fixate along the visual axis of the *dominant* eye; the other eye focuses *secondarily.*
6. *Try this experiment:*
   a. Place the tip of your right index finger upon your right lateral canthus, as shown in Fig. 2-5.
   b. Fixate on your left index finger held upright at arm's length.
   c. Gently press on your eyeball with your right index finger. By varying the pressure, you will be able to experience diplopia. If you do not get satisfactory diplopia when looking at your finger, look across the room at a distant object.

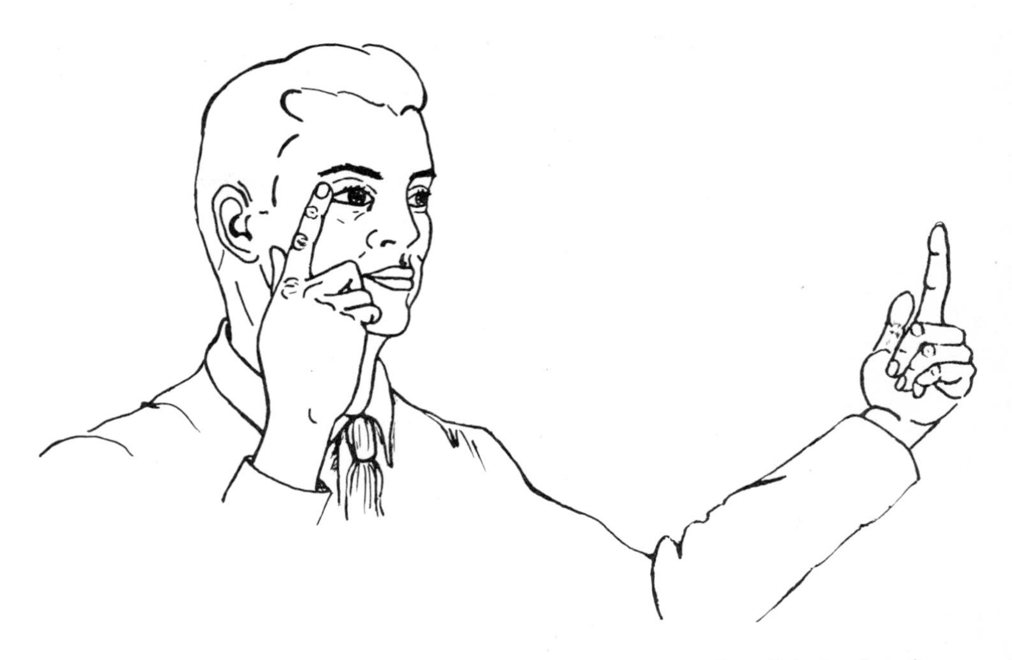

FIG. 2-5. Position of finger for lateral canthus compression to produce diplopia when the eyes gaze at the opposite finger.

d. Try the experiment again, holding the outstretched finger horizontally this time. With the finger vertical or horizontal, you should obtain diplopia. It may be greater with the finger in one position than another, and it may vary each time you try the experiment, depending on the amount of pressure. Also hold the outstretched finger horizontally and try to get diplopia by pressing on your eyeball through the upper lid with your other finger.

7. With your right finger compressing your lateral canthus, decide whether you get better diplopia with the finger vertical or horizontal and then move the finger from center to side or up and down, in whichever direction gives the most diplopia.

The distance between the diplopic images varies.

a. What happens to the distance between the diplopic images as you move your finger? ______________________________

____

b. While experiencing diplopia by pressing your lateral canthus, try to identify which image is faulty. It can be identified by:

(1) Alternating the pressure on the eye, causing the faulty image to move while the other image remains on target.

(2) Noticing which image is the sharpest. Can you explain why the image from the displaced eye is not as sharp as from the other eye? ______________________________

____

____

Ans: only the rays coming in along the visual axis strike directly on the fovea centralis, the part of the retina mediating the sharpest visual acuity.

8. The preceding experiment illustrates some laws of diplopia concerning the behavior of the diplopic image. In order to interpret it, we have to take a closer look at image formation. Consider first the *retinal*

image, which is based solely on *physical* optics. See Fig. 2-6 and draw the visual axis.

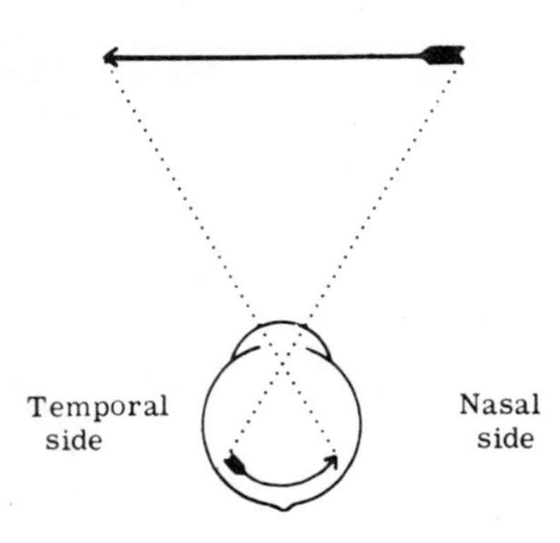

FIG. 2-6. Retinal image formed during monocular fixation with the left eye. Draw the visual axis.

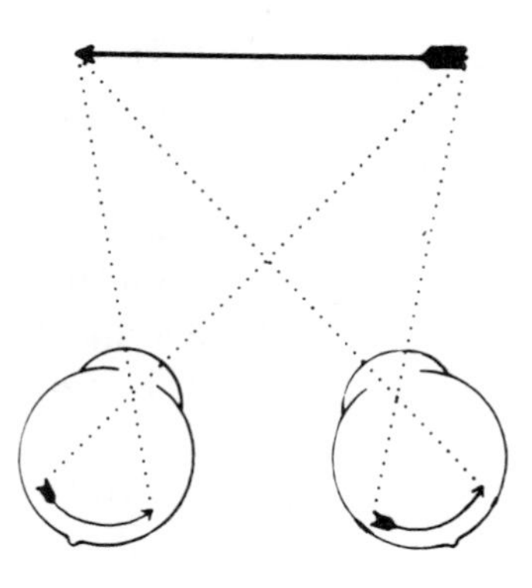

FIG. 2-7. Retinal image formed during binocular fixation. Rays along the visual axes strike the foveas. The remainder of the image falls on corresponding (but not precisely identical) temporal or nasal parts of the retina.

Note: Refer only to Fig. 2-6 until Fig. 2-7 is called for.

a. The image formed on the retina by the physical optics of the eye is a real image. It is called the *retinal* image.

b. The light rays which form the *nasal* half of the retinal image come from the ☐ temporal / ☐ nasal half of the object viewed.

temporal

9. The real image on the retina initiates afferent impulses which travel to the visual receptive area in the occipital lobe. By a process of learning, we associate the point of retinal stimulation with the reverse half of space. Hence, if light rays fall on the *temporal* half of a retina, the source will be perceived as in the ______________ half of space.

nasal (opposite)

10. We learn to reach to the nasal side for an object when its retinal image falls on the temporal side of the retina. Similarly, if the image falls on the *upper* half of the retina, we would reach for it in the ______________ half of space.

lower

opposite (reverse)

projects (refers)

retinal (real)

visual

11. The visual experience initiated by the retinal image is the product of the cerebrum. We call it the *visual image*. It is what the mind sees. The mind *projects* the visual image derived from one-half of the retina to the ______________ half of space.
12. The mind projects afferent impulses to their usual site of origin in all sensory systems. If your right auditory nerve were stimulated by an electrode, you would experience a sound as coming from the right side of space. If you bump your ulnar nerve at the elbow, you feel a shock-like sensation down your forearm into your little finger. In each case, we say that the afferent impulses have initiated a sensation which the mind ______________ to the usual site of origin of the stimuli.
13. The image formed by the physical optics of the eyeball is called the ______________ image.
14. The image which the mind projects as a result of the retinal image is called the ______________ image.
15. Work through Fig. 2-7 to understand how binocular fixation brings the retinal images onto corresponding parts of the retinas of the two eyes. Begin by drawing in the visual axes. After you think you understand the drawing, try to reproduce it.

visual

C. Explanation of diplopia produced by canthal compression

1. For description, the visual image of the normally functioning eye is called the *true* image; of the abnormal eye, the *false* image. Of course, one image is no more "true" or "false" than the other, because both are ______________ images imposed on the afferent data by the mind.
2. Canthal compression mechanically displaces the eye, deviating the visual axis from the fixation point. We will consider only the diplopia produced with the target finger vertical. (Although a few of you may fail to get diplopia this way, the explanation can still be followed.) With the finger vertical in the midline, you got one, or with practice, two results: one image was projected to the *right* or the *left* of the true position of the finger. Whichever direction the false image was projected depends on how the eyeball happened to be displaced. Study Figs. 2-8 and 2-9.
3. Explain why the false image appears to the right of the true image in Fig. 2-8. ______________

Ans: The retinal image falls on the nasal half of the retina and, by learning, the mind projects the visual image to the right.

II. Clinical tests for ocular malalignment

A. The canthal compression test shows that the eyes must be aligned properly to bring the retinal images onto corresponding retinal areas. The penalty for failure is diplopia. The best bedside method for detecting ocular malalignment is the *corneal reflection test:*

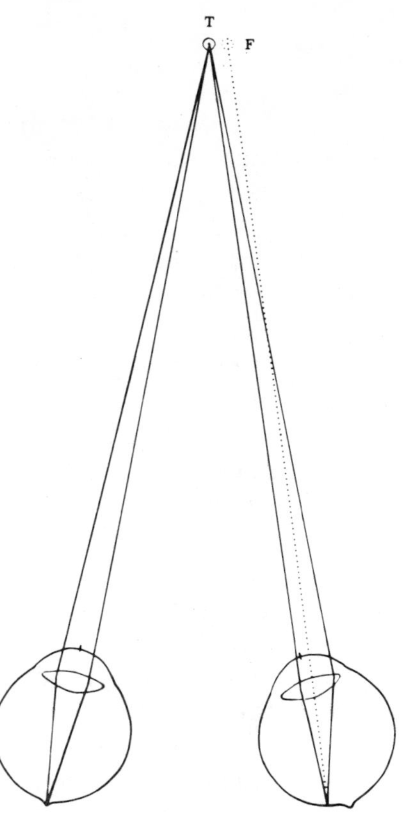

FIG. 2-8. Diagram to explain the projection of the false image to the right when the right eye is turned in (or fails to abduct). T = true image. F = false image. With a colored pencil, draw the visual axis of each eye.

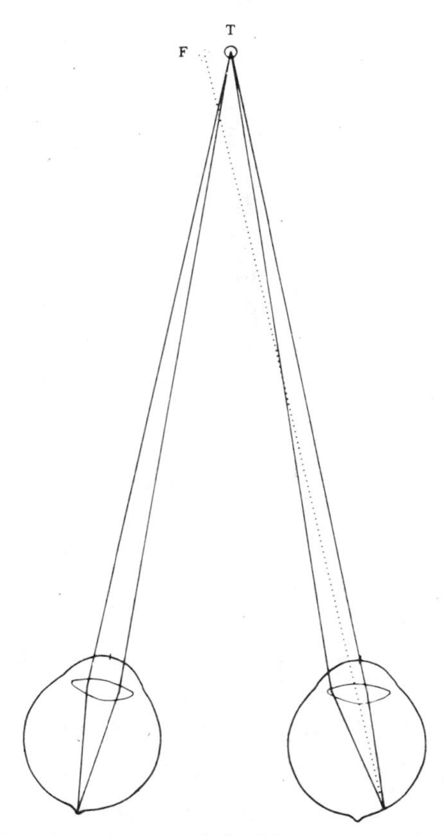

FIG. 2-9. Diagram to explain the projection of the false image to the left when the right eye is turned out (fails to adduct). Draw the visual axis of each eye.

1. Darken your room and locate a distant light source such as a window or a light bulb. (If you have a roommate, use him and the light of your otoscope.) The instructions will be given as though you have no partner.
2. As you gaze straight ahead into the mirror, observe that a single, bright diamond of light reflects off each cornea. By slight mirror movements try to center these diamonds simultaneously on the two corneas. What is the exact location of the corneal light reflections with respect to the true geometric center of each cornea? ____________

____

See next frame.

3. In most subjects, the points of corneal light reflection, after being centered as carefully as possible, will be slightly medial to the true corneal centers. The reason is that the visual axes and anteroposterior axes do not quite coincide. See Fig. 2-10.

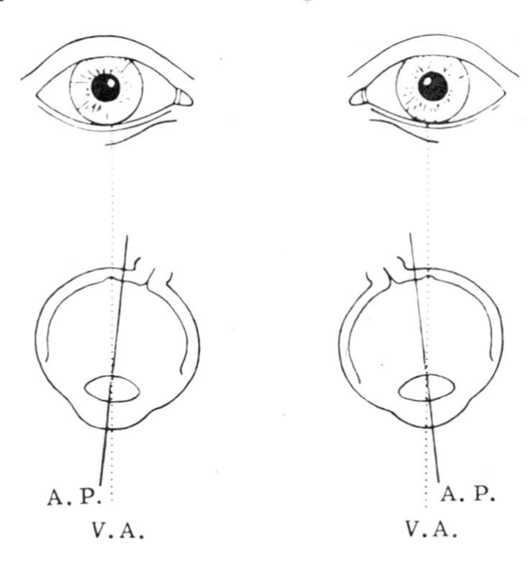

FIG. 2-10. Diagram to show why the corneal light reflections are slightly medial to the true geometric centers of the corneas. The patient is looking straight ahead. His fixation reflexes have automatically aligned the visual axes parallel to each other, to bring the parallel light rays from infinity onto the foveas. The true, geometric anteroposterior axes of the eyes now diverge slightly. A.P. = Anteroposterior axis. V.A. = Visual axis.

slightly divergent

4. Fig. 2-10 shows that when the person looks straight ahead, the anteroposterior axes of the eyes are ☐ slightly divergent / ☐ slightly convergent / ☐ parallel.
5. While watching your corneal light reflections, move the mirror slightly to one side (or have your partner move his eyes). The points of corneal light reflection are then displaced the same distance, to end on corresponding points of the corneas, provided the ocular movements are normal. Thus, the points of corneal reflection provide a means for determining ocular alignment. Move your mirror around full range, chasing the points of reflection over the surfaces of the corneas and noting the correspondence of the points.
6. While inspection of the relation of the limbus to the lid margins gives a quick impression of ocular alignment, the final court of appeals is the corneal reflection test. If the corneal light reflections are noncorresponding, the patient has a lesion of his ocular system. It is most

likely in the neuromuscular apparatus. If you rely only on the relation of limbus to lids, you may be misled if the lids are assymmetrical or if the patient has some degree of canthus dystopia, as do many young children.

7. Thus, you check for ocular malalignment in two ways:
   a. Noncorrespondence of the points of light in the ____________ ____________ test.
   b. Abnormality in the relation of ____________ to lid margins.

corneal reflection

limbus

8. Which of these two tests is the most decisive? ____________ ____________.

corneal reflection test

9. Why do you look for *non*correspondence and *ab*normality of the limbus relation rather than correspondence and normality? ____________ ____________

Ans: It is a fundamental principle of physical diagnosis to expect every function to be abnormal until proved otherwise. If you missed this answer, reread pages 27-28.

B. Procedure for testing the alignment and range of movement of the eyes

1. Ask the patient to look straight ahead at a distant object. Note the relation of the limbus to the lid margins. Compare the corneal light reflections.
2. Test the full range of ocular movements. See instructions in Sec. V-A, pages 66-67, and return to this page.
3. The finger should be moved through the fields of gaze as far as the patient's eyes can follow. When you have gotten the patient to follow your finger to the extreme of each field of gaze, have him hold the position for inspection. What is the best sign of slight deviation of the eyes? ____________ ____________

noncorresponding corneal light reflections

4. Why do you always have the patient follow your finger through a full range of movement? ____________ ____________

Ans: This is the same fundamental principle: you expect all ocular movements to be abnormal until proved otherwise. When the patient's eyes are in the primary position, the muscles are not displaying their capabilities. Ocular malalignment and diplopia sometimes appear only on forceful deviation of the eyes.

5. As you watch the patient's eyes converge, one eye normally "breaks" off target and returns to the primary position, while the other eye follows the finger.
   a. What happens to the pupils when the patient converges his eyes? ____________

Watch someone as he follows your finger to his nose.

Dilates

☑ c.

b. What happens to the pupil of the eye that undergoes the convergence break? ____________

6. After the patient has followed your finger around, you may have observed noncorrespondence of corneal light reflections during one movement. Since the patient may have diplopia, you should reproduce the movement and ask the patient about it. Select the best-phrased question:
   - ☐ *a.* You are seeing two fingers in place of one, aren't you?
   - ☐ *b.* Do you have diplopia?
   - ☐ *c.* How many fingers do you see?
7. Students frequently make type *a* and type *b* errors. The first question may force an erroneous answer, since the patient expects the doctor to know what will happen. The second question uses a technical term unfamiliar to the patient. What generalization can you make about the phrasing of questions? ____________
____
____

Ans: Your question should neither imply the answer nor use technical words like diplopia: it should be completely open to allow the patient to report his symptoms freely.

8. We have outlined two tests, maneuvers, or, as I would prefer to say, *operations* for detecting ocular malalignment.
   a. Inspection of the relation of the limbus to the lid margins, caruncles, and canthi.
   b. Inspection for noncorrespondence of the corneal light reflections.
9. A third method of investigating ocular malalignment is to ask the patient to report what is seen.
10. The first two methods (8*a* and *b*) of investigating disease are *operational.* They depend on the examiner performing the operation constituting the test and noting the result, the operation and the notation being done according to some generally agreed upon criteria. Any number of examiners, repeating the same operation, should obtain the same objective result. Once we inquire about symptoms, the result is out of our control. It depends on the subjective experiences and will of the patient. The difference between the objective manifestations of disease, the signs, and the subjective manifestations, the symptoms, must be clear at all times.

C. Manifest ocular deviations: what to call them

1. The terms *squint, manifest strabismus,* and *heterotropia* are synonymous. The layman speaks of "cross-eye" or "squint," the neurologist of "strabismus," the opthalmologist of "heterotropia." Well, you have to talk with all of them.
2. Heterotropia (manifest strabismus) is any ocular deviation detected by observing noncorrespondence of the corneal light reflections when the eyes are in any position. This is an ☐ operational/ ☐ interpretational definition.

Ans: Operational. Heterotropia is defined in terms of the maneuver or operation by which it is identified.

3. Suppose we stated that "Heterotropia is any deviation of the visual axis of an eye from the fixation point." This would be an ☐ operational / ☐ interpretational definition.

Ans: Interpretational. We do not, cannot, determine the visual axis in the living patient. We infer it.

4. Clearly distinguish operational from interpretational definitions, that is to say, description from interpretation. Sadly, most dictionaries uncritically mix operation and interpretation. Suppose you wish to find the length of a meter. Some dictionaries will advise you that a meter is one ten-millionth of the distance between the equator and the poles, measured on a meridian of the Earth. Well, don't try to pace that off. That obviously *interprets* the length of a meter. Try this definition: a meter is the distance between two transverse lines on a platinum-iridium bar kept at the National Bureau of Standards, when the bar is at 0° C. Now that tells you in operational terms the length of a meter. What you do is observe the distance between two lines. That simple operation gives you the length of a meter. An operational definition tells you the operation or circumstances you reproduce to verify and experience something through your own senses. In other words, if you do *this*, you will find out *that*.

5. As operationally defined by the best test for it, heterotropia means any manifest ocular deviation detected by ______________________

____

inspecting for non-correspondence of the corneal light reflections

6. According to the direction of deviation of the errant eye, the heterotropias can be named this way:

HETEROTROPIA
- → Exotropia — eye deviates outward (laterally)
- → Esotropia — eye deviates inward (medially)
- → Hypertropia — eye deviates upward
- → Hypotropia — eye deviates downward

7. To give the full name, the right or left eye is designated. Thus, left exotropia means that the left eye is deviated ☐ in / ☐ out / ☐ up / ☐ down.

out

8. If both eyes deviate outward, the patient would have bilateral ______________________.

exotropia

9. If the right eye deviated inward, the patient would have ______________________.

right esotropia

10. In Fig. 2-11 write down the proper diagnosis. The patient was asked to fixate straight ahead in each case. In designating whether it is the right or left eye, remember that you are looking *at* the patient. In subsequent ocular illustrations, the cornea will face you or be faced downward on the paper to simulate the actual circumstance of examining a patient.

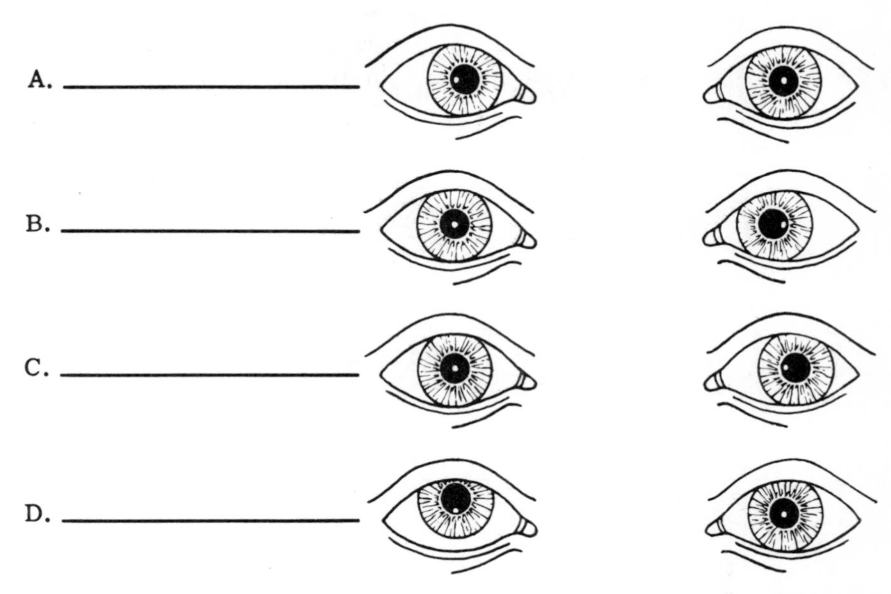

A. R esotropia
B. L esotropia
C. L exotropia
D. R hypertropia

FIG. 2-11. Location of the corneal light reflections in heterotropia. Write down your diagnoses in blanks *A* to *D*, and designate whether the abnormal eye is right or left.

D. The cover-uncover test for ocular malalignment

1. After you have inspected the eyes in the primary position and through the whole range of movement, do the cover-uncover test. See Fig. 2-12.

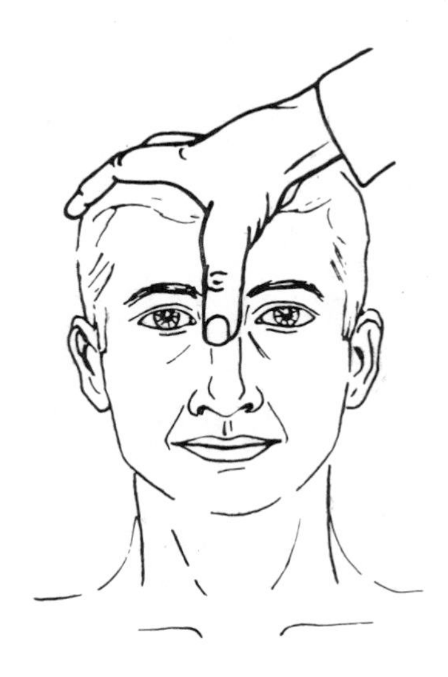

FIG. 2-12. Resting position of the examiner's thumb for the cover-uncover test.

2. *Method*
   a. Place your thumb between the patient's eyes, as shown in Fig. 2-12.

b. Instruct the patient to stare at a distant point. Some patients have difficulty in maintaining fixation, but it is essential to the test.

c. The thumb is swung first in front of one eye, then *back to the bridge of the nose* and then over the other eye. It is unnecessary to occlude all vision with your thumb, only *central* vision. You must watch for movement of *one* or *both* eyes and for noncorrespondence of the corneal light reflections.

3. *Interpretation.* If neither eye moves, they are presumed to be normally locked together in fixation; *the patient has no ocular malalignment.* If an eye moves when central vision is occluded, the eyes are not normally locked together in fixation.
4. The cover-uncover test is always done whether or not you find heterotropia. To analyze it, however, we will start with a patient who has heterotropia. Skip Figs. 2-14 to 2-16 until called for in the text.

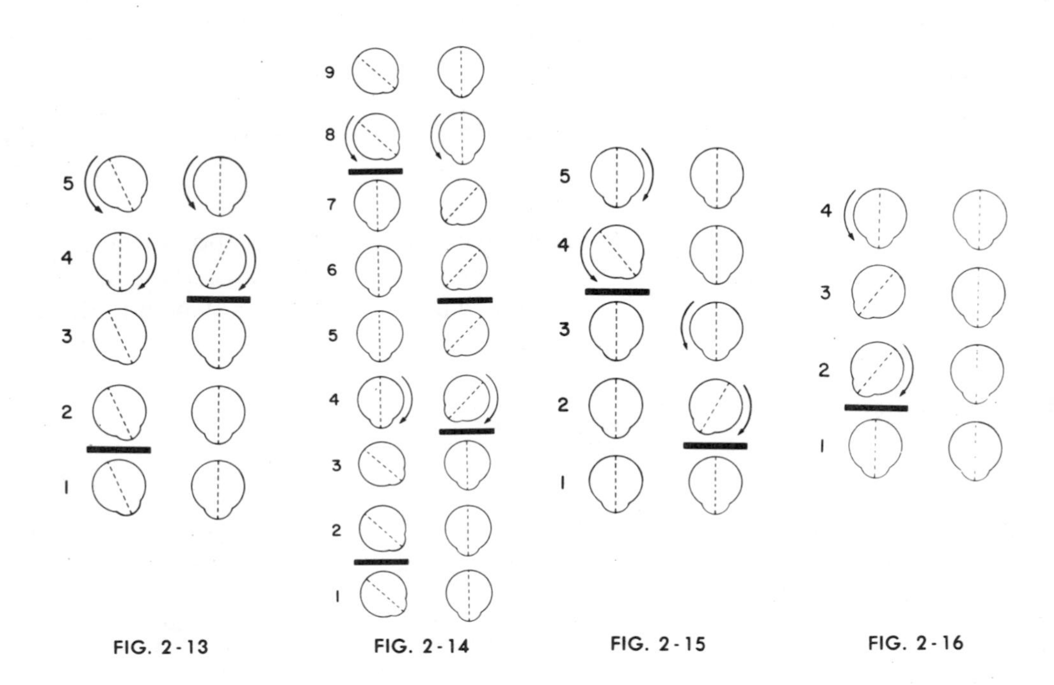

FIGS. 2-13 to 16: Results of the cover-uncover test for ocular malalignment. See text for explanation. *(After Jampolsky.)*

right esotropia

5. *Analysis of the cover-uncover test in monocular heterotropia*

a. Refer to Fig. 2-13, step 1. Notice that step 1 is at the *bottom* of the figure. The patient is instructed to look straight ahead, as for any part of the eye examination. In this case, the patient, being allowed free vision, fixates with his left eye, his dominant eye. This patient appears to have the ocular malalignment called ☐ right / ☐ left____________________________.

b. In step 2, the examiner occludes central vision with his thumb. No change is observed in ocular alignment.

c. In step 3, the thumb is replaced on the bridge of the nose. The eyes maintain the same angulation of the visual axes.

d. In step 4, the left eye was covered after the patient was again instructed to fixate on the same distant point. The right eye then shifts to bring the central light ray onto the fovea, and the left eye rotates inward. (An explanation will be offered later for this inward movement; for the moment, let us merely note the fact of it.)

e. In step 5, the examiner replaces his thumb on the bridge of the patient's nose. The eyes shift to return fixation to the dominant left eye.

f. A similar sequence of events could be observed in a patient with right exotropia instead of esotropia. If you would like, draw the events of right exotropia alongside Fig. 2-13, 1 to 5. At any event, go back through Fig. 2-13 without using the text instructions.

g. Suppose the patient in Fig. 2-13, 1 had diplopia when looking straight ahead.

(1) The parallel rays from the distant object would strike the ☐ nasal / ☐ temporal side of the retina of the right eye.

nasal

(2) Then the visual image would be projected into the field which would normally stimulate the nasal side of the retina. Thus, the false image would be projected to the ☐ right / ☐ left of the true image.

right

6. *Analysis of the cover-uncover test in alternating heterotropia*

a. In Fig. 2-14, follow through the sequence. Notice that at the start this patient ostensibly has the ocular malalignment called ☐ right / ☐ left ______________.

right
esotropia

b. After working through Fig. 2-14, you will see that the patient alternates fixation. In step 1 he fixates with the left eye, and in step 5, he fixates with the right eye. Since the right and left eyes alternately deviate inward, the heterotropia is called alternating ______________.

esotropia

c. Work through the sequence of Fig. 2-14, imagining that the patient's eyes deviated out rather than in. This abnormality would be called ______________.

alternating
exotropia

*******E. The cover-uncover test for latent ocular deviations, heterophorias*

1. When a normal person looks at infinity, his visual axes are parallel and he "fuses" the two retinal images into one mental image. Binocular fusion requires central vision and is developed with maturation of the infant. Fusion-fixation reflexes operate to keep both eyes "on target" whenever the normal person's eyes are open. In some patients, the eyes appear straight during preliminary testing, and show normal motility, but when central vision is covered in one eye, the eye deviates. When the cover is removed, reestablishing central vision, the fusion-fixation reflexes immediately realign the eye. Ocular deviations appearing only when central vision is blocked and disappearing when central vision is reestablished are called heterophorias.

2. An ocular deviation apparent when the patient is permitted free central vision is called *hetero* ______________, while a

hetero*tropia*

deviation apparent only when central vision is occluded is called *hetero* ________.

heterophoria

3. If the eye deviates only when the examiner is blocking central vision, the deviation is called ________.

heterophoria

4. The critical operation of the cover-uncover test is to ________ central vision.

block (cover)

5. What maneuver must always restore ocular alignment to distinguish heterophoria from heterotropia? ________.

uncovering the occluded eye

6. *Inward* deviation or *adduction* of the eye only during occlusion of central vision is called ☐ exophoria / ☐ hyperphoria / ☐ esophoria.

esophoria

7. *Abduction* of an eye *only* during occlusion of central vision is called ________.

exophoria

8. Manifest adduction of an eye when the patient has free central vision is called ________.

esotropia

9. Upward deviation of an eye *only* during occlusion of central vision is called ________.

hyperphoria

10. If you have trouble keeping your *t*ropias and *p*horias straight, try to remember *t* for *t*ropia for *t*urned eye.
11. Fig. 2-15 depicts the cover-uncover test in heterophoria. Work through it. The latent deviation in Fig. 2-15 is called alternating ________.

esophoria

Note: Since esophoria virtually always involves both eyes, the adjective *alternating* is not usually used.

a. Suppose in step 5 of Fig. 2-15 that the right eye had not been restored to proper alignment on removal of the cover. The manifest inward deviation, not corrected all the time by central vision, would be called ☐ right / ☐ left ________.

right esotropia

b. If one of the patient's eyes aligns sometimes when the cover is removed, but does not align at other times, the condition is called ☐ intermittent / ☐ alternating heterotropia.

intermittent

12. The general term for a latent ocular deviation occurring only during occlusion of central vision in one eye is ________.

heterophoria

13. The general term for a manifest ocular deviation not corrected all the time by free central vision is ________.

heterotropia

14. Complete the definitions in *a* and *b* by stating the clinical maneuvers that disclose heterophoria and heterotropia:

a. Heterotropia is a ☐ manifest / ☐ latent ocular deviation detected by inspection for ________.

manifest

Ans: noncorresponding corneal light reflections and abnormal relation of the limbus to lid margins.

b. Heterophoria is a ☐ manifest / ☐ latent ocular deviation detected by ________.

latent

Ans: seeing the eye shift when its central vision is blocked during the cover-uncover test.

15. Now try to name the abnormality in Fig. 2-16. Pay particular atten-

intermittent right exotropia

the right eye remained manifestly deviated even after central vision was restored

tion to step 3. Since the patient starts and finishes with apparently straight eyes, the deviation of one eye is only intermittent. Therefore, the abnormality in Fig. 2-16 is called ______________ ☐ right/ ☐ left ______________.

16. The abnormality in Fig. 2-16 is a *tropia* rather than a *phoria* because ______________

17. Figs. 2-13 to 2-16 show why you must do the cover-uncover test along with the other tests for ocular deviation: you may see nothing abnormal on inspection of the eyes at rest or on movement, but the abnormality is uncovered only by the cover-uncover test.

III. Ocular motility: Peripheral mechanisms

NOTE: This section describes the actions of the ocular rotatory muscles. Fig. 2-28 summarizes these actions. If it contents you, clip out Fig. 2-28 and paste it in your handbook, or if you have a bulldog memory, simply memorize it. Of course what you memorize quickly, you forget quickly. If you want permanent retention based on understanding, work through the text, which calls for you to make two simple models. One of the models uses paper tapes to simulate the ocular muscles, enabling you to reason out their actions and recall them when needed. I have found that many students automatically reject model-making as a waste of time. Let me say this: you will never really understand the ocular rotations unless you experience the actions by seeing them happen and feeling them with your own fingers. It might interest the skeptics among you to know that Leonardo da Vinci (1452–1519), who dissected many human bodies to study muscles, devised the method of tugging on tapes attached to the origin and insertion of muscles to teach himself their actions. To *experience* what you learn, get these things and make the models: 1. An olive, or small ball of clay, or even a wad of gum. 2. Toothpicks or applicator sticks. 3. Several straight pins. 4. Scissors. 5. A table tennis ball or similar ball that you can stick pins into.

A. Introduction

1. Within the limits set by the palpebral fissure, the ocular movements must be infinitely variable. The eye must be able to aim the visual axis to any point within the perimeter of movement.
2. The two eyes must move conjugately. Thus, when both fixate on any point in the visual field, the image falls upon corresponding parts of each retina.

B. Ocular rotation. The simplest way to achieve infinitely variable movement, to aim the visual axis to any point within the perimeter of movement, is to provide for rotation of the eye around three axes. See Fig. 2-17 and identify the vertical axis, *V;* the lateral axis, *L;* and the anteroposterior axis, *A-P.*

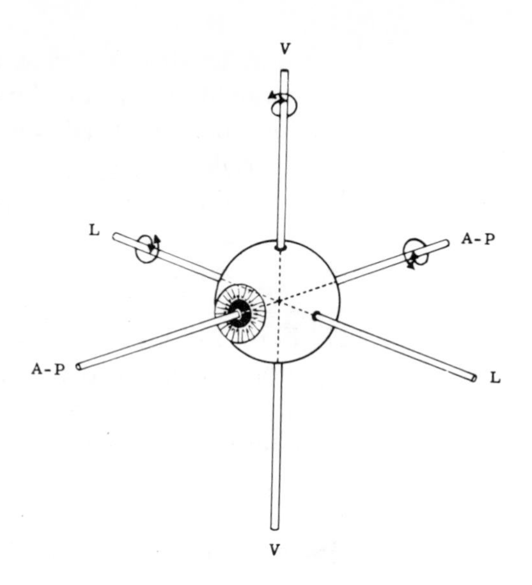

FIG. 2-17. The three rotational axes of the eye. V = vertical. L = lateral. A-P = anteroposterior.

C. Two teaching models

1. To visualize ocular rotation, get a stuffed olive, clay, or wad of gum and insert three toothpicks in it. Rotate each of the three toothpicks. Then and only then will you understand ocular rotation, that it is *axial* rotation. In Fig. 2-18 check the eye which shows the correct, axial rotation:

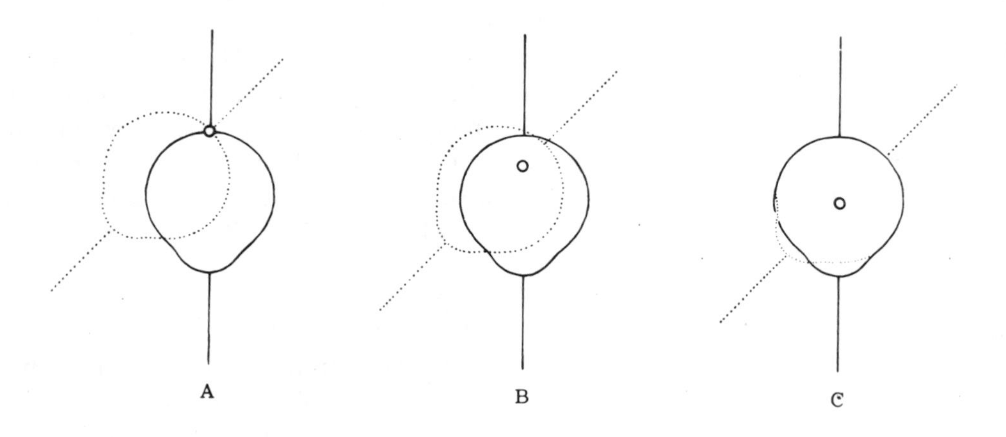

☑ C

FIG. 2-18. Diagram to show the possible methods of ocular rotation. Only one type of rotation, *axial* rotation, is correct. It is shown by ☐ A/ ☐ B/ ☐ C.

2. Get a table tennis ball. Using a lead pencil, mark a cornea and the points of emergence of the three axes (Fig. 2-17). Label the three axes. Then place the ball on the mouth of a bottle, as shown in Fig. 2-19. Subsequently we will pin on paper strips as eye muscles.

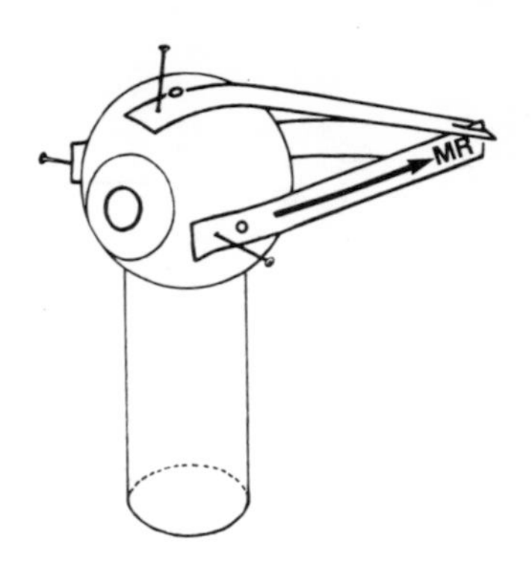

FIG. 2-19. Table tennis ball on a bottle mouth, with paper strips pinned in place to simulate ocular muscles.

D. *The four rectus muscles*

1. The simplest way to move the eyes around two axes is by four muscles. See Fig. 2-20. Label the axes, learn the names of the four rectus muscles, and note their insertion in relation to the axes.

Lateral

Vertical

A-P

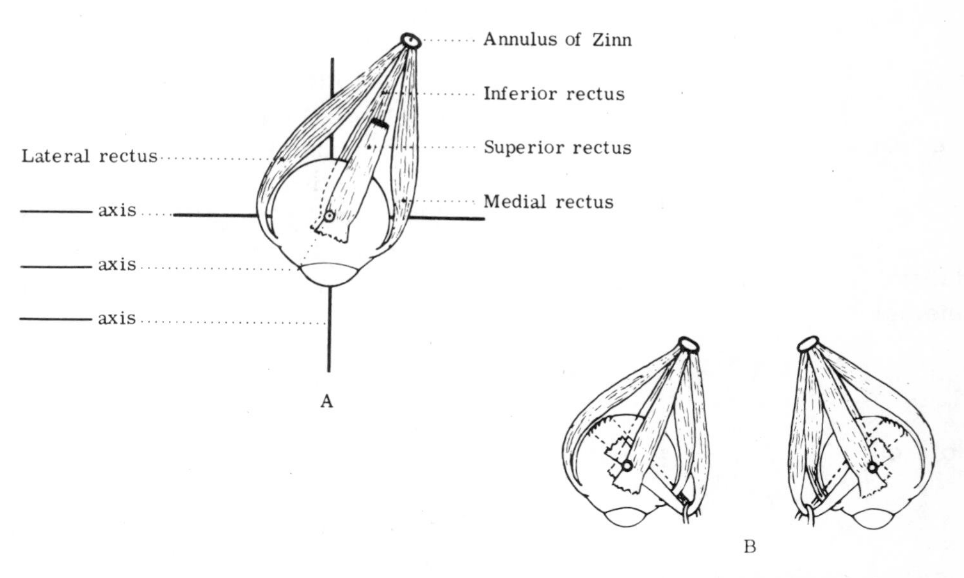

FIG. 2-20. Origin and insertion of the ocular muscles. *A.* Right eye as seen from above, showing the rectus muscles. *B.* Both eyes seen from above, showing all the ocular rotatory muscles and their direction of origin and insertion when the eyes are in the primary position.

E. *Action of medial and lateral rectus muscles*

1. Cut two strips of paper. Mark them MR and LR for medial and lateral recti. Draw an arrow along the strips to represent the vector or line of pull of the contracting muscle (see arrow in Figs. 2-19 and 2-21). Stick a pin through the anterior end of the strip, and stick it into the table tennis ball slightly anterior to but exactly in line with the lateral axis. Now put the ball on the bottle top. Align the strips to pull exactly straight back, as in Fig. 2-19. Pull and relax the medial and lateral recti strips

Vertical

A-P

Lateral

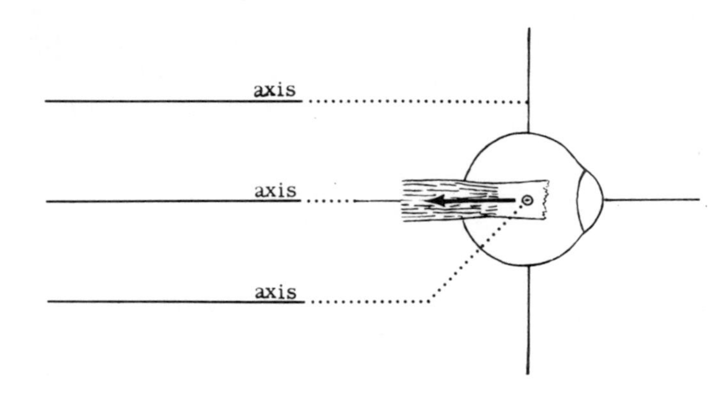

FIG. 2-21. Lateral view of the right eye to show the direct pull of the lateral rectus muscle over the lateral axis.

and observe the exact axial rotation of the ball around the vertical axis. Study Fig. 2-21 and label the axes.

2. From your model, and only from your model (have you made the model?), will you fully appreciate this fact: You have to pull exactly straight back, along the vector arrow in Fig. 2-21, or the eye will wobble around some other axis rather than showing precise rotation around the vertical axis.
3. Since the medial and lateral recti pull exactly straight back, they have one and only one action: to adduct or abduct the eye. The actions of the medial and lateral recti rotate the eye around the ______________ axis. The other ocular rotatory muscles have an oblique relation to the ocular axes and do display more than one effective action.
4. In order for the eyes to move conjugately to the right, the ____________ rectus of the right eye contracts in unison with the ______________ rectus of the left eye.

vertical

lateral
medial

F. Action of superior rectus muscle

1. From Fig. 2-20, it is apparent that when the superior rectus contracts it will rotate the eye upward around the ______________________ axis. This is the primary action of the muscle.
2. The angulation of the superior and inferior recti causes a difference in the strength of the primary action and permits secondary and tertiary actions, depending on the position of the eye. To understand how the actions of some of the ocular muscles change as the eyes rotate, you must know the origin and insertion of the muscles in relation to the axes of the eyeball.
3. The recti all originate from the *annulus of Zinn* which is attached to the optic foramen. In Fig. 2-20 note that from their origin, the recti run ☐ laterally/ ☐ medially.
4. Notice in Fig. 2-20 that the superior rectus runs somewhat ☐ medial to/ ☐ lateral to the vertical axis.
   a. We have already seen that the superior rectus has the primary action to rotate the eye ________________________ around the lateral axis.

lateral

laterally

medial to

upward

medial
adduction

b. To analyze the other actions of the superior rectus, pin another strip of paper to the ball, inserting the pin anteromedial to the vertical axis, as in Fig. 2-19. Angulate the strip along the normal line of pull of the muscle as shown in Fig. 2-25*B* and notice the effect on the ball when the strip is pulled.

c. Because its line of pull is slightly medial to the vertical axis, the superior rectus has a secondary action to rotate the eye medially around the vertical axis. The muscle whose sole action is medial rotation of the eye is the ______________ rectus and this action is also termed ________ duction.

5. To visualize the secondary action better and to see clearly the tertiary action of the superior rectus, imagine the eye in a position of extreme adduction as in Fig. 2-22. Pull on the superior rectus strip after the ball has been turned medially, as in Fig. 2-22.

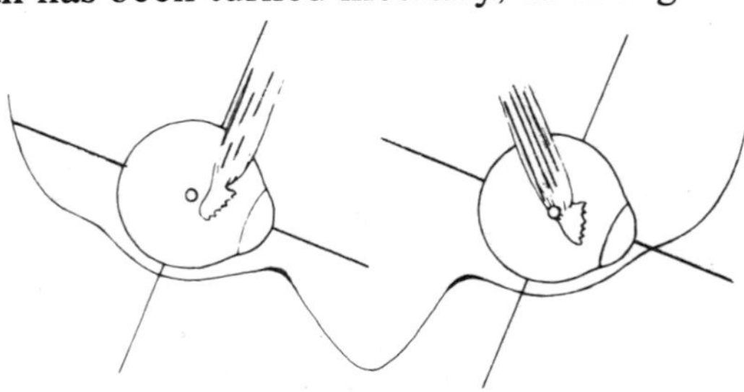

FIG. 2-22. Eyes as seen from above to illustrate the relation of the pull of the superior rectus muscle to the ocular axes when the eyes rotate to the left (rotation exaggerated).

6. Now it is observable that the superior rectus can elevate the eye, adduct it, and in addition can tilt the vertical axis inward. This action of intilting the vertical axis is called *intorsion*, as shown in Fig. 2-23.

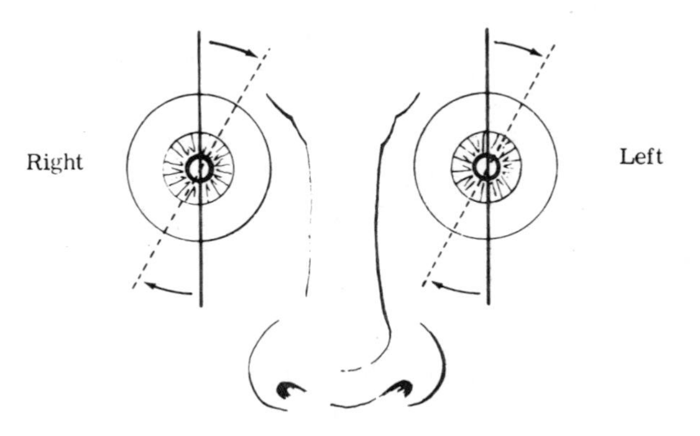

FIG. 2-23. Torsion of the eyes. The right eye is undergoing *in*torsion; the left, *ex*torsion. The torsions are named *in-* or *ex-*, depending on whether the top of the vertical axis tilts in (medially) or out (laterally).

intorsion

extorsion

7. In Fig. 2-23, the right eye has rotated around the A-P axis, tilting the top of the vertical axis *in*. Therefore, it is called ☐ intorsion/ ☐ extorsion.

8. In the left eye, the top of the vertical axis tilts *out*. Therefore, it is called ________ *torsion.*

A-P

9. The torsions involve rotation of the eye around the ______ axis. Use your toothpick model to visualize this action.
10. When the eye is *abducted,* the point of insertion of the tendon of the superior rectus shifts laterally, as shown in Fig. 2-24.

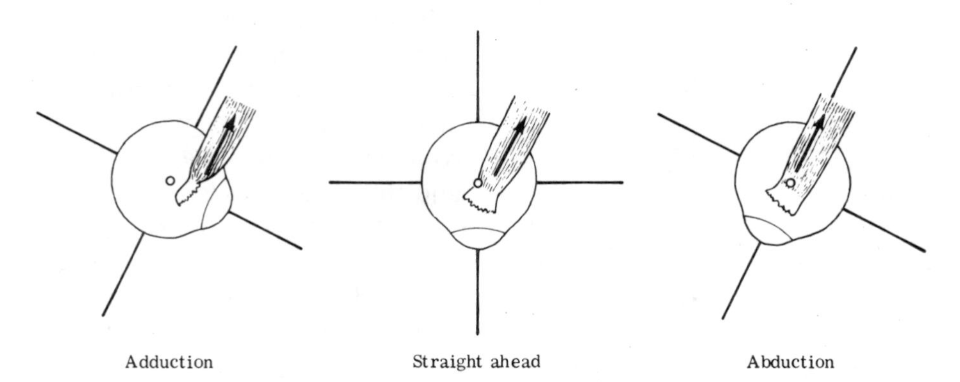

FIG. 2-24. Right eye and superior rectus muscle as seen from above. Notice how the position of the eye changes the relation of the muscle insertion to the vertical axis and, therefore, changes the effective action of the muscle.

Find out from your model.

11. Would the superior rectus act to adduct or intort when the eye is abducted? ☐ Yes / ☐ No.
12. With the eye abducted, the superior rectus pulls directly over the vertical axis. It dissipates none of its strength in adduction or intorsion. Therefore, the superior rectus elevates the eye most strongly when the eye is ☐ adducted / ☐ straight ahead / ☐ abducted.
13. In what position of the eye would the superior rectus have the weakest action of elevation? ______.
14. In summary, the primary action of the superior rectus is ______ of the eye. This action is strongest when the eye is ______.
    a. The secondary and tertiary actions are ______ and ______ the eye.
    b. In testing for the strongest elevating action of the right superior rectus you would ask the patient to look in what direction? ______ ______.

abducted

adduction
elevation
abducted
adduction
intorsion

up and to the right

G. *Action of the inferior rectus muscle*

1. The *inferior rectus* muscle has the same direction of origin and insertion as the superior rectus. See Fig. 2-20. The primary action of the inferior rectus is to ☐ depress / ☐ elevate the eye.
2. Its secondary action would be to ______ the eye.
3. You will have to analyze its tertiary action carefully. Pin a strip to the eye to represent the inferior rectus and consider its action with the eye *adducted.* Then when the inferior rectus contracts, the top of the vertical axis would be tilted ☐ internally / ☐ externally.
4. Internal tilting of the vertical axis is called ______, external tilting is called ______.

depress
adduct

externally
intorsion
extorsion

adduction

5. What is the only eye movement in which the superior and inferior recti could rotate the eye in the same direction? ______________.
6. The superior and inferior recti are not effective adductors unless the eye has already begun to adduct by action of the medial rectus, which is the critical muscle for adduction.

down and to the right

7. To test the strongest action of the right inferior rectus as a depressor, in what direction would you ask the patient to look? ______________ ______________.

depress
adduct
extort

8. In summary: The three actions of the inferior rectus are a primary action to ______________ the eye, a secondary action to ______________ the eye, and a tertiary action to ______________ the eye.

H. Action of the superior oblique muscle

1. The superior oblique originates from the lesser wing of the sphenoid bone, just above the annulus of Zinn. It threads its tendon through a trochlea (pulley) attached to the rim of the bony orbit. See Fig. 2-25*A*. When the tendon runs to the eye, it inserts *posteriorly* to allow the superior oblique to have an effective pull when contracting. In so attaching, it runs somewhat *medial* to the vertical axis, like the superior and inferior recti. Cut another paper strip and attach it correspondingly. (The concept of superior oblique action given here is the traditional one. A dissenting view is discussed later.)

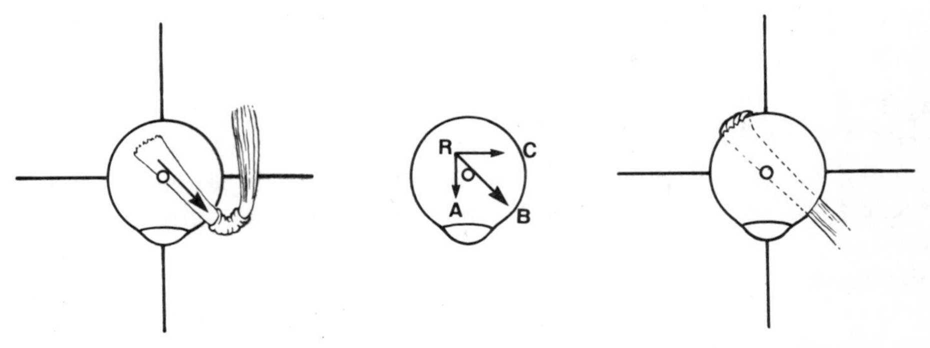

FIG. 2-25. Right eye, as seen from above, to illustrate the actions of the superior and inferior oblique muscles. The arrow in A represents the line of pull of both muscles, which is somewhat medial to the vertical axis. Notice that vector R-B originates posterolateral to the vertical axis.

depresses
lateral
abducts, V
intorts, A-P

depress
abduct
intort

2. The vector diagram of Fig. 2-25*B* resolves the arrow **R-B** into effective components.
   a. Vector **R-A** ☐ depresses / ☐ elevates the eye around the ______________ axis.
   b. Vector **R-C** ☐ abducts / ☐ adducts the eye around the ______________ axis, and ☐ intorts / ☐ extorts the eye around the ______________ axis.
   c. Therefore, vector **R-B** acts to ______________, ______________, and ______________ the eye.

depress
abduct

intort

3. To recapitulate. Contraction of the superior oblique, when the eye starts in the primary position, causes:
   a. A *primary* action to ☐ depress / ☐ elevate the eye.
   b. A *secondary* action to ☐ adduct / ☐ abduct / ☐ elevate the eye.
   c. A *tertiary* action to ☐ intort / ☐ extort the eye.
4. When the eye is in the primary position, the vertical axis is located *anterior* to the line of strongest pull of the superior oblique tendon (arrow in Fig. 2-25*A*). Complete Fig. 2-26 to show the relation of the vertical axis of the eye to the center of pull of the superior oblique tendon when the eye is *adducted.*

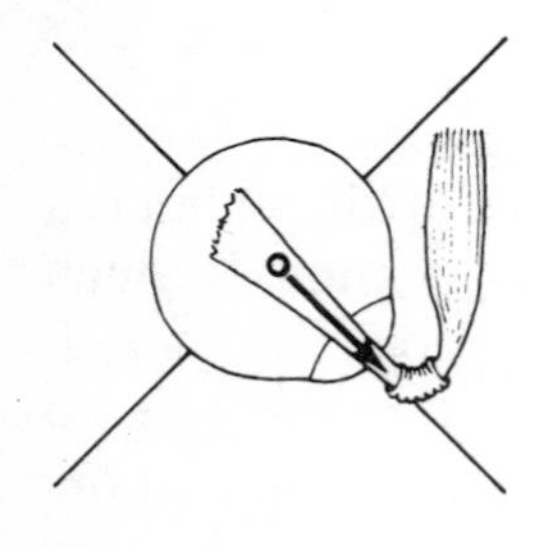

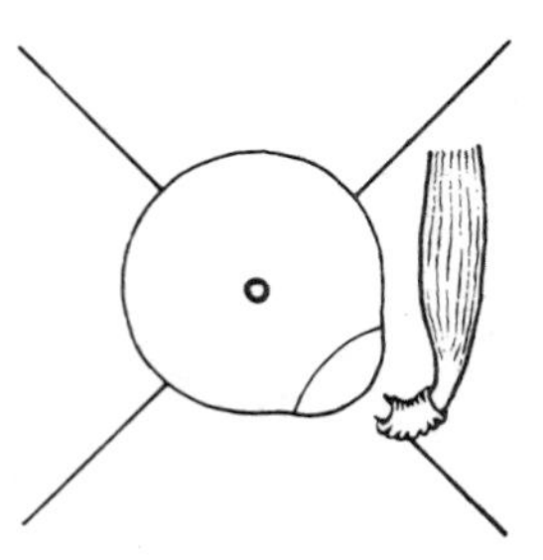

FIG. 2-26. Blank to be completed to show the relation of the vertical axis to the line of pull of the superior oblique tendon when the eye is adducted.

abduct
intort

adduction

in and down

5. When the eye is *adducted,* the line of pull of the tendon of the superior oblique is directly over the vertical axis. Therefore, none of the action of the muscle is dissipated in the other actions which are to ______________ ______________ and to ______________ the eye.
6. In what position of the eye does the superior oblique have the strongest *primary* action of downward rotation of the eye? ______________.
7. Hence, the clinical test for the strongest action of the superior oblique is to ask the patient to look ______________.
8. **Note:** The analysis of superior oblique action given here is the classical one advocated by most neuro-ophthalmologists. Jampel disagrees, suggesting that the *only* action of the superior oblique is to *intort* the eye. Whether the Establishment will tumble is unknown. It will be an interesting exercise in Academia. Jampel's idea is appealing. It would be nice to reduce the problem to one muscle, one action.

Bibliography

Jampel, R.: The action of the superior oblique muscle, *Arch. Ophthal.*, 75:535-544, 1966.

I. Action of the inferior oblique muscle

1. The inferior oblique muscle, in contrast to the other ocular muscles, originates from the medial inferior rim of the bony orbit. It is the only ocular muscle to originate anteriorly. It inserts on the posteri-

elevates

abduction

extorsion

abduction

or part of the eyeball. In order to attain sufficient length, it wraps further around the eye than the other muscles.

2. The inferior oblique passes posteriorly, somewhat *medial* to the vertical axis, and its obliquity and alignment with the vertical axis is like that of the superior oblique. See Fig. 2-25*C*.
   a. The *primary* action is exactly antagonistic to the superior oblique. The inferior oblique ____________________ the eye.
   b. The *secondary* action is ____________________, acting in harmony with the superior oblique.
   c. The *tertiary* action is ____________________, antagonistic to the superior oblique.
   d. What is the only action in which the superior and inferior oblique could pull with each other? ____________________.
3. The obliques can only be strong abductors after the eye has already started to rotate outward from the pull of the lateral rectus. When the lateral rectus is paralyzed, the obliques cannot initiate abduction and the eye cannot be abducted. We come squarely up against a problem. Intorsion, the so-called tertiary action of the superior oblique, is clinically one of its most important actions; according to Jampel, its only action. Therefore, in classifying intorsion as a tertiary action, we do not mean it is a negligible action.

J. A vector diagram of ocular muscle action

1. In the blanks of Fig. 2-27, place the initials of the muscles represented by the vector arrow numbers.

1. LR
2. IR
3. SR
4. MR
5. IO
6. SO

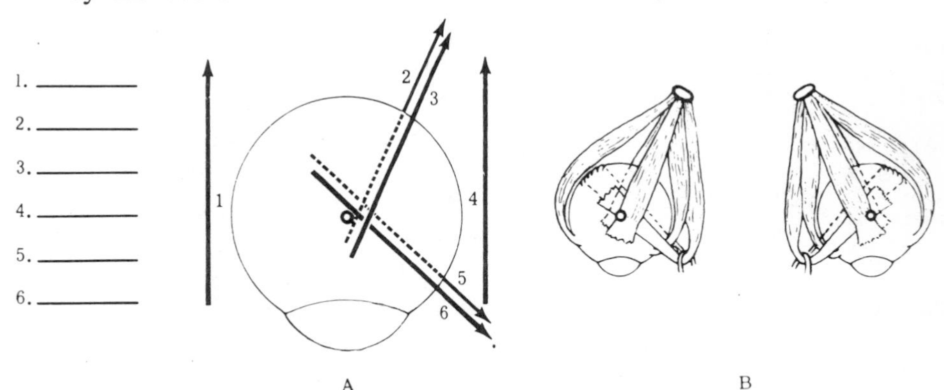

FIG. 2-27. Eyes, as seen from above. A. Composite vector diagram to show the effective direction of pull of the muscles when the right eye is in the primary position. Fill in blanks 1 to 6 with initials corresponding to the muscle represented by the vectors. *B.* Composite drawing of all of the ocular rotatory muscles. Match them with the vectors shown in *A*.

lateral rectus

2. The vector diagram combined with a knowledge of origin and insertion provides a basis for you to remember forever the actions of the ocular muscles. We can state that when the eye is in the primary position, the pull or vector of all the ocular muscles is medial to the vertical axis except for the ____________________ muscle.

superior and inferior oblique, and the superior and inferior recti

medial lateral recti

3. It is because four of the ocular muscles pull "off center," pull medial to the vertical axis, that the muscles have their particular secondary and tertiary actions. The four muscles that pull off center when the eye is in the primary position are the ____.
4. The two muscles that always pull "on-center" and therefore have only primary actions are the ________________ and ________________.
5. Cover the answers in Table 2-1 and recite them. Use drawings or the ball model where necessary to figure out the answer.

TABLE 2-1. Summary of Eye Movements of Individual Muscles

Muscle	Primary action	Secondary	Tertiary
Medial rectus	adducts		
Lateral rectus	abducts		
Superior rectus	elevates	adducts	intorts
Inferior rectus	depresses	adducts	extorts
Superior oblique	depresses	abducts	intorts
Inferior oblique	elevates	abducts	extorts

K. *Yoking of ocular muscles*

1. We have seen how the ocular muscles act alone; now we want to consider how they collaborate to keep the eyes aligned. If a patient has diplopia on looking to the left, you would suspect weakness of the *ad*ductor of the right eye or the *ab*ductor of the left eye.

lateral rectus

medial rectus

   a. The strongest *ab*ductor of the left eye is the muscle whose only function is abduction, ________________.
   b. The strongest *ad*ductor of the right eye is the muscle whose only function is adduction, ________________.
   c. Since these muscles must act in unison for lateral conjugate gaze of the eyes, we say they are yoked.
2. Suppose the patient complains of diplopia when he looks *up* and to the *left*.

superior rectus

adduction intorsion

inferior oblique

decreases increases

   a. When the left eye is *ab*ducted, the strongest elevator is the ________________.
   b. When the right eye is *ad*ducted the elevating power of its superior rectus is diverted to the secondary action of the muscle, ________________ and to the tertiary action of the muscle, ________________.
   c. As the superior rectus loses its elevator strength during adduction, another muscle converts its action solely to elevation. That muscle is the ________________.
   d. During adduction of an eye, the elevator action of the superior rectus ☐ decreases / ☐ increases while the elevator action of the inferior oblique simultaneously ☐ decreases / ☐ increases.
   e. Thus, for upward gaze to the left, the ________________

superior rectus
inferior oblique

________________ muscle, which elevates the left eye, is "yoked" to the ________________ muscle of the right eye, which replaces the vanishing elevator action of the right superior rectus.

superior rectus
inferior oblique

f. A patient with diplopia on looking upward and to the left would be expected to have weakness of either the ________________ muscle of the left eye or the ________________ muscle of the right eye.

superior oblique

g. Which muscle has the strongest *depressant* action when the eye is adducted? The ________________.

inferior rectus

h. Which muscle has the strongest *depressant* action when the eye is abducted? The ________________.

inferior rectus
superior oblique

i. A patient, looking to the right, has diplopia when he looks down. Which yoke muscles would you suspect of weakness: either the ________________ muscle of the right eye or the ________________ muscle of the left eye.

equal

3. It will now be apparent that the muscles yoked for conjugate eye movements must have equal stimulation by the nervous system. Thus, if the right lateral rectus is innervated (stimulated) to rotate the right eye to the right, the left medial rectus is innervated (stimulated) to an ________________ degree. This principle is called *Hering's law* (Ewald Hering, 1834-1918). State Hering's law in your own words:

____
____
____
____.

Ans: During conjugate eye movements, the yoke muscles are equally innervated (stimulated).

1. SR
2. LR
3. IR
4. IO
5. MR
6. SO
7. SR
8. LR
9. IR

4. *A summary of the yoke muscles.* Complete Fig. 2-28 by writing down the initials of the muscle most important for movement in the direction of the arrow.

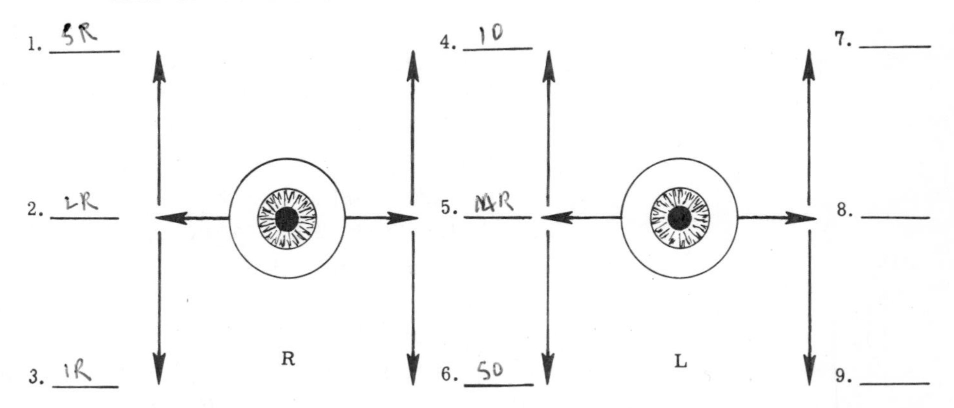

FIG. 2-28. Yoking of strongest actions of ocular muscles in moving the eyes in the cardinal directions of gaze. In blanks 1 to 9, place the initials of the muscle whose strongest action is indicated by the arrow. Then read *across* the diagram, e.g., 1 to 4 or 4 to 7, to see which muscles pair up. Thus, in looking to the right and up, the superior rectus muscle (1) of the right eye is yoked with the inferior oblique muscle (4) of the left eye.

	L. The laws of diplopia
	1. Repeat the canthal compression experiment and obtain diplopia with the finger vertical. Move the finger to the right and left, studying the distance between the true and false images. You should find a null point straight ahead where the images are virtually superimposed. Identify the false image by its haziness.
right	*a.* If the false image projects to the *right* of the finger, the distance between the images increases as you move the finger to the ______________ side.
left	*b.* If the false image projects to the left, the distance between the images increases as you move to the ______________ side.
	c. If you follow the images too far laterally, one disappears. Can you discover an explanation (look for the simplest one)? ______________ ______________

Ans: The nose blocks the light rays from entering one eye.

increases	2. As you move your finger away from the midpoint, the distance between the true and false images ☐ increases / ☐ decreases / ☐ stays the same. Go to the next frame for the explanation, unless you would like to try to work it out yourself.
	3. In Fig. 2-29*A*, the straight left eye receives the real image on its fovea. The mind projects the visual image back to the true target position (T1). The deviated right eye receives the real image on the nasal side of the fovea. The mind projects the visual image to the right of the true target position (F1). In Fig. 2-29*B*, the mobile left eye follows the target to the right (T2). The immobile right eye remains imprisoned in its original position, and as the target moves rightward, the real image moves leftward (nasally) on the retina. The mind projects the visual image more and more rightward. Thus D2 > D1.
peripheral	4. No matter which way the false image deviates, it moves away from the true image. The true image remains centered on target. This is the first law of diplopia: the false image is projected ☐ peripheral / ☐ central to the true image.
opposite	5. If the false image is to the right of the true image, as in Fig. 2-29*A*, the eye is deviated to the left (or has not rotated sufficiently to the right). The false image projects in the ☐ same / ☐ opposite direction of eye deviation.
downward	*a.* If the false image projects above the true image, the afflicted eye is deviated ☐ upward / ☐ downward.
right	*b.* If the false image is to the left, the afflicted eye is deviated to the ☐ right / ☐ left.
opposite	6. Thus, the second law of diplopia is that the false image projects in the ☐ same / ☐ opposite direction as the direction of eye deviation.
	7. State the first two laws of diplopia:
See frame 4	*a.* The law of peripheral projection: ______________ ______________.

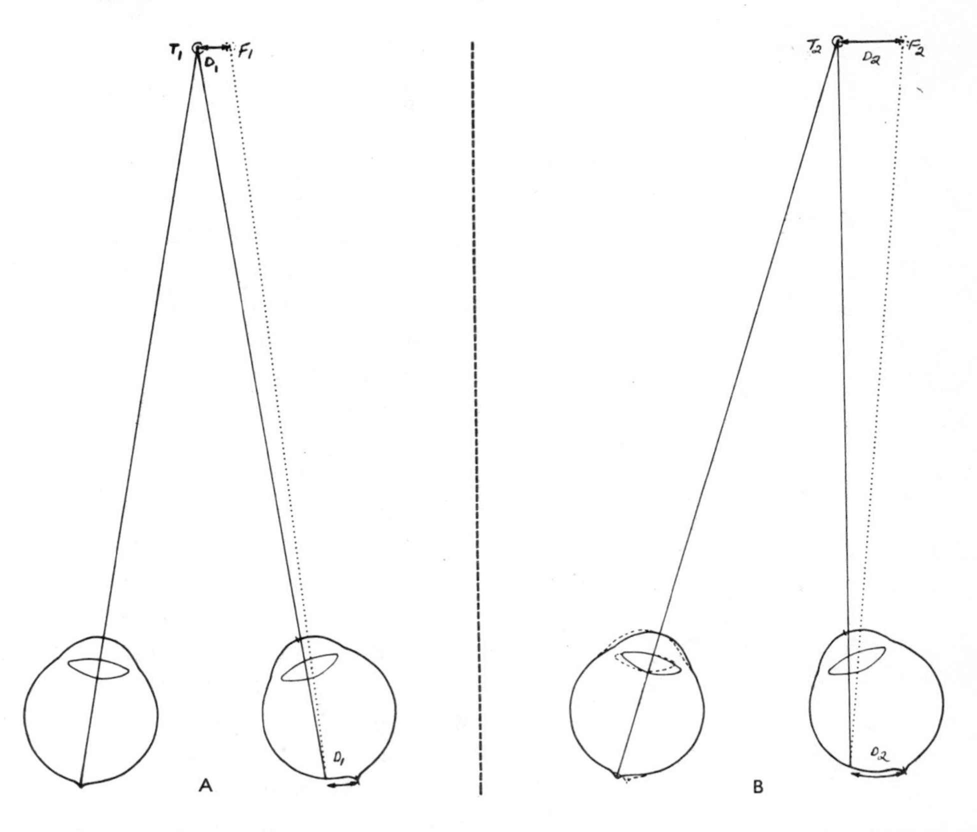

FIG. 2-29. Illustration of a law of diplopia—the distance between the true and false images increases when the patient looks in the direction of projection of the false image. T_1 = true image; F_1 = false image; D_1 = distance 1; D_2 = distance 2.

b. The law of opposite deviation of the false image: ______________________

____

See frame 6

8. In Fig. 2-29, with projection of the false image to the right, the right eye has failed to abduct to center its visual axis on target.
   a. Thus, the diagram simulates paralysis of the ______________________ ______________________ muscle.
   b. The false image is projected ☐ toward / ☐ away from the direction of action of the lateral rectus.

lateral rectus

toward

9. The third law of diplopia is that the false image projects ☐ toward / ☐ away from the direction of action of the paretic muscle, and when the patient looks in the direction of action of the paretic muscle, the distance between the diplopic images ☐ increases / ☐ decreases.

toward

increases

10. It should now be clear that the laws of diplopia, along with the corneal reflection test, permit you to diagnose the faulty muscle. These laws need not be memorized, since they can be recovered any time you need them by pressing on your lateral canthus.
11. State the three laws of diplopia:
   a. The law of peripheral projection: ______________________

   ____

   b. The law of opposite deviation: ______________________

   ____

frame 4

frame 6

frame 9

c. The law relating the false image to the paretic muscle: ____________
____
____
____

M. Procedure for testing a patient who has diplopia – a summary

1. *Observe the corneal light reflections.* This sign is checked when the eyes are straight ahead and when they are turned in the various directions of gaze. The ocular muscles of one eye are matched in agonist-antagonist pairs. When one member of the pair is paretic or paralytic, its antagonist acts unopposed. Hence the faulty eye deviates away from the direction of action of the faulty muscle, toward the pull of the intact member of the pair.
2. *Identify the position of maximum diplopia.* As you move your examining light through all fields of gaze, have the patient report when the two images are maximally separated.
3. *Identify the eye which produces the false image.* The eye which produces the false image has the faulty muscle. The false image is the peripheral image. It is identified by occluding vision alternately in the two eyes. When the normal eye is occluded, the sharp, central image disappears. When the abnormal eye is occluded, the hazy, peripheral image disappears. A colored glass placed over one eye helps to keep track of the two images during motility testing.
4. *Reason out the muscle responsible for the deficient ocular action.*
5. *In summary, the patient who complains of diplopia is examined this way:*
   a. Corneal light reflections are checked.
   b. The position of the eyes in which the diplopia is greatest is identified (one of the muscles which moves one of the eyes to this position is faulty).
   c. The eye which has the peripheral image is identified (it is the eye with the faulty muscle).
   d. The faulty muscle is reasoned out.

N. Analyze these patients

1. This patient complains of double vision on looking to the left. Testing discloses that image separation is greatest on left lateral gaze.
   a. Left lateral gaze is under control of the ____________ ____________ muscle of the right eye, and the ____________ muscle of the left eye.

   medial rectus
   lateral rectus

   b. On occlusion of the right eye, the central image disappears. On occlusion of the left eye the peripheral image disappears. Therefore, the afflicted eye is the ☐ left/ ☐ right eye and the afflicted muscle is the ☐ right/ ☐ left ____________ ____________ muscle.

   left
   left lateral rectus

2. This patient complains of double vision when looking up. The images separate greatest when the patient looks up and to the left.
   a. This direction of gaze is under control of the ____________ ____________ muscle of the left eye and

   superior rectus

inferior oblique	the ______________________ muscle of the right eye.
left left superior rectus	*b.* On occlusion of the right eye, the central image disappears. On occlusion of the left eye, the peripheral image disappears. Therefore, the afflicted eye is the ☐ right / ☐ left and the afflicted muscle is the ☐ right / ☐ left ______________________.

O. Clinical classification of heterotropia

1. *Introduction.* In determining the cause of heterotropia, the clinician tries to classify it into one of two types:
   a. The *paralytic* type caused by a neuromuscular lesion.
   b. The *nonparalytic* type usually caused by lesions which interfere with central vision in one eye: refractive errors, opacification of the cornea or lens (refracting media), or macular lesions.
2. *Effect of paralytic heterotropia caused by nerve or muscle lesions on yoke muscles*

away from	*a.* When an ocular muscle or group of muscles is paretic or paralytic, the intact muscles act unopposed. Hence, the eye deviates ☐ away from / ☐ toward the direction of pull of the afflicted muscle.
increase	*b.* When the patient looks in the direction of pull of the afflicted muscle, the normal eye moves more than the afflicted eye. Hence, the heterotropia and diplopia ☐ increase / ☐ decrease when the patient looks in the direction of action of the involved muscle.
left See next frame	*c.* When turning in the direction of pull of the afflicted muscle, the *weak* eye rotates too little, while the *normal* eye may rotate too far. With a lateral rectus paralysis on the *right,* the patient's ☐ right / ☐ left eye would adduct too far when the patient looks to the right. Explain this result by Hering's law. ______________________ ______________________.
strongly	*d.* According to Hering's law, the nervous system stimulates the yoke muscles equally. If a muscle is weak, the patient automatically overstimulates in an attempt to rotate the afflicted eye. The normal yoke muscle receives the same excessive stimulus and contracts too ______________.
	e. *Use of the cover-uncover test in the analysis of neuromuscular heterotropia.* The description by Scobee is so lucid that it is reproduced to introduce you to the concept of *primary* and *secondary* deviation of the eyes.

Primary deviation is the deviation of the eye with the paretic muscle when the sound eye is fixing. Secondary deviation is the deviation of the sound eye when the eye with the paretic muscle is fixing. In paresis, secondary deviation is greater than primary deviation.

As an example of primary deviation, supppose the left lateral rectus is paretic, right eye dominant, and the patient fixes upon some object straight ahead with the right eye. The right medial rectus and the right lateral rectus are normal muscles and require but a normal innervation to maintain fixation with the right eye. According to Hering's law, similar normal innervations go to the yoke muscles of the right lateral rectus and the right medial rectus — to the left medial rectus and the left lateral rectus. The left lateral rectus is paretic and responds in subnormal fashion to normal stimuli; the left medial rectus is normal and thus not properly opposed by the subnormal tonus of its paretic antagonist. The left medial rectus will, therefore, seem to overact since it will pull the left eye inward toward the nose in adduction. The deviation produced is small but definite and is a left esotropia. This is deviation of the paretic eye with the sound eye fixing — *primary deviation.*

As an example of secondary deviation, suppose the left lateral rectus is paretic, left eye dominant, and the patient fixes upon some object straight ahead with the dominant left eye. The left lateral rectus, in order to perform its usual functions, must be excessively innervated because it is paretic; its yoke muscle, the right medial rectus, receives the same excessive innervation according to Hering's law. The right medial rectus is a normal muscle receiving an excessive innervation and it makes an excessive response, pulling the right eye well inward in adduction. This is a deviation of the sound eye with the paretic eye's fixing—*secondary deviation.* In paresis, secondary deviation is greater than primary deviation and the reason should now be obvious.

— Richard Scobee

intorsion

left (If the answer is unclear review Fig. 2-23.)

3. *Effect of neuromuscular heterotropia on head position*
   a. The patient with heterotropia tends to compensate for an afflicted muscle by turning or tilting his head. The head posture compensates for or keeps the eyes in such a position as to avoid the action of the affected muscle. Thus, with a right superior oblique palsy, the patient has weakness of ☐ intorsion/ ☐ extorsion of the right eye, an action for which the superior oblique is mainly responsible.
   b. The unopposed action of the extortors would cause the eye to be in a position of extorsion. In compensation, therefore, the patient with a right superior oblique palsy tilts his head to the ☐ right/ ☐ left to prevent diplopia.
   c. A persistent head tilt is called *wryneck,* or *torticollis.* Oblique muscle palsy is only one of many causes for torticollis.
4. *Effect of heterotropia on vision.*
   a. An infant or young child with heterotropia of congenital or early onset learns to suppress vision from the errant eye. He does not complain of diplopia even though the heterotropia persists throughout life. On the other hand, if the heterotropia comes on in later childhood or adulthood, the patient usually has diplopia.
   b. In a young child, image suppression may become habitual. He loses any effective vision in the eye, even though the anatomic pathways are intact. If the suppression is untreated, sight can never be recovered. Such a loss of vision is called *suppression amblyopia* (amblyopia ex anopsia). Suppression amblyopia occurs not only with heterotropia but also with many monocular disorders of retinal image formation—refractive errors, opacification of the refracting media, or retinal lesions. Suppression amblyopia, if due to neglect, means one thing: malpractice. It is a preventable cause of monocular blindness. It is one of the reasons every infant and young child must have a complete ocular and funduscopic

examination. If the attending physician suspects any ocular abnormality, the patient should have the benefit of specialty consultation. Ocular deviations persisting beyond the first weeks of life should never be neglected because of a naive expectation that the infant will grow "out" of it. He may grow more and more "into" it.

P. *Nonparalytic or concomitant heterotropias*

1. With muscular paresis or paralysis, the eyes do not move concomitantly — one eye moves *more* or *less* than the other. Hence, we can classify paralytic heterotropia as *nonconcomitant.* In another type of heterotropia, the eyes are malaligned, but upon movement, they retain the same malalignment, the same degree of deviant angulation. These *concomitant* heterotropias are usually nonparalytic. As a general rule, then, *concomitant* heterotropia is nonparalytic, while nonconcomitant heterotropia is the result of muscular paralysis.

concomitant

2. If the eyes maintain the same degree of deviation in all directions of gaze, the heterotropia is ☐ concomitant / ☐ nonconcomitant.

The angle of deviation increases in the direction of action of the afflicted muscle

3. Concomitant heterotropia may be intermittent, but when present, the deviation is the same in all directions of gaze. What happens to the angulation of the eyes in heterotropia due to neuromuscular lesions, when the eyes move? ______________________________

____

____

4. The cause of concomitant heterotropia is usually a disturbance in image formation on one macula — cloudiness of the cornea, a severe refractive error, a cataract, or a macular lesion. In some cases, it is as if a new macula is established, off center from the true macula, and then the visual axis is aligned on the new macula. The patient alternates in fixating with the normal eye and the abnormal one. He learns to suppress vision from whichever eye he is not using at the moment for fixation, much as you can learn to use a monocular microscope with both eyes open. Thus, the patient alternately fixes with one eye and suppresses vision from the other eye. When fixation alternates between the two eyes, suppression amblyopia does not occur. (In fact, suppression amblyopia is treated by patching the eyes alternately to ensure that both are used for fixation.)
5. *The clinical characteristics of concomitant heterotropia*

same

   a. The deviation of the ocular axes is ☐ the same / ☐ different for the primary position and in all directions of gaze.

   b. In contrast to nonconcomitant heterotropia, the primary and secondary deviations disclosed by the cover-uncover test are ☐ equal / ☐ unequal in concomitant heterotropia.

Ans: Equal. (If they weren't equal the patient would have nonconcomitant heterotropia.)

   c. When either eye fixates alone, it shows a full range of motility. None of the individual muscles is paralyzed.

**Starred sections optional.

nonconcomitant
concomitant

d. The patient has no diplopia. Would he have a compensatory head tilt? ☐ Yes / ☐ No. Explain: ______________________________

Ans: No. The head tilt of the patient with paralytic heterotropia compensates for the action of the paralytic muscle. To avoid diplopia the patient tilts or turns his head to keep the eyes in a position not requiring the action of the affected muscle. In concomitant heterotropia there is no paralysis, no diplopia, and no head tilt.

6. The term *paralytic heterotropia* is essentially synonymous with ☐ concomitant / ☐ nonconcomitant heterotropia. The term *nonparalytic* heterotropia is essentially synonymous with ______________ heterotropia.

Q. Complete Table 2-2 by making a check in the left-hand columns (1 and 2) if the characteristic in column 3 applies.

P	N-P
✓	
	✓
✓	
	✓
	✓
✓	
✓	

TABLE 2-2. Differential Diagnosis of Paralytic and Nonparalytic Heterotropia

1	2	3
Paralytic (nonconcomitant)	Nonparalytic (concomitant)	Clinical characteristic
		Ocular deviation changes with eye movement.
		Full movement when each eye is tested after covering the other.
		Secondary deviation greater than primary.
		Secondary and primary deviations equal.
		Frequently has opacity or severe refractive error in one eye.
		Has diplopia if heterotropia comes on after early age.
		Often has compensatory head turning or tilting.

Note to Table 2-2. The rules given here cover the majority of the cases. When heterotropia is of long standing, fibrosis and contracture of the affected muscles may change the deviation patterns given here. Other confounding factors are eccentric fixation and fusional problems at the cortical level.

IV. Refraction and accommodation

A. Light refraction by the normal eye. The refracting media of the eye includes the cornea and lens. Study refraction by the emmetropic (normal) eye in Fig. 2-30.

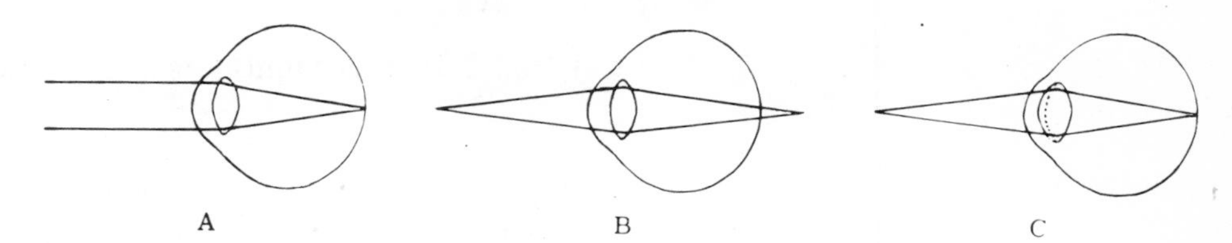

FIG. 2-30. Schematic cross sections of the eye to show focal point of light rays. *A.* Emmetropic eye. Parallel rays from a distant object focus on the retina. *B.* Emmetropic eye in which no adjustment has been made to accommodate for near vision. The light rays from the near point diverge as they travel to the eye. They focus behind the retina. *C.* Emmetropic eye accommodated for near vision. The lens has thickened, increasing its power of refraction. The divergent rays now focus upon, rather than behind, the retina.

B. Accommodation reflex

medial rectus

1. Near vision requires convergence of the visual axes onto the fixation point, an action accomplished by the ______________________ ______________ muscles.
2. The pupils constrict as the eyes converge. Cormiosis is caused by the sphincter action of the *pupilloconstrictor* muscle of the iris. The constricted iris produces a pinhole camera effect, screening off the more peripheral rays that require the most refraction to focus on the retina.
3. Convergence and cormiosis are two of the requisites for accommodation. The third is thickening of the lens, increasing its ability to refract the more divergent rays from the near fixation point. Lens thickening is accomplished by action of the *ciliary muscle*.

convergence
constriction
thickening

4. Thus, during accommodation for near vision, three distinct events occur: ______________________ of the visual axes onto the fixation point, ______________________ of the pupil, and ______________________ of the lens.
5. Although the act of looking at a near object is volitional, neural mechanisms lock the three events of accommodation into a single *accommodation reflex*. Thus, whenever a person voluntarily converges the eyes, neural circuits automatically complete the other two events of the accommodation reflex, pupilloconstriction and lens thickening.
6. *Complete Table 2-3.*

convergence / medial recti

cormiosis / pupilloconstrictor muscle

lens thickening / ciliary muscle

TABLE 2-3. The Accommodation Reflex and the Muscles That Accomplish It

List the three events of the accommodation reflex	List the responsible muscles
	(skeletal)
	(smooth)
	(smooth)

**C. *Myopia and hyperopia*

1. Study Fig. 2-31 in conjunction with Table 2-4.

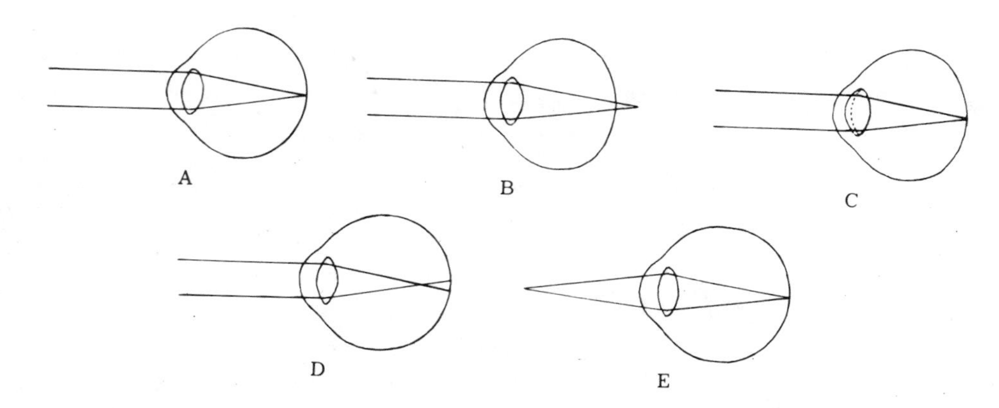

FIG. 2-31. Refraction. Notice the point of focus relative to the diameter of the eye in parts A to E and compare with statements *A* through *E* in Table 2-4.

TABLE 2-4. Focal Point of Light Rays Undergoing Refraction By Emmetropic, Myopic, and Hyperopic Eyes.

A. *Emmetropia.* The diameter of the normal eye is proper relative to its refracting power. Parallel rays from a distant source focus on the retina without accommodation. Divergent rays from a near source require lens thickening to be focused on the retina.

B. *Hyperopia.* The diameter of the eye is too short relative to its refracting power. Parallel rays focus behind the retina.

C. *Hyperopia with accommodation.* The lens of the hyperopic eye must thicken, increasing its focusing power, to bring parallel rays to focus on the retina. When the hyperopic person looks at a near object, he has no accommodation reserve.

D. *Myopia.* The diameter of the eye is too long relative to its refracting power. Parallel rays focus in front of the retina.

E. *Myopic eye focusing on near object.* Divergent rays from the near object focus properly on the retina with little or no accommodation.

2. A person with sharp vision for far away *and* close objects is ☐ emmetropic / ☐ myopic / ☐ hyperopic.
3. For far vision, the emmetropic person's muscles of accommodation are ☐ active / ☐ relaxed.
4. A person with sharp vision for far objects, but blurred vision for close objects, is said to be "farsighted." The technical term for farsightedness is ☐ emmetropia / ☐ myopia / ☐ hyperopia.
5. The hyperopic eye focuses parallel rays ☐ behind / ☐ in front of / ☐ upon the retina.

emmetropic

relaxed

hyperopia

behind

when looking at close and far objects	*a.* The hyperopic patient requires some activity of the accommodation reflex to thicken the lens ☐ only when viewing far objects / ☐ only when viewing close objects / ☐ when looking at close and far objects.
only during near vision	*b.* Normally, however, the accommodation reflex should be active ☐ at all times / ☐ only during far vision / ☐ only during near vision.
myopia	6. A person with blurred vision for distant objects, but sharp vision for near objects, is said to be "nearsighted." The technical term for nearsightedness is ☐ emmetropia / ☐ myopia / ☐ hyperopia.
in front of	*a.* The myopic eye focuses parallel rays from far objects ☐ in front of / ☐ upon / ☐ behind the retina.
less	*b.* Therefore during near vision, the myopic person needs ☐ more / ☐ less accommodation to bring the divergent rays onto the retina.
less	*c.* As compared to the emmetropic or hyperopic person, the myopic person places ☐ less / ☐ more demand on his accommodation reflex.

7. On scrap paper, draw three eyeballs and show the focal point of parallel rays in emmetropia, hyperopia, and myopia. Compare with Fig. 2-31*A, B,* and *D.*

****D.** *Relation of refractive errors to heterotropia and heterophoria.* (To be done only if optional section *C,* page 66, was completed.)

1. Young infants frequently have minor tropias. During the first several months of life, they develop binocular fixation and fusion of the images from the two eyes. In addition to the immaturity of the nervous system, another reason the young infant does not see well is that the eye is thought to be too short relative to its refracting power. With maturation, the eyeball expands.

hyperopic	2. Since the infant's eyes tend to be too short in relation to the focal point of the lens, he is ☐ myopic / ☐ emmetropic / ☐ hyperopic.
myopic	3. As the eyeball increases in diameter with maturation, the hyperopia tends to change to emmetropia. If the child is emmetropic at birth instead of hyperopic, he would become ________ as the diameter of the eye increases with growth.

4. Because of the small diameter of the eyeball relative to the focusing power of the lens, infants tend to keep their lenses thickened. In other words, they tend to accommodate all of the time. When 2 to 3 years old, the child turns its attention to the close, detailed inspection of near objects, which places extra demands on accommodation. The need for accommodation may overcome the hyperopic child's capacity for it.

esophoria	*a.* Since one of the accommodation mechanisms is convergence of the eyes, the hyperopic child at first will show only a latent tendency to crossing of his eyes, which would be called ☐ esotropia / ☐ esophoria.
esotropia	*b.* If the hyperopia is severe, the esophoria may convert to a manifest internal deviation of an eye, which would be called ________.
	c. Thus, refractive errors or neuromuscular lesions may cause crossed eyes. Two eyelid anomalies in children may give a spurious appear-

dystopic canthus
epicanthal folds

more

less

drift apart

exophoria
exotropia

hyperopia

myopia

ance of crossed eyes because the limbus appears to be too close to the medial eyelid margins. The anomalies are ________________ ________________ and ________________.

5. Consider the infant who is going to be myopic at maturity. As his eyeball enlarges with age, he becomes ☐ more / ☐ less myopic. Therefore, his accommodation mechanism tends to become ☐ more / ☐ less active.
   a. With an underactive accommodation mechanism, the child's eyes would tend to ☐ drift apart / ☐ converge too much.
   b. At first he might show only a latent tendency to drift apart, which would be called ________________ or later if manifest, ________________.
6. Tropias and phorias are very common with refractive errors.
   a. Esophoria or esotropia in a child would raise the question of ☐ myopia / ☐ emmetropia / ☐ hyperopia.
   b. Exophoria or exotropia in a child would raise the question of ☐ myopia / ☐ emmetropia / ☐ hyperopia.
   c. Clearly, tests for visual acuity, for hyperopia and myopia, must be included in the physical examination. These tests will be discussed in the section on visual fields.

V. Summary of Ocular Motility Examination

A. This chapter has prepared you to test the patient's ocular motility

1. Ask the patient to fixate on your finger, which you hold in front of him in the midline about 50 cm away. Start at point 1 on the H which your finger ultimately will describe. See Fig. 2-32.

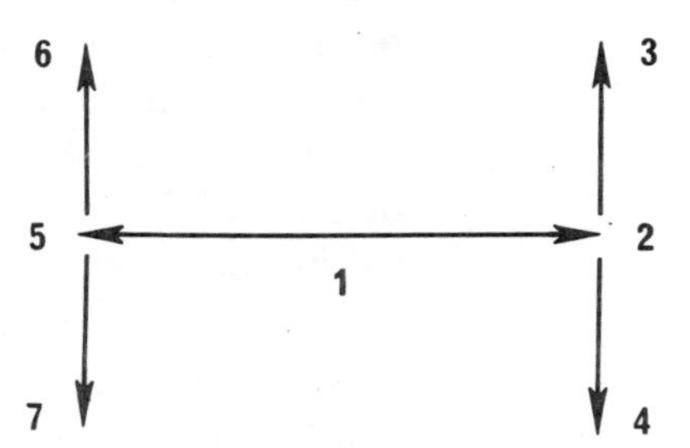

FIG. 2-32. The H through which the examiner moves his finger to test ocular motility, and the numbering of the stations.

2. Have the patient follow your finger horizontally to station 2, the extreme end of lateral gaze. Gently press on top of the patient's head with your other hand, fixing the head in position, permitting only the eyes to move.
3. Hold the finger at station 2 and inspect the eyes for the corneal light reflections and the relation of the limbus to lid margins, canthi, and caruncles. Look for nystagmus. If you see it, move your finger back a few cm toward station 1. If the nystagmus disappears, it probably is a nonpathological type called *pseudonystagmus.* This and other types of nystagmus are discussed later.

4. Next, move to stations 3 and 4 at the extremes of lateral upward and downward gaze. Repeat the observations of step 3.
5. Move your finger back to the horizontal plane and across to station 5 and repeat all observations and maneuvers at 6 and 7.
6. Finally, move your finger back to station 1 and instruct the patient, "Look right at my finger," and move it in to touch the bridge of the nose, observing convergence and pupilloconstriction. Usually, one eye breaks off of convergence when the finger is several cm away from the nose.

B. Inquire whether the patient saw double at anytime during the maneuvers.

C. If the patient saw double or you observed ocular malalignment, proceed with the steps of section M, page 58 for the analysis of diplopia.

D. Do the cover-uncover test.

Bibliography

Bach-y-Rita, P., and Collins, C. (ed): *The Control of Eye Movements,* New York, Academic Press, 1971.

Bender, M.: *The Oculomotor System,* New York, Hoeber Medical Division, Harper & Row, 1964.

Burger, L., Kalvin, N., and Smith, J.: Acquired lesions of the fourth cranial nerve, *Brain,* 93:567–574, 1970.

Davson, H.: *The Eye,* vol. 3, 2nd ed., Muscular Mechanisms, New York, Academic Press, Inc., 1970.

Duke-Elder, W.: *Text-book of Ophthalmology,* vol. IV, The Neurology of Vision Motor and Optical Anomalies, St. Louis, C. V. Mosby, 1949.

Gay, A., and Newman, N.: Eye movements and their disorders: an analytical evaluation, from *Scientific Foundations of Neurology,* M. Critchley (ed), Philadelphia, F. A. Davis, 1972.

Helveston, E.: A two-step test for diagnosing paresis of a single vertically acting extraocular muscle, *Amer. J. Ophthal.,* 64:914–915, 1967.

Hoyt, W., and Nachtigaler, A.: Anomalies of ocular motor nerves, *Amer. J. Ophthal.,* 60:443, 1965.

Jampolsky, A.: Strabismus, chap. 20, in L. Holt (ed.), *Pediatric Ophthalmology,* Philadelphia, Lea & Febiger, 1964.

Leibman, S., and Gellis, S.: *The Pediatrician's Ophthalmology,* St. Louis, C. V. Mosby, 1966.

Reinecke, R., and Miller, D.: *Strabismus. A Programmed Text,* New York, Appleton-Century-Crofts, 1966.

Scobee, R.: *Disturbances of Ocular Motility.* Section in Instruction, Home Study Courses, American Academy of Ophthalmology and Otolaryngology, Omaha, Douglas Printing Co., 1951.

Walsh, F. and Hoyt, W.: *Clinical Neuro-ophthalmology,* 3rd ed., Baltimore, The Williams & Wilkins Co., 1969.

Weaver, R., and Stanley, J.: *The Neuro-Ophthalmologic Examination* in Special Techniques for Neurologic Diagnosis, Toole, J. (ed), *Contemporary Neurology Series,* vol. 3, Philadelphia, F. A. Davis, 1969.

3

The Brainstem and Cranial Nerves. A Brief Review of Their Clinical Neuroanatomy

But chieflye the anatomye
Ye oughte to understande:
If ye will cure well anye thinge,
That ye doe take in hande.

— John Halle (1529 - 1566)

I. Gross subdivisions of the neuraxis

A. *The neuraxis (central nervous system) Learn Fig. 3 - 1*

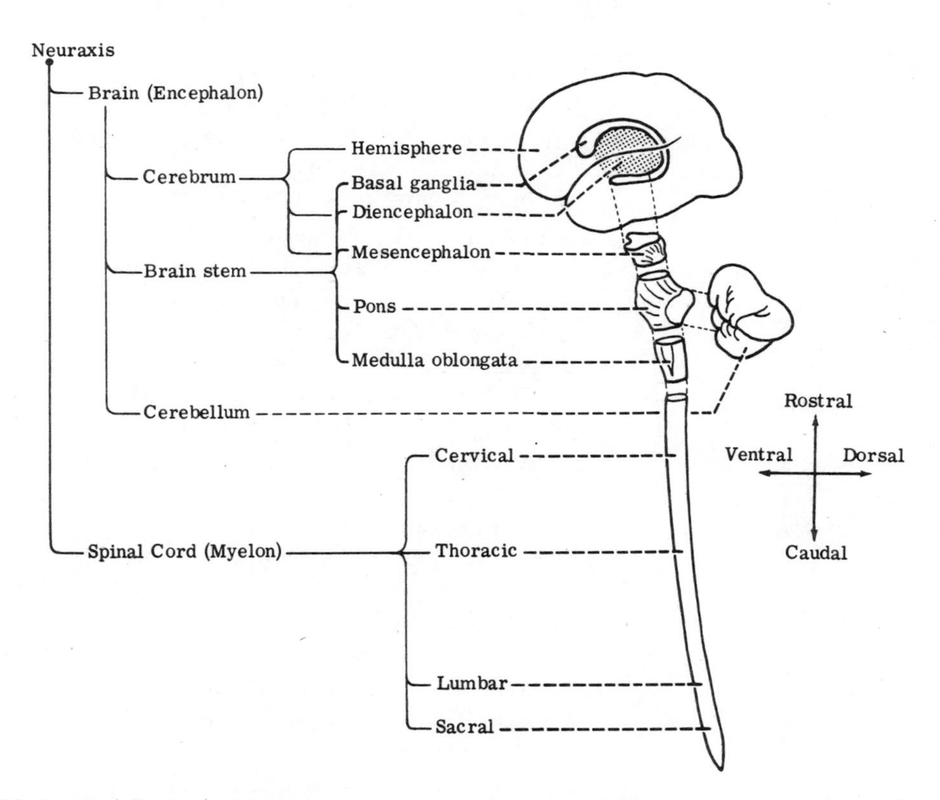

FIG. 3 - 1. Subdivisions of the neuraxis (central nervous system). Notice how the definitions of the terms *brain, brainstem,* and *cerebrum* overlap but are not synonymous.

B. Basic definitions, or how to get the part of the neuraxis you want

1. The *spinal cord* is strictly defined: transect the neuraxis at the level of the foramen magnum. That part of the neuraxis caudal to the cut is the spinal cord.
2. The *cerebrum* is strictly defined: transect the neuraxis at the junction of pons with mesencephalon: What is rostral is the cerebrum.
3. The *brainstem* is elastic. Some authors include basal ganglia, diencephalon, mesencephalon, pons and medulla oblongata. Others mean only the mesencephalon, pons, and medulla. We are in the first group. Hence, here is how to get a brainstem as we shall define it:
   a. Cut off the spinal cord at the foramen magnum.
   b. Scrape away the cerebral cortex and the underlying white matter.
   c. Scrape away the cerebellar cortex and the underlying white matter. What is left are the basal ganglia and four transverse subdivisions: the *diencephalon,* the *mesencephalon, pons,* and *medulla oblongata.* Label these four transverse subdivisions of the brainstem in Fig. 3-2, in rostrocaudal sequence.

1. Diencephalon
2. Mesencephalon
3. Pons
4. Medulla

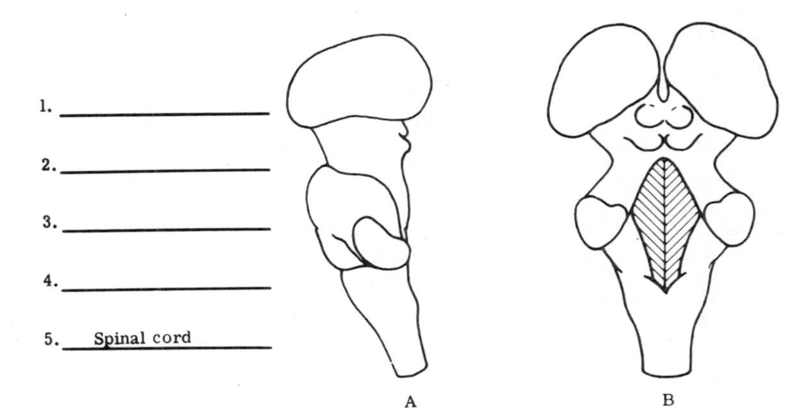

FIG. 3-2. The four transverse subdivisions of the brainstem and the junction with the spinal cord. Complete labels 1 to 4. A. Left lateral view. B. Dorsal view.

II. Somites, spinal nerves, and the theory of nerve components. A review, or how to get to the neurology clinic through the muck and slime of phylógenesis, the controlled cataclysms of embryogenesis, and a little help from set theory.

A. Somites

1. During phylogeny and ontogeny, the body wall develops from serially homologous segments called *somites.* See Fig. 3-3*A* only.
2. Each somite is a block of mesoderm in continuity with its neighbors. The somite differentiates into a dermatome, myotome, and sclerotome. The dermatome spreads out under the ectoderm to form the dermis. Thus, the products of a single somite consist of:
   a. A ________ *tome* which produces dermis.
   b. A ________ *tome* which produces muscle.
   c. A ________ *tome* which produces bone.

dermatome
myotome
sclerotome

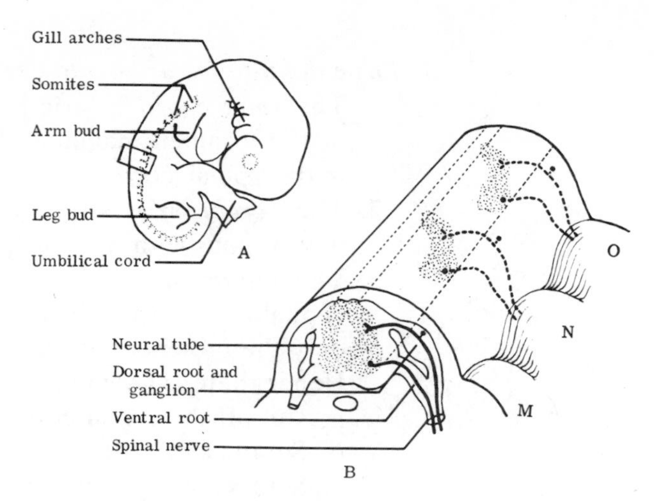

FIG. 3-3. Somites in a 5-week-old human embryo. *A*. Serial arrangement of the somites lateral to the neuraxis. *B*. Enlargement of neuraxis and somites blocked off in *A*. Notice that each somite (M, N, and O) receives only one nerve.

3. Elaboration of head and limbs requires radical transformations in the original somites of these regions. The only part of the adult body to retain somite simplicity is the thorax, where nerves, muscles, ribs, and intercostal vessels preserve the primordial segmental pattern in obvious form.

B. Spinal nerves and the theory of nerve components

1. Each spinal nerve innervates the skin, muscle, and bone directly derived from one somite, and it innervates the viscera which originally were directly covered by the somite.
2. Each spinal nerve is formed by the union of dorsal and ventral roots. Each dorsal root provides somatic afferent (SA) fibers for somatic sensation and visceral afferent (VA) fibers for visceral sensation. Locate these components in Fig. 3-4.
3. Each ventral root provides somatic efferent fibers (SE) for skeletal muscle, and visceral efferent (VE) fibers for smooth muscle and glands. Locate these components in Fig. 3-4.

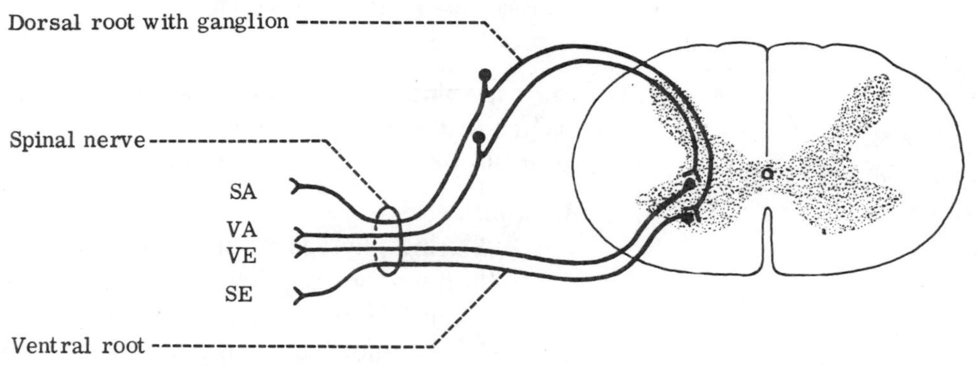

FIG. 3-4. Cross section of spinal cord and typical spinal nerve to show the classification of the axons into SA (somatic afferent), VA (visceral afferent), VE (visceral efferent), and SE (somatic efferent) components.

only sensory

4. Each dorsal root contains ☐ only sensory (afferent) / ☐ only motor (efferent) / ☐ motor and sensory nerve fibers.

motor (efferent)

dorsal
ventral

dorsal root

5. Each ventral root contains only ________________ nerve fibers.
6. All afferent nerve fibers enter the spinal cord through the ________________ roots. The efferent fibers leave the spinal cord through the ________________ roots.
7. The diagrams of neuronal connections in this text should always be read by tracing along the course of the nerve impulses. In Fig. 3-4, the nerve impulse would start at one of the somatic or visceral receptor endings, let us say the SA. The impulse would then travel centrally past the ________________ ________________ ganglion.
8. In the gray matter of the spinal cord, the SA axon synapses on a motor neuron. A synapse is represented in Fig. 3-5.

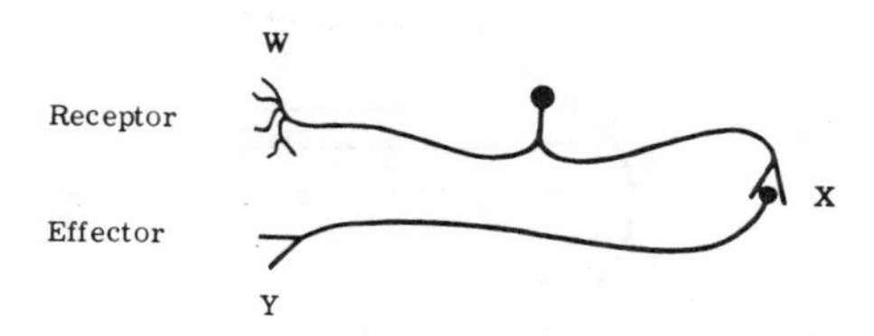

FIG. 3-5. Conventional representation of a synapse at X. A receptor is any sensory nerve ending. An effector is any motor nerve ending on a secretory cell or a muscle fiber.

WXY

   a. The flow of nerve impulses at a synapse is *from* the incoming axon *to* the next neuron. It is a one-way valve.
   b. In Fig. 3-5, the flow of impulses is □ WXY / □ YXW.
9. Draw and label a cross section of the spinal cord showing the dorsal and ventral roots and their components. By means of arrows, indicate the course of impulse flow, beginning at a receptor and ending at an effector.

Check drawing against Fig. 3-4.

C. The fate of the spinal dermatomes

1. The phylogenetic specializations leading to limb and head development disturb the simplicity of the serial segmentation of the body into somites. See Fig. 3-6.

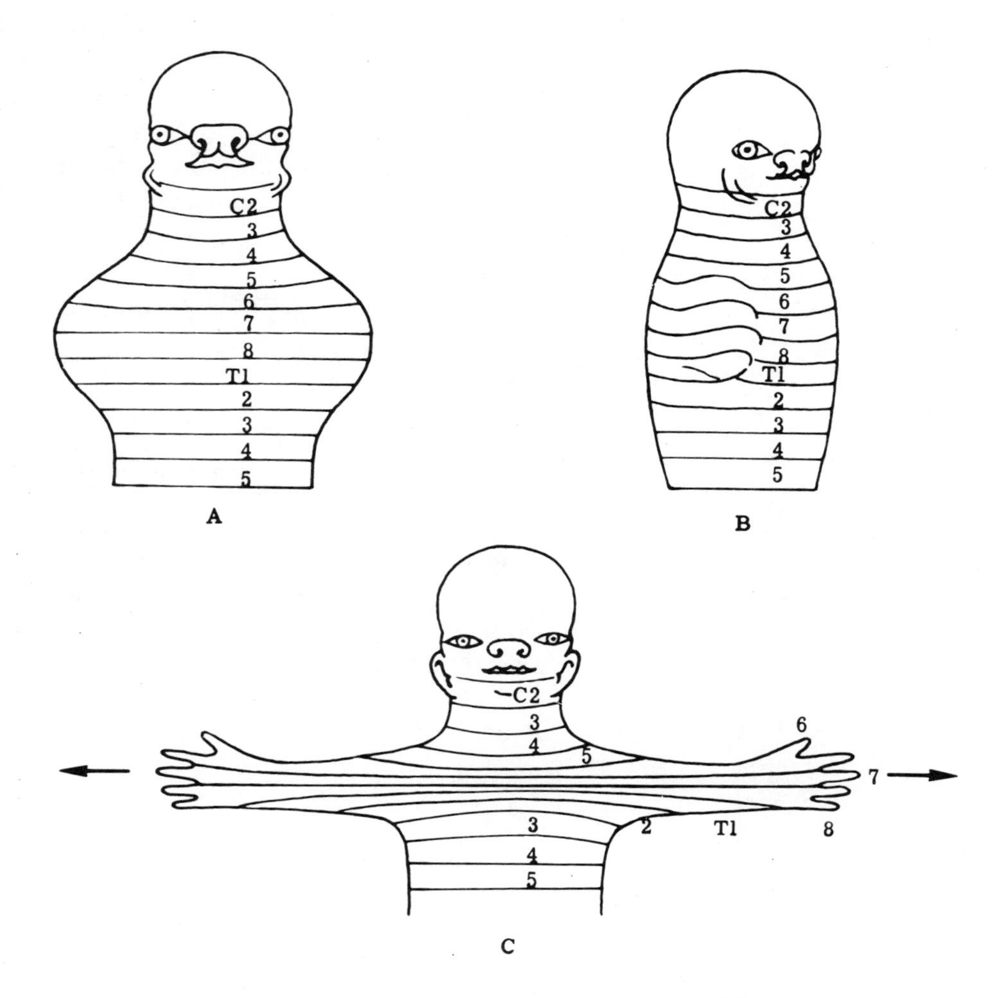

FIG. 3-6. Representation of dermatomal dislocation caused by development of the limbs. Notice that no dermatomes are represented rostral to C_2.

2. Notice in Fig. 3-6 how the proximal portions of the dermatomes attenuate. Finally they are stretched so thin that C_4 abuts on T_2 in the final state of the dermatomes, as shown in Fig. 3-7A.
3. Wherever a dermatome migrates, it drags its original nerve supply with it. The same rule holds for the myotomes and sclerotomes which also migrate out during proplasia of the limbs. Although the somite nerve remains attached to its original site on the spinal cord, the spinal nerves anastomose in the brachial and lumbosacral plexuses to share common peripheral nerves in getting to their original terminal fields. Since the spinal nerve retains its original spinal cord attachment and innervates its original somite components no matter where they go, we will call this principle the *law of original innervation*.

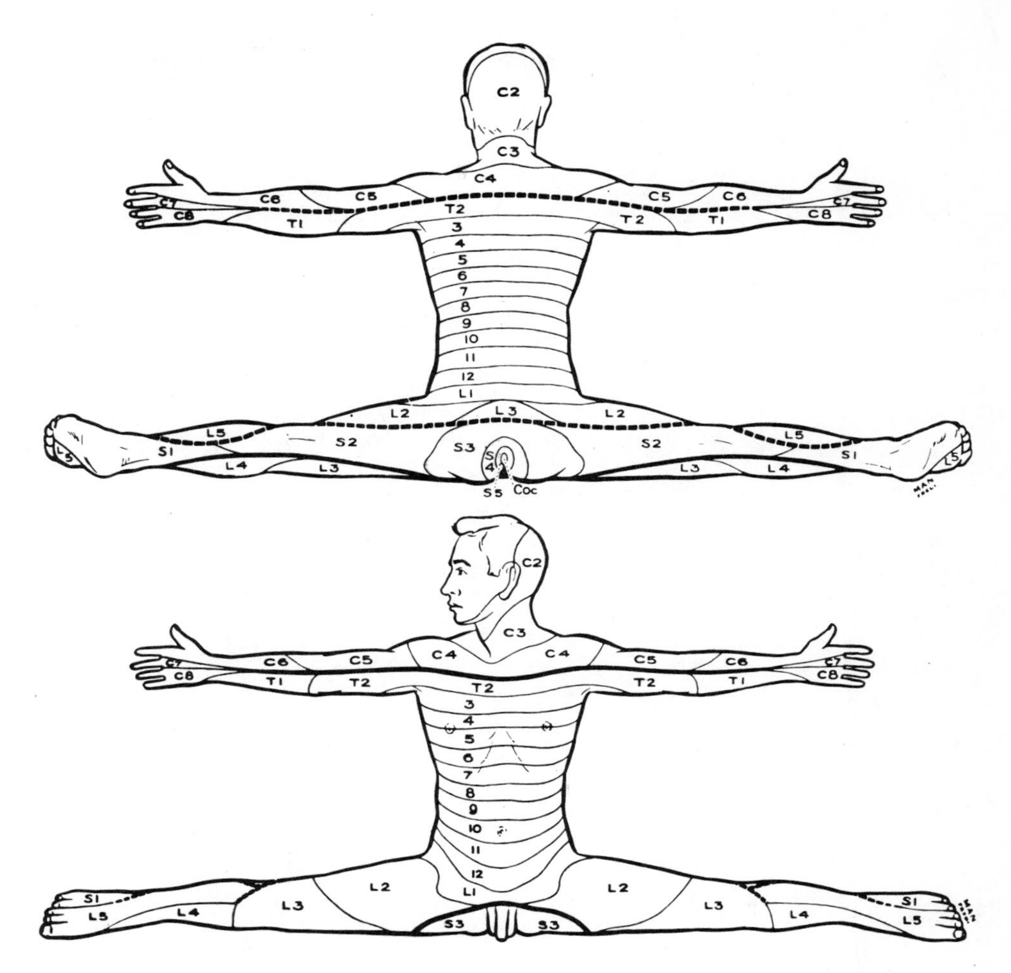

FIG. 3-7A. Contrasting cutaneous innervation areas of dermatomes and peripheral nerves. *A. Dermatomal areas:* The numbers correspond to the spinal cord level of the dermatome. C = cervical, T = thoracic, L = lumbar, S = sacral. (*From W. Haymaker and B. Woodhall: Peripheral Nerve injuries, 2d ed., Philadelphia, W. B. Saunders Company, 1962.*)

4. Because somite axons detour in the plexuses, the peripheral nerves distal to the plexus have more or less than the dorsal and ventral root axons from one spinal cord segment. A lesion in or distal to a plexus thus causes deficits that do not conform to somite boundaries. By mapping the area of sensory loss, the clinician can decide whether the patient suffers from a dorsal root (dermatomal), plexus, or a peripheral nerve lesion. Compare in principle the dermatomal and peripheral nerve distributions in Fig. 3-7*A* and *B*, but do not memorize them. Notice that only in the thoracic region do the somite and peripheral nerve distributions conform exactly.
5. *The fate of the cranial somites*
   From C_2 to the sacral region of the spinal cord, all somites are retained in unbroken continuity, although some are radically altered. In the cephalic region, somite continuity is interrupted. Some become useless and disappear, while others are renovated until they are scarcely recognizable. Before we discuss the cranial nerve somites, it will be felicitous to review the cranial nerves more generally. If I just heard a groan from the audience, let me affirm that I know the dif-

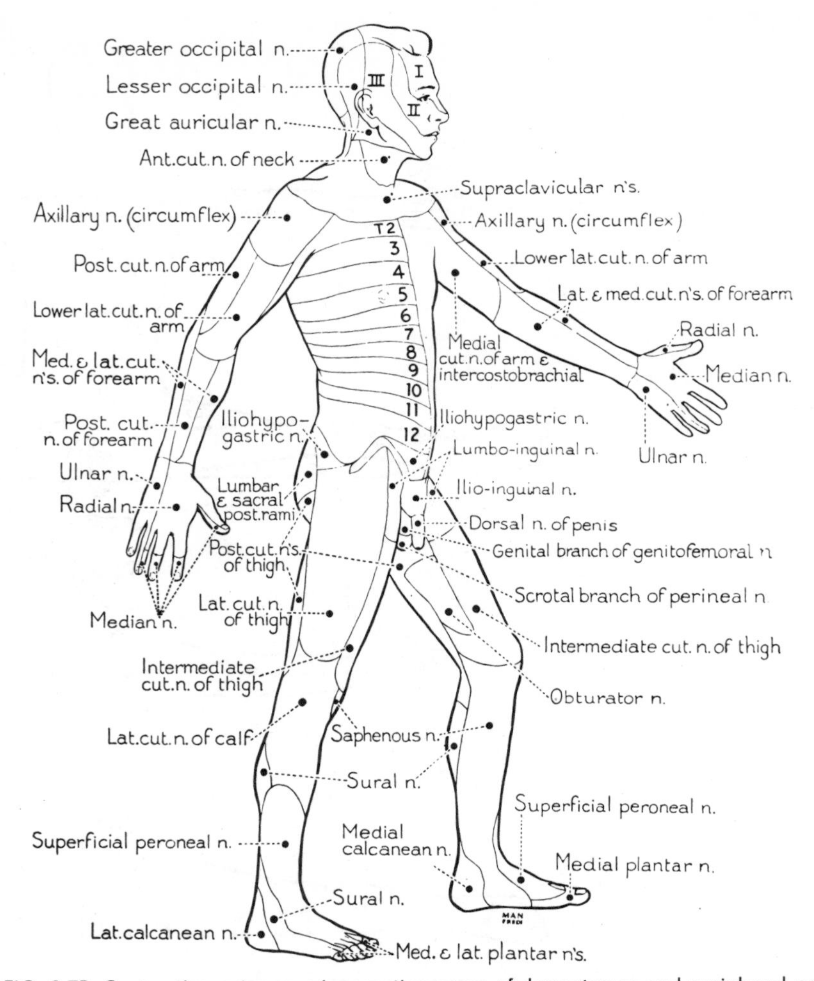

FIG. 3-7B. Contrasting cutaneous innervation areas of dermatomes and peripheral nerves. *B. Areas of sensory innervation by peripheral nerves:* Dermatomal axons may travel by more than one peripheral nerve, and a peripheral nerve may carry axons from more than one dermatome. Clinically, the important task is to decide whether the patient's sensory complaint falls into a dermatomal or peripheral nerve distribution. *(From K. Poeck: Einführung in die klinische Neurologie, Berlin, Springer-Verlag, 1966.)*

ference between bump and crevice anatomy and clinical anatomy. What is here must be known to practice medicine and to enjoy clinical diagnosis. If it won't make you a great neurologist, it will at least keep you from being dangerous to your patients.

III. Anatomic review of the brainstem and cranial nerves

So the present classification of the cranial nerves into 12 numbered pairs was devised by a German medical student [Samuel Soemmering, 1755-1830] nearly two centuries ago. Its basis is the holes in the floor of the skull through which nerves extend out from the cranial cavity to organs as diverse as the eyes and the bowels. Only in part does it sort the nerves according to their function or ultimate distribution. Although rather arbitrary and awkward, it seems likely to be with us for some time.

— C. Wilbur Rucker

A. For clinical neurology you must know

1. The name and number of the cranial nerves.
2. The fiber components of the cranial nerves.

3. The point of attachment of the cranial nerves to the brain.
4. The location of the cranial nerve nuclei.
5. The longitudinal and transverse subdivisions of the brainstem and its plan of internal organization.
6. The location of the major tracts on cross section of the brainstem.

B. *Nomenclature.* At best, the cranial nerves are difficult to learn; at worst impossible. Therefore, you need to utilize every aid offered by the erratic and unprincipled nomenclature.

1. You must know the *number* and the *name* of the nerve.
   a. The *number* tells you the sequence of the nerve along the rostrocaudal axis of the brain (XI excepted).
   b. The *name* tells you at least something about the components, function or distribution of the nerve. Learn Table 3-1.

TABLE 3-1. Relation of Cranial Nerve Name to Anatomy or Function. Learn This Table.

Number and name of nerve	Functional or anatomic significance of name
I Olfactory	It smells
II Optic	It sees
III Oculomotor	Its muscles move the eyeball
IV Trochlear	Its muscle moves the eyeball after running through a trochlea or pulley
V Trigeminal	It has three large sensory branches to the face
VI Abducens	It abducts the eye
VII Facial	It moves the muscles of all facial orifices
VIII Vestibulocochlear	It equilibrates, hears
IX Glossopharyngeal	It supplies taste fibers to the tongue and activates the pharynx during swallowing
X Vagus	It is a vagrant, wandering from the pharynx to the splenic flexure of the colon
XI Spinal accessory	It arises in the cervical spinal cord, runs into the skull, out again, and conveys accessory fibers to the vagus
XII Hypoglossal	It runs under the tongue

2. *Function of cranial nerves.* It is helpful to be able to express in one or a few words the function of the nerves. In fact, the function of all cranial nerves can be compressed into 47 little words. This is the ultimate distillation: it can't be any simpler. Learn Table 3-2.
3. From Table 3-2, and phylogenetic and embryologic data, we can begin to construct sets of cranial nerves which tie them into memory packages.
   a. The *first* and simplest set, the *somitic* set, is directly homologous with the spinal nerves because it innervates derivatives of cranial somites. It consists of cranial nerves III, IV, VI, and XII.
   b. The *second* set, the *Solely Special Sensory Set,* (SSSS), is of diverse embryologic origin. It contains nerves I, II, and VIII. One special sense, taste, is included with the third set of nerves.

TABLE 3-2. Function of Cranial Nerves. Learn this table.	
Number and function	
I:	Smells
II:	Sees
III, IV, and VI:	Move eyes; III constricts pupils
V:	Chews and feels front of head
VII:	Moves the face, tears, tastes, salivates
VIII:	Hears, equilibrates
IX:	Tastes, salivates, swallows, monitors carotid body and sinus
X:	Tastes, swallows, lifts palate, phonates, afferent and parasympathetic efferent to thoracico-abdominal viscera
XI:	Turns head, shrugs shoulders
XII:	Moves tongue

c. The *third* set, the *branchial* set, is phylogenetically derived from branchial (gill) arches. Since the branchial arches are all rostral, no spinal nerves contain branchial arch components. Five of the twelve cranial nerves are branchial nerves: V, VII, IX, X, and XI.

C. The somitic set of cranial nerves: III, IV, VI, and XII

1. Of the original dozen or so cranial somites, only a few survive the travail of evolution. All cranial dermatomes are lost. The first cervical dermatome (C_1) also disappears. Hence, the most rostral dermatome present is ______________.

C_2 (Review Fig. 3-6 if you missed.)

2. Three of the rostral myotomes survive, wondrously rehabilitated into the ocular muscles.
   a. According to the law of original innervation, these three myotomes must retain their original innervation. Thus, there are three motor nerves to the eye muscles, nerves number ______________, ______________, and ______________. (If you have trouble recalling, sort through the cranial nerves one by one, I to XII.)

III, IV, VI

   b. Supplying skeletal muscle derived from somites, these nerves must all have a ☐ VA / ☐ SE / ☐ VE component.

SE

   c. Although a point of some dispute, we will assume that any nerve supplying SE fibers to a *skeletal* muscle also returns afferent fibers from it. Hence, cranial nerves III, IV, VI, and XII *all* have a ☐ SA / ☐ VE / ☐ VA component.

SA

   d. Of the three somitic nerves to the eyeball, only III innervates visceral (smooth) muscles. These muscles are the pupilloconstrictor muscle and the ciliary muscle, which adjusts lens thickness.
   e. Hence, the only motor nerve to the eye to have a VE component is ______________. Apparently no VA fibers return to the neuraxis in this nerve.

III

3. While three of the rostralmost cranial somites produce ocular muscles, some cranial somites intermediate between the rostralmost

and caudalmost disappear completely. Of dermatome, myotome, and sclerotome, not a trace. What would you expect to happen to their nerve supply? Explain: ______________________________
____
____
____

Ans: According to the law of original innervation, somites retain their own nerve supply. If the somite disappears, the nerve disappears.(As we shall see, it is for this reason that the SE nuclei of the brainstem are discontinuous, unlike the spinal cord where all somites are retained and the ventral horn is one continuous SE nucleus.)

SE, SA

4. The *caudal* cranial somites donate their *myotomes* to form the tongue muscle, their *sclerotomes* to the base of the skull, and their *dermatomes* to oblivion. Although we say that XII is one nerve, its rootlets neatly erupt serially from the medulla, in original somite order. See nerve XII in Fig. 3-10. Then, like somite nerves to the extremities, the rootlets unite into a common trunk to reach their original somites. XII is a plexus with only one nerve leading out! Don't be misled by the common trunk: the law of original innervation holds. Without any viscera to innervate, XII has only two components, ☐ SE/ ☐ VE/ ☐ VA/ ☐ SA.
5. Put checks in Table 3-3 to show the components of the somitic set of cranial nerves.

	III	IV	VI	XII
SA	✓	✓	✓	✓
VA				
VE	✓			
SE	✓	✓	✓	✓

TABLE 3-3. Nerve Components of the Somitic Cranial Nerves

	III	IV	VI	XII
SA				
VA				
VE				
SE				

6. *A recapitulation of the somitic set of cranial nerves*
Because of their common ontogenetic and phylogenetic origin, III, IV, VI, and XII form a *set* of cranial nerves, the simplest set by far, because they reflect *somite* simplicity. In fact, having lost *all* their dermatomes, *most* of their viscera, and *much* of their sclerotomes, they might be considered retrogressive. If you need a final mnemonic, notice that all somite cranial nerves are integer multiples or divisors of XII. No other *motor*, no *branchial* cranial nerves are (but I and II of the SSSS are). The one difficulty in remembering this set is that only cranial nerve ____________ has a VE component.

III

D. The set of branchial cranial nerves . . . "or human face divine"

1. To the poet Milton, it was the human face divine, handed down ready-made, without a history, from a deity and passed along from man

to man. But the biologist, William Gregory, "charged that the real [ancestral face belonged not to a precreated man but to] a poor mud-sucking protochordate of pre-Silurian times; that when in some far-off dismal swamp a putrid prize was snatched by scaly forms, their facial masks already bore our eyes and nose and mouth."

2. The branchial arches usurped the task of the retrogressive cranial somites. Thus, the history of the face, from fish to man, is in large part the history of the branchial arches. See Fig. 3-8.

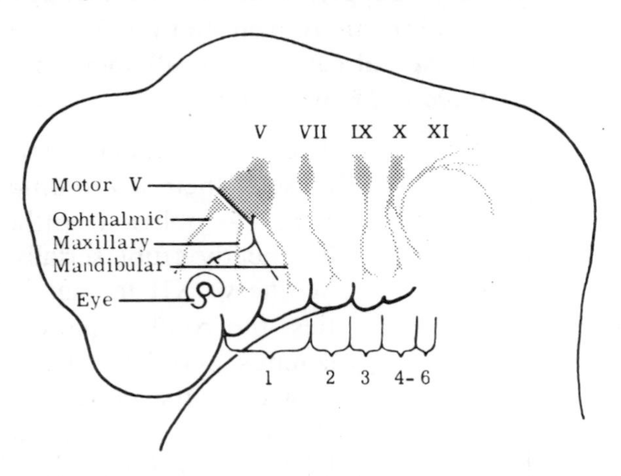

FIG. 3-8. Phantom view of a 6-week-old human embryo to show the innervation of the branchial arches by the branchial set of cranial nerves. The cranial nerves are numbered above in Roman numerals. The branchial arches are numbered below in Arabic numerals. The first arch divides into two processes, a maxillary and a mandibular. Learn this figure.

3. On close inspection, the branchial arches are remarkably similar to somites in fundamental plan.
   a. Thus, each branchial arch has only ________________ nerve and artery.
   b. Each arch has a skin covering, analagous to the ________________ of a somite.
   c. Each arch has a mesodermal core which produces skeletal muscle and bone, analogous to the ________ *tome* and ________ *tome* of the somite.

4. As you can imagine, the law of original innervation holds throughout the migrations and transformations of the branchial arch derivatives. The branchial nerves are complicated and will be defined in the context of clinical testing. For the present you should know their names, numbers, and general function, as in Table 3-4.

TABLE 3-4. Summary of Branchial Set of Cranial Nerves

Arch number	Cranial nerve number	Name	General function
1			
2			
3			
4			
5-6			

one

dermatome

myotome
sclerotome

V trigeminal
VII facial
IX glossopharyngeal
X vagus
XI spinal accessory
For function, check Table 3-2

E. *The solely special sensory set (SSSS) of cranial nerves: I, II, and VIII*

1. In contrast to the *transverse* segmentation of the solid body wall into somites and branchial arches, the viscera, including the neuraxis, are *longitudinal* tubes. The mechanism of elaboration of the hollow tubes is *diverticulation*. See Fig. 3-9.

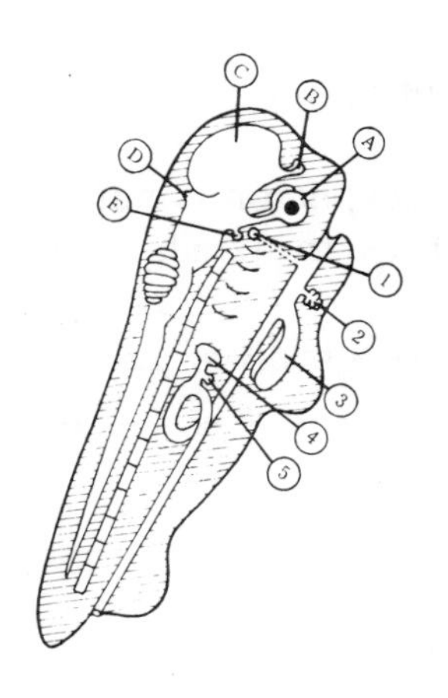

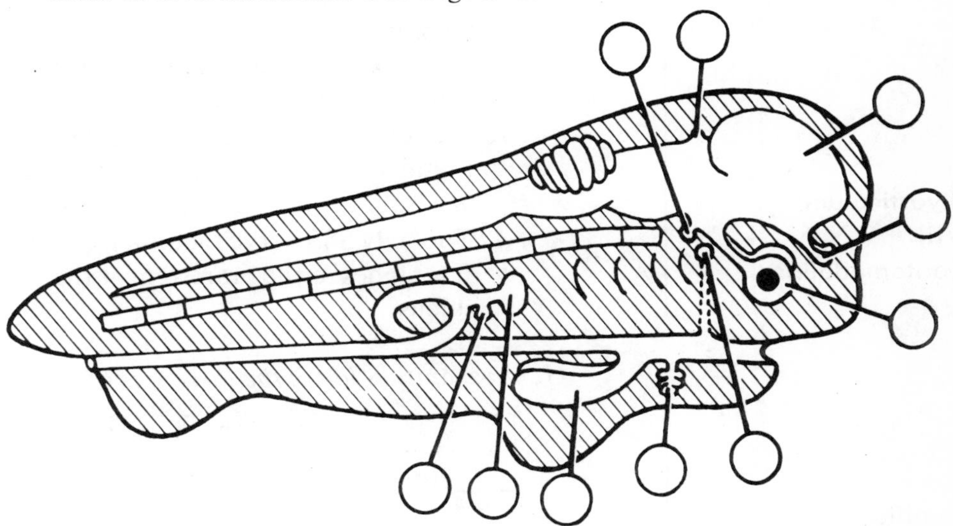

FIG. 3-9. Phantom view of a generalized vertebrate to show how the neural and alimentary tubes undergo *diverticulation*, their common mode of elaboration of accessory organs.

   a. Along the alimentary tube in Fig. 3-9 place numbers in rostrocaudal sequence to label the *diverticulae* that form the: (1) adenohypophysis, (2) thyroid gland, (3) lungs, (4) gallbladder and liver, and (5) pancreas.
   b. Along the neural tube in Fig. 3-9, place letters in sequence to label diverticulae that form the: (1) optic bulbs, (2) olfactory bulbs, (3) cerebral hemispheres, (4) pineal body, and (5) neurohypophysis.

2. The mechanisms of body wall and facial evolution are *migration, proplasia,* or *atrophy* of somites and branchial arches. In contrast, the mechanism of evolution of the visceral tubes is the out-pouching of ______________________.

diverticulae

3. *Cranial nerve I* consists only of axons from olfactory neurons located in the nasal mucosa. See Fig. 9-1. These axons penetrate the skull to synapse on the olfactory diverticulum. These axons tear away from the olfactory bulb upon removal of the brain. Hence you do not see them with the other cranial nerves on the base of the brain.
4. So-called cranial nerve II is neither developmentally nor histologically a peripheral nerve. Instead it is the retained stalk of the optic diverticulum that extended out to form the retina. The retina constitutes a portion of the brain wall brought to the surface to detect light rays. The optic stalk—the optic "nerve"—consists of brain wall, thus central, not peripheral nervous tissue. See the optic nerve, cranial nerve II, where this stalk attaches to the diencephalon in Fig. 3-10, at its original site of embryologic origin.
5. *Cranial nerve VIII* differentiates with the cochlear apparatus for detecting sound and the vestibular apparatus for detecting motion

and position. Of the three solely special sensory cranial nerves, VIII is the only true nerve histologically. It attaches to the brainstem at the *pontomedullary* sulcus, a crevice between the pons and the medulla. See nerve VIII, Fig. 3-10.

F. In summary

I

II
diverticulum
VIII
pontomedullary

1. The only cranial nerve synapsing on a diverticulum from the cerebrum is number ________.
2. The only cranial nerve attaching directly to the diencephalon is nerve number ________. It is not a true nerve. It is the stalk of a ________________ from the diencephalon.
3. The only SSS nerve that is a true peripheral nerve histologically is ____. It attaches to the brainstem at the ________________________ sulcus.

G. A recapitulation of the three sets of cranial nerves: Do Table 3-5

Somitic: III, IV, VI, XII
Branchial: V, VII, IX, X, XI
Solely special sensory: I, II, VIII

TABLE 3-5. The Three Sets of Cranial Nerves		
Name of set	Characterized by:	Nerves in set
1.	(1 per body segment)	
2.	(1 per gill arch)	
3.	(no motor axons)	

H. The point of attachment of the cranial nerves to the brain

1. Learn now, once and for all, this one fact about the attachment sites of the cranial nerves: nerves VI, VII, and VIII—and thus a somite, branchial, and special sensory nerve—attach, in that order, at the pontomedullary sulcus. Observe this fact in Fig. 3-10. This fact plus knowing the special embryology of the olfactory and optic bulbs means that you fairly well know where all cranial nerves attach. Nerves III to V must be caudal to II, yet rostral to the pontomedullary sulcus. Nerves IX to XII must be caudal to the pontomedullary sulcus. Study Fig. 3-10 as follows: learn the labels on the left and right sides, color each set of cranial nerves with a different color, do the test frames 2-10, and then draw Fig. 3-10 from memory.

I
II
III
mesencephalon

III, IV

V

2. Cranial nerve number ________ synapses on the olfactory bulb.
3. The stalk of a diencephalic diverticulum forms cranial nerve ________.
4. The rostralmost *motor* cranial nerve is ________. It attaches to the ☐ diencephalon / ☐ mesencephalon.
5. The site of attachment of IV is not shown in Fig. 3-10 because it comes off dorsally from the mesencephalon. It is the only cranial nerve to do so. Thus, the two cranial nerves attached to the mesencephalon are ________ and ________.
6. Only one cranial nerve attaches to the lateral sides of the bulging belly of the pons, ________.

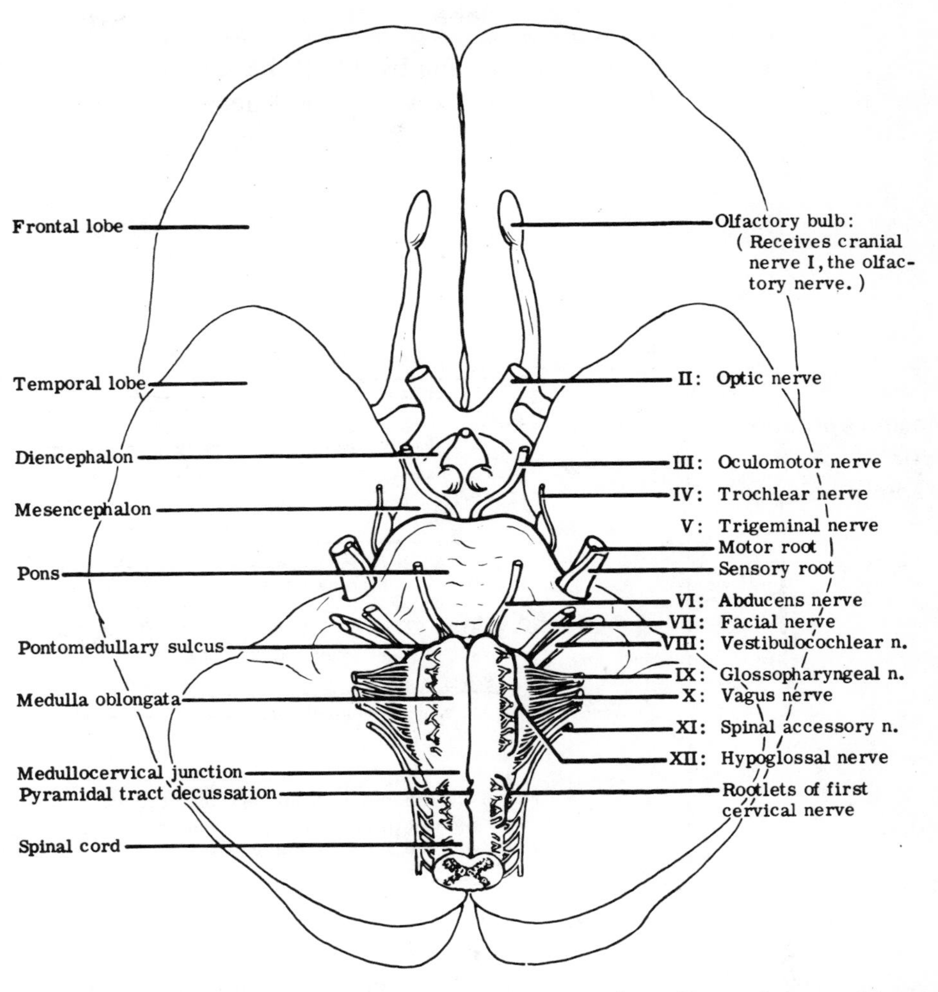

FIG. 3-10. Ventral view of the brain to show the sites of attachment of the cranial nerves. Only the attachment of cranial nerve IV, which exists from the dorsal surface of the mesencephalon, cannot be shown in this view.

VI, VII, VIII	7. The three cranial nerves attaching at the pontomedullary sulcus are ________, ________, and ________, in *ventrodorsal* order.
IX, X, XII XII	8. Three additional cranial nerves attach to the medulla: ________, ________, and ________. Of these, ________ is the most ventral.
XI	9. The only cranial nerve originating from the spinal cord is ________.

10. In Fig. 3-10, notice that cranial nerves III, VI, XII and the first cervical nerves line up along the parasagittal plane of the brainstem.

a. To emphasize this fact, use the same color as for the somite set of nerves and pencil in a line connecting C_1 with cranial nerve III.

lateral to	*b.* Discounting that IV is a maverick, attaching dorsally, we can say that the somite cranial nerves are anatomically linear with the somite spinal nerves, just as they are phylogenetically homologous. The nerves of the branchial set then all attach ☐ lateral to / ☐ medial to / ☐ in line with the somitic set.

I. Location of the cranial nerve nuclei in the caudal three brainstem units Learn Fig. 3-11. Begin by labeling the caudal three brainstem units on the left. Then color the sets of cranial nerve nuclei, using the same colors as for Fig. 3-10. After learning Fig. 3-11, try the program following it.

1. Mesencephalon
2. Pons
3. Medulla oblongata

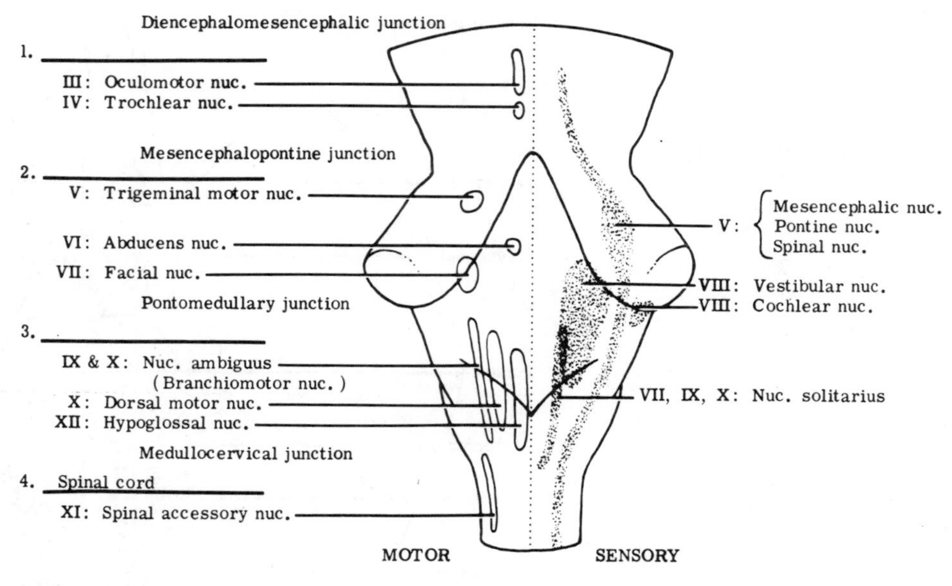

FIG. 3-11. Phantom dorsal view of the cranial nerve nuclei in the brainstem and rostral portion of the cervical cord. Cranial nerve *motor* nuclei on the left, *sensory* nuclei on the right. Fill in blanks 1 to 3 with the proper name for the subdivision of the brainstem.

J. A summary of the location of cranial nerve nuclei. In thinking out the answers to Frames 1 to 9, sort through the cranial nerves one by one, I to XII, for each question.

III, IV,

1. The cranial nerve nuclei limited to the mesencephalon are ______.

IX, X, XII,

2. The cranial nerve *motor* nuclei limited to the medulla are for cranial nerves number ______.

V (sensory)
V(sensory)
XI (motor)

3. The one cranial nerve nucleus extending from the spinal cord to the mesencephalon belongs to cranial nerve ______.
4. The two cranial nerve nuclei found in the rostral part of the cervical cord are ______ (sensory) and ______ (motor).

nucleus solitarius
IX, X

5. The sensory nucleus limited solitarily to the medulla is called nucleus ______. It serves the sensory functions of the medullary branchial nerves, ______.

V, VI, VII
vestibular
cochlear
VIII
XI

6. The cranial nerve motor nuclei limited to the pons are ______.
7. The cranial nerve sensory nuclei which straddle the pontomedullary junction are the ______ and ______ nuclei of cranial nerve ______.
8. The caudal three brainstem units contain the *motor* nuclei for all cranial nerves exclusive of ______, which originates in the spinal cord.

I, II

9. The only cranial nerves attaching to the brain rostral to the mesencephalon are ______.

III, IV, VI, XII. (Did you automatically list them in rostrocaudal sequence? — let's learn that habit.)

K. Internal relations of the cranial nerve nuclei

1. Along the parasagittal plane are the motor nuclei of cranial nerves ______, ______, ______, and ______, all members of the somitic set.

2. The somitic set of cranial nerve motor nuclei are linear with and homologous with the SE neuronal column of the spinal cord. The spinal cord SE column extends in unbroken continuity to the rostral end of the spinal cord. Why is the column of SE nuclei in the brainstem discontinuous? ______________________________

Ans: Some of the cranial nerve somites disappear and their nerves likewise disappear.

X

3. The *VE* column is represented in the medulla by the dorsal motor nucleus of nerve ______. While scattered nuclei of the VE column also occur along the more rostral part of the brainstem, they are not shown in Fig. 3-11.

lateral to

4. Notice that the branchial efferent column, like the sites of attachment of the branchial nerves to the brainstem, is ☐ medial to / ☐ lateral to / ☐ in line with the SE column. Using the appropriate color, draw a line connecting the nuclei of the branchial set in Fig. 3-11.
5. In column 1 of Table 3-6 list, in rostrocaudal sequence, the numbers of the *branchial* cranial nerves. Then complete the rest of the table.

V (trigeminal), pons.
VII (facial), pons
IX (ambiguus), medulla
X (ambiguus), medulla
XI (spinal accessory), spinal cord

TABLE 3-6. Number, Name, and Location of Branchial Efferent Nuclei

Number of cranial nerve	Name of branchial motor nucleus	Anatomic subdivision of neuraxis containing the nucleus

medial to

medial to

6. We have seen that the nuclei of the somitic cranial nerves are all ☐ medial to / ☐ lateral to / ☐ in line with the branchial set.
7. We have seen that the point of attachment of the somitic set to the brainstem is ☐ medial to / ☐ lateral to the branchial set.
8. Write a general law stating how the nuclei and sites of brainstem

attachment of the two sets of cranial motor nerves are located with respect to the midsagittal plane.

____

____

____

Ans: The somitic nuclei are all paramedian, that is, adjacent to the midsagittal plane, and the nerves attach in a paramedian line along the brainstem. The branchial nuclei are aligned more laterally and their nerves attach more laterally. (As will be shown in the next section, the actual location of the branchial nuclei in respect to the somitic nuclei is ventrolateral.)

L. Longitudinal organization of the brainstem

1. The mesencephalon, pons, and medulla, the three caudal transverse divisions of the brainstem, can be divided into three longitudinal units, a *tectum, tegmentum* and *basis.* See the labels on the left side of Fig. 3-12.

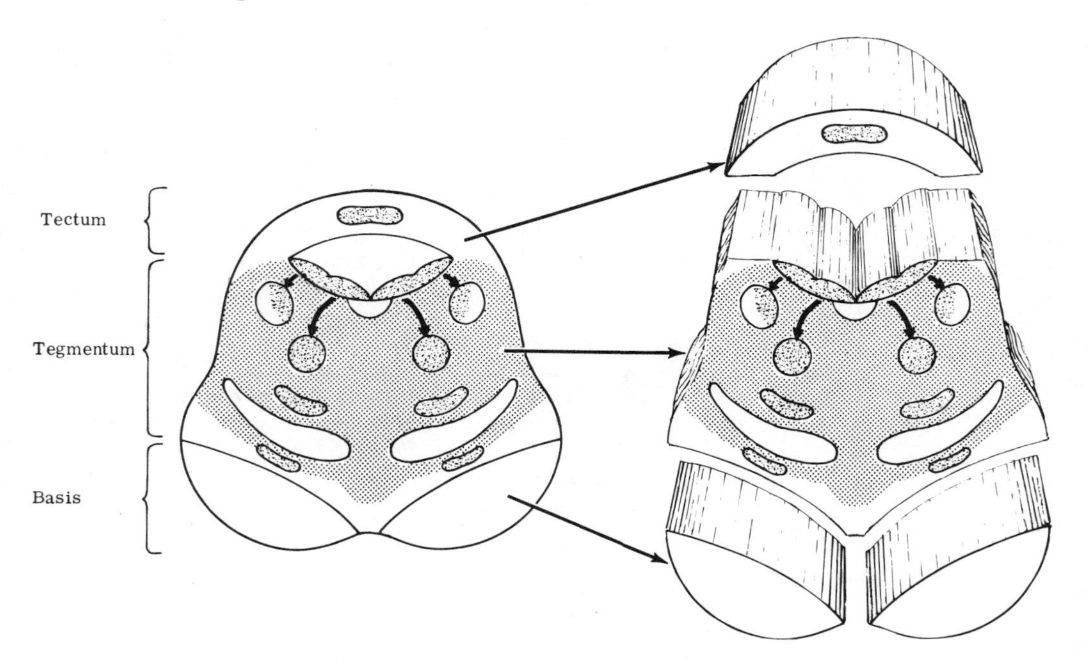

FIG. 3-12. Exploded view of a generalized cross section of the brainstem to show the three longitudinal subdivisions.

2. *The tectum (literally: roof), the roof of the brainstem*
   a. All brainstem structures dorsal to the plane of the aqueduct and fourth ventricle are included in the tectum.
   b. The tectum of the mesencephalon is the quadrigeminal plate, a coordinating center for auditory and visual reflexes.
   c. The caudal part of the tectum is the anterior and posterior medullary vela, curtains which form the immediate roof of the fourth ventricle.
   d. As we have defined the brainstem, would the cerebellar cortex and white matter form part of the tectum? ☐ Yes / ☐ No.
   e. After removal of the cerebellar cortex and deep white matter, the

☒ No

quadrigeminal

deep cerebellar nuclei remain in the tectum as the pontine homologue of the ________________ plate of the mesencephalon.

3. *The tegmentum (literally: covering), the cover of the basis*
   a. The tegmentum can be regarded as a block of tissue extending from the rostral end of the spinal cord to (and slightly into) the caudal end of the diencephalon. It consists of gray matter and tracts.
   b. The gray matter of the tegmentum:
      (1) Motor and sensory nuclei of the cranial nerves.
      (2) Reticular formation.
      (3) Supplementary motor nuclei, within or just ventral to the tegmentum: red nucleus, substantia nigra, pontine nuclei of the basis pontis, and olivary nuclei of the medulla.
   c. The tracts of the tegmentum consist of many short ascending and descending pathways, some cerebellar pathways which cut through, and the major sensory pathways to the diencephalon and cerebral cortex.
4. *The basis (literally: the bottom of anything)*
   a. The basis consists of corticofugal pathways: corticobulbar and corticospinal (pyramidal), and corticopontine tracts.
   b. An exception to the rule that the basis is white matter is in the pons, where the nuclei of the basis pontis, which receive the corticopontine tracts, swell the brainstem enormously. In the medulla, the basis is the medullary pyramids. Hence, we have a basis mesencephali, basis pontis, and basis medulli.

tectum
tegmentum
basis

5. In summary, the three longitudinal subdivisions of the mesencephalon, pons, and medulla are the ________________, ________________, and ________________.
6. The division into tectum, tegmentum, and basis does not extend into the diencephalon, which has a different embryologic origin and a different plan.

M. Internal organization of the brainstem

1. If the clinician has a sound basic concept of the general structure of the brainstem, he need not fret over local variations, which can be looked up when needed. Fig. 3-13 is a generalized cross section of the brainstem. Notice how it illustrates these general rules:
   a. The cranial nerve nuclei cluster in the dorsal half of the tegmentum, below the aqueduct or fourth ventricle. The branchial efferent nuclei are always lateral (ventrolateral) to the somitic efferent nuclei.
   b. The supplementary nuclei cluster in the ventral half of the tegmentum or encroach into the basis.
   c. The long ascending tracts, the sensory tracts to the diencephalon, run in the ventral part of the tegmentum.
   d. The long descending tracts, the corticofugal tracts, run in the basis.
   e. The cerebellar tracts cluster along the dorsolateral aspect of tectum and tegmentum.

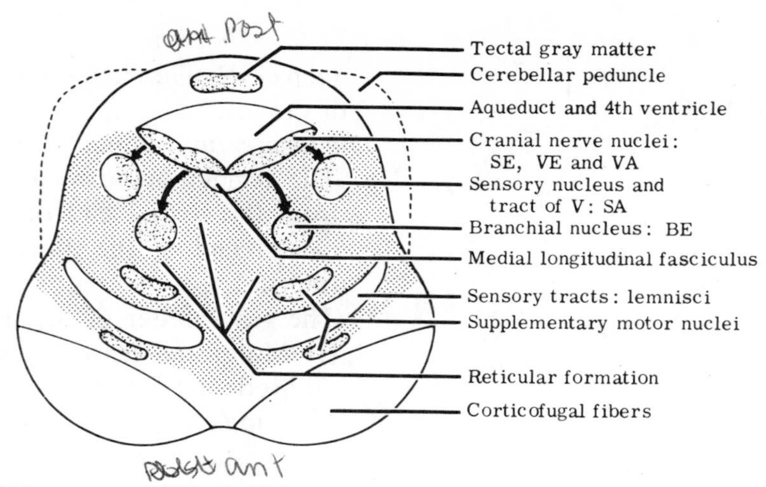

FIG. 3-13. Generalized cross section of the brainstem. Nuclei are heavily stippled, reticular formation is lightly stippled, and white matter is white. Learn this figure.

f. The reticular formation fills in the space not occupied by nuclei or tracts.

2. On scrap paper, trace the perimeter of Fig. 3-13. Then from memory draw in and label the white matter: cerebellar tracts, sensory tract of V, medial longitudinal fasciculus, sensory and corticofugal tracts. Compare your drawing with the original.
3. Trace another outline, draw the gray matter from memory, and compare with the original.
4. From memory, draw the outline of the generalized brainstem and insert and label the white and gray matter. Does yours look like the original?
5. *Functional significance of tectal and tegmental gray matter*

a. Like the spinal cord, which is little more than a reflex center, the cranial nerve nuclei with their afferent and efferent connections can carry on simple tactile and muscle stretch reflexes. The integrated activity for elaborate reflexes, such as respiration and swallowing, requires more gray matter, the reticular formation.

b. Reticular formation, sufficient to some tasks but not all, condenses into nuclei, including the supplementary motor nuclei.

c. But reticular formation and supplementary nuclei are not enough either. The tectum evolves the quadrigeminal plate and cerebellum. The quadrigeminal plate is an integrative center for reflex behaviors associated with hearing and seeing. It is a quasicortex. A cortex is a layer of gray matter on the surface of the neuraxis. Cortex always signifies a more complex, a more plastic neural activity than the simple reflexes of nuclei or the more complex reflexes of the reticular formation. In the pontine tectum, a few simple nuclei were sufficient at first to assist the evolving vestibular apparatus, but as the vestibular apparatus in particular evolved with the proprioceptive system in general, more plastic and elaborate control was necessary. The answer was a cortex, the cerebellar cortex, which smothered over and elaborated upon the roof nuclei as an integrative mechanism for proprioception.

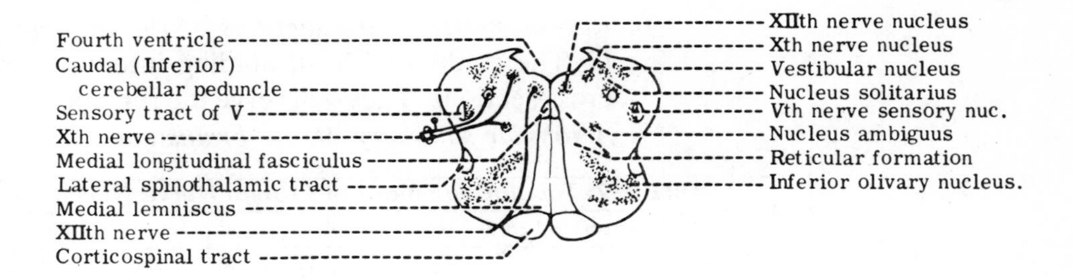

FIG. 3-14. Transverse section of medulla oblongata.

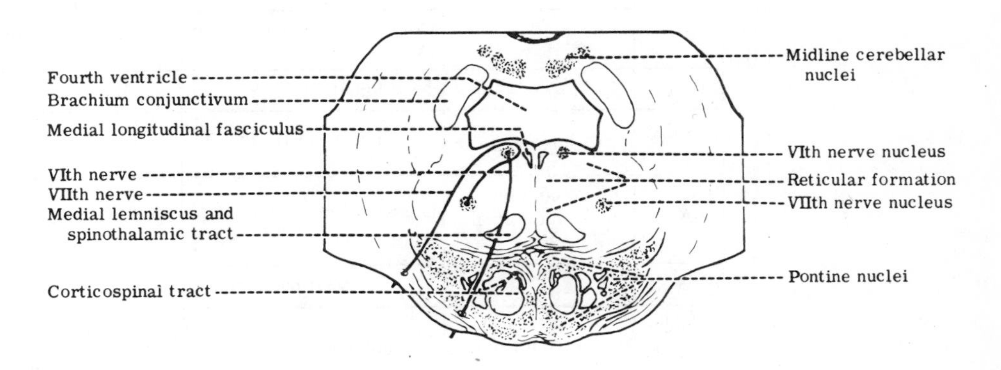

FIG. 3-15. Transverse section of pons, VIIth nerve (caudal) level.

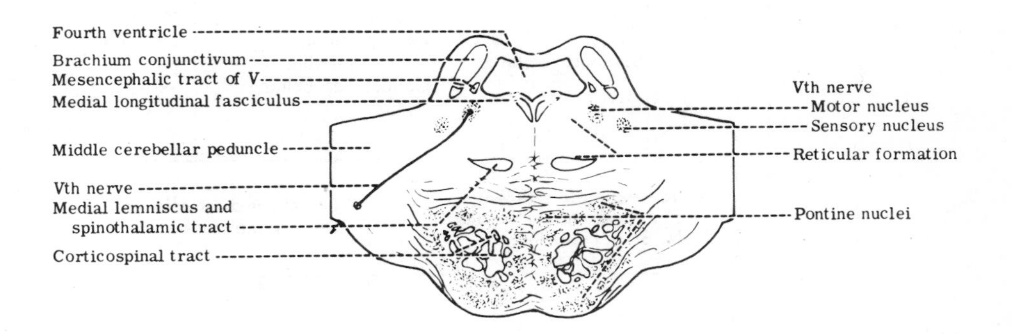

FIG. 3-16. Transverse section of pons, Vth nerve (rostral) level.

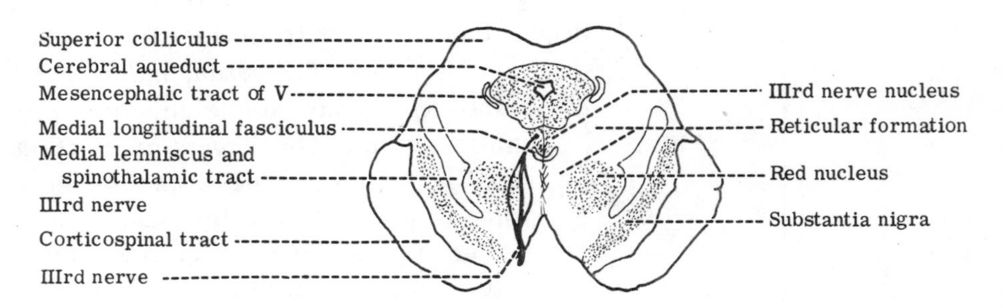

FIG. 3-17. Transverse section of mesencephalon.

6. *Representative cross-sections of the mesencephalon, pons, and medulla.* The student with an abiding interest in neurology will learn these cross-sections. They will serve the remaining students for reference.

**7. *A tabular summary of the brainstem*

TABLE 3-7. *Tabular Summary of Cranial Nerve Nuclei and Tracts of the Brainstem*

	Upper cervical cord	Medulla	Pons	Mesencephalon
Tectum	....	Roof of 4th ventricle	Roof of 4th ventricle & deep cerebellar nuclei	Quadrigeminal plate
SE	Ventral horn cells of C_1	Hypoglossal n. (XII)	Abducens n. (VI)	Oculomotor n. (III) Trochlear n. (IV)
BE	Spinal access. n. (XI)	Ambiguus n. (IX, X, XI)	Facial and trigeminal n. (VII, V).	....
VE	....	Dorsal motor n. of vagus (X)	Salivatory nucleus of VII	Pupilloconstrictor n. (III)
VA	....	N. solitarius (IX, X)	....	....
SVA (Taste)	....	N. solitarius (VII, IX, X)	....	....
SA	Dorsal column nuclei and spinal root of V	Dorsal column nuclei. Root of V	Main sensory n. of V	Mesencephalic root of V
SSA	....	Vestibular and cochlear n. (VIII)		....
Supplementary motor nuclei	Reticular formation	Reticular formation Olivary n.	Reticular formation. Pontine n. of basis pontis	Reticular formation Substantia nigra, red n.
Long tracts in transit	Corticospinal Medial longitudinal fasciculus Lat. spinothalamic Spinocerebellar Dorsal columns	Corticospinal Medial longitudinal fasciculus Lat. spinothalamic Spinocerebellar Caudal cerebellar peduncle Medial lemniscus	Corticospinal Medial longitudinal fasciculus Lat. spinothalamic Rostral and middle cerebellar peduncles Medial lemniscus	Corticospinal Medial longitudinal fasciculus Lat. spinothalamic Rostral cerebellar peduncle Medial lemniscus

SE = somatic efferent
SVA = special visceral afferent
N. or n. = nucleus
BE = branchial efferent
SA = somatic afferent
VA = visceral afferent
SSA = special somatic afferent

**N. *Some further facts about the composition of cranial nerves, for the purely curious student*

1. A tabular summary of the components of the cranial nerves is given in Table 3-8. Nerves I and II are omitted since their unique embryologic origin removes them from the category of true cranial nerves.
2. *The common plan of the branchial nerves VII, IX, and X*
   a. V and XI are as simple in composition and distribution as the somitic nerves. The accessory portion of XI quickly joins X to carry BE axons to the branchial muscles of the larynx and VE axons, probably to the thoracic or abdominal viscera. Nerves VII, IX, and X are the most complicated of the cranial nerves. They pursue radically different peripheral courses, but they all have the same components and adhere to a common plan. Hence, to learn a great deal about one of them is to learn a great deal about

all of them. As a prototype, refer to Fig. 9-6, the VIIth cranial nerve, as you study these common features of VII, IX, and X:

TABLE 3-8. Tabular Summary of Cranial Nerve Components

	Somitic (somatic) set				Branchial set					
	III	IV	VI	XII	V	VII	IX	X	XI	VIII
SE	+	+	+	+						
BE					+	+	+	+	+	
VE	+					+	+	+	+	
VA						+	+	+		
SVA						+	+	+		
SA	*+	*+	*+	*+	+	+	+	+	*+	
SSA										+

*The only SA component is presumed to be proprioceptive axons from the muscles innervated.

(1) Each conveys BE axons to striated muscle derived from a gill arch.

(2) Each conveys VE (preganglionic parasympathetic) axons to a peripheral ganglion located in or near one of the large exocrine glands of the head or to glands in mucous membranes or viscera.

(a) *VII* sends VE axons to the lacrimal glands, to the mucous glands of the nasal mucosa via the sphenophalatine ganglia, and to the submandibular and sublingual glands via the submandibular ganglia. VII does not innervate the parotid gland, through which it runs.

(b) *IX* sends VE axons to the parotid gland via the otic ganglion and to the glands of the pharyngeal mucosa.

(c) *X* sends VE axons to the glands of the pharyngeal and laryngeal mucosa and to the smooth muscle and glands of the thoracico-abdominal viscera, as far as the splenic flexure of the colon.

(3) Each conveys VA fibers from the pharyngeal mucosa. The Xth nerve also carries afferents from the thoracico-abdominal viscera.

(4) Each conveys SVA fibers for taste. VII from the anterior two-thirds of the tongue, IX from the posterior third, and X from the palatal orifice: rostrocaudal sequence.

(5) Each conveys SA fibers from the skin of the external auditory canal. The contribution of twigs from these nerves to the ear serves to emphasize the complex origin of the ear, which is formed from the branchial arches. The skin area of V on the face, and the skin twigs of VII, IX, and X, serve to emphasize that the skin of the branchial arches is rehabilitated while the skin of cephalic somites is lost.

(6) Summarize the nerve components of VII, IX, and X. ____________ ____________.

BE, VE, VA, SVA, and SA

3. Table 3-9 summarizes the peripheral distribution of nerves VII, IX, and X. Study in rostrocaudal sequence: VII, IX, and X.

TABLE 3-9. Nerve Components of Cranial Nerves VII, IX, and X and Their Peripheral Distribution

	Branchiomotor (BE)	Visceromotor (VE) (all parasympathetic)	VA	Taste (SVA)	SA
VII	To all muscles of face and facial orifices and to stapedius muscles.	To lacrimal, submandibular, and sublingual glands: all large exocrine glands of head except parotid. To nasal mucosa.	From posterior nasopharynx and soft palate.	Anterior two-thirds of tongue	Twig to ear
IX	To pharyngeal plexus for swallowing.	Parotid gland and pharyngeal mucosa.	Soft palate and upper pharynx, carotid body and sinus.	Posterior two-thirds of tongue	Twig to ear
X	To pharyngeal plexus and laryngeal muscles (via accessory branch of XI)	To glands of pharyngeal and laryngeal mucosa and to glands and smooth muscle of thoracico-abdominal viscera. Inhibitory axons to the heart	Pharynx and larynx and thoracico-abdominal viscera.	From region of epiglottis.	Twig to ear

Bibliography

Ariens Kappers, C., Huber, G., and Crosby, E.: *The Comparative Anatomy of the Nervous System of Vertebrates,* New York, The Macmillan Company, vols. 1 and 2, 1936.

Barr, M.: *The Human Nervous System,* New York, Harper & Row, 1972.

Blechschmidt, E.: *The Stages of Human Development Before Birth,* Philadelphia, W. B. Saunders Company, 1961.

Carpenter, M.: *Core Text of Neuroanatomy,* 2nd ed., Baltimore, The Williams & Wilkins Co., 1978.

Crosby, E. C., Humphrey, T., and Lauer, E.: *Correlative Anatomy of the Nervous System,* New York, The Macmillan Company, 1962.

Elliott, H.: *Textbook of Neuroanatomy,* 2nd ed., Philadelphia, J. B. Lippincott Co., 1969.

Grant, J.: *An Atlas of Anatomy,* 5th ed., Baltimore, The Williams & Wilkins Co., 1962.

Gregory, W.: *Our Face from Fish to Man,* New York, G. P. Putnam's Sons, 1929.

Krieg, W.: *Functional Neuroanatomy,* 3d ed., Evanston, Ill., Brain Books, 1966.

Noback, C. R., and Demarest, R. J.: *The Human Nervous System,* 2nd ed., New York, Blakiston Division, McGraw-Hill Book Company, 1975.

Olszewski, J., and Baxter, D.: *Cytoarchitecture of the Human Brain Stem,* Philadelphia, J. B. Lippincott Co., 1954.

Peele, T. L.: *The Neuroanatomic Basis for Clinical Neurology,* 3rd ed., New York, Blakiston Division, McGraw-Hill Book Company, 1977.

Riley, H. A.: *An Atlas of the Basal Ganglia, Brain Stem and Spinal Cord,* New York, Hafner Publishing Company, 1960.

Rucker, C. W.: History of the numbering of the cranial nerves, *Mayo Clin. Proc.,* 41:453, 1966.

Shaeffer, J. P.: *Human Anatomy,* 11th ed., New York, Blakiston Division, McGraw-Hill Book Company, 1953.

Truex, R., and Carpenter, M.: *Strong and Elwyn's Human Neuroanatomy,* 5th ed., Baltimore, The Williams & Wilkins Co., 1964.

**IV. The blood supply of the brain

A. The four major blood vessels of the brain are shown in Fig. 3-18

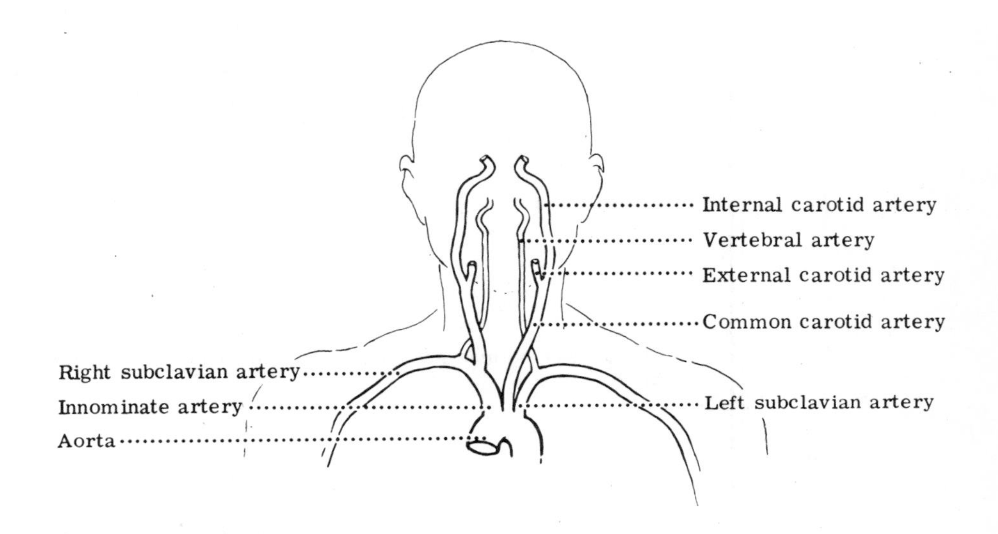

FIG. 3-18. Major arteries supplying the brain. Color them red and learn them.

B. An insect figurine to remember the arteries at the base of the brain: On scrap paper, make a drawing as described in steps 1 to 11, as related to Fig. 3-19:

1. Draw a pair of eyes (with hypertelorism).
2. Complete the facial outline, completing the circle of Willis.
3. Add a trunk and a pair of hind legs.
4. Draw four forelimbs (all insects have six legs).
5. Add antennae (feelers).
6. Put a tube in each ear and striate it (the lenticulostriate arteries).
7. Create a few irregular ribs.
8. Put on a belt.
9. Attach some feelers to his hind legs. (Feelers to the front of him and feelers to the back of him — see step 5 also.)
10. Label the arteries — see Fig. 3-20.
11. Put the brainstem in place behind (dorsal to) the arteries. See Fig. 3-21. Mentally connect the four arteries of Fig. 3-21 with those of Fig. 3-18.

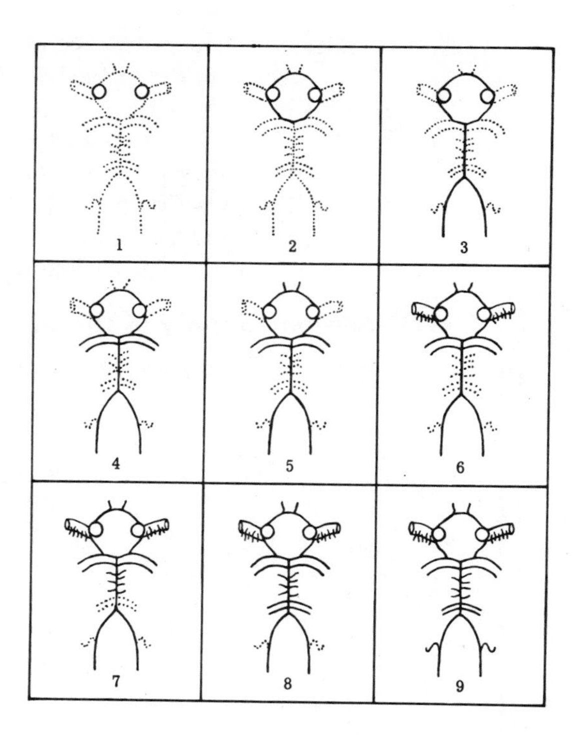

FIG. 3-19. Progressive drawing of the insect figurine which outlines the arteries at the base of the brain.

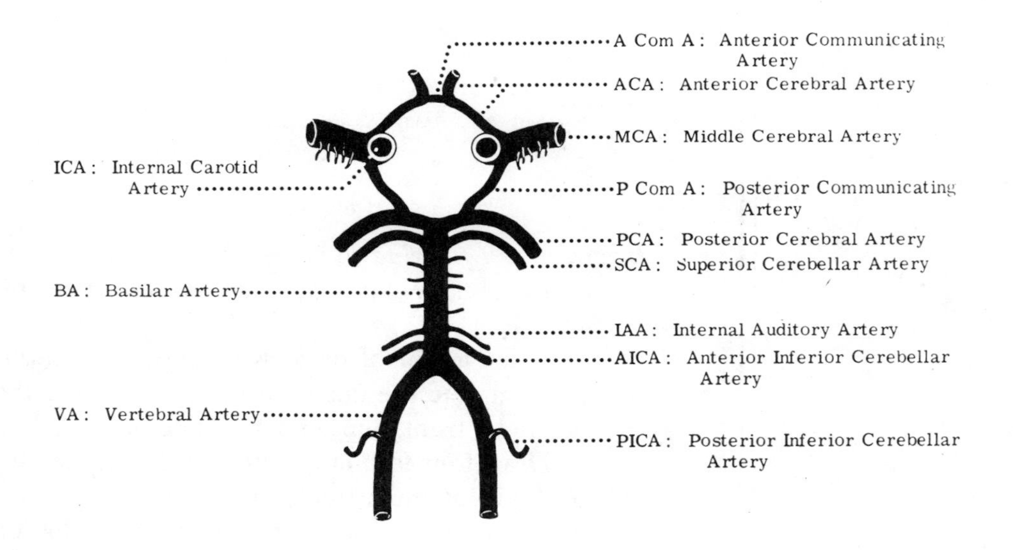

FIG. 3-20. Names of the arteries at the base of the brain.

C. A handy method for remembering the irrigation area of ACA, MCA, and PCA, the three major cerebral arteries

1. *ACA:*
   a. Put your hands together back-to-back in front of your forehead.

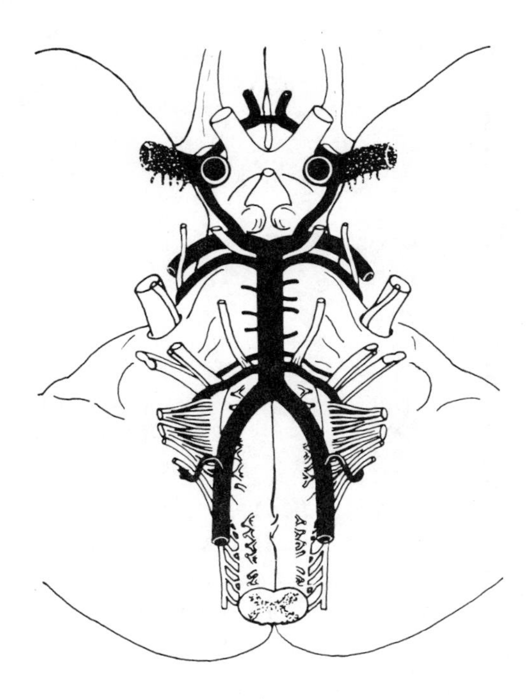

FIG. 3-21. Relation of the arteries to the base of the brain. Notice that the vertebral arteries unite at the pontomedullary junction and that the length of the basilar artery is the length of the pons.

b. Insert them into the interhemispheric fissure and pick up the cerebral hemispheres. The area you cover when picking up the hemispheres is the irrigation area of ACA. See Fig. 3-22.

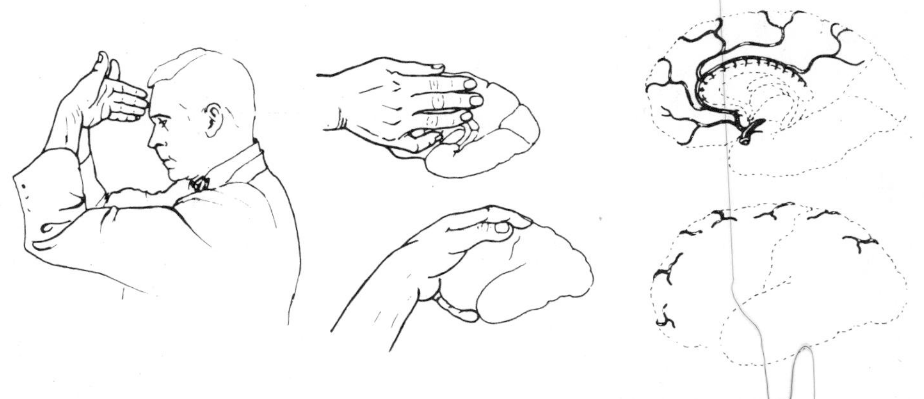

FIG. 3-22. Position of the hands for remembering the irrigation area of the anterior cerebral artery (ACA). Notice that the top hemisphere is a medial view of the right cerebral hemisphere and that it has been picked up by the right hand. Notice that the bottom hemisphere is a lateral view of the left cerebral hemisphere and that it has been picked up by the left hand. The same relationship holds for Figs. 3-23 and 3-24.

2. *MCA:*
   a. Clasp the sides of your head as though to pick up the cerebrum by squeezing on its sides.
   b. The area of the cerebrum your hands cover is the irrigation area of MCA. See Fig. 3-23.

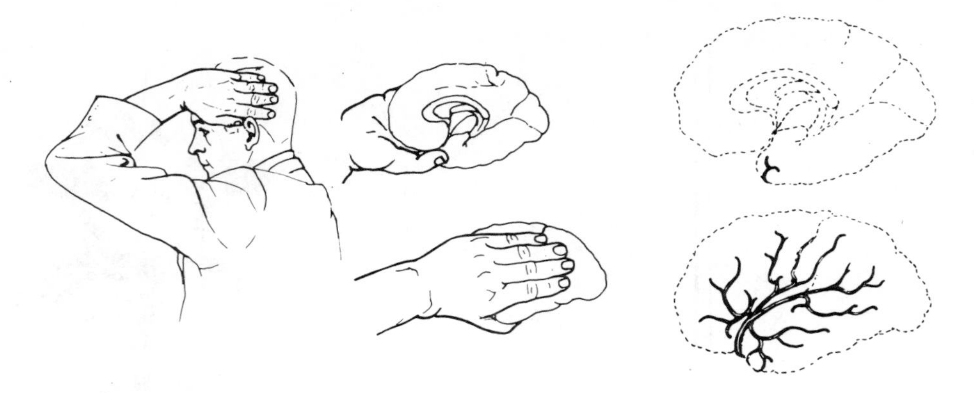

FIG. 3-23. Position of the hands for remembering the irrigation area of the middle cerebral artery (MCA).

3. *PCA:*
   a. Put your hands together, back-to-back, behind your head. You will find that your thumbs must be down, when your hands are in position.
   b. Insert your hands into the interhemispheric fissure and pick up the cerebral hemispheres. The area you cover when picking up the hemispheres is the irrigation area of PCA. See Fig. 3-24.

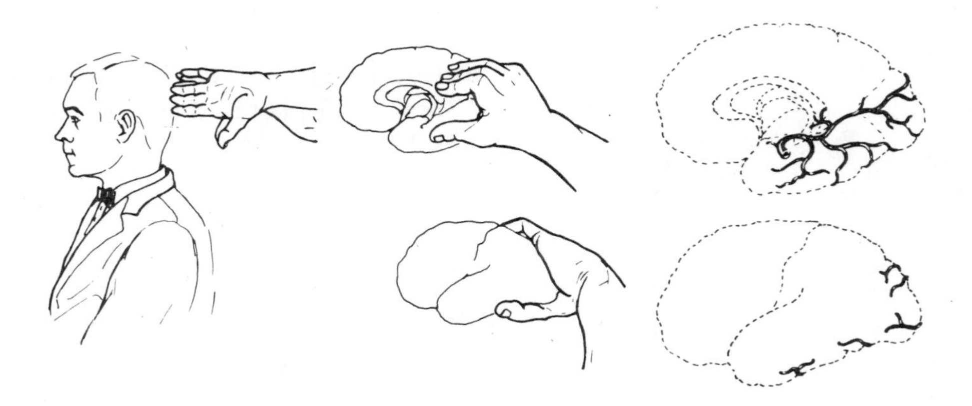

FIG. 3-24. Position of the hands for remembering the irrigation area of the posterior cerebral artery (PCA).

above
below
below

4. The secret to the use of the hand lies in remembering where to lay the thumbs. For ACA, the hands are back-to-back with the thumbs ☐ above / ☐ below. For MCA, the hands are palm-to-palm with the thumbs ☐ above / ☐ below. And for PCA, the hands are back-to-back with the thumbs ☐ above / ☐ below.
5. Trace the medial and lateral views of the hemisphere on scrap paper and, using three colors, shade the irrigation areas of the three major cerebral arteries.

D. Irrigation of the interior of the brain

1. Fig. 3-25 shows the irrigation of the interior of the cerebral hemispheres.

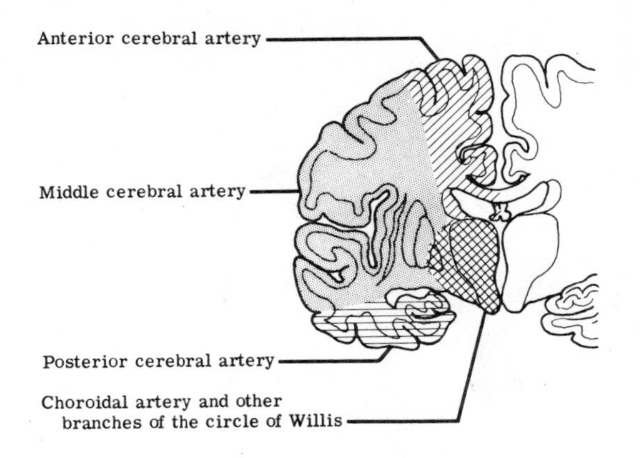

FIG. 3-25. Coronal section of the cerebrum to show the irrigation areas of the major cerebral vessels in the interior.

2. Fig. 3-26 shows the irrigation of the brainstem.

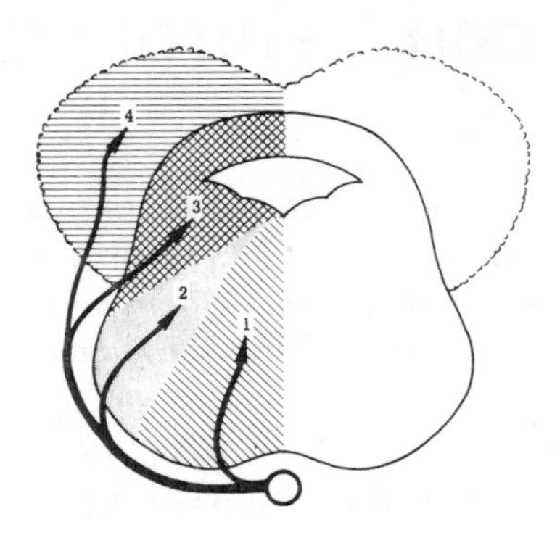

FIG. 3-26. Transverse section of the brainstem to show the irrigation areas of the branches of the vertebral-basilar system. (1) Paramedian branch of basilar artery. (2) Short circumferential branch of basilar artery. (3 and 4) Long circumferential branches of basilar artery. ACA, MCA, and PCA can all be regarded as long circumferential arteries of the cerebrum, in direct analogy to SCA, AICA, and PICA, which are long circumferential arteries of the brainstem and cerebellum.

Bibliography

Fields, W. S., and Moosy, J.: *Stroke: Diagnosis and Management: Current Procedures and Equipment,* St. Louis, Green, 1973.

Goldensohn, E. S., and Appel, S. H. (eds.): *Scientific Approaches to Clinical Neurology,* Philadelphia, Lea & Febiger, 1977.

Kaplan, H., and Ford, D.: *The Brain Vascular System,* Amsterdam, Elsevier Publishing Company, 1966.

Meyer, J. S. (ed.): *Modern Concepts of Cerebrovascular Disease,* New York, Spectrum Publications, 1975.

Stephens, R. C., and Stilwell, D. L.: *Arteries and Veins of the Human Brain,* Springfield, Charles C Thomas, Publishers, 1969.

Toole, J., and Patel, A.: *Cerebrovascular Disorders,* 2nd ed., New York, McGraw-Hill Book Company, 1977.

Vinken, P., and Bruyn, G. (eds.): *Vascular Diseases of the Nervous System,* New York, American Elsevier Publishing Company, Part I, vol 11, 1972; Part II, vol 12, 1975.

4

The Visual System: Clinical Examination for Lesions in the Peripheral Nerves and Central Pathways

Seasons return; but not to me returns
Day, or the sweet approach of even or morn,
Or sight of vernal bloom or Summer's rose,
Or flocks, or herds, or human face divine.

— John Milton (on his own blindness, at age 43)

I. Peripheral innervation of the eye muscles

A. *The extraocular muscles, the skeletal muscles of the eye*

1. The six ocular rotatory muscles are innervated by three nerves. Two nerves supply one muscle each, the muscle supplied being signaled by the name of the nerve.
2. *The IVth cranial nerve*
   a. IV is called the ______________ nerve.
   b. It innervates the ______________ muscle, the only muscle to have a trochlea.
   c. This muscle has three actions, ______________, ______________, and ______________ of the eye.
3. *The VIth cranial nerve*
   a. VI is called the ______________ nerve. It innervates the ________ ______________ muscle.
   b. The only action of this muscle is to ______________ the eye.
4. *The IIIrd cranial nerve*
   a. III is called the ______________ nerve.
   b. III innervates all ocular rotatory muscles, except for the ________ ______________ and the ________ ______________.

trochlear
superior oblique

depression
abduction, intorsion

abducens
lateral rectus
abduct

oculomotor
lateral rectus
superior oblique

medial, superior inferior recti (and) inferior oblique

c. The ocular rotatory muscles innervated by III are the ______ ______, the ______ and the ______.

d. In addition, III innervates one muscle, which elevates the eyelid, the *levator palpebrae* muscle.
   (1) If this muscle is weak, what sign will the patient show? ______ ______.

ptosis

   (2) When you watched the surface area of your upper lid in the mirror as you moved it up and down, you were testing the action of the ______ ______ muscle.

levator palpebrae

5. *The 11 ocular muscles: eight extraocular and three intraocular:* Of the eight extraocular muscles, seven are skeletal, comprising the six ocular rotatory muscles and the levator palpebrae muscle, and one—the superior tarsal muscle—is smooth. The three intraocular muscles, all smooth, consist of the pupillodilator, pupilloconstrictor, and ciliary muscles.
6. Like all skeletal muscles, the skeletal muscles of the eye act by cholinergic neuromuscular transmission. The smooth muscles of the eye, as will be emphasized, act either by cholinergic or adrenergic transmission.

B. The visceral or smooth muscles of the eye

1. The eyeball contains three intraocular muscles, all smooth muscles.
   a. The pupilloconstrictor and pupillodilator muscles of the iris adjust the diameter of the pupil.
   b. Being a circular muscle which surrounds and adjusts the diameter of a body aperture, the pupilloconstrictor muscle can be classed as a sphincter.
   c. The ciliary muscle, a ring of smooth muscle, adjusts the diameter of the lens, to alter its refracting power.
   d. Encircling the lens and acting to adjust its diameter, the ciliary muscle can likewise be classed as a sphincter.
   e. The three intraocular smooth muscles are the ______, ______ and ______ muscles.

ciliary, pupilloconstrictor pupillodilator

2. The eyelid has one extraocular smooth muscle of clinical importance, the *superior tarsal* muscle. Like levator palpebrae, it elevates the eyelid. We can say that the superior tarsal muscle adjusts the diameter of the palpebral fissure.
3. If we consider the role of smooth muscle in the bowel, bronchi, blood vessels, ureters, bladder, etc., we can generalize that the function of smooth muscle is to adjust the ______ of the apertures or passageways of the viscera.

diameter

4. Curiously, however, the one viscus whose *sole* function is to change its diameter, the heart, is striated, not smooth muscle. Striated muscle is specialized for quick, powerful contractions, smooth muscle for slow, *tonic* contractions.

levator palpebrae

superior tarsal

superior tarsal

equal

dilation (*corectasia*)

constriction (*cormiosis*)

sympathetic
parasympathetic

parasympathetic

a. Which muscle of the upper eyelid would be expected to act during voluntary activity to make quick adjustments in the diameter of the palpebral fissure? ______ ______.

b. The muscle which responds slowly, tonically, to set the diameter of the palpebral fissure is the ______ ______ muscle.

c. Of these two muscles, ☐ levator palpebrae / ☐ superior tarsal is innervated by VE axons of the autonomic nervous system.

5. Smooth muscles are sometimes paired, as the pupillo*constrictor* and pupillo*dilator* muscles of the iris. When paired in such a way, the two smooth muscles act in *tonic opposition* to each other.
6. The pupilloconstrictor muscle is *parasympathetic* and *cholinergic*; the pupillodilator is *sympathetic* and *adrenergic*. Normally sympathetic and parasympathetic tone balance each other. When the pupil is held at one size, the vector acting to increase pupillary diameter is ______ to the vector acting to decrease it.
7. If a lesion or drug interrupts one autonomic system, either sympathetic or parasympathetic, the other acts unopposed. Parasympathetic denervation results in pupillo ______ (cor ______).
8. Sympathetic denervation results in pupillo______ (cor______).
9. The ophthalmologist never presumes to be able to do a complete funduscopic examination without dilating the pupil. The pupil can be dilated by stimulating the ☐ sympathetic / ☐ parasympathetic nervous system, or by blocking the ☐ sympathetic / ☐ parasympathetic nervous system.

   a. The pupillodilator muscle is sympathetic, the pupilloconstrictor and ciliary muscles are parasympathetic. With sympathomimetic or parasympathetic blocking drugs, the pupil will dilate, and exposure to light will make the patient uncomfortable. Which drug would also interfere with lens thickening by paralyzing the ciliary muscle? ☐ sympathomimetic / ☐ parasympathetic blocking agent?

   b. Although pupillodilator drugs will inconvenience the patient, they must be used routinely for an adequate funduscopic examination. The pupils of infants respond slowly to the drugs:

   For infants: Cyclopentolate (Cyclogyl) 1% ophthalmic solution. Two drops in each eye every 15 min for three doses.
   Older patients: One or two drops in each eye. May be repeated in 15-20 min.

10. Since pupillodilation increases intraocular pressure, you should never dilate the pupils until you have checked the intraocular pressure. For accurate measurement of intraocular pressure, a tonometer is used. Tonometry is part of the routine physical examination for all adults. The most frequent cause of increased pressure is glaucoma. Two percent of all adults over 40 years of age have glaucoma.

C. The syndrome of parasympathetic paralysis of the eye

1. In accordance with the general plan of the parasympathetic system, the pupilloconstrictor pathway begins in the VE column of the brainstem, exits with a peripheral nerve, synapses in a ganglion located near the end organ, and then enters the end organ. Trace the flow of impulses through Fig. 4-1. Begin at the IIIrd nerve nucleus in the mesencephalon.

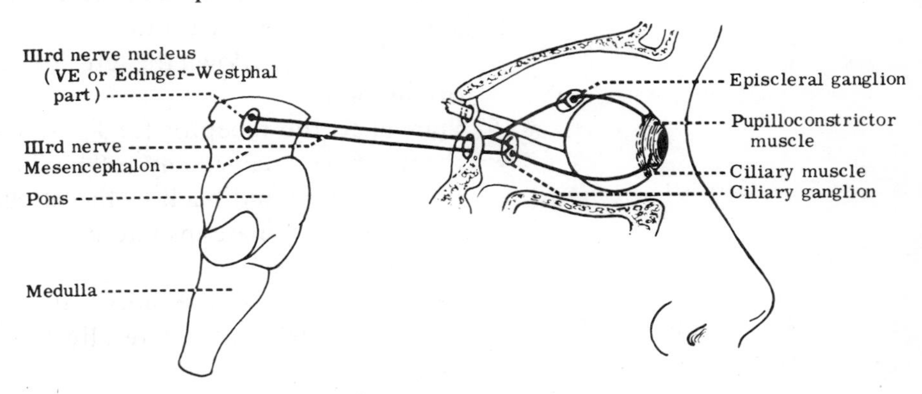

FIG. 4-1. Pathway of parasympathetic (VE) axons from the IIIrd nerve nucleus to the pupilloconstrictor muscle via the IIIrd nerve.

2. The muscles supplied by the VE axons of III are:
   a. ☐ intraocular / ☐ extraocular.
   b. ☐ smooth / ☐ skeletal.
   c. named ________________ and ________________ muscles.

intraocular
smooth
ciliary
pupilloconstrictor

3. The VE axons of III are the only efferent pathway for reflex pupiloconstriction. Since the VE and SE axons of III have a virtually synonymous nuclear origin and peripheral pathway, lesions affecting one set of axons usually affect both, but some important exceptions occur. State the clinical deficits of a patient with a pure parasympathetic IIIrd nerve syndrome: ________________
____

Corectasia and absence of reflex pupilloconstriction to light or accommodation, and blurring of near vision (ciliary muscle paralysis)

D. The pupillary light reflexes

1. For this exercise, get a flashlight and a ruler. If possible, test another person; if not use a mirror. Darken your room or go into a closet.
2. Using only slight background illumination, estimate the size of the pupil in mm ________.
3. Now shine the flashlight into one eye. Do both pupils constrict equally when you shine your light in one? ________________
____

Don't look here for the answer: do the experiment

4. The difficulty in doing this test on yourself is that when you look into the mirror, you will accommodate. You will have difficulty separating the pupillary constriction of accommodation from the pupillary constriction of light. This, in itself, is a valuable lesson: In testing for the pupillary light reflexes, the patient should be looking at a ☐ distant / ☐ close object.

distant

5. Direct constriction of the pupil in the eye stimulated by light is called the *direct light reflex.* The *consensual* constriction of the opposite pupil when light stimulates only one eye is the *consensual light reflex.*
6. Fig. 4-2 shows the pathway for the direct and *consensual light reflexes.* Learn this pathway as if your life depended on it: someone else's may sometime. Knowledge of pupillary reflexes is essential for evaluating coma, cerebrovascular disease, brain tumors, and injuries—a large segment of medical practice. Study Fig. 4-2 this way:
   a. Learn the names down the left side. Those on the right are for general orientation.
   b. Start at R, the receptor for light. We will always start at the receptor when we analyze any reflex. Trace the path of impulses through the brainstem and back to the effector muscles.
   c. Notice the alternate ipsilateral-contralateral course of axons through the optic chiasm.
   d. Notice that once the nerve impulses reach the mesencephalon, they are distributed bilaterally to the VE nucleus of III (Edinger-Westphal nucleus) and back out over both IIIrd nerves. Hence light stimulation in one eye will cause both pupils to contract equally. The consensual pupillary constriction equals the direct.
   e. Notice that according to the general plan of the parasympathetic system, the ganglion of synapse of the VE axon is near the end organ, the ciliary and pupilloconstrictor muscles.

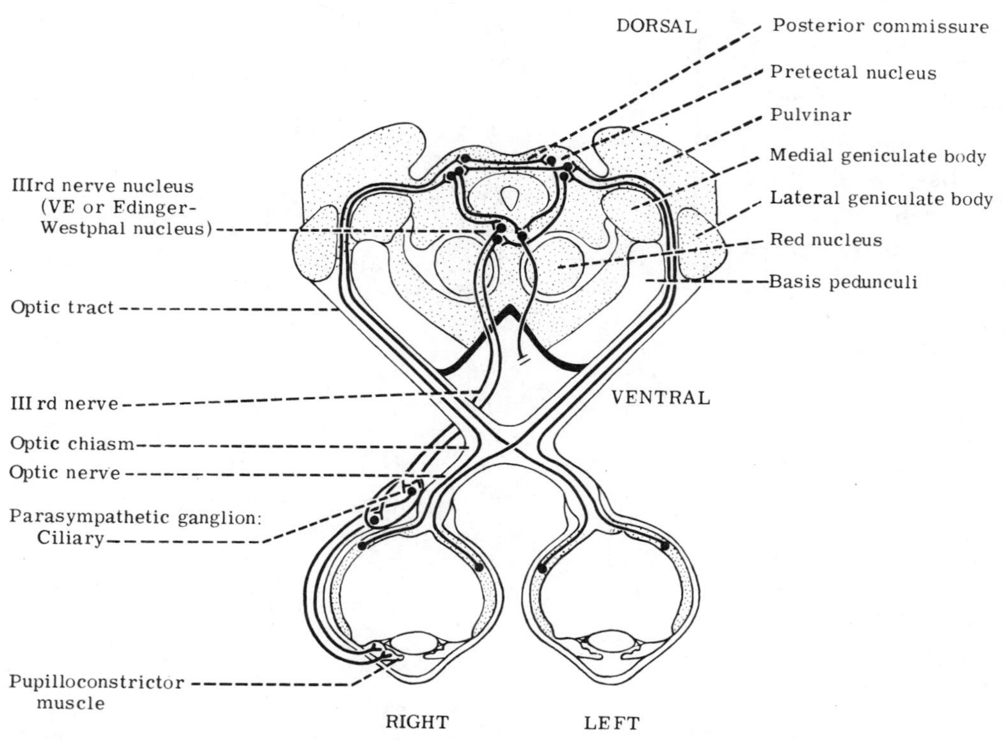

FIG. 4-2. Diagram of afferent (optic nerve) and efferent (IIIrd nerve) pathway for pupilloconstriction. R stands for the receptor which, in this case, is the retina. The mesencephalon has been transected through its rostral part, encroaching on the geniculate bodies and pulvinar, nuclei of the diencephalon. Learn this diagram. *(Adapted from E. Crosby, T. Humphrey, and E. Lauer: Correlative Anatomy of the Nervous System, New York, Macmillan Company, 1962.)*

optic

mesencephalon

ganglion

left optic nerve

☑ c.

See next frame

7. The afferent limb of the pupillary light reflex consists of the __________ nerve and tract.
8. The IIIrd nerve nucleus is located in the ☐ mesencephalon / ☐ pons / ☐ medulla.
9. As is typical of the parasympathetic system, the VE axons of III synapse in a peripheral __________________ located near the muscle to be innervated.
10. As is typical of reflex arcs, the pupillary reflex arc has a *receptor, afferent limb, central nuclear synapse(s),* an *efferent limb,* and an *effector.* Can you name all of them? If not, trudge back to Fig. 4-2.
11. On scrap paper draw the axonal pathways for the pupillary light reflex.
12. If a patient has no direct light reflex in the left eye, but has a consensual light reflex on the left when the right eye is illuminated, the lesion is in the ☐ right optic tract / ☐ left IIIrd nerve / ☐ left optic nerve.
13. *Analyze this patient:* He was admitted to the hospital because of hypertension. You examine him a few hours after the initial examination by the intern. The patient has had no visual complaints, and the intern recorded normal eyes. You find a dilated right pupil, but no ptosis, heterotropia, fundus lesions, loss of vision, or other ocular signs. He has no direct or consensual pupillary light reflex on the right, and no pupilloconstriction in accommodation. The direct and consensual response of the left pupil to light is normal and it constricts during accommodation. The best inference is:
    a. ☐ The patient is blind in the right eye and has a right IIIrd nerve lesion.
    b. ☐ The patient has an intact right optic nerve, but has complete interruption of the right IIIrd nerve.
    c. ☐ The patient has had eyedrops placed in the right eye to dilate the pupil.
14. **Answer:** *a* is excluded because the patient is not blind and has a consensual reflex on the *left*, proving that the afferent pathway, the optic nerve, from the right retina is intact, *b* is excluded because of no ptosis or ocular malalignment; *c* is all that is left. The reason for this frame is that the commonest cause of dilated, nonreactive pupils (in medical student practice in teaching hospitals) is that the intern or resident has used – properly – eyedrops to dilate the pupil for an adequate funduscopic examination. The intern erred however in dilating only one pupil. The more general implication of the frame is that in "thinking through" a reflex arc, you must include both receptor *and* effector as possible sites of mischief. And the final lesson – always record on the chart that the pupils have been dilated.
15. This next patient is somnolent because of a head injury, but he is arousable. His left eye is turned down and out and does not turn on command although the other eye moves on command. When the patient attempts to look to the right and down, the left eye intorts strongly, but remains turned down and out. His left pupil is dilated

	and fixed (nonreactive) to light or in accommodation. No eye drops were used. The right pupil shows a direct and a consensual response to light and reacts normally in accomodation. This patient most likely has a lesion of his: ☐ left optic nerve / ☐ right optic nerve / ☐ left IVth nerve only / ☐ left IIIrd nerve / ☐ the ocular findings cannot be explained by a single nerve lesion.
left IIIrd nerve	
	16. Because of the importance of pupillary signs, corectatic (mydriatic) drugs should not be used in patients with impaired consciousness.
glaucoma and impaired consciousness	17. Name two contraindications to pupillodilator drugs: ______________

18. *Abnormal pupillary responses to light and accommodation*
   a. Two important syndromes of abnormal or dissociated pupillary response to light and accommodation are the Argyll Robertson pupil (Douglas Argyll Robertson, 1837-1909) and Adie's pupil (William Adie, 1886-1935). I do not consider it necessary to memorize the distinction between these syndromes; hence, they are presented in Table 4-1 for reference only.
   b. What you must know is how to recognize abnormal pupillary responses and be able to consult a reference for the implication. The basic issue is compulsive thoroughness in the examination. After reading through Table 4-1, you will see why you must routinely test pupillary constriction to light *and* in accommodation.

TABLE 4-1. Differential Diagnosis of Argyll Robertson and Adie's Pupils

Characteristic	Argyll Robertson pupil	Adie's myotonic pupil
Laterality	Usually bilateral	Usually unilateral (aniscocoria)
Size	Cormiosis	Mild corectasia
Pupillary outline	Irregular	Regular (normal circle)
Response to light	None (neither direct nor consensual).	Very slow direct and consensual response and remains myotonically contracted after light is removed.
Response to dark	No pupillodilation	Slow pupillodilation, with delay in constriction on reexposure to light.
Response to accommodation	Constricts	Constricts very slowly and remains myotonically constricted after accommodation is relaxed.
Response to mydriatics	Poor or none	Responds normally.
Systemic features.	Virtually pathognomonic of syphilis. If the patient has tabes dorsalis, his muscle stretch reflexes will be absent.	Benign disorder, often associated with absent muscle stretch reflexes — "Adie's syndrome."

E. The syndrome of sympathetic paralysis of the eye and face (Bernard-Horner; or Horner's syndrome)

1. As is typical of the sympathetic system, the *central* pathway begins in the hypothalamus. It sends axons to the VE column of the spinal cord.

2. As is typical of the sympathetic system, the *peripheral* pathway begins in the VE column of the spinal cord. The VE column extends from T_1 to L_{2-3}. Mnemonic: T_1-L_{2-3}. The primary VE axons exit with a spinal nerve to synapse in one of the ganglia of the paravertebral chain. The secondary axons, from the paravertebral ganglion, then hitchhike along blood vessels or nerves to their effectors. Trace a sympathetic nerve impulse to the eye in Fig. 4-3, starting at the hypothalamus.

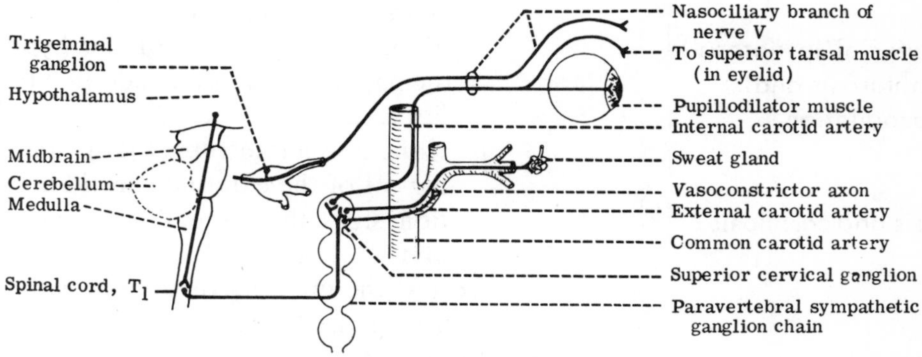

Trigeminal ganglion
Hypothalamus
Midbrain
Cerebellum
Medulla
Spinal cord, T_1
Nasociliary branch of nerve V
To superior tarsal muscle (in eyelid)
Pupillodilator muscle
Internal carotid artery
Sweat gland
Vasoconstrictor axon
External carotid artery
Common carotid artery
Superior cervical ganglion
Paravertebral sympathetic ganglion chain

FIG. 4-3. Diagram of sympathetic pathway from the hypothalamus (part of the diencephalon) to the pupillodilator and superior tarsal muscles, sweat glands of the face, and the smooth muscle of the carotid arteries.

3. A fundamental difference in the anatomy of the sympathetic and parasympathetic systems is the location of the ganglion for synapse of the primary VE axon.
   a. The ganglia of the sympathetic nervous system are located ________________.

in the paravertebral chain

   b. By contrast, the ganglia of the parasympathetic nervous system are located ________________.

in or near the end organ to be innervated

4. The ocular muscles innervated by sympathetic axons are ________________.

superior tarsal and pupillodilator

5. The carotid sympathetic plexus provides vasoconstrictor control for the carotid system and innervates the sweat glands of the face.
6. From the anatomy of sympathetic innervation of the face, list the signs you would expect to see in a patient who had a stab wound in the neck, interrupting the cervical sympathetic chain. To compile your list, run down the right-hand labels of Fig. 4-3. ________________

cormiosis, ptosis, anhidrosis (lack of sweating), and vasodilation

7. These four features of sympathetic facial denervation: ________, ________, ________, ________ constitute the Bernard-Horner syndrome.

cormiosis, ptosis, anhidrosis, and vasodilation

Note: Enopthalmos is said to be part of this syndrome. In man this sign is inconstant and more apparent, because of ptosis, than real.

8. Explain why miosis occurs after sympathetic denervation of the eye: ________________

Ans: the pupillodilator muscle is in tonic opposition to the pupilloconstrictor muscle. When the pupillodilator muscle is paralyzed, the pupilloconstrictor muscle acts unopposed.

9. After sympathetic paralysis, the miotic pupil will constrict further in response to light or accommodation, because then the muscle is given a "maximal" rather than a "tonic" stimulus.
10. The number of signs of sympathetic facial denervation vary depending on the location of the lesion along the sympathetic pathway:
    a. If the lesion interrupts the sympathetic pathway *proximal* to the carotid artery, between the hypothalamus and the carotid artery, the patient will show, in addition to ptosis and cormiosis, __________ __________ and __________.
    b. If the lesion interrupts the sympathetic pathway *distal* to the branching off of the external carotid artery, the only sympathetic denervation signs the patient will show are __________ and __________.
11. To test the integrity of the sympathetic pathway to the eye, pinch the skin over the face or neck firmly for 5 sec. Both pupils should dilate briskly—the *spinociliary* (*ciliospinal*) reflex. Do the test in subdued light and with the patient looking in the distance to avoid the pupilloconstricting effect of the light and accommodation reflexes.

hemifacial (ipsilateral) anhidrosis and vasodilation

ptosis and cormiosis

Bibliography

Adie, W.: Tonic pupils and absent tendon reflexes: A benign disorder sui generis; its complete and incomplete forms, *Brain,* 55:98–113, 1932.

Beard, C.: Ptosis, 2nd ed., St. Louis, C. V. Mosby and Co., 1976.

Green W., Hacket, E., and Schlezinger, N.: Neuro-ophthalmologic evaluation of oculomotor nerve paralysis, *Arch. Ophthalmol.,* 72:154-167, 1964.

Hollenhorst, R.: The pupil in neurologic diagnosis. *Med. Clin. N. Am.,* 52:871-884, 1968.

Lucy, D., Van Allen, M., and Thompson, H.: Holmes-Adie syndrome with segmental hypohidrosis, *Neurology,* 17:763–769, 1967.

Reeves, A., and Posner, J.: The ciliospinal response in man, *Neurology,* 19: 1145–1152, 1969.

Zinn, K.: *The Pupil,* Springfield, Charles C Thomas, 1972.

F. The differential diagnosis of ptosis

1. The muscles which elevate the eyelid are:
    a. A smooth muscle called the __________ muscle innervated by the __________ nervous system.
    b. A skeletal muscle called the __________ __________ muscle, innervated by the __________ nerve.
2. The rise and fall of the eyelid on volitional vertical eye movements is caused by the ☐ superior tarsal / ☐ levator palpebrae muscle.
3. Since either a IIIrd nerve lesion or a sympathetic lesion may cause ptosis, it is wise to be able to distinguish the two. Complete Table 4-2 by placing a + sign in column 2 *or* 3.

superior tarsal
sympathetic

levator palpebrae
III

levator palpebrae

III	Symp.
	+
+	
	+
+	
	+
+	

TABLE 4-2. Differential Diagnosis of IIIrd Nerve and Sympathetic Ptosis

1	2	3
Feature	Present with IIIrd nerve lesion	Present with sympathetic lesion
Cormiosis		
Corectasia		
Reaction to light and accommodation		
Usually have heterotropia		
Elevation of eyelid on upward gaze		
Normal sweating		

4. *The differential causes of ptosis*
   a. Sometimes ptosis is neither the result of a IIIrd nerve lesion nor the result of a sympathetic denervation. The IIIrd nerve has a neurohumoral transmitter, acetylcholine. In myasthenia gravis, levator palpebrae weakness results from defective impulse transmission at the neuromyal junction. Ptosis from nerve or neurohumoral transmission lesions is called *neuropathic* ptosis. Ptosis may occur in muscle diseases such as dystrophy, *myopathic* ptosis. Sometimes ptosis is congenital and may or may not be associated with other anomalies. After injury or inflammation, ptosis may be caused by lid edema.
   b. The point is this. In analyzing ptosis, you must "think through" the possible lesion sites and integrate the sign with other physical signs and the history. The lesion may be:
   (1) *Central:* at the hypothalamus, brainstem, or spinal cord.
   (2) *Peripheral:* along the course of the IIIrd or sympathetic nerves.
   (3) *Neuromyal:* at the nerve-muscle junction.
   (4) *Local:* congenital, inflammatory, or traumatic.
   c. Thus ptosis is not simply one thing or another: it is a puzzle to be solved. The function of any sign is to generate the differential diagnostic possibilities in the mind of the physician.
5. The 34-year-old woman in Fig. 4-4*A* suddenly noticed double vision. The patient in Fig. 4-4*A* was unable to adduct, elevate, or depress her right eye, but it did intort when she attempted to look down and to the left. The right eyelid did not elevate on volitional upward gaze. The right pupil neither reacted directly nor consensually to light. The left pupil did react directly and consensually. All other neurologic functions were intact. These findings indicate a lesion affecting the ________________.

   right IIIrd nerve

   Cerebral angiograms showed an aneurysm of the right posterior communicating artery, which had compressed the IIIrd nerve after its exit from the midbrain.
6. The 21-year-old woman in Fig. 4-4*B* complained of deep pain behind her left eye for several months. For some weeks her left eyelid had

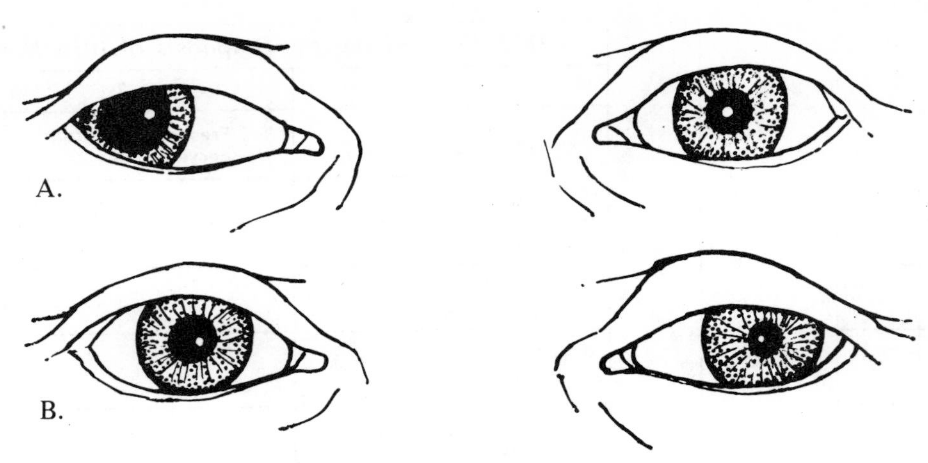

FIG. 4-4. Two patients with ocular abnormalities. Describe and diagnose them.

drooped. Examination showed only ptosis and miosis. All other neurologic findings remained intact. At her doctor's request, the patient brought in old facial photographs which proved that the ptosis was new. Thus a lesion had recently interrupted the ______________________ ______________________ to her eye. Because she had only ptosis and miosis without hemifacial anhidrosis, the lesion must have affected the pathway distal to origin of the ______________________ ______________________ artery.

sympathetic pathway

external carotid

Normal eye movements and the absence of exophthalmos tend to exclude a lesion in the orbit. The pain location and the neurologic findings implicated a lesion at the base of the skull. Inspection of the nasopharynx disclosed a suspicious mass. Radiographs of the skull base showed bony erosion. A biopsy of the mass disclosed a nasopharyngeal carcinoma infiltrating the base of the skull. It had encircled the internal carotid artery.

II. The visual fields

The visual field is . . . "an island of vision surrounded by a sea of blindness."

—Harry Traquair

A. The normal visual fields

1. Close one eye and stare fixedly straight ahead. The entire area of vision is called the *visual field.*
2. *Try this experiment*
   a. Position yourself a meter from a long row of books or get close to a short row, so that the books extend beyond the perimeter of your visual fields. Take great pains to stare fixedly at one book title, without moving your eyes at all. Can you read more than one book title? ______________________.

   If you can, you shifted fixation. Try again.

   b. The central area of sharpest visual acuity is called the *central* field. The experiment showed how small it is.
3. Now fixate on the same book. Make sure you position yourself so that the row of books extends to the peripheral limit of your field. While staring at a book directly in front of you, try to determine the color of the most distant book you can see. After trying to determine the color, shift your gaze to look straight at the book. How does the

color of the book differ when seen in your central field of vision as contrasted to its color when seen in the peripheral field? ________________

________________.

Ans: Peripherally, the book is drab, nearly colorless. With central vision it immediately becomes bright and vivid.

Visual acuity and color are functions of the central fields.

4. What do you conclude about the relation of visual acuity and color vision to the peripheral and central fields of vision? ________________

____

____

B. Anatomic basis of central and peripheral vision

1. The receptors for the central fields are the *cone* neurons of the retina. You can remember this by the mnemonic of the 5 C's: the *c*ones mediate *c*olor and a*c*uity for the *c*entral fields and are located around the fovea *c*entralis, but it is easier just to repeat the experiment. The cones are most efficient in bright light.
2. The receptors for the *peripheral* fields are the *rod* neurons of the retina. The rods are efficient for detecting form and movement, even in dim light, but they are poor for color and acuity.

cones

peripheral

cones

peripheral
rods

acuity and color vision

3. The □ cones/ □ rods tend to cluster around the fovea centralis of the macula.
4. In the retina, the rods are □ central to/ □ peripheral to the cones.
5. If a patient complained of decreasing visual acuity and had no opacities such as a cataract, you would suspect a lesion of the □ cones/ □ rods in the retina or in their axonal pathway to the cerebrum.
6. If the patient complained of inability to see in dim light, but acuity was preserved, you would expect a lesion of the □ central/ □ peripheral part of the retina which contains the □ rods/ □ cones.
7. What are the two outstanding characteristics of central vision?

____

C. Clinical testing of central vision. Acuity is tested at the bedside by having the patient read fine print, held at a distance. For a small child or mentally defective patient, use a large *E* printed on a card and have him point in the direction of the bars as you rotate the card. Test the eyes separately. If the patient is partially blind, test the ability to count the number of fingers held up at various distances. If the visual loss is so severe that the patient cannot see fingers, find out whether light perception remains. That is to say, push the analysis to the limit.

D. Clinical testing of peripheral vision by confrontation

1. Fixate straight ahead with one eye. Close or cover the other eye. Extend the arm ipsilateral to the fixating eye straight out to the side, and point your index finger up. Now, keeping the elbow extended, rotate the arm forward. The point at which you first see the finger defines the perimeter of your visual field.
2. Repeat the foregoing experiment, fixating with one eye and covering or closing the other. This time use the arm contralateral to the fixating

Yes

Eyebrow (or lid, if ptotic)

eye, and rotate the finger forward until it just becomes visible. Did you have to move it farther forward than the ipsilateral arm? □ Yes/ □ No.

3. Ostensibly the nose would seem to limit the nasal part of the visual field. Developmentally and phylogenetically this may be true. Apparently, however, the extent of the retina limits the nasal field (Tate and Lynn, 1977).
4. To locate the vertical perimeters of the visual field, fixate straight ahead with one eye, while bringing your index finger down from above and, next, up from below. What structure limits the height of the visual field? ______________
5. If the lid is ptotic, it should be held up when you test the patient's visual fields.
6. Learn the nomenclature of the visual fields in Fig. 4-5.

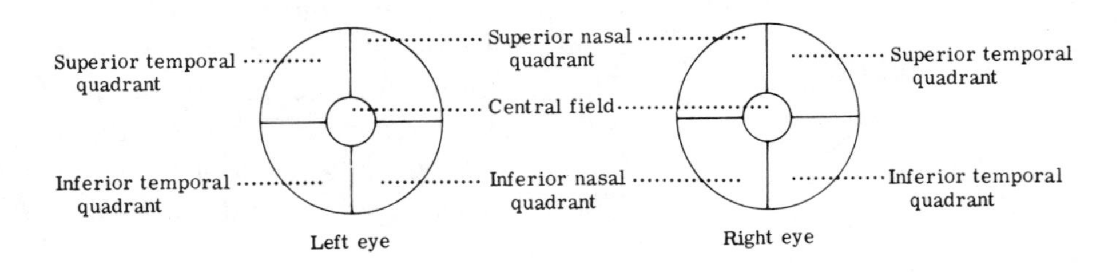

FIG. 4-5. Nomenclature of the normal visual fields.

E. Technique for confrontation testing of visual fields. See Fig. 4-6.

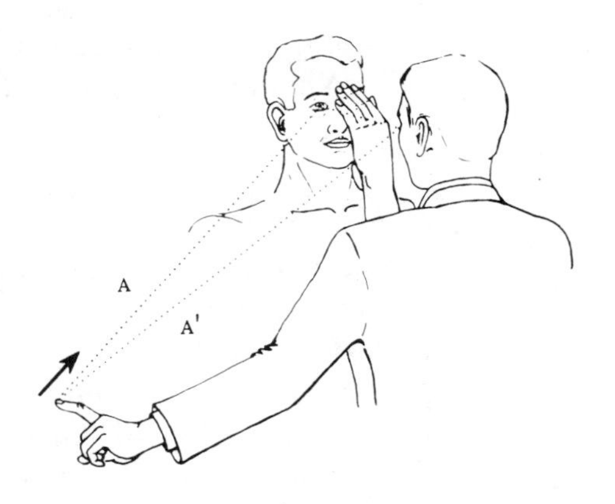

FIG. 4-6. Position of doctor and patient for testing the visual fields by confrontation.

1. Station yourself directly in front of the patient to confront him at a distance of about 50 cm. Start with your left eye directly in line with the patient's right eye, eye to eye but not breath to breath. The patient covers his left eye with his hand. Hold up your index finger just outside your own peripheral field, in the inferior quadrant. It is held equidistant between your eye and the patient's; as shown in Fig. 4-6, A = A'. Wiggle the finger slowly and move it toward the central field. The patient signifies when he first sees the finger wig-

gling. Test all quadrants of each eye separately, starting at the limit of your own vision. *You titrate the patient's field against your own.*

2. *Technical pointers*
   a. *Point 1.* Get yourself and the patient in the proper position. Both of you should be comfortable.
   b. *Point 2.* Establish communication with the patient so that he knows what to do. The best instructions are: "I want you to look directly into my eye. Don't look away. Now I want to find out what you can see out of the corner of your eye. Say, 'now' when you see my finger moving."
3. Confrontation is suitable for detecting large erosions of the island of vision by the sea of blindness. If a defect in the visual field is detected or an ocular or cerebral lesion suspected, the patient should be further tested with a *tangent screen*, to be discussed later.
4. Practice confrontation testing of the visual fields, using a normal subject.

F. Nomenclature of visual field defects

quadrantanopia

1. Visual field defects tend to fall into patterns of one-quarter or one-half of the visual fields. See Fig. 4-7*A*. Blindness in one-quarter of a field is called *quadrantanopia* (literally: quadrans =1/4; an = without; opia = vision). Since the superior temporal quadrant in Fig. 4-7*A* is completely blind, the full name is *complete left superior temporal* __________________.

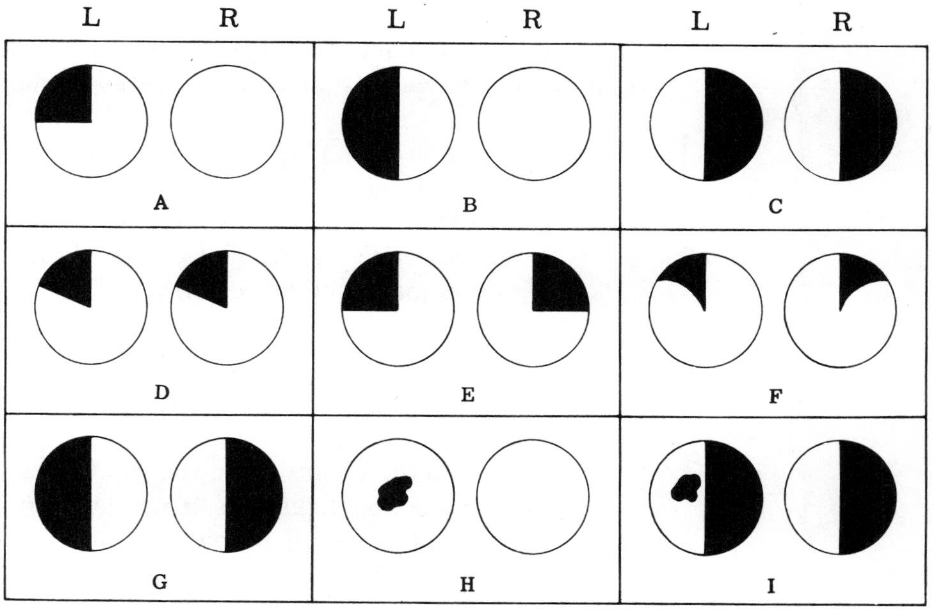

L R	L R	L R
A	B	C
D	E	F
G	H	I

FIG. 4-7. Patterns of visual field defects. The darkened area is the area of blindness. The left eye of the patient is to the reader's left. Imagine that you are looking through the patient's eyes.

hemianopia

2. Blindness in one-half of a field, or a *hemi* defect, as in Fig. 4-7*B*, would be called __________________*anopia.* The complete name for the field defect is complete temporal hemianopia of the left eye.

complete right homonymous hemianopia

3. When corresponding quadrants or halves of the fields, e.g., the right halves, are affected, the defect is termed *homonymous*, and it is described as *right* or *left*. What is the complete name for the field defect in Fig. 4-7*C*?
____

right
left

4. The terms *homonymous* or *corresponding* as applied to visual field defects, thus, mean that the defect corresponds to the way that visual space is represented by the retinal and visual images during binocular vision. Refer to Fig. 4-8. When the patient with a complete right homonymous hemianopia looks straight ahead, he would be blind in the ☐ right/ ☐ left half of space and see in the ☐ right/ ☐ left half.

incomplete left superior homonymous quadrantanopia

5. Name the defect in Fig. 4-7*D*. _______________

quadrantanopia

6. *Noncorresponding* field defects are sometimes called *heteronymous* to contrast them with homonymous. See Fig. 4-7*E*. It is simpler to describe them directly. Thus, the defect in Fig. 4-7*E* would be called complete superior bitemporal _______________.

incomplete superior bitemporal quadrantanopia

7. Fig. 4-7*F* is called _______________

complete bitemporal hemianopia

8. In Fig. 4-7*G* the defect is called _______________
9. The field defects of Figs. 4-7*E, F,* and *G* would not be homonymous because _______________
____

Ans: the defect is not in corresponding parts of the fields according to the way the right and left halves of space are recorded by the visual system (as in Fig. 4-7C).

central

10. An irregular field defect, not approximating a quadrantic defect is called a *scotoma*. A scotoma may be *central, paracentral* or *peripheral*. See Fig. 4-7*H*. The defect would be called a _______________ scotoma of the left eye.

G. *Anatomic basis of visual field defects.* Use these instructions to study Fig. 4-8
   1. Learn the names down the right side.
   2. Notice that light rays from the *right half* of space fall on the *nasal* side of the *right* retina, and on the *temporal* side of the *left* retina.
   3. At the chiasm, axons from the *nasal* half of the right retina decussate to travel through the optic tract with the axons from the *temporal* half of the left retina.
   4. The retinal axons synapse on neurons of the lateral geniculate body, a thalamic nucleus which relays sensory impulses to the cerebral cortex. The thalamus is part of the diencephalon. The tract of axons formed by geniculate body neurons is called the *optic radiation* or *geniculocalcarine tract.*

5. Using a colored pencil, draw in the retinal pathway from the *nasal* half of the left retina and *temporal* half of the right. Include the geniculate body synapse. Make sure you draw a mirror image of the corresponding axons already in the drawing.
6. Bars are drawn across the optic pathways at A to G to simulate lesions at various sites. At the left, label the field defects resulting from the lesions.
7. Note that lesions of the *superior* fibers, F, of the geniculocalcarine tract cause contralateral inferior homonymous quadrantanopia.
8. Practice drawing the entire optic pathway from the retina to the occipital cortex.

A Complete blindness, L eye.
B Complete bitemporal hemianopia
C Complete nasal hemianopia, L eye
D Complete R homonymous hemianopia
E Complete R superior homonymous quadrantanopia
F Complete R inferior homonymous quadrantanopia
G Complete R homonymous hemianopia

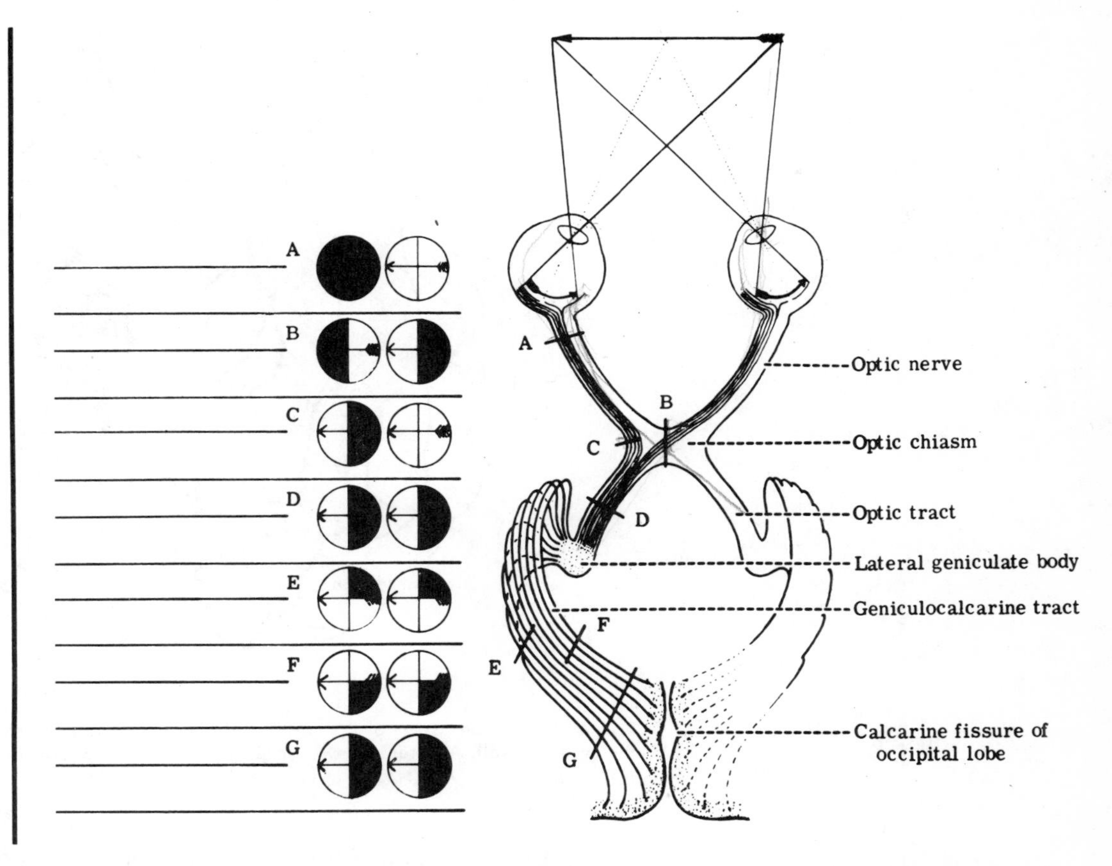

FIG. 4-8. Visual pathway from retina to occipital cortex. The blanks A to G are to be filled in according to the lesion represented at A to G in the figure. The optic axons, originating in retinal neurons, synapse at the lateral geniculate body. The small scale of the drawing precludes showing this feature.

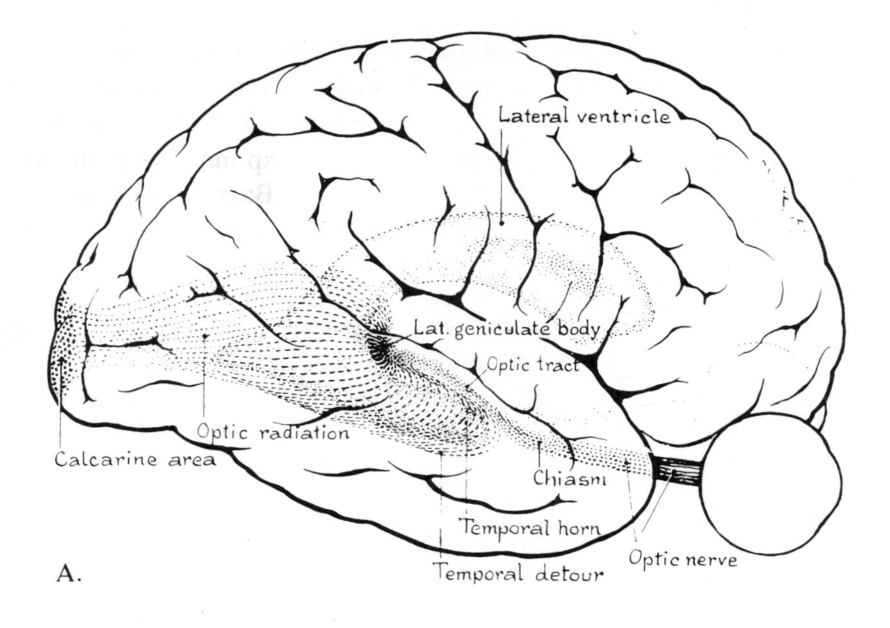

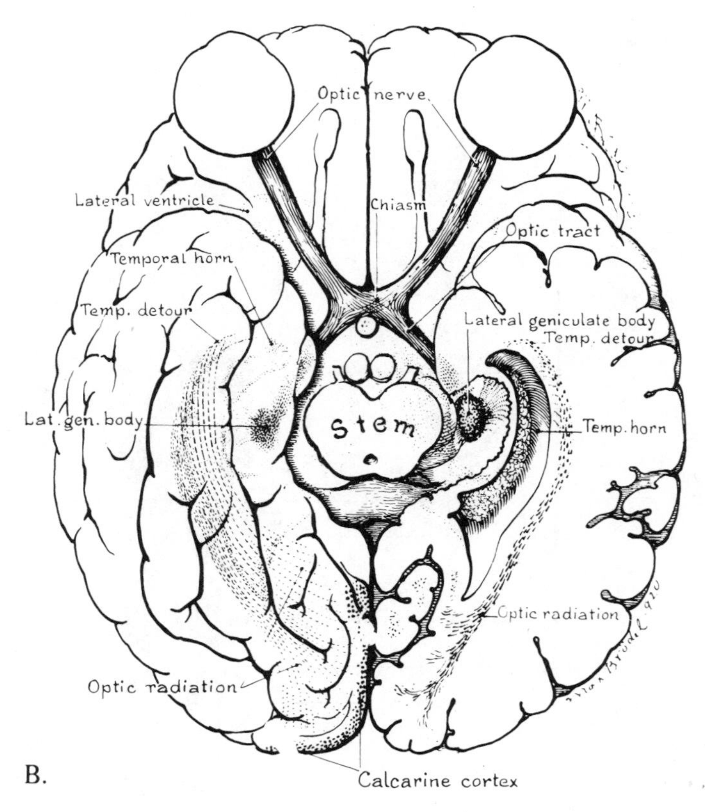

FIG. 4-9. Phantom views of the cerebrum to show the anatomic relation of the optic pathways to the cerebral wall. A. Lateral view of right cerebral hemisphere. B. Ventral view of cerebrum. (*From H. Cushing: Trans. Am. Neurol. Assoc.*, 47:374-423, 1921.)

9. See Fig. 4-9*A* and *B* for the actual course of the optic pathways through the cerebrum. Note that visual field testing assays the integrity of large parts of the temporal, occipital, and inferior margin of the parietal lobes.

H. Quantitative mapping of the visual fields and blind spot. Confrontation testing discloses gross fields defects. With a *perimeter,* the examiner can plot the periphery of the fields more accurately than with confrontation. Then the fields have the slightly irregular outline of Fig. 4-10, rather than being exactly round as we have depicted them. For detailed mapping of central vision, the examiner uses a *tangent screen.* The patient sits 1 or 2 meters away from a black screen 1 or 2 meters square, fixating on its center (with one eye covered). The examiner moves a 1 to 5 mm white spot through the field of vision. After mapping the physiologic blind spot, he systematically searches the central field for pathologic blind spots, called *scotomas.* The chart he makes becomes part of the medical record. See Fig. 4-11. These valuable methods only supplement, but do not supplant, confrontation testing by the attending physician.

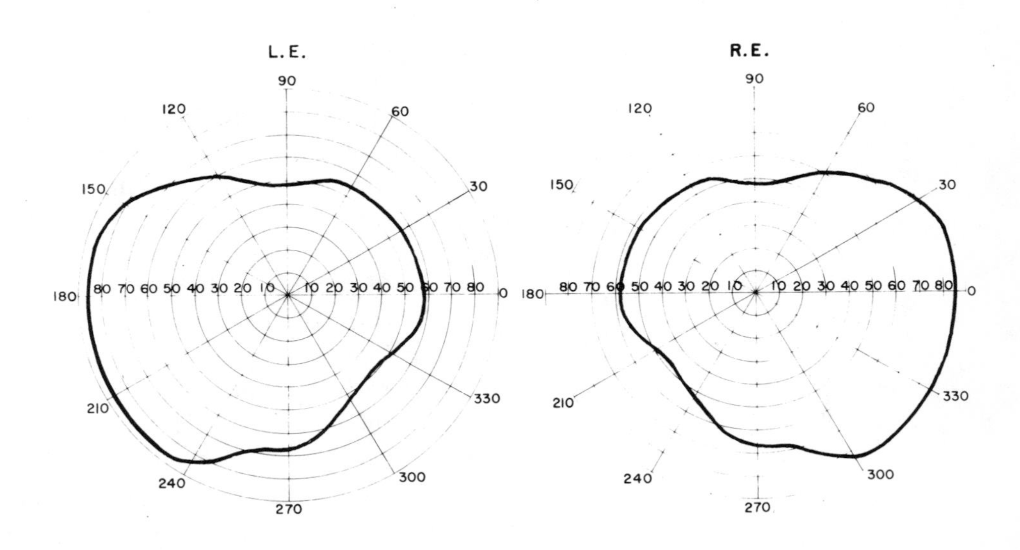

FIG. 4-10. Actual outline of visual fields charted by perimetry. The numbers are readings in degrees.

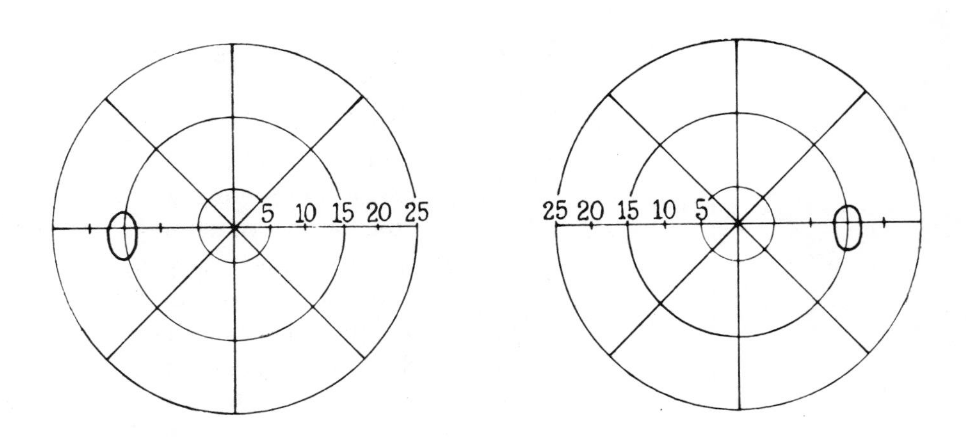

FIG. 4-11. Chart for recording the central portion of the visual fields, as determined by tangent screen examination.

I. The physiologic blind spot

1. Do this experiment with Fig. 4-12.

FIG. 4-12. Demonstration of the blind spot. See the text.

   a. Hold the page about 30 cm away.
   b. Cover your left eye.
   c. Fixate on the left cross. Make sure you do not break fixation at any time, but you should be able to make out the right cross also.
   d. Move your face slowly toward the page. As you maintain fixation on the left cross, attend to the image of the right cross.
   e. At some point the right cross disappears. As you continue to move closer, it reappears. If this does not happen you broke your fixation on the left cross — try again.
   f. Again cover your left eye, fixate on the left cross, and position your head so that the right cross disappears. Put your pencil point in the blind spot and move it very slowly toward the left cross. Make a mark on the paper when the point just becomes visible. By working around the blind spot, you can map out its perimeter. Be careful: if your fixation wavers, you will have a blind spot with very irregular borders. The blind spot is mapped more accurately on a distant tangent screen than with the short target distance of this experiment.
2. Get a test subject. Draw an *x* on a piece of paper for a fixation target and fasten the paper to a wall, making your own tangent screen. Seat the subject 100 cm away and map out the blind spot, moving the test object from the far right through the blind spot, toward the fixation point. Then work from the center of the blind spot to its periphery.
3. We do not ordinarily recognize the blind spot. We attend to the fixation point of the visual axes and ignore the blind spot, just as we ignore physiologic diplopia.
4. *Anatomic basis of the blind spot.* See Fig. 4-13.
5. Blind spot measurements are of some importance in detecting early papilledema, or in confirming that the papilledema is getting worse. The optic papilla of many normal subjects is not sharply outlined on ophthalmoscopic examination. If these patients have a neurologic complaint, the examiner may be uncertain whether the patient has papilledema or *pseudo*papilledema, a normal disc with indistinct margins. Serial measurement of the size of the blind spot will help distinguish the conditions. In pseudopapilledema, the blind spot remains the same, while in papilledema, the blind spot ________________ in size.

increases

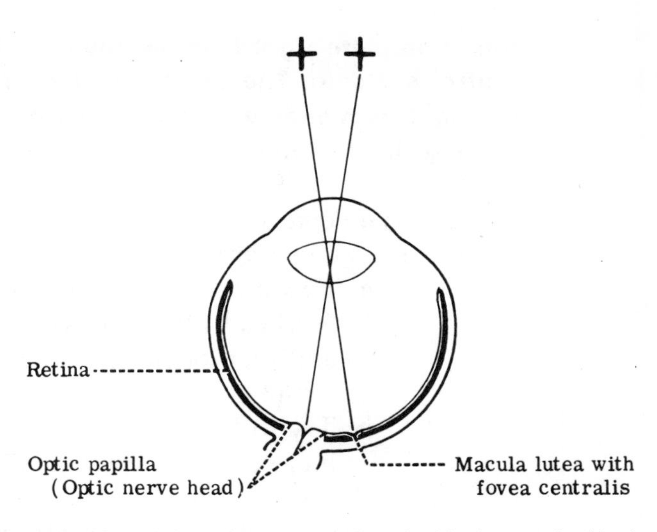

FIG. 4-13. Horizontal section of the right eye to explain the blind spot. The blind spot is caused by the absence of receptor neurons at the optic papilla (optic nerve head). Normally, the size of the blind spot depends on the diameter of the papilla.

Bibliography

Lyle, T.: Optic disc oedema; the differential diagnosis of its causes, *J. Neurol. Sci.,* 1:309-324, 1964.

J. Pathologic blind spots

1. Retinal lesions such as hemorrhages or exudates may prevent light penetration to the receptor neurons or destroy them. The pathologic blind spot produced depends on the size and location of the lesion.
2. A patient who had sudden loss of visual acuity without blindness would be expected to have a ☐ macular/ ☐ peripheral lesion, if the lesion is in the retina. If the field defect is large, it can be detected by confrontation. Ophthalmoscopic examination, of course, will disclose a retinal lesion. If the lesion is in the optic nerve, the retina may look normal. The evidence for an organic cause of the loss of acuity will be the demonstration of a scotoma by ______________ screen examination.
3. Although in theory quadrantic or hemianopic field defects could result from retinal or optic nerve lesions, in practice this virtually never occurs. These field defects appear only when the lesion affects the chiasm, optic tract, geniculocalcarine tract, or occipital lobe. Lesions of the pathways from the chiasm to the occipital lobe usually cause *patterned* defects, while lesions of the retina or optic nerve, if not so severe as to cause blindness, cause scotomas, *irregular* field defects.
4. Fig. 4-7*I* is the field defect found in a 53-year-old hypertensive patient who complained of headaches, sudden loss of vision on the right side and blurring of vision in the left eye. Write out the name of the defects.

____

macular

tangent

Ans: Complete right homonymous hemianopia with left superior quadrant paracentral scotoma. The patient had an infarct of the left occipital lobe, causing the right hemianopia, and a recent hypertensive hemorrhage in the left retina, causing the scotoma.

K. Physiologic suppression of vision

1. *Try this experiment:*
   a. Fixate on a distant point straight ahead. Place your palm on your forehead with your wrist directly between your eyes. Close one eye and then open it. Under which condition do you see more of your wrist? ______________________.
   b. Try to look at the tip of your nose. Then close one eye. You see more of your nose with ☐ one eye / ☐ both eyes open.

one eye closed

one

2. By closing one eye, you prove that the light rays from the wrist are striking photosensitive areas of the retina, yet the wrist is visible to one eye but vanishes when both eyes are open. We interpret the experiment to mean that the medial, overlapping portions of the visual fields are suppressed during binocular vision. See Fig. 4-14. This is another example of physiologic suppression to rid the visual image of confusing elements.

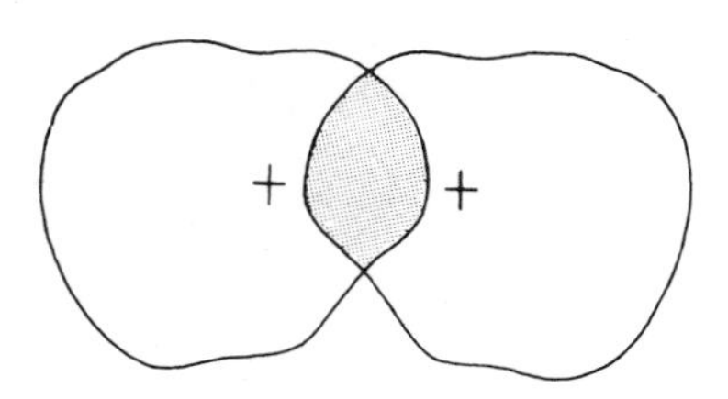

FIG. 4-14. The overlapping, shaded area of the visual fields undergoes physiologic suppression.

L. Pathologic suppression of vision

1. *Suppression amblyopia:* If someone has heterotropia from infancy, he would be expected to have diplopia, if we apply the laws of adult neurology. However, the infant learns to suppress the image from the errant eye. If he is allowed to continue to suppress the image for the first few years of life, he ultimately becomes completely blind in the deviating eye, even though the retina and visual pathways are structurally intact. So strong are the suppressive forces that rid the visual image of confusing elements that the child can rarely be made to see again once he has suppression blindness.
2. *Pathologic visual suppression from cerebral lesions* (visual inattention, visual extinction)
   a. Hold your arms straight out to the sides.
   b. Fixate straight ahead.
   c. Rotate your arms forward until you can see the tips of your fingers. Notice that you can make out both fingertips at the periphery of your fields, even though you look straight ahead. The presenta-

tion of two stimuli, such as the two fingers, on opposite sides, is called *simultaneous stimulation.*

d. Technique for simultaneous stimulation of visual fields. Assume the same position as for regular confrontation, but the patient has both eyes open. Extend your fingers into your inferior temporal quadrants near, but not beyond, the periphery of your own visual fields. Wiggle one finger and request the patient to point to *the* finger that moves. Then wiggle both fingers simultaneously and ask him to point to *any* finger that moves. If he perceives both stimuli, he will point to both fingers. Repeat the test in the upper temporal quadrants and then simultaneously stimulate nasal and temporal quadrants of one eye at a time.

e. Results and interpretation

(1) Patients with parietal or parieto-occipital lobe lesions, particularly on the right side, when presented with simultaneous stimuli, will not attend to the stimulus from the *contralateral* side. If, as in the usual case, the patient does not attend to stimuli from the left half of space, the lesion is in the ☐ right/ ☐ left parietal lobe.

(2) However, when the patient is tested by confrontation, using a single finger in the left visual field, no defect is demonstrated. The patient is then said to have *visual inattention* for the left side of space.

f. Hemianopia is detected by using a single stimulus, while visual inattention is detected by using ________________ stimuli.

g. If the patient is blind in one-half of the visual field, it is called ________________. If he does not recognize simultaneous stimuli in one-half of a visual field when both halves are stimulated, it is called ________________ ________________.

h. Explain the difference between hemianopia and visual inattention.

____

____

____

____

right

simultaneous (double)

hemianopia

visual inattention
(visual suppression)

Ans: hemianopia means that the patient is blind for single and double stimuli in one visual field. Visual inattention means that the patient does not perceive one of simultaneous right- and left-sided stimuli, but has no hemianopia when tested with a single stimulus.

Bibliography

Bender, M. B., and Bodis-Wollner, I.: Visual dysfunctions in optic tract lesions, *Ann. Neurol.,* 3:187-193, 1978.

Critchley, M.: *The Parietal Lobes* (reprint), New York, Hafner Publishing Co., Inc., 1966.

Ellenberger, C., Jr.: Modern perimetry in neuro-ophthalmic diagnosis, *Arch. Neurol.,* 30:193-201, 1974.

Gassel, M., and Williams, D.: Visual function in patients with homonymous hamianopia, Part II: Oculomotor mechanisms, *Brain,* 86:1–36, 1963.

Harrington, D.: *The Visual Fields: A Textbook and Atlas of Clinical Perimetry,* 2d ed., C. V. Mosby Co., 1971.

King, E.: The nature of visual field defects, *Brain,* 90: 647–668, 1967.

Leicester, J., Sidman, M., Stoddard, L., and Mohr, J.: Some determinants of visual neglect, *J. Neurol. Neurosurg. Psychiat.,* 32:580–587, 1969.

Smith, J.: *Neuro-ophthalmology VI,* St. Louis, C. V. Mosby Co., 1972.

Tate, G. W., and Lynn, J. R.: *Principles of Quantitative Perimetry: Testing and Interpreting the Visual Field,* New York, Grune and Stratton, 1977.

Williams, D., and Gassel, M.: Visual function in patients with homonymous hemianopia, Part I: The visual fields, *Brain,* 85:175–250, 1962.

M. Ophthalmoscopy

1. By now, you know what I would have you do to learn ophthalmoscopy. Sit down with a normal person and, using colored pencils, draw the optic fundus and draw it faithfully, precisely and in exquisite detail. Listen, you will never, *never,* do competent ophthalmoscopy unless you can draw the fundus. Moreover, you often should use drawings in your clinical notes rather than laborious written descriptions.
2. Making a drawing forces you to search the fundus systematically. Do it this way the first time and this way every time for the rest of your career:
   a. Remove your and your partner's glasses, unless one or both of you have a severe refractive error. Darken the room.
   b. Ask your partner to fix his gaze on a specific object straight ahead. Hold the ophthalmoscope in your right hand and use your right eye to your partner's right eye; hold the scope in your left hand and use your left eye to his left eye. When looking through the scope, keep both eyes open, attending only to the image from the eye behind the scope. Learn this art. It well repays the time required.
   c. Start with the ophthalmoscope 10 to 15 cm from your partner's eye, and with a strong positive lens focus on the media in succession from cornea to lens to vitreous, using successively weaker lenses. Inspect the cornea both with and without the scope for opacities and for a circular ring near the limbus, which if grayish-white is an arcus senilis, or if greenish-brown, a Kayser-Fleischer ring pathognomonic of Wilson's hepatolenticular degeneration.
   d. Next focus on a retinal vessel using whatever lens setting from 0 to a strong minus that is necessary to overcome refractive errors.
   e. After locating a retinal vessel, follow it along until you find the optic disc (optic papilla). Now study Figs. 4-15 and 4-16 before continuing.
   f. Returning to your partner, identify the pigment ring around the disc, note the disc color, and the presence or absence of a physiologic cup. If present, the physiologic cup is white as compared to the rest of the disc. Identify the arteries, the thin, brighter appearing vessels and the thicker, duller appearing veins. Look for venous pulsations where

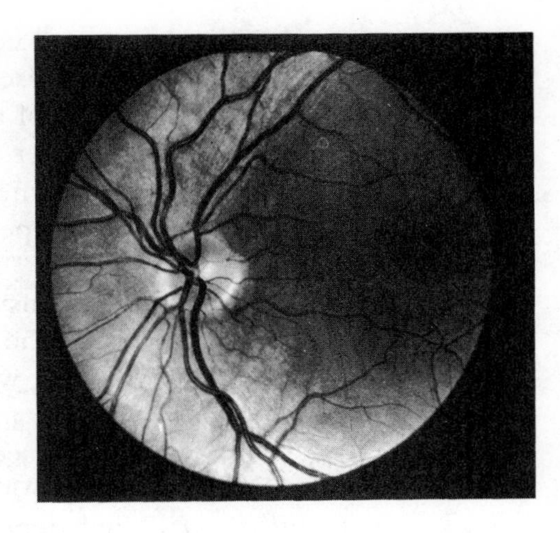

FIG. 4-15. Optic fundus as seen through an ophthalmoscope. Notice the optic disc with the vessels radiating from it and the avascular, dark oval area two disc diameters lateral which is the macula.

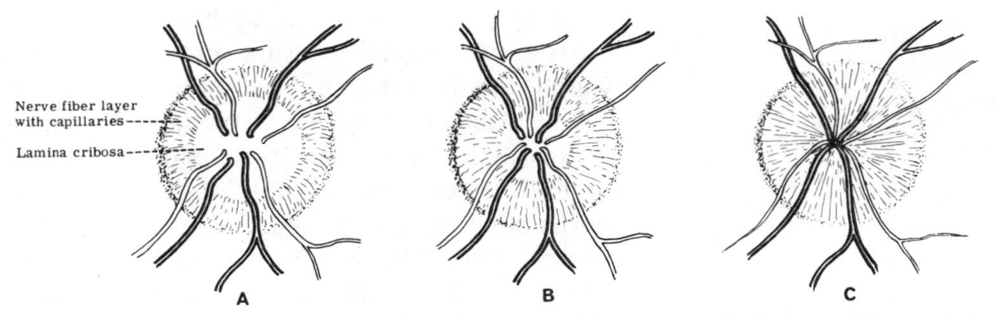

FIG. 4-16. Normal variation in the size of physiologic cup of the optic papilla. The size of the cup depends on whether the nerve fibers perforate the lamina cribrosa only at its periphery or all over its surface. A. Large cup. See the large white ring of lamina cribrosa showing around the vessels and the spread of the vessels where they perforate the disc. B. Medium-sized cup. Notice the small white ring and the more compact relation of the vessels. C. Absence of a physiologic cup in an otherwise normal disc. The vessels originate as from a point.

the veins bend over the edge of the physiologic cup. Press on the patient's sclera through his eyelid and watch the veins collapse. Follow each artery out as far as possible. Locate the macula, a darker, avascular area 2 disc diameters lateral to the disc. Note the pearl of light reflecting from its center, the fovea centralis. Study the texture of the retina.

3. Now make your drawing, and to check how observant you have been, answer these questions. Put your answers in the left-hand column and you will have written your own program.
   a. What is the normal ratio of arterial diameter to venous (A-V ratio)?
   b. What is the width of the stripe of light reflection from the arteries?
   c. Do the arteries nick or indent the veins where they cross?
   d. Between the superior and inferior temporal branches of the retinal artery, how many blood vessels can you count coursing over the disc? Be sure to have the disc sharply in focus.
   e. Which margin of the disc shows the most pigment?
   f. Which borders of the disc—the superior, inferior, nasal, or temporal—normally look more blurred than the other borders?

g. What is the normal color of the disc?
h. Which half of the disc, the nasal or temporal, is the palest?
i. What is the range of normal variability in the diameter of the physiologic cup? (Answer only after you have looked at several eyes.)
j. How many disc diameters away from the disc is the macula?
k. Does the fundus appear perfectly smooth or does it have a leathery texture?

4. Now, after trying to answer the questions, decide whether you should repeat the drawing. The questions cannot be bluffed. Should you try again? While wrestling with your conscience, listen to Walt Whitman:

   > Failing to fetch me at first keep encouraged,
   > Missing me one place, search another,
   > I stop somewhere waiting for you.

5. *Papilledema:* Papilledema is a blurred or elevated optic papilla (optic nerve head or optic disc), resulting from edema fluid in the nerve fibers as they cross the disc to perforate the lamina cribrosa and enter the optic nerve. Most often, papilledema results from transmission of increased intracranial pressure into the eye via the subarachnoid space which extends out along the optic nerve. See Fig. 4-17.

   The retinal veins converge on the optic papilla to form the ophthalmic vein, which enters the retinal end of the optic nerve. If the pressure around it increases, the ophthalmic vein, being thin-walled, collapses, obstructing the retinal veins. The retinal veins and papillary capillaries distend, leak fluid into the nerve fibers on the optic papilla and into the surrounding retina, and may rupture, causing visible hemorrhages on or around the papilla. Thus, the ophthalmoscopic features of papilledema are: Blurring of the nerve fibers as they converge on the disc,

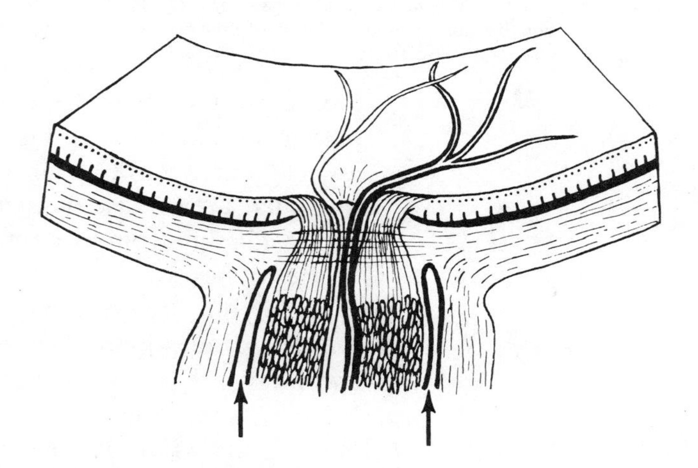

FIG. 4-17. Section of optic papilla and optic nerve. The arrows show how the subarachnoid space extends out around the optic nerve.

venous engorgement with loss of venous pulsations, then obliteration of the physiologic cup, and later disc elevation and hemorrhages. From Fig. 4-18, pick out the retina which shows papilledema (and one hemorrhage) ☐ A / ☐ B / ☐ C / ☐ D / ☐ E / ☐ F.

☒ B (Hemorrhage is at vein bifurcation just inferior to disc.)

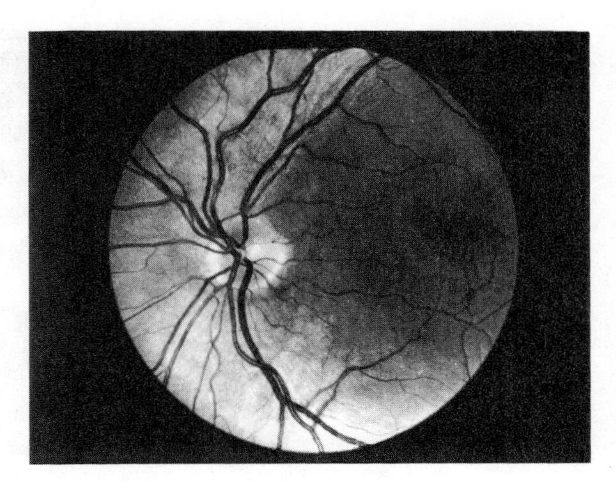

FIG. 4-18A

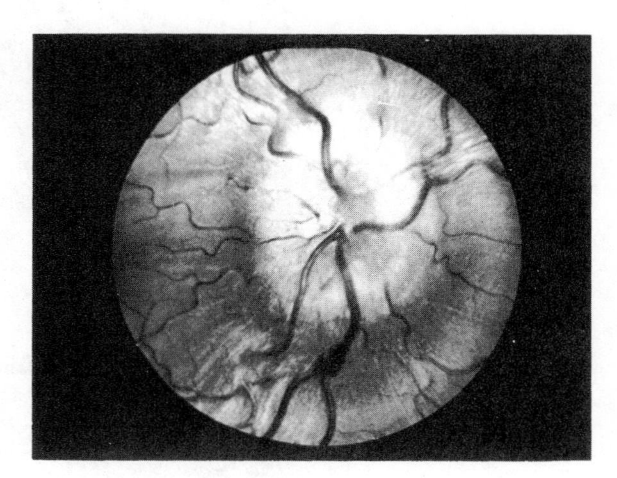

FIG. 4-18B

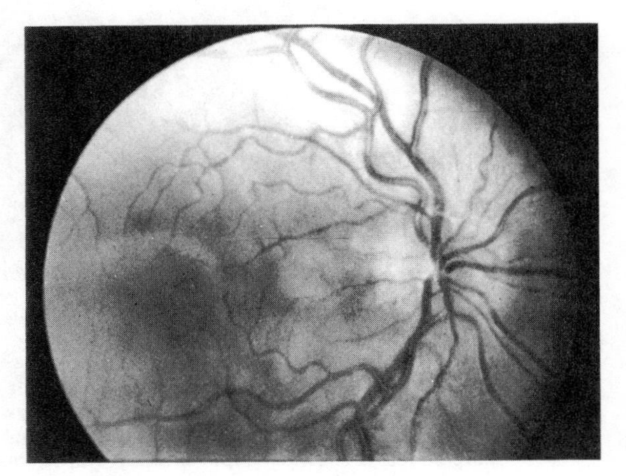

FIG. 4-18C

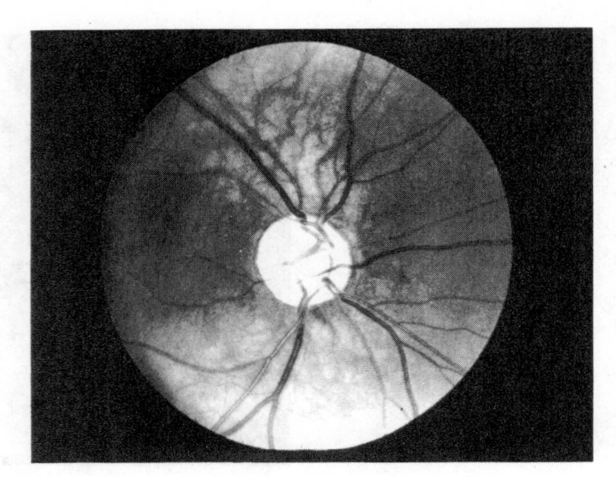

FIG. 4-18D

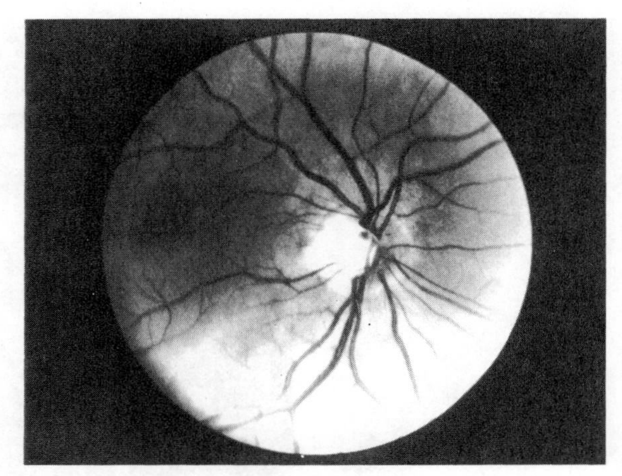

FIG. 4-18E

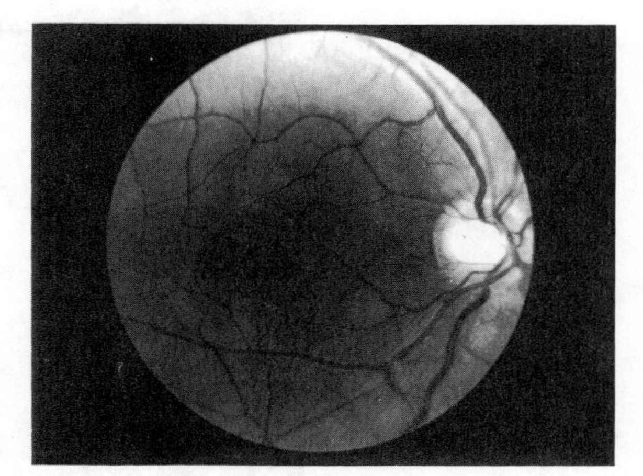

FIG. 4-18F

FIG. 4-18. Photographs of optic papilla in various conditions. *(Courtesy of Dr. Eugene Helveston.)* A. Normal. B. Papilledema. Notice how the edematous swelling engulfs and obscures the proximal segments of many vessels. Also notice the hemorrhage along the course of the vessel just inferior to the disc. C. Pseudopapilledema. D. Primary optic atrophy. Notice the chalk-white disc with cooky-cutter sharp edges. E. Secondary optic atrophy. Notice the pale, gray-white color laterally (to the reader's left) and the shaggy margins. F. Large physiologic cup, a normal variation.

Increased intracranial pressure, ophthalamic vein compression, leakage of edema fluid into and around optic papilla.

a. Describe the steps in the pathogenesis of papilledema: ______________________________
____
____
______________________________.

b. *Differential diagnosis of papilledema:* Although true papilledema is always pathologic, not all that looks like papilledema is papilledema. See Table 4-3.

TABLE 4-3. Optic Disc Anomalies Confused with Papilledema. (Reference only.)

Medullated nerve fibers: a whitish-yellow patch of fibers which radiates into the retina from the disc.
Congenital vascular anomalies of the vessels with glial overgrowth.
Small scleral aperature: the disc appears protruded; usually seen in an hyperopic eye with a short sagittal axis.
Drusen (waxy appearing bodies which push up beneath and may protrude through the disc).
Pseudopapilledema: see next section.
Papillitis: see later section.

6. *Differential diagnosis of true and pseudopapilledema*

a. Perhaps 5 percent of normal individuals have some blurring and even elevation of the optic papilla, a condition called *pseudopapilledema.* Pseudopapilledema often unduly alarms the clinician and leads to unnecessary, painful, and even harmful diagnostic investigations, when in most instances careful clinical observations, based on drawings and periodic assessment of the disc, would lead to the correct, benign diagnosis of pseudopapilledema. The difficulty arises in distinguishing early papilledema from pseudopapilledema. You will have little difficulty recognizing advanced papilledema when it shows extreme papillary swelling and hemorrhages. In pseudopapilledema, the disc margins look blurred, but the central portion of the disc protrudes rather than the peripheral as in true papilledema, and the vessels show preretinal branching. See Fig. 4-19.

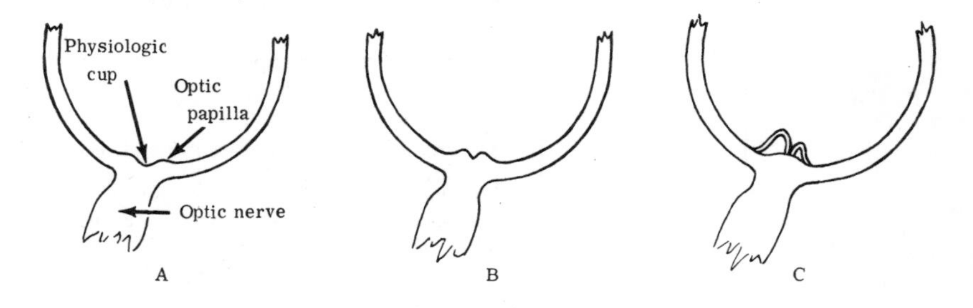

FIG. 4-19. Optic papilla in horizontal sections of the eye. A. Normal optic papilla, showing slight elevation of the papillary margins and normal depth of the physiologic cup. B. Early true papilledema, showing elevation of the papillary margins and beginning obliteration of the physiologic cup. C. Pseudopapilledema, showing pre-retinal branching of the vessels, central elevation of the optic papilla, and absence of a physiologic cup.

b. The elevated disc of pseudopapilledema may come from Drusen (hyaloid bodies) pressing up from beneath the nerve fiber layer.

Drusen and pseudopapilledema occur most frequently in blond Caucasians. Also, pseudopapilledema most often occurs in hyperopic rather than myopic patients. If you suspect pseudopapilledema in a blond Caucasian or hyperopic patient, inspect the fundi of family members. Since these conditions often are hereditary, the answer becomes clear if other family members also have blurred discs. From Fig. 4-18, select the disc which shows pseudopapilledema: ☐ A / ☐ B / ☐ C / ☐ D / ☐ E / ☐ F.

☑ C

c. Two further tests help identify papilledema in doubtful cases:

(1) *Measurement of the blind spot*
The optic papilla causes a blind spot in the visual field because it contains no light-receptive neurons. Since papilledema encroaches on the surrounding retina, reception of light rays by the peripapillary retina suffers. Thus, as the papilledema advances the blind spot ____________ in size. What type of visual field examination would you order to measure the blind spot? ________________________.

increases

tangent screen examination of central fields

(2) *The fluorescein dye test:* After injection of fluorescein into an arm vein, the fundus is photographed. Fluorescein can be visualized in the papilla and surrounding retina after it passes through the leaky walls of the distended retinal vessels. Thus the two tests in addition to ophthalmoscopic examination to diagnose papilledema are ________________________
________________________.

measure blind spot
fluorescein dye test

d. To summarize the differential features of papilledema and pseudopapilledema, complete Table 4-4.

TABLE 4-4. Differentiation of True and Pseudopapilledema. (Reference only).

	Papil-ledema	Pseudo-Papil
Disc characteristics		
Hyperemic, pink color (vascular distension).	____	____
Physiologic cup present (early).	____	____
Sparing of temporal margin (early).	____	____
High point of elevation central. (See Fig. 4-19.)	____	____
Drusen (hyaline bodies) submerged in children, exposed in adults, gray-yellow translucent color of disc. Applies only to blond Caucasians.	____	____
Vessel characteristics		
Dilated veins.	____	____
Venous pulsation present.	____	____
Disc obscures origin of vessels.	____	____
Arteries appear tortuous, show preretinal branching, and the disc does not obscure the origin of the vessels.	____	____
Prominent choroidal vessels (from lack of retinal pigment).	____	____
Hemorrhages.	____	____
Hyperopia	____	____
Enlarged blind spot	____	____
Fluorescein dye test: shows leaky vessels on and around disc.	____	____

PAPIL-LEDEMA	PSEUDO-PAPIL
+	0
+	0
+	0
0	+
0	+
+	0
0	+, 0
+	0
0	+
0	+
+	0
0	+
+	0
+	0

7. Summary of procedures to diagnose papilledema.
   a. Make careful clinical notes, drawings or photographs describing:
      (1) The color of the disc.
      (2) Degree of blurring of disc margins and location of blurring.
      (3) Condition of the physiologic cup.
      (4) Venous congestion and pulsation.
      (5) Peripapillary wrinkles and folds.
      (6) Hemorrhages or exudates.
      (7) Measurable elevation of disc.
   b. Measure the patient's visual acuity.
   c. Chart the blind spot in the visual field.
   d. Consider the common anomalies confused with papilledema, as outlined in Table 4-3.
   e. Do the fluorescein dye test.
   f. Make careful serial examinations.
8. *Optic atrophy, primary and secondary*
   a. If a lesion destroys retinal neurons or their optic nerve fibers as they course to the optic papilla, the fibers degenerate and disappear. If a lesion interrupts optic fibers in the optic nerve, the fibers degenerate and disappear back to their retinal neurons of origin. Thus, with either retinal or optic nerve lesions, the optic papilla becomes denuded of nerve fibers, which brings us to a profound secret: the optic nerve fibers and retinal neurons are transparent and colorless. Why then doesn't the optic disc appear white, being backed by the white lamina cribrosa of the sclera? The answer is that the color of the disc is the color of the capillaries which accompany the nerve fibers and nourish them. Why does the physiologic cup appear white?
   ____
   ____
   ____.

No nerve fibers and, therefore, no capillaries cover the white lamina cribrosa

   b. *Primary* optic atrophy: when nerve fibers disappear from the disc, the condition is called *optic atrophy.* In optic atrophy, when the nerve fibers degenerate, the capillaries undergo retrogression and disappear. This is a general rule: whenever the parenchymatous elements of an organ degenerate, so does its blood supply. Compare the capillarity of the pre- and post-menopausal ovary. In severe optic atrophy or retinal destruction, the arteries and veins also become smaller. Disappearance of the nerve fibers and capillaries exposes the chalk-white lamina cribrosa which then appears as a flat white disc with a cooky-cutter sharp border against the retina, a condition called *primary* optic atrophy. From Fig. 4-18, select the disc which shows primary atrophy: ☐ A/ ☐ B/ ☐ C/ ☐ D/ ☐ E/ ☐ F.

☑ D

   c. *Secondary* optic atrophy follows long-standing disc lesions such as chronic papilledema or papillitis. The optic nerve fibers disappear, but connective tissue proliferation incited by the lesion causes the disc to become gray and shaggy appearing, with ragged borders. In both primary and secondary optic atrophy, the nerve fibers cross-

secondary

☑ E

ing the disc disappear, but connective tissue proliferates on the disc only in ______________________ optic atrophy.

d. Table 4-5 summarizes the differential features of primary and secondary optic atrophy. From Fig. 4-18, select the disc which shows secondary optic atrophy: ☐ A/ ☐ B/ ☐ C/ ☐ D/ ☐ E/ ☐ F.

TABLE 4-5. Differential Diagnosis of Primary from Secondary Optic Atrophy

Primary Optic Atrophy	Secondary Optic Atrophy
Follows acute or chronic lesions of optic nerve or retina.	Follows chronic lesion of optic papilla, usually papilledema or papillitis.
Disc is chalk-white with cooky-cutter sharp borders.	Disc is gray with shaggy borders from connective tissue proliferation.
Lamina cribrosa exposed.	Lamina cribrosa obscured.
Arteries and veins reduced in size if optic atrophy is severe and prolonged.	Arteries thin, veins may be dilated.
May affect only one sector of the disc.	Usually affects entire disc.

9. *Differential diagnosis of papilledema, papillitis, and acute retrobulbar neuritis.* Inflammatory or toxic processes may involve the optic papilla, so-called *papillitis.* Inflammatory, toxic, or demyelinating processes may affect the optic nerve behind the optic bulb, so-called *acute retrobulbar neuritis.* See Fig. 4-20.

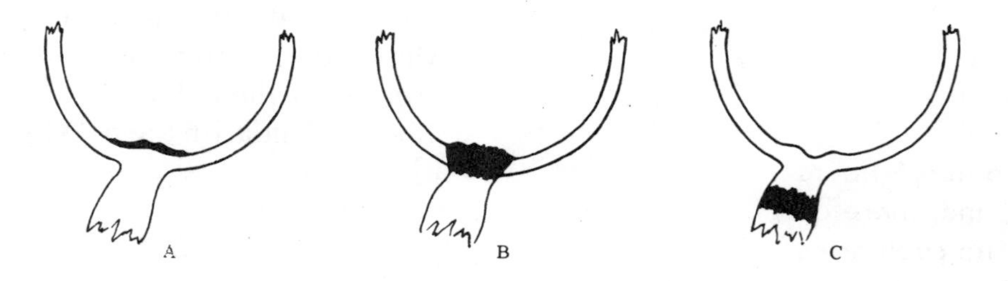

FIG. 4-20. Sites of lesions in the optic papilla and nerve. A. Papilledema. B. Papillitis. C. Retrobulbar neuritis.

They degenerate and disappear

primary optic

a. The ophthalmoscopic appearance of papillitis may be indistinguishable from papilledema, but with papillitis the patient lacks vision whereas with *papilledema* he retains vision. With acute retrobulbar neuritis, the disc and vessels look normal early in the course, but if the process destroys nerve fibers in the optic nerve, what happens to the nerve fibers and capillaries on the disc? ______________________

______________________.

The optic disc then has the ophthalmoscopic appearance called ______________________ atrophy.

b. *Notice this critical fact:* the degeneration of optic nerve fibers and capillaries takes many days to several weeks to occur. Thus, if you look at the optic papilla in acute retrobulbar neuritis, you will not see atrophy. Even though the patient has no vision, his optic disc may look normal: the patient sees nothing and neither do you.

c. The differential effects of papilledema, papillitis, and acute retrobulbar neuritis on ophthalmoscopic appearances and visual acuity summarize as follows:
   (1) If the physician sees a swollen disc, and the patient sees as usual: papilledema.
   (2) If the physician sees a swollen disc, and the patient doesn't see as usual: papillitis.
   (3) If the physician sees nothing abnormal, but the patient's vision is abnormal: acute retrobulbar neuritis.

d. Thus, to put these statements in their tersest form:
   (1) If both the patient and physician see something: ________________.
   (2) If the physician sees something, and the patient doesn't: ________________.
   (3) If neither sees anything: ________________.

papilledema

papillitis

acute retrobulbar neuritis

Bibliography

Atlee, W., Jr.: Talc and cornstarch emboli in eyes of drug abusers, *JAMA,* 219:49-51, 1972.

Chester, E.: *The Ocular Fundus in Systemic Disease,* Chicago, Year Book Medical Publishers, 1973.

Hayreh, S. S.: *Anterior Ischemic Optic Neuropathy,* New York, Springer-Verlag, 1975.

Hoyt, W., and Pont, M.: Diagnosis of optic disk anomaly, *JAMA,* 181:191-196, 1962.

Levin, B. E.: The clinical significance of spontaneous pulsations of the retinal vein, *Arch. Neurol.,* 35:37-40, 1978.

Miller, S., Sanders, M., and Ffytche, T.: Fluorescein fundus photography in the detection of early papilledema and its differentiation from pseudopapilledema, *Lancet,* 2:651-654, 1965.

Nover, A., and Glodi, R.: *The Ocular Fundus,* Philadelphia, Lea and Febiger, 1966.

O'Day, D., Crock, G., and Galbraith, J.: Fluorescein angiography of normal and atrophic optic discs, *Lancet,* 1:224-226, 1967.

Rosen, E. and Savir, H.: *Basic Ophthalmoscopy: Ophthalmoscopic diagnosis in systemic disorders,* New York, Appleton-Century-Crofts, 1971.

Wise, G., Dollery, G., and Henkind, P.: *The Retinal Circulation,* New York, Harper & Row, 1971.

5

Central Mechanisms of Body Motility, Ocular Motility, and Nystagmus

It would seem, therefore, that we may look upon the pyramidal system as an internuncial, a common, pathway by which the sensory system initiates and continuously directs, in willed movements, the activities of the nervous motor mechanisms. This sensory afflux is a condition of willed movements, and unless we consider both in association we cannot hope to see the purpose of either.

—F. M. R. Walshe

I. The innervation of movement

A. *The concept of lower motor neurons (LMNs) and upper motor neurons (UMNs)*

1. LMNs are *all* neurons of the somatic, visceral, and branchial efferent cell columns which send motor axons into the peripheral nerves.
2. UMNs are *all* motor neurons which send axons from the cerebral cortex or the brainstem to activate *LMNs*. No *UMN* axons leave the neuraxis.
3. Peripheral nerves contain motor axons from ☐ UMNs only / ☐ LMNs only / ☐ both UMNs and LMNs.

LMNs only

4. If you cut a peripheral nerve, the paralysis affects *all* and *only* the individual muscle(s) supplied by the nerve. This type of paralysis is called ☐ LMN / ☐ UMN paralysis.

LMN

B. *The pyramidal tract, the UMN pathway for volitional movement*

1. For willed movements, the most important UMN pathway is the pyramidal tract. This tract begins in neurons of the motor cortex, located in the precentral and, to a lesser extent, the postcentral gyri. Study Fig. 5-1.
2. Axons from the cortical motor neurons traverse the white matter of the cerebrum and descend to the LMNs of the brainstem and the spinal cord.
   a. The cortical motor pathway to the brainstem nuclei, both branchial and somatic nuclei, is called the *corticobulbar* tract.

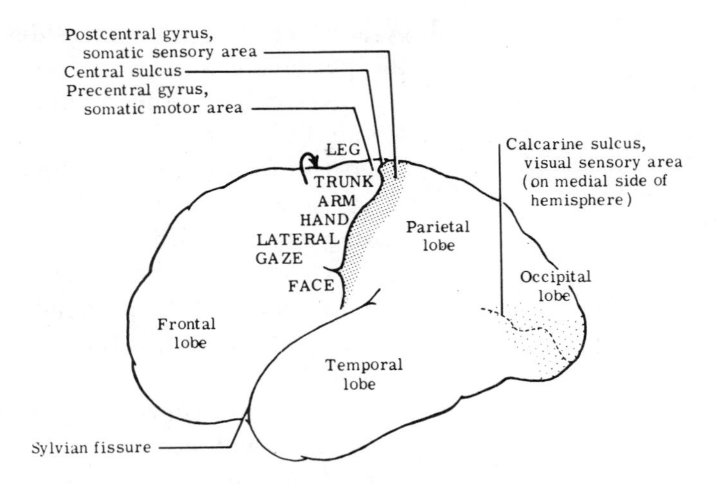

FIG. 5-1. Lateral view of the left cerebral hemisphere. Notice the location of the somatic motor, somatic sensory, and visual sensory areas. A center for lateral movement of the head and eyes (conjugate gaze center) is located just anterior to the motor strip of the precentral gyrus. The leg portion of the motor and sensory cortex extends over onto the medial aspect of the hemisphere.

b. The cortical motor pathway to the spinal cord is the *corticospinal* tract. Follow these pathways in Fig. 5-2 and learn the names along the left side.

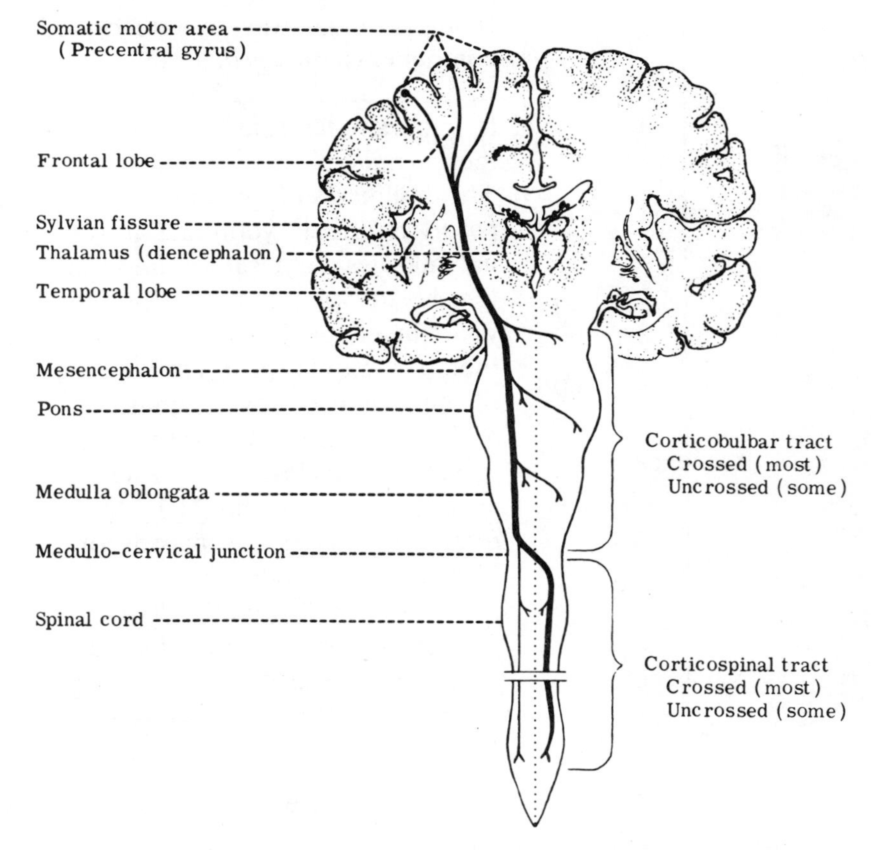

FIG. 5-2. Coronal section of the neuraxis to show the pyramidal tract pathway from the cerebral motor cortex to the LMNs of the brainstem and spinal cord.

	3. According to its original definition by Ludwig Turk (1810-1868), the pyramidal tract would include only the axons descending through the pyramids of the medulla oblongata. The corticobulbar system would be excluded. By usage, however, the pyramidal tract is defined to include corticobulbar and corticospinal components.
corticobulbar corticospinal	*a.* As shown in Fig. 5-2, the two components of the pyramidal tract decussate at different levels of the neuraxis. Decussating at various levels of the brainstem is the *cortico* ______________ component of the pyramidal tract, while decussating at the medullocervical junction is the *cortico* ______________ component.
contralateral (Review Fig. 5-2 if you erred.)	4. If a lesion interrupts the pyramidal tract in the cerebrum, volitional movement will be paralyzed on the ☐ ipsilateral / ☐ contralateral side of the body.
	a. Complete or near complete paralysis on one side of the body is called *hemiparalysis* or *hemiplegia.*
*hemi*paresis	*b.* Paresis or incomplete paralysis on one side of the body is called ______________.
contralateral	5. If a pyramidal tract is interrupted rostral to its decussation, the hemiplegia is ☐ ipsilateral / ☐ contralateral to the lesion.
ipsilateral	6. If a pyramidal tract is interrupted caudal to its decussation, the hemiplegia is ☐ ipsilateral / ☐ contralateral to the lesion.
cortico*bulbar* cortico*spinal*	7. If a pyramidal tract is interrupted in the cerebrum, both pyramidal components, the *cortico* ______________ and *cortico* ______________ tracts, are affected.
cortico*spinal*	8. If a pyramidal tract is interrupted caudal to the decussation, only the *cortico* ______________ tract is affected.
	9. The hallmark of pyramidal tract interruption is that the paresis or paralysis affects volitional movements of the parts, not the individual muscles or a set of muscles. Volitional movements, even if ostensibly simple, require the action of more than one muscle. Flex your finger, pucker your lips, or wink your eye — in every case more than one muscle springs into action. Movements, then, are compounded of the action of several muscles.
LMNs	*a.* If the patient has paresis or paralysis of one muscle or a restricted set of muscles, while other movements of the limbs are normal, the lesion is in the ☐ UMNs / ☐ LMNs.
UMNs	*b.* If the patient has paresis or paralysis of the movements of one side of the body, sparing the other side, the lesion is most likely in the ☐ UMNs / ☐ LMNs.
movements muscles	*c.* Taking some poetic license, we may epitomize this conclusion by saying that UMN lesions paralyze ☐ movements / ☐ muscles, while LMN lesions paralyze ☐ movements / ☐ muscles.

II. The relation of sensory pathways to movement

A. Introduction: If you intend to reach up to scratch your nose, the muscles to be activated and their sequence of activation depend on where your hand starts from and the obstacles it might encounter on the way. Information by which a cerebral hemisphere guides movement comes from two great afferent systems, the *visual* and *position* sense systems. By crossing of their axons, these systems bring their messages to the proper hemisphere.

B. Crossing of the visual afferent system

The wiring diagram of the brain shows that one occipital lobe receives information from the ☐ ipsilateral / ☐ contralateral half of the visual field. The partial decussation of axons at the chiasm is a very deliberate arrangement to insure just this result.

contralateral (Review Fig. 4-8 if you missed.)

C. Crossing of the somatic afferent system

1. In common with the special sense of vision, the somatic pathways for skin sensation and position sense also cross the midline to reach the opposite hemisphere. Study Fig. 5-3.

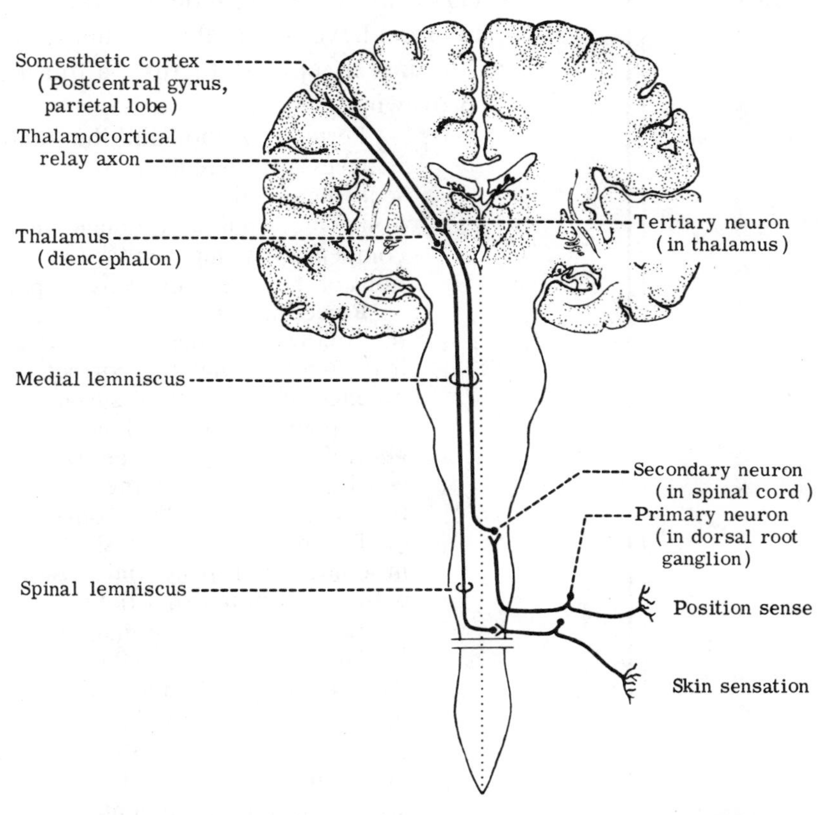

FIG. 5-3. Coronal section of the neuraxis to show how the somatic sensory systems of the cord decussate to innervate the contralateral hemisphere. Notice that the sensory pathways decussate at different levels.

2. Thus, visual and somatic afferent pathways innervate mainly the ☐ ipsilateral / ☐ contralateral cerebral hemisphere.
3. The visual and somatic sensory data necessary to guide movement in the right half of space are brought to the ☐ right / ☐ left cerebral hemisphere.
4. The left cerebral hemisphere, which receives sensory information from the right half of space, controls movement in the ☐ right / ☐ left half of space.

contralateral

left

right

medullocervical

5. The decussation by which the pyramidal tract from one hemisphere directs movement of the contralateral limbs occurs at the ____________ ____________ junction.
6. Using a colored pencil, superimpose the pyramidal pathway of Fig. 5-2 onto Fig. 5-3. Then, mentally follow a nerve impulse from a somatic sensory receptor through to the cerebral cortex and back to the LMNs via the pyramidal tract.
7. After the diagram is completed as requested, it will represent a distinct concept, a unity of structure and function. It can be described as the *law of contralateral hemispheric sensory-motor innervation.*

**D. *Explanation for decussations.* The basic reason for the contralaterality of pathways, according to Santiago Ramon y Cajal (1853-1934), is found in an analysis of the visual decussation. Submammalia (fish, amphibia, reptiles, and birds) have no cerebral visual cortex. Their optic impulses are brought to the mesencephalic tectum, a quasi-cortex. Here are Cajal's explanation and drawings:

> Perhaps, I thought, the fundamental crossing of the optic tracts is necessarily bound up with the physical mechansim of vision. Let us seek then in this Mechanism for the logical reason of such an organization. Once it is ascertained, nothing will be easier than to explain as compensatory and corrective arrangements, the primordial decussations of the motor and sensory pathways.
>
> Rejecting other conjectures, I became possessed obsessively by the following thought: Everything will have a simple explanation if it is admitted that the correct perception of an object implies the congruence of the cerebral surfaces of projection, that is those representing each point in space. Hence, in order that the mental perception may be unified and may agree exactly with the external reality, or, in other words, in order that the image conveyed through the right eye may be continuous with that conveyed through the left eye, the intercrossing of the optic paths from side to side is quite necessary; a total crossing in animals with panoramic vision, a partial crossing in animals endowed with a common visual field.
>
> The accompanying diagrams explain the foregoing theory clearly.
>
> The first diagram [Fig. 5-4] shows the form and direction which the mental visual image would have had on the supposition that the optic nerves had not crossed.
>
> The incongruity of the two images is evident: that projected through the right eye does not fit with that from the left eye, and it would be impossible for the animal to synthesize the two images into a continuous representation. The horizon would be presented as a panoramic view formed from two photographs, the right and left ones being laterally inverted.
>
> Let us now examine the mental image resulting from the intercrossing of the optic nerves, an intercrossing adopted by nature in the case of lenticular eyes. [Fig. 5-5] shows with the greatest clearness that, thanks to the crossing, the two images, right and left, correspond and make a continuous panorama, the lateral inversion disappearing.
>
> Things take place somewhat differently in the mammals, in which the double visual projection reproduces the same region of space. In these animals there exists the uncrossed tract [Fig. 4-8], through which the duplication of visual images is ingeniously avoided, while the advantages of the crossing are retained.

[Fig. 5-5] shows also that the visual decussation has brought about the decussations of the principal voluntary motor and of the sensory paths.

— Santiago Ramon y Cajal

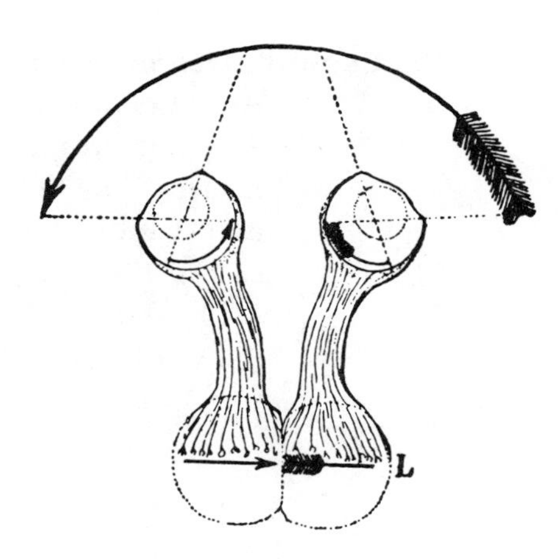

FIG. 5-4. The discontinuous representation of the visual images from the two eyes when there is no optic decussation. (*From S. Ramon y Cajal: Recollections of My Life, Memoirs of the American Philosophical Society*, vol. 8, 1937.)

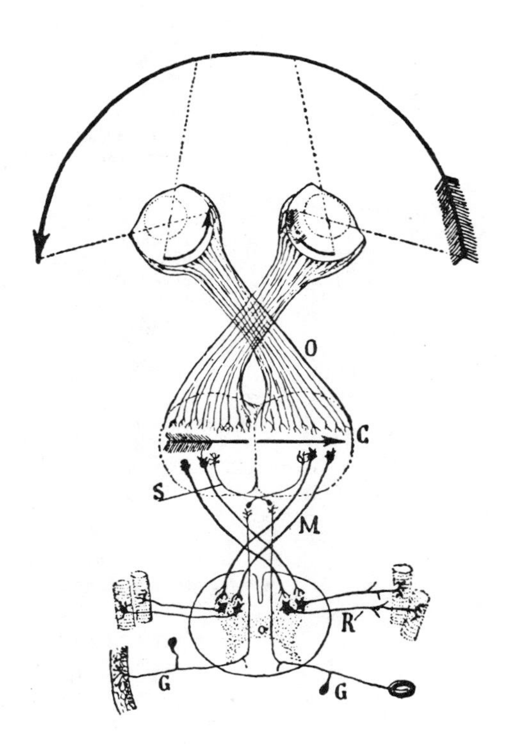

FIG. 5-5. Diagram to show how the optic decussation permits continuous representation of the visual images from the two eyes in lower animals with panoramic vision. Compare with Fig. 4-8 to see how continuous central representation of the visual images is achieved by partial decussation of optic axons in animals with binocular stereoscopic vision. (*From S. Ramon y Cajal: Recollections of My Life, Memoirs of the American Philosophical Society*, vol. 8, 1937.)

Bibliography

Ramon y Cajal, S.: *Recollections of My Life* (translated by E. Horne Craige), *Memoirs Amer. Phil. Soc.*, vol VIII, 1937.

III. Central mechanisms of ocular motility

A. Brainstem connections

1. A special brainstem pathway, the *medial longitudinal fasciculus,* (MLF), insures that the yoke muscles for lateral conjugate gaze receive equal innervation. The MLF connects the VIth and IIIrd nerve nuclei. Fig. 5-6 shows the corticobulbar pathway for lateral conjugate gaze and the MLF. Trace along this pathway from the electrode on the cortex to the ocular muscles.

1. VIth
2. IIIrd
3. IIIrd
4. Medial rectus
5. VIth
6. Lateral rectus

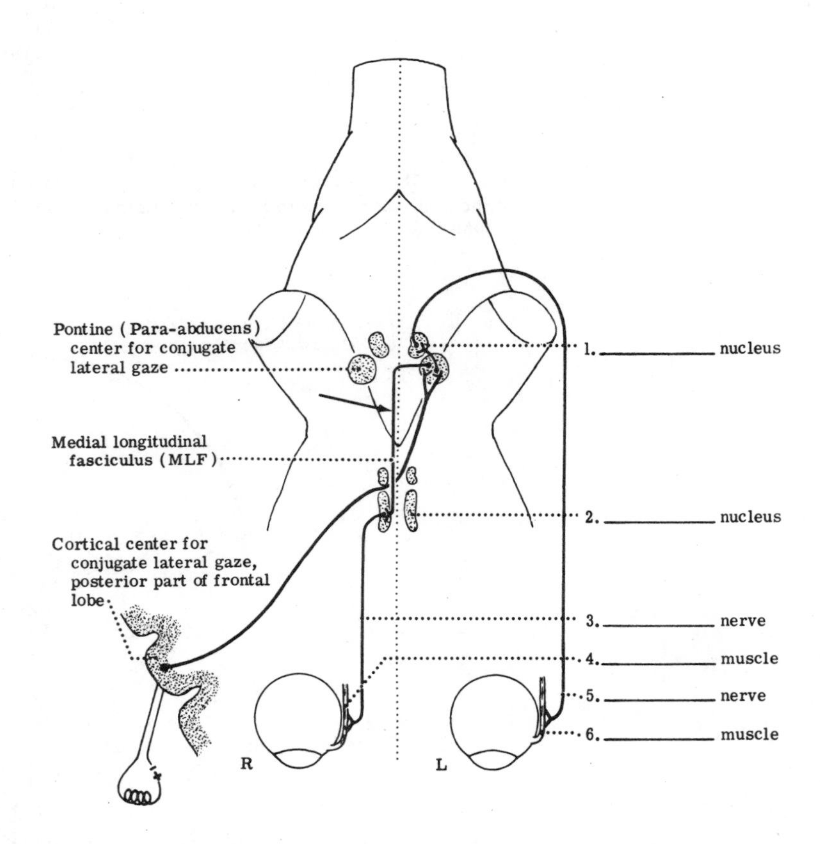

FIG. 5-6. Dorsal view of the brainstem to show corticobulbar pathways for voluntary conjugate lateral eye movements. Complete blanks 1 to 6.

left

accordance

2. If a stimulating electrode or volitional impulses activate the conjugate gaze center in the *right* frontal lobe, the eyes (and head) turn ☐ right/ ☐ left/ ☐ straight ahead.
3. Is the result in frame 2 in accordance with or contradictory to the law of contralateral innervation? Explain: ______________________
____
____
____

Ans: In terms of the law of contralateral innervation you should expect this result. If the right cerebral hemisphere receives visual impulses from the left side of space and if the individual is attracted to some visual stimulus from the left side, shouldn't the right hemisphere turn the eyes, and as we shall see, the head to the left?

the right eye will not adduct

4. Suppose a unilateral lesion has interrupted the MLF at the tip of the arrow in Fig. 5-6. When the patient attempts to look to the left: ☐ the left eye will not abduct/ ☐ the right eye will not abduct/ ☐ the right eye will not adduct/ ☐ neither eye will move.
5. In addition to adductor paralysis on left lateral gaze, the patient would also show an oscillation of the left eye, a feature which cannot be deduced from the diagram. Such oscillatory movements of the eyes are called *nystagmus*. Hence, a second sign of the MLF syndrome is monocular nystagmus of the *abducting* eye. At rest the eye has no nystagmus. It occurs only during abduction.
6. These two signs, paralysis of the *adducting* eye and nystagmus of the *abducting* eye, appear *only* on gaze to the opposite side of the MLF lesion. The eyes adduct normally on convergence or on vertical gaze. The corticobulbar pathways for convergence and vertical eye movements, thus, run directly into the mesencephalon to the LMNs of the IIIrd and IVth nuclei, rather than in the MLF.

looking to the right

7. What would be the only direction of gaze in which the patient with a *left*-sided MLF lesion would have heterotropia? (Reason out the answer from Fig. 5-6, remembering that in the previous example we used a right-sided lesion. It may be helpful to draw in the pathway from the left cerebral hemisphere with colored pencil.) ____________ ____________.

adduct

nystagmus
abducting

normal

8. *To summarize:* the signs of a unilateral MLF lesion occur only when the patient attempts to look away from the side of the lesion.
   a. The patient is unable to ____________ the eye ipsilateral to the lesion.
   b. The patient shows monocular ____________ of the ____________ ducting eye, contralateral to the lesion.
   c. All other eye movements, including conjugate vertical gaze, and pupillary responses are ____________.
9. What are the signs of a bilateral MLF lesion at the level indicated by the arrow? ____________
____
____
____

Ans: Monocular nystagmus of the leading eye on attempted gaze to either side. Paralysis of adduction of the following eye on attempted gaze to either side. All other eye movements and pupillary responses are preserved.

through the MLF
directly to the IIIrd and IVth nerve nuclei

10. The pathway for voluntary lateral conjugate eye movements runs ☐ through the MLF/ ☐ directly to the IIIrd and IVth nerve nuclei, while the pathway for convergence and for voluntary vertical conjugate eye movements runs ☐ through the MLF/ ☐ directly to the IIIrd and IVth nerve nuclei.

Yes

11. Would a patient with a bilateral MLF lesion be able to converge his eyes during accommodation? ☐ Yes / ☐ No.

B. Clinical signs of lesions in the cortical centers for lateral eye and head movement

1. Just as movements of one side of the body are controlled by the contralateral hemisphere, head and eye turning to one side are controlled by the contralateral hemisphere.
2. Normally, the head and eyes are maintained straight ahead by rather powerful vectors generated by the centers of both hemispheres. The vector generated by one hemisphere is counterbalanced by a vector from the other hemisphere. See Fig. 5-7*A*.

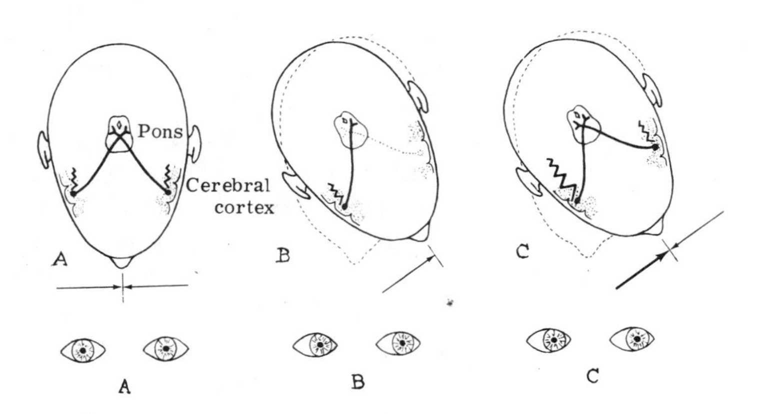

FIG. 5-7. The head-and-eye-turning center (conjugate gaze center) in the posterior part of the frontal lobe. The arrows beneath the figures represent the strength of the vector originating in one center, acting to turn the head and eyes to the opposite side. Below each head is shown the position of the eyes. Notice the corticobulbar pathway to the pons and that it decussates. Relate this pathway to the MLF in Fig. 5-6. A. Normal resting condition. The vectors are equal and the head and eyes are straight ahead. B. A lesion has destroyed the conjugate gaze center on the left. The right center acts unopposed. The head and eyes deviate to the left. C. An epileptogenic lesion has caused an excessive discharge of impulses from the right conjugate gaze center. The vector from the right hemisphere overpowers the one from the left. The head and eyes deviate to the left.

3. The tendency for centering of the eyes and head is very strong. Try to keep your eyes turned completely to one side even for as little as 30 sec. You will feel a considerable relief when they are returned to the midline. In fact many mentally defective subjects are unable to sustain deviation for 30 sec. It is hard to sustain the eyes in any position, horizontal or vertical, off of the midline.
4. Under normal resting conditions, the vectors for lateral deviation of the head are opposite and equal: the head and eyes remain in the midline. Suppose you have examined a patient who had the sudden onset of complete *left* hemiplegia involving the movements of the mouth as well as of the extremities. He must, therefore, have a lesion of corticobulbar and corticospinal tracts at a rostral brainstem or cerebral level on the ☐ right / ☐ left side.
   a. What would you expect to be the position of the head and eyes in this patient? ☐ midline / ☐ turned to the left / ☐ turned to the right.

right

turned to the right

b. Explain the answer to part *a:* ______________________________
____
____
____.

Ans: The head and eye turning center of the right cerebral hemisphere or its corticobulbar fibers have been destroyed by the lesion. The center for head and eye turning of the left hemisphere would be acting unopposed. Therefore, the head and eyes would be turned to the right, opposite to the hemiplegic side. This example again shows the unity of visual and motor space. The same center, the right motor cortex, which guides extremity movement in the left half of space, also turns the head and eyes to the left. Review Fig. 5-1.

right

5. Some cerebral lesions act as irritants to the cortical neurons. They cause an excessive discharge of impulses, akin to stimulation by an electrode. Such an irritative lesion is called an *epileptogenic focus* because it initiates epileptic seizures. Suppose you have observed a patient with an epileptic seizure which began by turning of the head and eyes to the *left*. You would anticipate that he had an epileptogenic focus in the ☐ right/ ☐ left frontal lobe. See Fig. 5-7*C*.

right

6. After the epileptic cataclysm has subsided, the cortical neurons which have been discharging excessively are metabolically exhausted and temporarily nonfunctional. Immediately *after* an epileptic seizure caused by a right-sided cerebral lesion, to which side would the head and eyes be turned? ☐ right/ ☐ left? Explain:
____
____
____

Ans: Since the *right* eye and head turning center is exhausted, the *left* acts unopposed. The head and eyes turn to the right, opposite to the direction they turned during the seizure.

movements
muscles

7. Cortical or corticobulbar pathway lesions, as we have seen, paralyze conjugate eye movements. The group of muscles participating in the movements are not paralytic. A nerve lesion, on the other hand, such as of the VIth nerve, paralyzes a muscle, leaving other movements intact. In special cases, such as the MLF syndrome, where the lesion is in an internuclear (internuncial) axonal system, the muscle is paralyzed during only one movement and acts during others. Apart from a few special cases such as the MLF syndrome, we can conclude that ocular movements illustrate the epigram that UMN lesions paralyze ☐ movements/ ☐ muscles, while LMN lesions paralyze ☐ movements/ ☐ muscles.

8. In fact, the MLF syndrome helps to emphasize that when an individual muscle is paralytic for only one movement and participates in others, the responsible lesion cannot be in the LMN.

Bibliography

Hoyt, W. F., and Daroff, R. B.: Supranuclear disorders of ocular control systems in man, in *The Control of Eye Movements,* Bach-y-Rita, P., and Collins, C. C. (eds), New York, Academic Press, 1971.

Ross, A., and DeMyer, W.: Isolated syndrome of the medial longitudinal fasciculus in man, *Arch. Neurol.,* 15:203-205, 1966.

Rothstein, T. L., and Alvord, E. C., Jr.: Posterior internuclear ophthalmophlegia, *Arch. Neurol.,* 24:191–202, 1971.

C. *Eye-hand coordination in visuosensory space and the tonic neck reflexes (TNRs)*

1. The tonic neck reflex (TNR) is elicited this way: With the infant or child *supine* and *quiet*, the examiner gently but forcefully turns the head to one side, holding it there for at least 30 sec. The result is shown in Fig. 5-8.

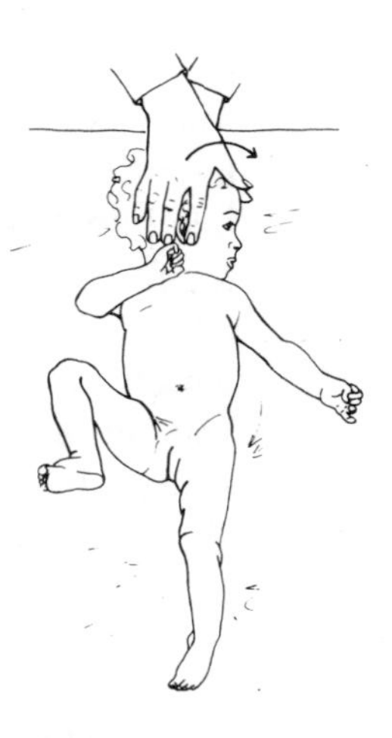

FIG. 5-8. Posture of the extremities during a tonic neck reflex. The examiner has forcefully turned the infant's head to the left.

2. The normal infant shows the posture of Fig. 5-8 to some degree, but quickly struggles out of it. TNRs are most prominent between the ages of 2 to 4 months, at a time when the infant is learning to fixate and reach for objects. Careful observation of normal infants of this age discloses that they spend much time in the TNR posture.
3. The expected result of the head-turning maneuver can be remembered by the rule that the *head looks to the side of the extended extremities.* Since the head and eyes look to the side of the extending hand, we can interpret the TNR as the forerunner of eye-hand coordination. One's eyes discover one's hand moving in space. The eyes then learn to direct the hand as it explores space and learns to grasp visual targets.
4. The TNR is set into action when head turning stimulates position sense receptors in the neck. The afferent pathway of the reflex runs *rostrally* into the brainstem and then *caudally* into the cord by extrapyramidal UMN pathways of the brainstem. The reflex is interpreted as a primitive movement pattern. It disappears as cerebral pathways establish dominance over the primitive reflexes during maturation. Any undue persistence of the TNR posture, either when spontaneously assumed by the infant or induced by an examiner, predicts poor motor development. It indicates that UMN dominance over

the primitive reflexes is not proceeding according to the normal developmental timetable. UMN control of movement will be faulty.

5. The TNRs may reappear in older children or adults who suffer high brainstem lesions interrupting corticobulbar and other descending motor pathways: cerebral dominance over the stem is lost.
6. When the head of an infant is turned to one side, the ipsilateral extremities ☐ flex / ☐ extend, while the contralateral extremities ☐ flex / ☐ extend. This reflex is called the ________.
   a. The foregoing definition is ☐ operational / ☐ interpretational.
   b. An operational definition states fact (or an agreed upon procedure). Give an interpretational definition of the TNR: ________

extend
flex
TNR
operational

Ans: An interpretational definition of the TNR is that it is a primitive brainstem reflex underlying normal visuomotor development. It disappears during maturation as the UMNs establish dominance over primitive reflex mechanisms.

7. What is the pathophysiologic interpretation and prognostic significance of undue persistence of the TNR after the fourth month? ________

Ans: Persistence of the TNRs indicates that UMN dominance over the brainstem reflexes is not proceeding according to the developmental timetable. The infant is likely to show permanent deficits in UMN control of movement.

Bibliography

Magnus, R.: Cameron Prize Lectures on some results of studies in the physiology of posture, *Lancet,* 2:531-536; 585-588, 1926.

Roberts, T.: *Neurophysiology of Postural Mechanisms,* New York, Plenum Pub. Corp., 1967.

IV. Nystagmus

A. Introduction

1. Eye position at any time is the result of many competing forces:
   a. The activity of cortical head and eye turning centers.
   b. The position of the head in relation to space, movement, and gravity.
   c. The illumination and conditions of vision.
   d. The refractive error of the eyes.
   e. The demands of binocular fixation and image fusion.
   f. The survival and advantage-seeking possibilities of the circumstances and the intent of the bearer of the eyes.
2. The incessant counterplay of these forces requires intricate feedback circuits. The exquisite control afforded by feedback circuitry encumbers a peril: feedback circuits oscillate when something goes awry.

a. Involuntary to-and-fro oscillations of the eyes are called *nystagmus.* The types and causes are many, perhaps not infinite, but many.

b. It is unimportant to know all the possible types of nystagmus. What you must be able to do is describe what the patient shows and trace through a dendrogram, which will lead you to the probable diagnosis.

B. *Symptoms of nystagmus*

1. The *symptoms* are:
   a. Nausea (with or without vomiting).
   b. Vertigo: a sensation of movement, frequently rotation of self or environment.
   c. Oscillopsia: oscillating vision, oscillation of objects viewed.
2. The presence of *symptoms* depends on age of onset and type of nystagmus. Recall that heterotropia of congenital or early origin usually causes no diplopia. Similarly, nystagmus of congenital or early origin usually is asymptomatic.

C. *The signs of nystagmus*

1. *The form of nystagmus:* In analyzing the signs of nystagmus, the *initial* step is to classify the nystagmus as to the *form* of eye movement.

Nystagmus form
→ Horizontal
→ Vertical
→ Rotatory
→ Mixed

a. The major forms of nystagmus are easy to remember if you will ask yourself this: What are the *possible* forms of eye movement? They all occur around one of the ocular axes.
(1) Horizontal (lateral) eye movements are rotations around the ______ ______ axis.
(2) Vertical movements are rotations around the ______ ______ axis.
(3) Rotatory movements (torsions) are rotations around the ______ ______ axis.

b. Hence, the *forms* of nystagmus are:

Nystagmus forms
→ ______
→ ______
→ ______
→ ______

2. *The types of eye excursions*
   a. The *second* step is to observe whether the eye excursions are of *jerk* or *pendular* type. Jerk nystagmus has a *fast* and *slow* component.

vertical

lateral

A-P

Horizontal
Vertical
Rotatory
Mixed

pendular
jerk

pendular
jerk

Pendular nystagmus is like a pendulum: the excursions are of equal velocity. It is a tick-tock or metronomic movement.

b. If to = fro, the patient has ______________________ nystagmus.

c. If to ≠ fro, the patient has ______________________ nystagmus.

3. *The direction of nystagmus*

a. The *third* step, if the patient has jerk nystagmus, is to identify the *direction* of the nystagmus. The direction is usually named according to the direction of movement of the fast component.

right

b. If the nystagmus has the fast component to the right side, we say the direction is to the ______________________.

c. If the direction of the fast component is always to one side, the nystagmus is said to be *unidirectional.* If the direction of the fast component changes with the direction of eye movement, the nystagmus is *bidirectional.*

4. *The effect of eye movement:* determine whether the nystagmus changes in rate, amplitude or direction when the eyes are moved through the various fields of gaze. The data from direct observation of the patient, when integrated with the history, permits you to enter the dendrograms of Figs. 5-10 and 5-11. The basic data are summarized in Fig. 5-9.

1. Form:
Horizontal
Vertical
Rotatory
Mixed

2. Type:
Pendular
Jerk

3. Direction:
*Uni*directional
*Bi*directional

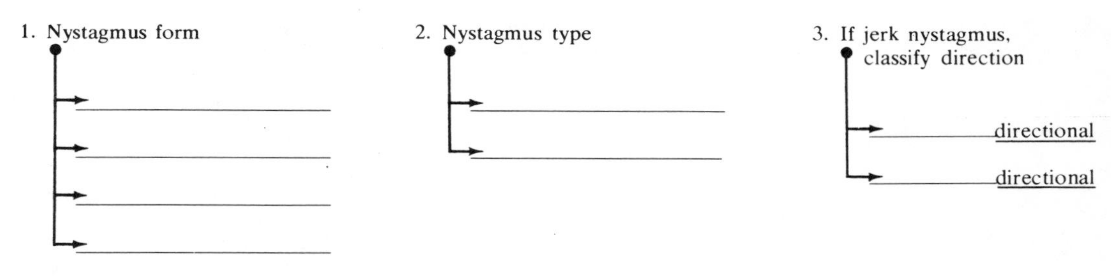

FIG. 5-9. The observations required for diagnosing the cause of nystagmus. You must note the form, type, and direction of the nystagmus.

5. Spontaneous nystagmus or that induced by caloric irrigation or positional change can be recorded electrically, electronystagmography. However, this specialized procedure is not widely available.

D. The dendrograms for nystagmus, Figs. 5-10 and 5-11.

1. After the nystagmus has been classified, the dendrograms lead you to the probable diagnosis. Notice that *pendular* nystagmus implies an ocular cause or lesion. *Jerk* nystagmus implies a *vestibular* or *neural* lesion. The dendrograms are for reference only. Trace through them, but do not attempt to memorize.

2. *Dendrogram for jerk nystagmus, Fig. 5-10.*

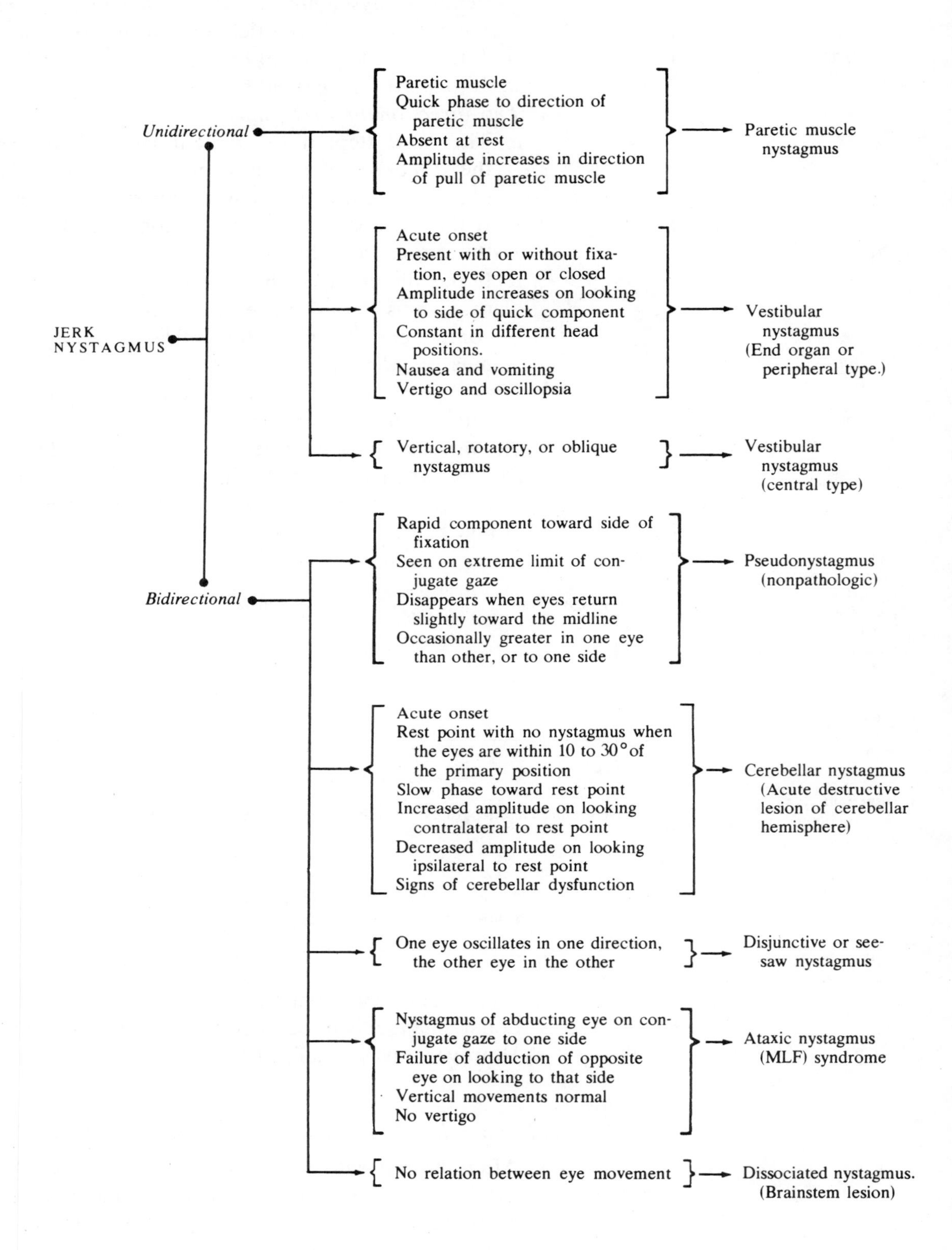

FIG. 5-10. Differential diagnostic dendrogram for jerk nystagmus. (Reference only.)

3. *Dendrogram for pendular nystagmus, Fig. 5-11.*

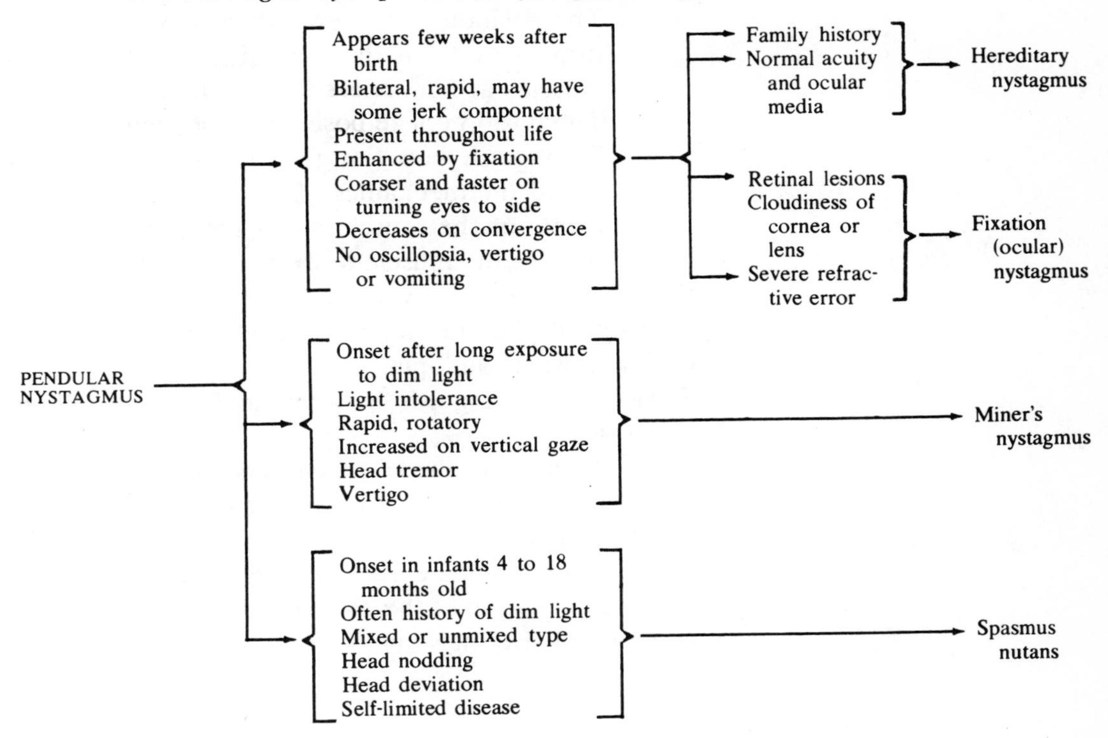

FIG. 5-11. Differential diagnostic dendrogram for pendular nystagmus. (Reference only.)

Bibliography

Carpenter, R. H. S.: *Movements of the Eyes,* London, Pion, 1977.

Kornhuber, H. H., and Fredrickson, J. M.: Recent clinical and experimental results concerning vestibular and oculomotor mechanisms. *Internat. J. Neurol.,* 8:23-33, 1970.

Korres, S.: Electronystagmographic criteria in neuro-otological diagnosis. 1: Peripheral lesions. 2: Central nervous system lesions, *J. Neurol. Neurosurg. Psychiatry,* 41:249-253, 254-264, 1978.

Walsh, F. and Hoyt, W.: *Clinical Neuro-ophthalmology,* 3rd ed., Baltimore, The Williams & Wilkins Company, 1969.

V. Summary of ocular motility. Sit down with another student and go over these points, which you must know:

A. The three axes of ocular rotation, corresponding to the three major anatomic planes of the body.

B. The three ocular nerves, their nuclei of origin, and terminal muscles.

C. The six muscles, their origin and insertion in relation to the axes of ocular rotation.

1. The muscles (or the tendon in the case of superior oblique) all insert *distal* to the way they approach the globe. See Fig. 2-20.
2. Only one muscle, the inferior oblique, arises anteriorly.
3. Only one muscle, lateral rectus, has its vector pulling *lateral* to the vertical axis. See Fig. 2-27.

D. For clinical application, think through these things:
1. The position of the eye when only one nerve is interrupted. The eyes turn away from the pull of the paralytic muscle because the intact muscles act unopposed.
2. The position of the eye when only one nerve is functioning.
3. Distinguish between the *possible* movements of the muscle according to the mechanics of origin and insertion, and the *strongest* movements of the muscle when the eye is rotated into the optimum position for the muscle to exert the strongest pull.

E. The role of the cover-uncover test in analyzing heterotropia (and heterophoria if you did the optional section).

F. The laws of diplopia.

G. How to distinguish between and identify sympathetic and IIIrd nerve ptosis.

H. The location of the UMN centers and LMN nuclei for conjugate eye movement and the concept of an eye-centering mechanism.

I. The different course of the corticobulbar fibers for conjugate lateral gaze and conjugate vertical gaze and convergence.

J. An explanation of the role of the MLF in lateral conjugate eye movements, based on Hering's law of equal innervation of yoke muscles.

VI. Summary of the eye examination

A. Now we have to unite the individual fragments of the eye examination into a coherent routine. I would have no trouble convincing you to practice if you were a tennis player wanting to improve his strokes or an actor. If a great actor were to play the role of a physician, he would practice hour after hour to capture the exact nuances of professional behavior. Ours, too, is a performing art. Do you always want to look like a beginner? If not practice with another student until you can offer a professional performance to your patient. Then you can say, with Blaise Cendrars:

> I have deciphered all the confused texts of the wheels and I have assembled the scattered elements of a most violent beauty

B. Part V, A, 1-5 of the Summarized Neurologic Examination organizes the scattered elements of the eye examination. Practice, *practice,* until they unite into one beautiful, flowing sequence for testing cranial nerves II, III, IV, and VI. Prove to yourself that you know this sequence by rehearsing with another student.

C. The five steps that you have just rehearsed constitute a minimum routine examination. Patients with ocular complaints or in whom you suspect a brain disorder may need a more thorough analysis of ocular motility mechanisms. Use Table 5-6 as a reference as needed to supplement Part V, A of the basic examination. Notice that steps 1-3 apply to the conscious, cooperative patient, while steps 4-5 depend on reflex or associated movements not under conscious control.

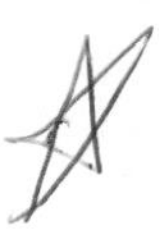

TABLE 5-6. *Outline of Clinical Tests for Central Eye Movement Disorders*

Type of Eye Movement	Method of Examination
1. Spontaneous movements during ordinary behavior and ordinary environmental stimuli.	Inspection while taking the history. Look for malalignment, range and persistence of eye movements, and for hyperkinesias such as nystagmus.
2. Volitional fixation and volitional movements.	Examiner observes steadiness and range of eye movements after commanding patient to fixate on a distant, straight ahead object and then to move the eyes to the *right, left, up,* and *down.*
3. Visual reflex ocular movements:	
a. Smooth pursuit	The patient's eyes pursue the examiner's finger as it moves through the full range of ocular movements.
b. Vergences	The examiner directs the patient to look at near and distant objects and to follow the examiner's moving finger in toward the patient's nose.
c. Reflex fixation	The patient fixates straight ahead and the examiner turns the patient's head slowly to the right, left, up, and down.
d. Alignment lock	As the patient fixates straight ahead the examiner alternately covers and uncovers first one, then the other eye and looks for deviation in alignment from monocular occlusion of vision (cover-uncover test).
*e. Optokinetic nystagmus (OKN)	Patient fixates on rotating drum or a moving striped strip.
4. Nonvisual reflex ocular movements:	
†a. Caloric nystagmus	Irrigation of ears with hot or cold water.
†b. Positional nystagmus	Placing the patient's head in various postures.
†c. Contraversive eye turning test (Doll's eye test, oculocephalic test).	Quick turning of the patient's head by the examiner's hands. Used in comatose patients.
†5. Associated eye movement (Bell's phenomenon).	The examiner holds the patient's eyelids open and observes the involuntary upward movement of the eyes that occurs when the patient attempts to close the eyes.

*Not discussed in this text
†Discussed later in text

6

Motor Examination of Cranial Nerves V, VII, IX, X, XI, and XII

"To those I address, it is unnecessary to go farther, than to indicate that the nerves treated of in these papers are the instruments of expression, from the smile upon the infant's cheek to the last agony of life. . ."

— Charles Bell (1774-1842)

I. Vth nerve

A. Functional anatomy

1. The Vth nerve chews. Chewing requires not only jaw closure but also a grinding, lateral movement.
2. Place your fingertips over the posterior part of your cheeks, about 2 cm above and in front of the angle of the mandible. Bite hard and relax several times. The muscle you feel is the *masseter. Masseter, temporal*, and *medial pterygoid* muscles close the jaw, but only the masseter can be adequately palpated. The pull of these muscles is relatively direct and uncomplicated.
3. Move your jaw from side to side. *Lateral* movement is caused by contraction of the *lateral* pterygoid muscles. It can only be understood by knowing the origin and insertion of the muscles.
4. In Fig. 6-1, study the origin and insertion of the lateral pterygoid muscle and the effect of its contraction on the tip of the mandible. Notice that the origin of the muscle from the base of the skull is immobile. When the muscle acts, only the mandible can move. The vector diagram indicates the movement of the tip when both muscles contract equally.
5. If only the right lateral pterygoid muscle contracts, the tip of the mandible moves to the ☐ right / ☐ left.
6. If the patient can move his jaw to the right but not to the left, he has paralysis of ☐ the right / ☐ the left / ☐ both lateral pterygoid muscle(s).

left

right

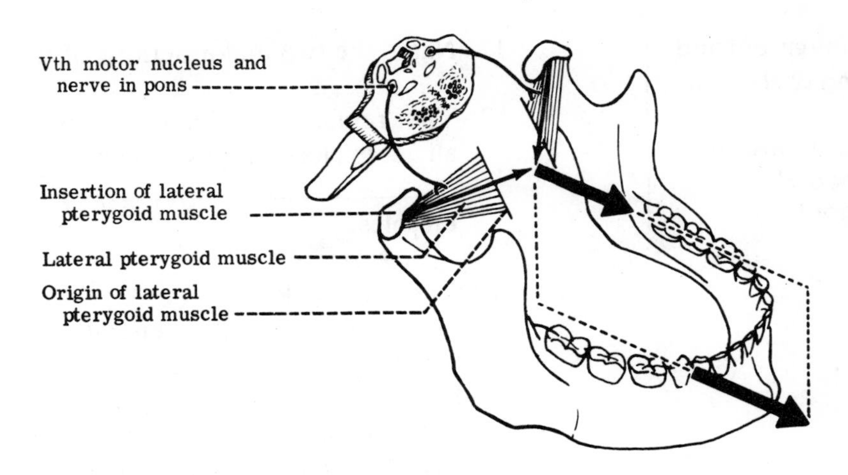

FIG. 6-1. Innervation and action of the lateral pterygoid muscles. If both muscles contract equally, the tip of the mandible moves forward in the midline. If only one muscle contracts, the tip moves forward and to the opposite side. Study the vector diagram (arrows between the muscles).

7. A second action of the lateral pterygoid muscle is to aid in opening the jaw by its insertion on the neck of the mandible. Study Fig. 6-2 for an understanding of this action.

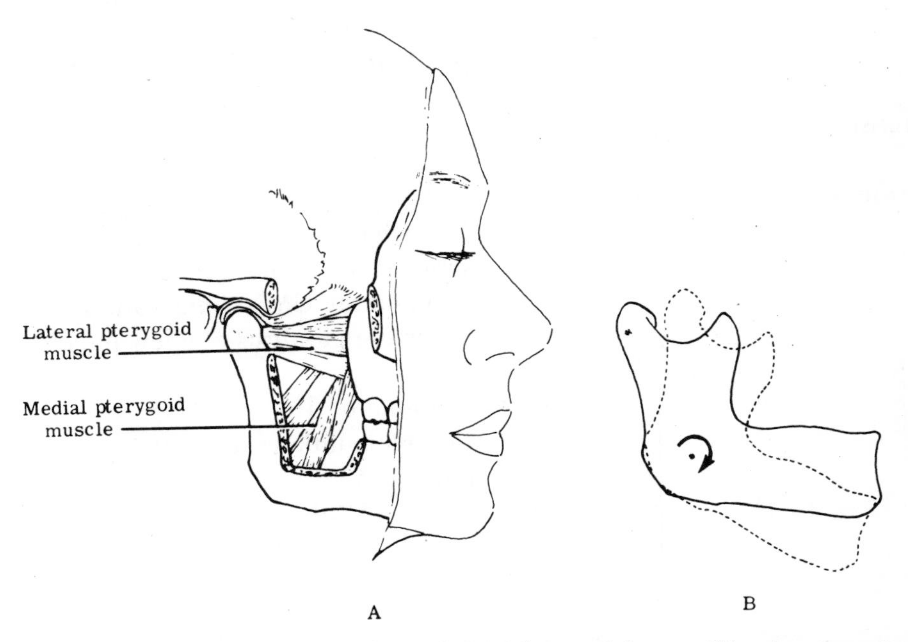

FIG. 6-2. Action of lateral pterygoid muscles to depress the tip of the mandible when the patient forcefully opens his jaw. The forward pull of the lateral pterygoid muscles acts to open the jaw because the jaw is suspended so as to rotate around an axis, as shown in B.

lateral pterygoid

right
down

left

8. If the patient's mandible moves forward and down in the *midline* on jaw opening, both ________ ________ muscles are contracted equally.
9. If the left lateral pterygoid muscle acts alone, the tip of the mandible moves not only to the ☐ right / ☐ left but also ☐ up / ☐ down.
10. If the patient's jaw deviates to the left on forceful opening, there is weakness of the ☐ right / ☐ left lateral pterygoid muscle.

lateral movement and opening of the jaw

11. Name the two major actions of the lateral pterygoid muscles: ______

masseter, temporal, and medial pterygoid

12. The remaining mandibular muscles innervated by the Vth nerve all act to close the jaw. The names of these muscles are: ______ ______ muscles.

B. UMN lesions of V

UMN = upper motor neuron

1. In accordance with general principles of UMN innervation, each Vth nerve nucleus receives axons from the contralateral hemisphere. However, the principle of contralateral motor innervation requires some qualification, because not all movements are carried out unilaterally. Many movements, such as trunk flexion, vertical head movements, chewing, and swallowing, are carried out by proximal muscles which act with bilateral symmetry much or all the time. Try to contract half of your diaphragm, half of your anal sphincter, and half of your abdomen. It is not to be denied that you can learn to make some of these movements unilaterally, such as abdominal muscle contraction, but it is not the customary action of these muscles. The law of contralateral innervation holds for movements such as those of the hand, which have as their outstanding characteristic free, independent unilateral mobility. Hence, we can say that:

bilateral

a. The muscles which ordinarily act symmetrically have ☐ only ipsilateral/ ☐ bilateral/ ☐ only contralateral UMN innervation.

contralateral

b. The distal muscles which ordinarily act unilaterally have mainly ☐ ipsilateral/ ☐ bilateral/ ☐ contralateral UMN innervation.

2. The trigeminal motor action falls between the two extremes of bilateral symmetrical movement and unilateral, independent movement. Because of bilateral UMN innervation, unilateral UMN lesions do not cause complete paralysis of chewing, only a mild and transitory paresis.

C. LMN lesions of V

1. Complete unilateral paralysis of the chewing muscles with other muscles intact implicates an LMN lesion. Explain in terms of general principles of UMN and LMN innervation. ______ ______ ______ ______

Ans: LMN. Since each trigeminal motor nucleus receives numerous UMN fibers from each motor cortex, a unilateral corticobulbar tract lesion does not denervate the nucleus. In a more general sense, UMN lesions do not selectively paralyze individual muscles or sets of muscles innervated by one peripheral nerve.

masseter

2. With LMN lesions, either of the neuron body or the nerve trunk, the axons may die. If the axons to a muscle die, we say the muscle is *denervated.* When a muscle is denervated, it undergoes atrophy. Atrophy of muscle, then, is one characteristic of LMN lesions. Which muscle innervated by the Vth nerve can be most readily palpated to check for atrophy? ______

D. Clinical tests of Vth nerve motor function

Note: Do each of the tests on yourself as they are described.

1. The temporal muscle fills out the temple. Check for atrophy by inspecting the temple. Even when the patient bites, the muscle is difficult to palpate. But if the muscle is atrophic from a LMN lesion, the temple is sunken.
2. The masseter is tested by palpation, just as you have already done on yourself. To test the patient's masseter, palpate the region of the muscle and ask the patient to bite hard.
3. The strength of jaw closure is tested by having the patient bite hard. Place the heel of one hand on the tip of the patient's mandible and the other on his forehead. Press hard on the tip of the mandible. You must help support his head with your opposite hand because jaw closure is a very strong movement and you do not want to test the strenth of head extension and jaw closure at the same time. You want to test only one muscle or set of muscles at a time.
4. Lateral pterygoids are tested by having the patient forcefully open his jaw as you note how its tip aligns with the notch between the upper, medial incisor teeth. Then you ask him to move his jaw from side to side. Finally ask him to hold his jaw forcefully to the side as you try to push it back to the center with the heel of your palm. What do you do with your opposite hand to avoid straining his neck? ________________________

Press against the opposite cheekbone

5. To be certain you know what to do, test Vth nerve motor function on yourself and on your guinea pig roommate. Don't just sit there: get up off of your ________________ and do it! I can't tell you the relative strength of movements. You have to begin to build up your own catalog of standards.

censored

E. Analyze this patient, a 46-year-old man with difficulty in chewing. Examination disclosed atrophy and complete paralysis of the left temporal and masseter muscles. When he opened his jaw, it deviated to the left. He could not move it forcefully to the right. He had no motor deficits involving the other cranial or somatic muscles.

The evidence points to ☐ an LMN/ ☐ a UMN lesion on the ☐ right/ ☐ left/ ☐ both side(s). Explain. ________________________

LMN
left

Ans: An LMN lesion is indicated because the paralysis affects only the muscles of a single nerve, V, the paralysis is complete, and the muscles are atrophic. Since the atrophic and paralyzed muscles are on the left, the left Vth nerve is involved.

Bibliography

Ramfjord, S., and Ash, M., Jr.: *Occlusion,* Philadelphia, W. B. Saunders Co., 1966.

II. The motor function of the VIIth cranial nerve

A. *Functional anatomy*

1. Look into a mirror and make every facial movement you can, including wiggling your ears. Every facial movement (excluding mandibular movements) tests the integrity of the VIIth cranial nerve. Work through Table 6-1.

TABLE 6-1. Clinically Important Movements and Muscles Innervated by the VIIth Cranial Nerve

Movements	Muscles
1. *Wrinkle up* your forehead, as in looking up as far as possible	Frontalis
2. *Close* your eyes as tightly as possible	Orbicularis oculi, the sphincter of the palpebral fissure
3. *Close* your lips as tightly as possible	Orbicularis oris, the sphincter of the oral fissure.
4. *Pull back* the corners of your mouth strongly, as in smiling. At the same time palpate your cheeks	Buccinator
5. *Pull down* the corners of your mouth strongly, as in pouting. At the same time palpate the anterolateral aspect of your neck and observe it in the mirror	Platysma

Vth

2. VII thus innervates *all* muscles of facial expression, the "mimic" muscles. These muscles stand guard around every facial aperture: the palpebral fissures, oral fissure, nares, and external auditory canals. In generalizing that VII innervates all facial muscles, we mean only the facial muscles proper. Mandibular muscles are innervated by the ____________ cranial nerve.
3. If we conceive of VII and its muscles as the guardian of the size and expression of the facial apertures, we can extend the notion of a guardian function to the middle ear. Here, VII innervates the *stapedius* muscle. Stapedius acts to dampen excessive movement of the ossicles during loud sounds. When it is paralyzed, the patient may report that ordinary sounds are uncomfortably loud.
4. The only clinically testable sensory function of VII is taste, to be studied later.
5. As is typical of peripheral nerves, the VIIth nerves do not cross the midline. Study only the LMNs of VII in Fig. 6-3. We will return to the UMN innervation later.

ipsilateral

ipsilateral

6. If the left VIIth nerve is cut, the patient would be unable to move the ☐ lower half / ☐ upper half / ☐ ipsilateral half of his face. Thus, if a patient has paralysis of all facial muscles on the right or left half of his face, he has an ☐ ipsilateral / ☐ contralateral LMN lesion of the VIIth nerve.

B. *LMNs of VII.* Study Fig. 6-4, learn the names, and compare it with the generalized brainstem section in Fig. 3-13

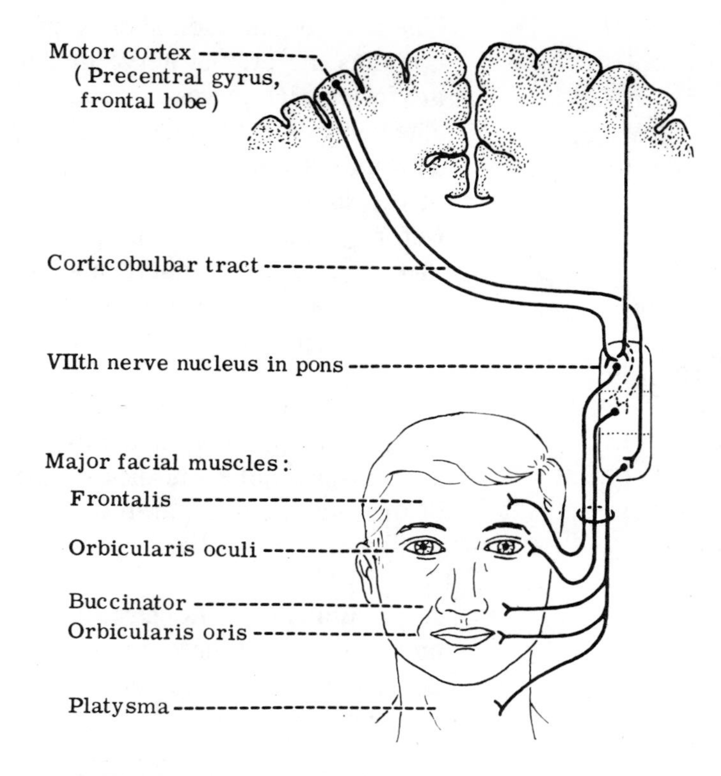

FIG. 6-3. UMN and LMN innervation of the facial muscles. The dotted lines indicate that the orbicularis oculi muscles receive a variable number of crossed and uncrossed axons. Therefore, the degree of weakness of the muscle varies with UMN lesions.

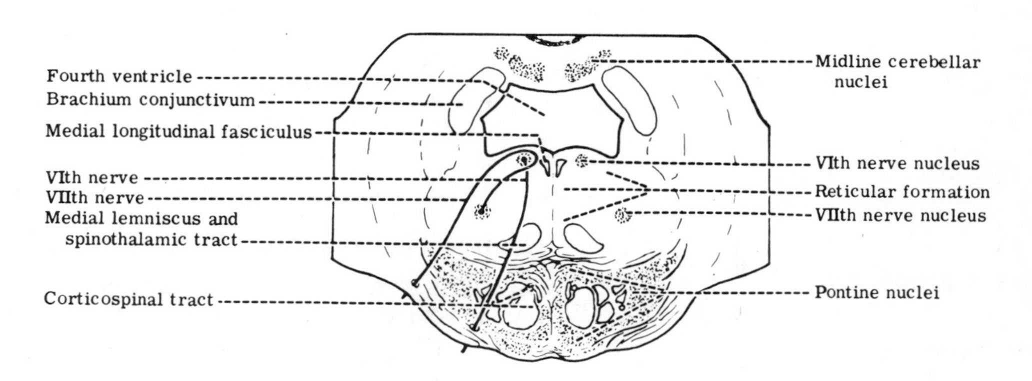

FIG. 6-4. Transverse section of the pons at a caudal level to include the VIth and VIIth cranial nerve nuclei. The VIth and VIIth nerves, along with the VIIIth, exit at the pontomedullary sulcus.

1. Notice the peculiar internal loop of VII around the VIth nerve nucleus. Using a colored pencil, draw in the course of the VIth and VIIth nerves on the opposite side of Fig. 6-4.

tectum
cerebellar

2. In accordance with general principles of brainstem anatomy, the roof of the pons is called the ______________. It contains the ______________ nuclei.

tegmentum

V, VI, VII

basis
corticospinal

VIth

VI, VII, VIII
(Review Fig. 3-10 if you erred.)

ipsilateral
LMN

3. The second longitudinal division of the pons, the ______________, contains the cranial nerve nuclei. The three motor nuclei of the pons are for cranial nerves ______________, ______________, and ______________.
4. The ventralmost longitudinal zone is the ______________. Through it run the ______________ tracts to the LMNs of the spinal cord.
5. Before exiting from the pons, the VIIth nerve fibers loop around the ______________ nerve nucleus.
6. Three cranial nerves exit at the pontomedullary sulcus. In ventrodorsal order, these nerves are ______________, ______________, and ______________.
7. No matter whether a lesion destroys the VIIth nerve nucleus, the intra-axial course of the axons, or the peripheral nerve trunk, the result is paralysis of the muscles of the ☐ ipsilateral / ☐ contralateral side of the face. Such a paralysis is called ☐ LMN / ☐ UMN paralysis.

C. UMNs of VII

1. A preliminary demonstration of the degree of unilaterality of facial movements will help to unravel the pattern of UMN paralysis and will fix it for easy recall forever. Try these movements as you watch in your mirror:

TABLE 6-2. Tests for Unilaterality of Facial Movements

Movement	Result
a. Retract one corner of your mouth at a time.	*Every* normal person can do it: The movement is *unilateral*.
b. Wink one eye at a time. Watch in your mirror for simultaneous contraction of the opposite orbicularis oculi muscle.	*Most* can do it, but some will be unable to wink one eye without the other. When one eye winks, the opposite orbicularis oculi contracts to some degree.
c. Elevate one eyebrow at a time.	*Few* will be able to do it, but everyone can elevate them together. The movement is essentially *bilateral*.

lip retraction

forehead elevation

2. The freest unilateral facial movement usually is ☐ forehead elevation / ☐ eyelid closure / ☐ lip retraction.
3. The least free unilateral facial movement usually is ☐ forehead elevation / ☐ eyelid closure / ☐ lip retraction.
4. The utility of the various facial movements provides a plausible explanation for the gradient of unilaterality. Notice when eating that you make unilateral lip movements to manipulate food and clear it from your cheeks. Indeed, one of the chief discomforts of a facial palsy is that food lodges in the cheek. Unilateral forehead movements offer no such utility. Although usually the eyes blink together, sometimes you need to close only one. Thus, the utility of lid closure falls between that of lid retraction and forehead wrinkling.

opposite

5. Body parts such as the hand and lip which have the freest, most independent unilateral movements derive their UMN innervation ☐ equally from each hemisphere / ☐ mainly from the opposite hemisphere.

6. Proximal customarily synchronous movements, such as chewing, swallowing, esophageal constriction and sphincter contraction, receive about the same number of UMN axons from each hemisphere, let us say 50/50. Free, independent unilateral movements are innervated by crossed and uncrossed axons in ratio of, let us say, 90/10. For movements with an intermediate degree of unilateral independence, the ratio might be 60/40, 70/30, and so on.

lip retraction
forehead wrinkling

7. Now predict the pattern of facial muscle weakness after unilateral destruction of one corticobulbar pathway. The patient would show *most* paralysis of ☐ forehead wrinkling / ☐ eyelid closure / ☐ lip retraction and *least* paralysis of ☐ forehead wrinkling / ☐ eyelid closure / ☐ lip retraction.
8. When the UMN lesion is large and acute, such as with a massive cerebral infarct, eyelid closure is usually paretic (incompletely paralyzed), along with paralysis of lip retraction. Because such a patient has weakness of eyelid closure, the physician who does not understand the gradient of unilaterality of facial movement frequently errs in thinking that the patient has an LMN VIIth nerve lesion.
9. Since lip retraction is the movement most affected by UMN lesions, the clinician must watch carefully for it during his interview and examination. The most reliable way to detect unilateral weakness of lip retraction is to watch for asymmetry of the depth and movement of the nasolabial folds, the prominent skin creases beginning just lateral to the lips and bowing upward to the nose. Using your mirror, observe these two creases when your lips are at rest, and during speaking.
10. Shortly after a UMN lesion, lip retraction contralateral to the lesion will be paralytic both during volitional movement *and* during emotional expression, such as smiling. In the chronic phase of the UMN lesion, especially if the patient has bilateral UMN lesions, lip retraction may remain weak during volitional action, but may be prominent or even exaggerated during emotional expression. Thus, the pathways for emotional expression differ from those for volitional, but we do not know their course.

D. *Clinical testing*

1. Inspection begins as you meet the patient and talk with him. Notice the play of facial muscles during ordinary speech and during emotional expression. Many disorders, such as muscular dystrophy, parkinsonism, and depression, reduce facial movement, a condition called "masked facies," in which the face is immobile—as though the patient wore a mask. Look for asymmetry of facial movements, asymmetry of blinking, and asymmetry of the movement and depth of the nasolabial folds.
2. Work through Table 6-4 with a partner. Often it is quicker for the examiner to illustrate the desired movements as he gives the commands. In working through Table 6-4, pay particular attention to the strength of eyelid closure. Can you open your partners eyelids against his maximum effort at closure? ____
____
____
____.

Don't go to Aristotle for the answer: answer the question after you try the test.

TABLE 6-4. Summary of Methods for Testing the Motor Function of Cranial Nerve VII

Command	Test	Muscle tested
(1) "Wrinkle up your forehead," or "Look up at the ceiling."	Inspect for asymmetry	Frontalis
(2) "Close your eyes tight and don't let me open them."	Inspect for asymmetry of wrinkles; try to pull eyelids apart	Orbicularis oculi
(3) "Pull back the corners of your mouth."	Inspect for asymmetry of nasolabial fold	Buccinator
(4) "Wrinkle up the skin on your neck," or "Pull down hard on the corners of your mouth."	Inspect for asymmetry	Platysma

3. Fig. 6-5 shows two patients with facial palsies. Each patient was asked to close her eyes tightly and to pull back the corners of her mouth as in smiling. Carefully inspect both sides of each face for asymmetry of facial movement and for differences in the bulk of the chewing muscles.

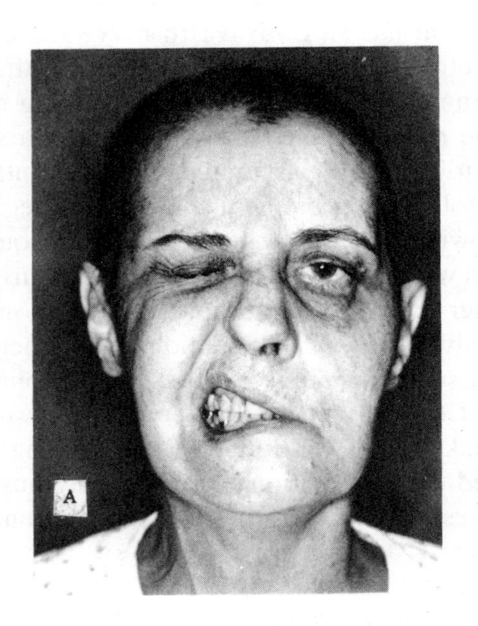

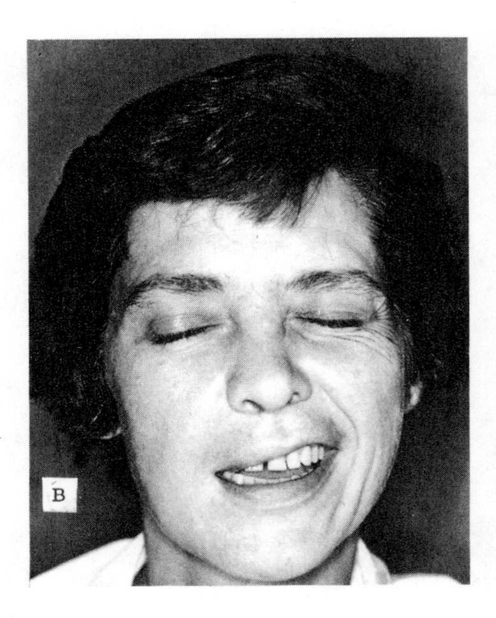

FIG. 6-5. Two patients with facial palsies. Each had been asked to close her eyes tightly and to pull back the corners of her mouth as in smiling.

See next frame.

4. Describe the abnormalities in the face of Patient A of Fig. 6-5: ________________________________.

left VIIth nerve

5. Patient A has weakness of eyelid closure on the left, as shown by lack of contraction of the orbicularis oculi muscle and absence of any wrinkles around her eye. The mouth retractors on the left are paralyzed. When this patient was asked to look up, the left half of her forehead failed to wrinkle. This pattern of total paralysis of all facial muscles on one side implicates a lesion of the ☐ right/ ☐ left ☐ VIIth nerve/ ☐ corticobulbar tract.

6. The cognoscente* of physical diagnosis will also have noticed on the left side of Patient A the hollowing of her temporal fossa and the concavity over the masseter muscle, indicating atrophy of the muscles and thus a

* A person having or claiming expert knowledge
CONNOISSEUR

V

VI

See next frame

☑ corticobulbar
☑ left
UMN

lesion of the ______________________ *th* cranial nerve. If you missed this finding, remember that you must compare both halves of the body, specifically looking for such asymmetries. Patient A had been operated on for removal of an acoustic nerve tumor, a neurofibroma. The tumor, expanding in the cerebellopontine angle, had already destroyed the Vth and VIIth cranial nerves, but since she had no weakness of abduction of her left eye, the ______________________ *th* cranial nerve was spared.

7. Describe the abnormalities in the face of Patient B of Fig. 6-5. ____________ ______________________.

8. The right side of her mouth failed to retract, and she has weakness of eyelid closure on the right, as shown by the wider exposure of the upper lid and lack of wrinkling around the right eye. This wrinkling on the normal side results from the purse-string, sphincter action of the orbicularis oculi muscle. When Patient B looked up, her forehead acted equally on both sides. Thus, on the right side of the patient's face, forehead movements were active, eyelid closure was weak, and mouth retraction was paralyzed. This gradient of involvement of the facial movement on the right side of the patient's face indicates a lesion of the: ☐ right/ ☐ left ______________________ nerve / ☐ corticobulbar tract originating from the ☐ right / ☐ left cerebral hemisphere. This is a(an) ☐ LMN / ☐ UMN facial palsy.

9. Patient B had suffered a cerebral infarct from occlusion of the middle cerebral artery to her left cerebral hemisphere.

III. Motor functions of the IXth and Xth cranial nerves

A. Functional anatomy. Learn Figs. 6-6 and 6-7

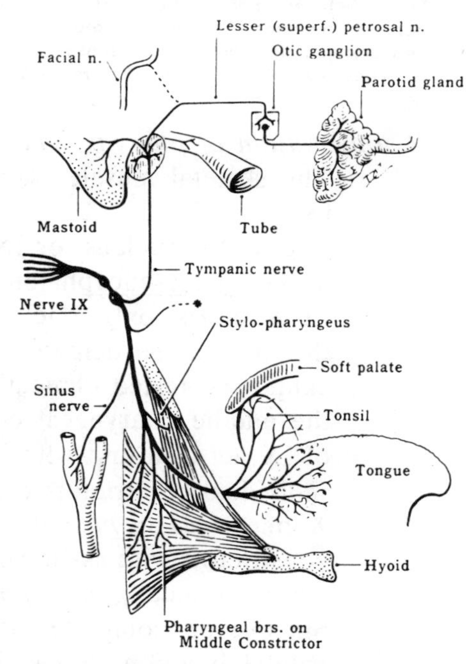

FIG. 6-6. Innervation of the palate, tongue, and pharynx by cranial nerve IX. Motor axons innervate the stylopharyngeus and middle pharyngeal constrictor. Sensory axons mediate taste sensation from the tongue, the afferent arc of the swallowing reflex, and the vasomotor, cardioinhibitory, and respiratory reflexes of the carotid body and sinus. (*From J. C. B. Grant: An Atlas of Anatomy, 5th ed., Baltimore, Williams and Wilkins Co., 1962.*)

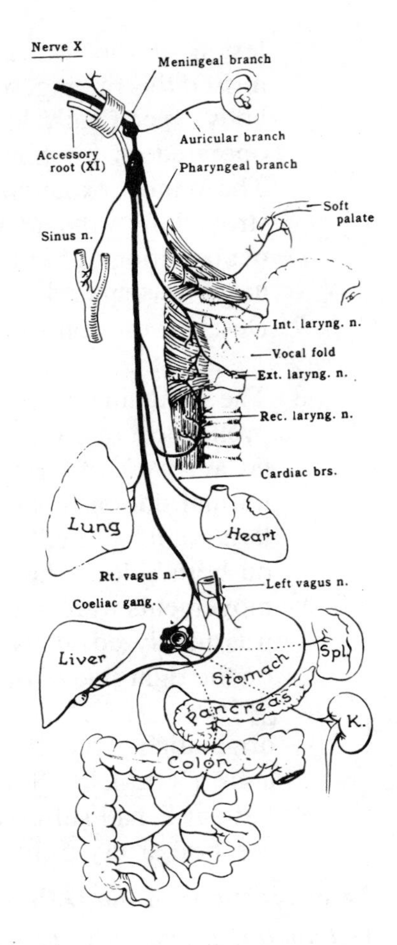

FIG. 6-7. Innervation of the palate, pharynx, larynx, and thoracicoabdominal viscera by cranial nerve X. The palatal branch innervates the levator palati muscles which lift the palate. The pharyngeal and laryngeal branches mediate sensory and motor functions of these structures. (*From J. C. B. Grant: An Atlas of Anatomy, 5th ed., Baltimore, Williams and Wilkins Co., 1962.*)

B. Innervation of pharynx and larynx.

gill or branchial

medulla

1. The skeletal muscles supplied by IX and X originally were derived from ______________ arches.
2. The motor nucleus for IX and X, called *nucleus ambiguus,* is located in the ☐ mesencephalon / ☐ pons / ☐ medulla.
3. IX supplies only one muscle exclusively (stylopharyngeus). Since this muscle participates with X in swallowing, its *isolated* function cannot be tested clinically. The remaining motor fibers of IX supply the middle pharyngeal constrictor. Since the pharyngeal constrictors of IX act as a unit with X in swallowing, the isolated function of the individual constrictors cannot be tested.
4. X innervates the *palatal* muscles, with assistance from V, the *pharyngeal* constrictors with assistance from IX, and the *laryngeal muscles* without any assistance: *palate, pharynx, larynx.*
5. Since even complete interruption of V has little clinical effect on palatal function, V can be disregarded. Hence, the clinically important motor functions of the palate, pharynx, and larynx are innervated by cranial nerves ______________ and ______________ .
6. Sensation from the palate and pharynx is mediated by IX and X and

IX, X

X

from the larynx by X alone. Hence, IX and X are both the *motor* and *sensory* sentinels of the palatal orifice, but ________ alone is the sentinel of the larynx.

XII

7. Swallowing is a complex act involving coordination of respiration with cranial nerve action. The act of swallowing is initiated when the tongue throws a food bolus back into the palatal archway. Tongue motility is exclusively a function of the ________ *th* cranial nerve (if you don't know, sort through the nerves I to XII until you come to the right one).

VII
V

8. Try to swallow when your lips are open. You may be able to do it after a struggle, but normal swallowing requires the lips and jaw to be closed. The lip muscle is innervated by the ________ *th,* and jaw closure by the ________ *th* cranial nerve.

V, VII, IX, X, XII.
X

9. Thus, swallowing requires the collaboration of cranial nerves ________ ________, while phonation by the larynx requires only cranial nerve ________ .

C. Clinical physiology of the soft palate

1. Under the influence of X, the soft palate swings upward and backward to contact the posterior wall of the pharynx, sealing off *oro*pharynx from *naso*pharynx. See Fig. 6-8*A* and *B.*

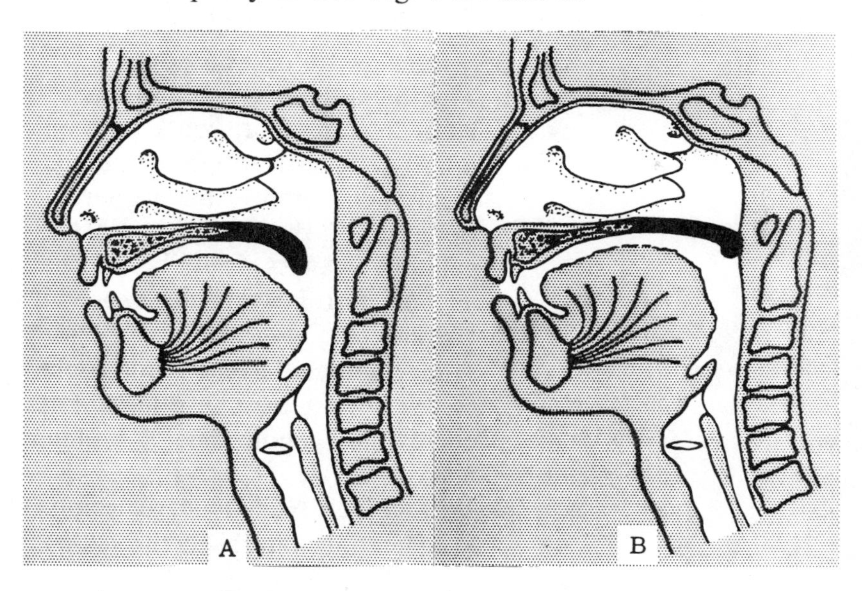

FIG. 6-8. Sagittal section of the head. *A.* Position of the soft palate when it is relaxed. *B.* Position of soft palate when it is elevated, occluding the nasopharynx from the oropharynx.

liquid
air

2. Unless the soft palate elevates properly, ________ will escape into your nose when you drink, and ________ will escape into your nose when you speak. The result is "nasal" swallowing and "nasal" speech.
3. Since physicists define both liquids and gases as fluids, we can agree that the function of the soft palate is to rightly divide the flow of fluids between the oral cavity and oropharynx, and between the oropharynx and nasopharynx. Looking further, we can say that the branchial

IX and X

V, VII

musculature of the throat controls the fluid traffic at the laryngeal and pharyngeal openings.

a. Thus, the fluid dynamics of the *oro*pharyngeal, *naso*pharyngeal, laryngeal, and esophageal orifices are mainly controlled by cranial nerves ________________ (with some assistance from V, VII, and XII).

b. Cranial nerves IX and X innervate the internal apertures of the head much as cranial nerves ____________(sensory) and __________ (motor) innervate the external apertures.

4. The palate elevates whenever it would be advantageous to keep anything which is in your oropharynx from getting into your nasopharynx. Thus, the palate elevates when you
   a. Swallow
   b. Whistle or trumpet
   c. Speak
5. Although palatal weakness causes nasal speech, the palate does not completely seal off the nasopharynx during most speech sounds. Instead, it merely reduces the nasopharyngeal aperture, detouring the air through the mouth, the path of least resistance. Complete palatal elevation is required for only a few sounds, such as:
   a. Gutturals: *K* or hard *G,* as in good.
   b. Vowels: sustained "EEEEE . . ." or "Ah . . ."

D. UMN innervation of IX and X

equal

UMN
LMN

contralateral

ipsilateral

1. The palate, pharynx, and vocal cords act with bilateral synchrony. Knowing this fact, you can predict that the number of crossed and uncrossed UMN fibers would be about ________________ from each cerebral hemisphere.
2. Because of the bilateral UMN innervation, a severe and enduring palatal weakness would be unusual after unilateral ☐ UMN / ☐ LMN lesions, but it would be expected after unilateral ☐ UMN / ☐ LMN lesions.
3. Some patients have a much higher percentage of crossed UMN axons to the brainstem than others. These patients show some palatal weakness which would be ☐ ipsilateral / ☐ contralateral to the UMN lesion.
4. With an LMN Xth nerve lesion, the palatal paralysis is ☐ ipsilateral / ☐ contralateral to the lesion.

E. Pseudobulbar palsy: The nomenclature of muscular paralysis from LMN and UMN lesions of the cranial nerves

1. Unfortunately, clinical jargon includes many different terms for UMN and LMN paralysis, terms which bear the imprint of medical history. The medulla was visualized by older anatomists as a bulb-like expansion of the spinal cord. Thus, the medulla was called the "bulb." LMN paralysis from a lesion of the bulb or its nerves was called "bulbar paralysis." UMN lesions paralyzing bulbar speech and swallowing mechanisms were called "pseudobulbar," or "false" bulbar paralysis, because the lesion was not truly in the bulb or its nerves. The UMN's were called "corticobulbar" fibers. By usage, the term *corti-*

cobulbar fibers has come to mean all cortical efferent fibers to cranial nerve motor nuclei III to XII. But we do not say bulbar paralysis when we mean LMN paralysis of cranial nerves other than those of the bulb. Well, "A foolish consistency is the hobgoblin of little minds." – Emerson.

LMN
IX to XII

2. Thus, "bulbar paralysis" means only an ☐ LMN / a ☐ UMN lesion of cranial nerves ☐ IX to XII / ☐ III to XII.
3. *The syndrome of pseudobulbar palsy*
   a. If a patient suffers acute, severe bilateral lesions of the corticobulbar fibers, as with bilateral cerebral infarction, he becomes comatose, mute, severely demented, and loses the ability to speak or swallow at all. In the recovery phase or with gradual lesions of the corticobulbar tracts, the patient shows a characteristic, virtually pathognomonic syndrome termed *pseudobulbar palsy.* He initiates speaking or swallowing very slowly. He slurs his words. His voice has a peculiar strained pitch and quality. He exhibits extreme emotional lability, crying one moment, laughing the next, like turning on and off a faucet. His face, most of the time, appears immobile as though it were a wooden mask, but when he cries or laughs, the facial movements expressing the emotion become exaggerated and prolonged, yet strangely, when queried he does not feel the emotion being expressed.

both volitional and emotional movements
volitional
emotional

   b. LMN lesions of cranial nerves would cause loss of ☐ emotional movements only / ☐ volitional movements only / ☐ both volitional and emotional movements.
   c. Bilateral UMN lesions would cause loss of ☐ volitional / ☐ emotional facial movements with preservation or exaggeration of ☐ volitional / ☐ emotional facial movements.

Check against frame 3. Did you miss something?

4. Summarize the clinical features of pseudobulbar palsy and state the pathways affected. ______________________________________
____
____
____
5. The many different terms for UMN and LMN paralysis are collected in Table 6-5. It is perfectly clear that the terms *UMN* and *LMN* cover the concept concisely, informatively, and universally. They are the terms to be used in this text.

TABLE 6-5. Synonyms or Near Synonyms for Muscular Paralysis from UMN and LMN Lesions

UMN paresis or paralysis	LMN paresis or paralysis
Central	Peripheral
Pseudobulbar	Bulbar
Suprasegmental	Segmental
Supranuclear	Nuclear, infranuclear

Bibliography

Langworthy, O., and Hesser, F.: Syndrome of pseudobulbar palsy. Anatomic and physiologic analysis, *Arch. Intern. Med.,* 65:106-121, 1940.

Lieberman, A., and Bensen, D.: Control of emotional expression in pseudobulbar palsy. *Arch. Neurol.,* 34:717-719, 1977.

F. The five basic mechanisms of speech

1. Speech requires a *bellows,* provided by the lungs and respiratory muscles—diaphragm, intercostal, and abdominal.
2. Speech requires *phonation* by the vocal cords.
3. Speech requires *articulation* by palate, tongue, lips, and to some extent the mandible.
4. Speech requires *resonance,* provided by the pharyngeal, oral, and nasal passages.
5. Speech requires *cerebral direction* of the lower mechanisms. Cerebral function in speech, other than the corticobulbar system, will be presented in a later chapter.

G. Phonation, role of cranial nerve X

1. Galen (130-200 A.D.) of Pergamum was troubled by the squealing of piglets when he did surgical experiments on them. But he was troubled even more by his own ignorance, which drove him to continue his experimentation. Since he had no anesthetic, he solved the squealing piglet problem and dispelled a share of his own ignorance with one stroke. After verifying that the voice came from the larynx, he found that it could be silenced by cutting the recurrent laryngeal nerves — and that is how we learned what these nerves do.
2. Only the larynx phonates. After phonation, speech sounds must be *articulated.* Hence, to make sounds is to ____________ *ate,* to shape the sounds into speech is to ____________ *ate.*

phonate
articulate

3. Whisper a sentence, for it clarifies the distinction between phonation and articulation. When whispering, you make no voice sounds with the larynx. Whispering shows that you can articulate with perfect clarity even though you do not phonate at all.

H. Articulation of speech

1. Articulate speech may be regarded as a mixture of voiced and nonvoiced sounds.
2. *Plosive sounds.* Try this experiment.
   a. Cup your palm and hold it about 3 cm in front of your mouth. Loudly say, "Puh, puh, puh, . . . guh, guh, guh, . . . M, M, M, . . . and kuh, kuh, kuh."
   b. In all but one of these sounds, you felt a *strong* puff of air in your hand. The sound not requiring forceful air expulsion was ____________.
   c. In order for you to expel air through your mouth, the ____________ ____________ must elevate to close off the nasopharynx from the oropharynx.
   d. Therefore, if the patient articulates plosives well, the soft palate elevates strongly.

M ("em")

soft palate

e. If the patient articulates plosives poorly, with escape of air through the nose, what would you suspect about the action of the palate?

____

____.

Ans: It does not seal off the nasopharynx. However, it does not have to be paralyzed. Mechanical defects, like a cleft palate, may prevent an effective seal of the nasopharynx.

3. *Sibilants and fricatives*

   a. Try the previous experiment, making a sustained, forceful "S . . ." sound. Do you feel a strong stream of air against your hand? ☐ Yes / ☐ No.

   Yes

   b. Fricatives involve frictional or rustling sounds. Try the experiment again, forcefully pronouncing "V, V, V, . . . Z, Z, Z, . . . and F, F, F."

   c. Try the sibilants and fricatives again, without using tongue or lips at all. Can you say them? ☐ Yes / ☐ No.

   No

   d. For the production of sibilants and fricatives, a strong stream of air must be forced through a small aperture formed by lips, tongue, and teeth. In order that air be diverted from the nose into the mouth, the ______________________________ must close strongly.

   soft palate

   e. Many speech sounds, such as sibilants and plosives, require no phonation. *Sh, P, T,* and *K* are examples. These sounds are called *voiceless consonants.* Hence, all speech sounds require ☐ articulation / ☐ phonation, but not all speech sounds require ☐ articulation / ☐ phonation.

   articulation
   phonation

4. *Labials.* While watching your lips in a mirror, recite each letter of the alphabet, and after each one try to make the sound without any lip movement. In Table 6-6, check the sounds which require strong labial action.
5. *Linguals.* Complete Table 6-7 by reciting the alphabet loudly and checking the sounds which require the tongue to touch the roof of the mouth. These sounds require strong lingual actions.
6. *Vowel sounds*

   a. Compare the tongue action of the *D, G,* and *J* sounds with the position of the tongue during vowel sounds. To understand tongue action during vowel sounds, do this: Press down on your tongue with a tongue blade as you recite the vowels.

   b. Vowels also require palatal elevation. The traditional clinical test for palatal elevation is to have the patient say, "Ah . . ." A vowel requiring tighter palatal closure is *E*, but the patient cannot say it with his mouth open to permit palatal inspection.

   c. A good test sentence for palatal function is one combining consonant and vowel sounds: "We see three geese."

I. Speaking of speech and swallowing disorders

1. Absence of any phonation is called ____________*phonia.*

   aphonia

2. A patient with faulty articulation as a result of a UMN, an LMN, or

Compare your chart with another student's.

TABLE 6-6. Letter Sounds Requiring Strong Lip Action (Labials)			
	Strong labial		Strong labial
A		N	
B		O	
C		P	
D		Q	
E		R	
F		S	
G		T	
H		U	
I		V	
J		W	
K		X	
L		Y	
M		Z	

TABLE 6-7. Letter Sounds Requiring Strong Tongue-tip Elevation (Linguals)			
	Strong lingual		Strong lingual
A		N	
B		O	
C		P	
D		Q	
E		R	
F		S	
G		T	
H		U	
I		V	
J		W	
K		X	
L		Y	
M		Z	

anarthria

a muscular lesion is said to have *dysarthria.* If he cannot speak at all because of a neural or muscular lesion, he has ________________.

a. The key to the definition of dysarthria is a defect in articulation of speech sounds, not the content of speech, not the words, and not the vocabulary. Dys- and an-arthria are not used for speech defects caused by emotional disorders or cerebral lesions which do not directly affect LMNs or UMNs for speech articulation.

b. The effect of emotional disorders and cerebral lesions on the content of speech, choice of words, and vocabulary will be discussed later.

3. A patient who is unable to speak because of dementia, deafness, or emotional illness is said to be *mute*. Mutism implies that the neuromuscular mechanism for speech production is intact. The block is at the level of the mind, not the UMN, LMN, or muscle.

dysphagia
aphagia

4. A patient with difficulty swallowing because of a UMN, an LMN, or a muscular lesion is said to have ________________ *phagia;* if he cannot swallow at all, ____________ *phagia.*
5. A patient who has an excessive escape of air into his nose during speech is said to have *hypernasal* speech. It indicates that the palate has not closed off the oropharynx, either because of palatal weakness or mechanical interference, such as from a cleft palate.
6. A patient who has too little nasal escape of air is said to have *hyponasal* speech.

a. Pinch your nostrils together and say "Good morning."

hyponasal

incompetent palatal closure

nasal obstruction

b. Lack of nasal escape of air transforms "Good morning" into "Good bordig." This would be ☐ hypernasal / ☐ hyponasal speech.

c. A patient with hypernasal speech would have ☐ incompetent palatal closure / ☐ nasal obstruction, while a patient with hyponasal speech would have ☐ incompetent palatal closure / ☐ nasal obstruction.

7. Review the definitions: *Aphonia, dysarthria, mutism, dysphagia, hypernasal,* and *hyponasal* speech.

J. An unfortunate, common, but preventable error

hyponasal

hypernasal

worse

1. Failure to distinguish between hyper- and hyponasal speech leads to serious errors in treatment. When the palate elevates, it comes into apposition with the dorsal pharyngeal wall. In children, the adenoid is often hypertrophied, bulging into the pharyngeal lumen. Hypertrophy of the adenoid would tend to cause ☐ hyponasal / ☐ hypernasal speech.

2. Some patients with neurogenic palatal weakness or submucous palatal clefts will have palatal escape of air, which is ☐ hyponasal / ☐ hypernasal speech. If the examining physician sees enlarged adenoids, he may decide he has found the culprit. Actually, in a patient with palatal weakness, the adenoid *reduces* the need for palatal elevation. Removal of the adenoids of a patient with hypernasal speech will make it ☐ better / ☐ worse. Explain.

____

____

____

Ans: Worse! Removal of the adenoid tissue increases the distance the palate has to elevate to shut off the nasopharynx. The weak palate is now even less capable of preventing nasal escape of air.

3. This example shows what happens if you put a knife in the wrong person's hand: he'll remove adenoids for hypernasal speech, snip a lingual frenulum for "tongue-tie," extract a uterus for backache, or pop out tonsils for fifty dollars.

K. Stuttering.

1. All of us suffer from pauses and repetitions when we speak, the toddler more than the adult. When the pauses and repetitions are unduly severe, the patient is a stutterer. He usually falters and repeats the first syllable of words, sometimes the middle or last. He is worse during emotional stress.

2. While the cause of stuttering is debated, it is usually regarded as a psychogenic disorder. Certainly no clear-cut evidence of neurologic dysfunction can be found in the majority of stutterers.

L. Clinical testing of the motor function of cranial nerves IX and X

1. *Speech*

a. In taking the history, you appraise the patient's speech automatically. If it is perfectly normal in all respects, you need do no further speech testing. If you suspect a defect, test the articulation mechanisms individually.

b. Test competency of articulation by the soft tissues, the soft palate, tongue and lips, with the KLM test. "Kuh, Kuh, Kuh," tests the ______________________________. "La, La, La," tests the ________________________. "Mi, Mi, Mi," tests the __________.

soft palate,
tongue
lips

2. *Swallowing:* If the patient has dysarthria or dysphagia, give him a glass of water to swallow.
3. *Inspection:*

a. Request the patient to open his mouth and sustain an "Ah. . . ." Inspect the tonsillar pillars for asymmetry as they arch upwards and medially to form the palate. Look at the arch, the arch above, not the uvula. Students commonly mistake an asymmetrically hung uvula for palatal palsy. Let the uvula hang as it will. See Fig. 6-9, and then study your own palatal action in the mirror.

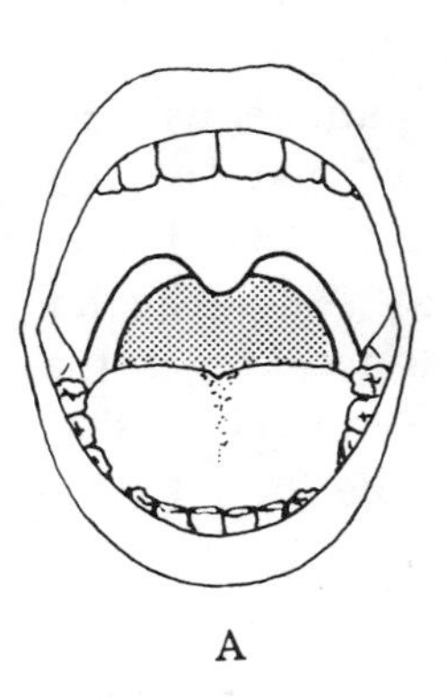

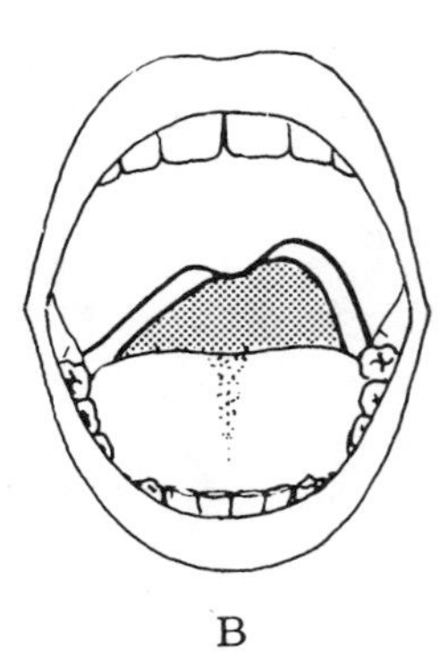

FIG. 6-9. Palatal arch. *A.* Appearance of palatal arch when a normal subject says, "Ah. . . ." *B.* Appearance of palatal arch when a patient with unilateral palatal weakness says, "Ah. . . ."

b. In Fig. 6-9*A*, a normal subject is saying "Ah . . . ," in *B*, a person with a palatal palsy. Which side is paralyzed in *B*? ☐ right / ☐ left.

right

c. The final test for anatomic elevation of the palate is the *gag reflex*. A tongue blade is touched against first one, then the other pillar of the palatal arch. The afferent arc of the gag reflex is primarily cranial nerve __________. The efferent arc is cranial nerve __________.

IX
X

d. If the palate fails to elevate when the patient says "Ah," but does elevate during the gag reflex, the patient would have to have ☐ a UMN / ☐ an LMN lesion. This is an important principle, the dissociation between volitional and reflex activity. If both reflex and volitional activity are abolished, the patient would have ☐ a UMN / ☐ an LMN, or a muscle lesion.

UMN

LMN or muscle

e. Incompetency of palatal elevation may result from UMN or LMN lesions, congenital malformations, such as cleft palate, myopathies, or local lesions in the soft tissue. Palatal incompetence is not simply one thing *or* another. Like every sign, it is a puzzle to be solved.

4. Many speech disorders can be learned only by listening to patients,

rather than from a text: disorders in rhythm, force, and timber of the voice. The speech affliction is often characteristic and even pathognomonic of some diseases. In the *cat's cry syndrome* (cri du chat), the infant sounds like a cat in heat. The diagnosis is confirmed from the patient's karyotype: the short arm of the fifth chromosome is absent. In *hypothyroidism*, the voice is deep and raspy. In *paralysis agitans* (Parkinsonism), the muscles are rigid, and the voice fails to show normal inflections and modulations: the sound is all on one plane, "plateau speech." *Cerebellar disease* causes the opposite; some sounds are overaccentuated, others underaccentuated: "scanning speech" as though the voice scanned from one peak of volume to another.

5. *Hoarseness and unilateral vagal lesions*
   a. Hoarseness is caused by a number of mechanical or neurogenic disorders. Its persistence always demands direct inspection of the cords by laryngoscopy. Both vocal cords may be completely paralyzed with little hoarseness. Therefore, merely listening to the voice or examining the palate constitutes an incomplete examination for Xth nerve function.
   b. What is the only diagnostic procedure that will definitely identify a vocal cord paralysis? ______________

laryngoscopy

Bibliography

Gordon, N., and Taylor, I.: The assessment of children with difficulties of communication, *Brain,* 87:121-140, 1964.

Lechtenberg, R., and Gilman, S.: Speech disorders in cerebellar disease. *Ann. of Neurol.,* 3:285-290, 1978.

Lillywhite, H.: Doctor's manual of speech disorders, *J.A.M.A.,* 167:850-858, 1958.

McWilliams, B., and Musgrave, R.: Differential diagnosis and management of hypernasal voices in children, *Trans. Amer. Acad. Ophthal. Otolaryng.,* 69:322-331, 1965.

Perkins, W.: *Speech Pathology: An Applied Behavioral Science,* St. Louis, The C. V. Mosby Company, 1971.

Silverstein, A., and Faegenburg, D.: Cineradiography of swallowing, *Arch. Neurol.,* 12:67-71, 1965.

Svien, H., Baker, H., and Rivers, M.: Jugular foramen syndrome and allied syndromes, *Neurology*, 13:797-809, 1963.

Travis, L. E. (ed): *Handbook of Speech Pathology and Audiology,* New York, Appleton-Century-Crofts, 1971.

Van Riper, C.: *Speech Correction, Principles and Methods,* 6th ed., Englewood Cliffs, N.J., Prentice-Hall, 1978.

IV. Motor function of the XIth cranial nerve

A. Functional anatomy

1. XI has two components, a spinal and an accessory part. Hence, it is called the ______________ ______________ nerve.
2. The spinal part supplies the sternocleidomastoid and rostral portions of the trapezius muscles. The accessory part is accessory to the vagus,

spinal accessory

supplying fibers which merely hitchhike along the proximal part of XI before joining X for distribution. When we say we test the function of XI, we mean we test the spinal part. Study Fig. 6-10.

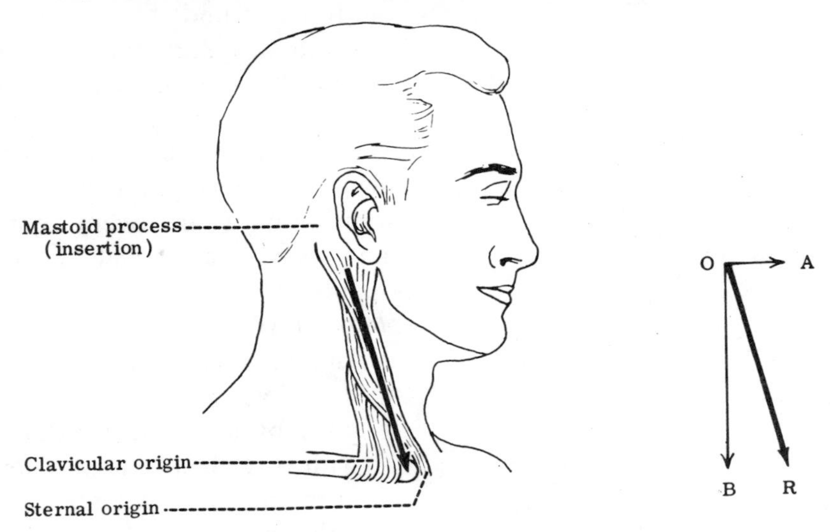

FIG. 6-10. Origin and insertion of the sternocleidomastoid muscle. On the right is a vector diagram of its action. The oblique arrow (O-R) is the actual line of pull. It can be resolved into a *horizontal* vector (O-A) acting to thrust the head forward and turn it to the opposite side, and into a *vertical* vector (O-B) acting to tilt the head to the same side as the muscle.

Answers	
sternum clavicle mastoid	*B. The sternocleidomastoid (SCM) muscle* 1. The SCM muscle originates from the ______ and the ______ and inserts into the ______ process.
right	2. Palpate both SCMs as you forcefully turn (turn, not tilt) your head to the *left*. Which SCM contracts most? ☐ right / ☐ left / ☐ neither.
left	3. Forcefully tilt (tilt, not turn) your head to the left. Which SCM contracts most? ☐ right / ☐ left / ☐ both equally.
Yes	4. Press back on your forehead with one hand while you thrust your head forward. Palpate both SCM muscles with your other hand. Do they both contract? ☐ Yes / ☐ No.
opposite same forward	5. You see, you don't have to memorize anything about the SCM action. You'll always take your head along. Each SCM has three actions: *a.* Turning head to ☐ same / ☐ opposite side. *b.* Tilting head to ☐ same / ☐ opposite side. *c.* Thrusting head ☐ forward / ☐ backward.
away from	6. The action of one SCM muscle in turning the head, like the action of one lateral pterygoid muscle in turning the mandible, results in turning ☐ toward / ☐ away from the side of the muscle.

C. The trapezius muscle

1. The trapezius *originates* in the midline from the occiput and the spinous processes of all cervical and thoracic vertebrae. It *inserts* into the clavicle and scapula.
2. Only the rostral part of the trapezius is innervated by XI. Its action is to elevate the shoulders.

contralateral

ipsilateral

moderate and transient

D. UMN innervation

1. Since SCM and trapezius may act unilaterally their LMNs receive a considerable percentage of UMN axons from the ☐ ipsilateral / ☐ contralateral motor cortex.
2. Since they are also proximal muscles which frequently act symmetrically, they also receive many UMNs from the ☐ ipsilateral / ☐ contralateral motor cortex.
3. As with any muscles receiving ipsilateral and contralateral UMN axons, SCM and trapezius show ☐ moderate and transient / ☐ severe and permanent weakness after an UMN lesion.

inspection

palpation

E. Clinical testing of XI

1. The first step in appraising any part of the body is ________________.
2. The SCM and trapezius muscles are inspected for size and asymmetry.
3. The second step in clinical investigation is ________________.
4. Palpate the muscles at rest and as they go through their actions.
5. Table 6-8 lists the methods for testing the strength of SCM and trapezius muscles. Try the maneuvers on yourself and another person.
6. In step 1, why were you asked to use the patient's cheek, rather than his mandible? ________________
____
____

Ans: You do not want to test lateral pterygoid *and* SCM. Test only one muscle at a time whenever possible.

right SCM

Press forward over vertebra prominens (C_7)

SCM

TABLE 6-8. Clinical Tests of the Motor Function of Cranial Nerve XI

Commands to patient	Examiner's maneuver
1. "Turn your head to the left; hold it there, and don't let me push it back."	Place your right hand on the left cheek of the patient, your left hand on his right shoulder to brace him and try to force his head to the midline. Repeat with the patient's head turned to the right. With the patient's head turned to the left, you test the ☐ right SCM / ☐ left SCM / ☐ trapezius muscle when you try to return the head to the midline.
2. "Push your head forward as hard as possible."	Place one hand on the patient's forehead and push backwards. What do you do with your other hand to brace the patient? ________________ ________________ In this maneuver you test the action of both ☐ SCM / ☐ trapezius muscles, which thrust the head forwards.
3. "Try to touch your ears with the tips of your shoulders."	Place your hands on both of the patient's shoulders and press down. Observe from in front and in back, and watch for scapular winging which may occur with trapezius or serratus anterior weakness.

V. Motor function of cranial nerve XII

A. LMN innervation and action of the tongue

hypoglossal
runs under the tongue

1. XII is called the ________________ nerve because it ________________________________.

2. XII controls all tongue movements. To understand the effect of nerve lesions on tongue movement, you must understand the action of the genioglossus muscles.

3. Notice in Fig. 6-11 that each genioglossus muscle is triangular. Its *apex* originates from the apex of the mandible, which is hard, unyielding, and immobile. Its *base* inserts into the base of the tongue, which is soft, fleshy, and mobile.

backward
forward

4. When genioglossus contracts, it tends to pull the mandible ☐ backward/ ☐ forward, and the base of the tongue ☐ backward/ ☐ forward.

very little

5. With your mandible in its normal resting position, how much are you able to *re*tract it? ________________.

forward

6. Hence, the mandibular origin of genioglossus is relatively immobile. Genioglossus contraction, therefore, must pull the base of the tongue ☐ forward/ ☐ backward.

genioglossus

7. If the tongue protrudes in the midline, both right and left ________________ muscles contract equally.

right (if the answer is unclear, review Fig. 6-12)

8. If the patient attempts to protrude his tongue in the midline and it deviates to the right, the ☐ right/ ☐ left genioglossus muscle is weak.

opposite

9. Compare the action of genioglossus in Fig. 6-11 with that of the lateral pterygoid muscle in Fig. 6-1. It is now clear that the mechanics of tongue and jaw protrusion are identical. Midline protrusion is the result of balanced muscular action. Compare the action of these two muscles with the SCM. All three muscles, when contracting unilaterally, move the part they operate to the ☐ same/ ☐ opposite/ ☐ neither side.

left genioglossus

10. The muscle which turns the tongue to the *right* is the ☐ right/ ☐ left ________________ muscle.

right lateral pterygoid

11. The muscle which turns the mandible to the *left* is the ☐ right/ ☐ left ________________ ________________ muscle.

left SCM

12. One muscle which turns the head to the right is the ☐ right/ ☐ left ☐ SCM/ ☐ trapezius muscle.

B. Effect of LMN lesions on muscular size and electrical activity

hypertrophy

1. Although we have mentioned only genioglossus, the bulk of the tongue is muscle. The size of normal muscle depends on *use*. If a muscle is used, it undergoes *use hypertrophy*. If not used, muscle undergoes *disuse atrophy*. The best example is a limb put in a cast for days or weeks. The muscle undergoes disuse atrophy. When the cast is removed and the muscles put back to work they undergo *use* ________________.

denervation

2. If deprived of axons, muscle fibers undergo *denervation* atrophy. If a XIIth nerve is interrupted, the muscle fibers on the ipsilateral half of the tongue undergo ________________ atrophy.

3. A normal muscle put at rest for prolonged periods of time under-

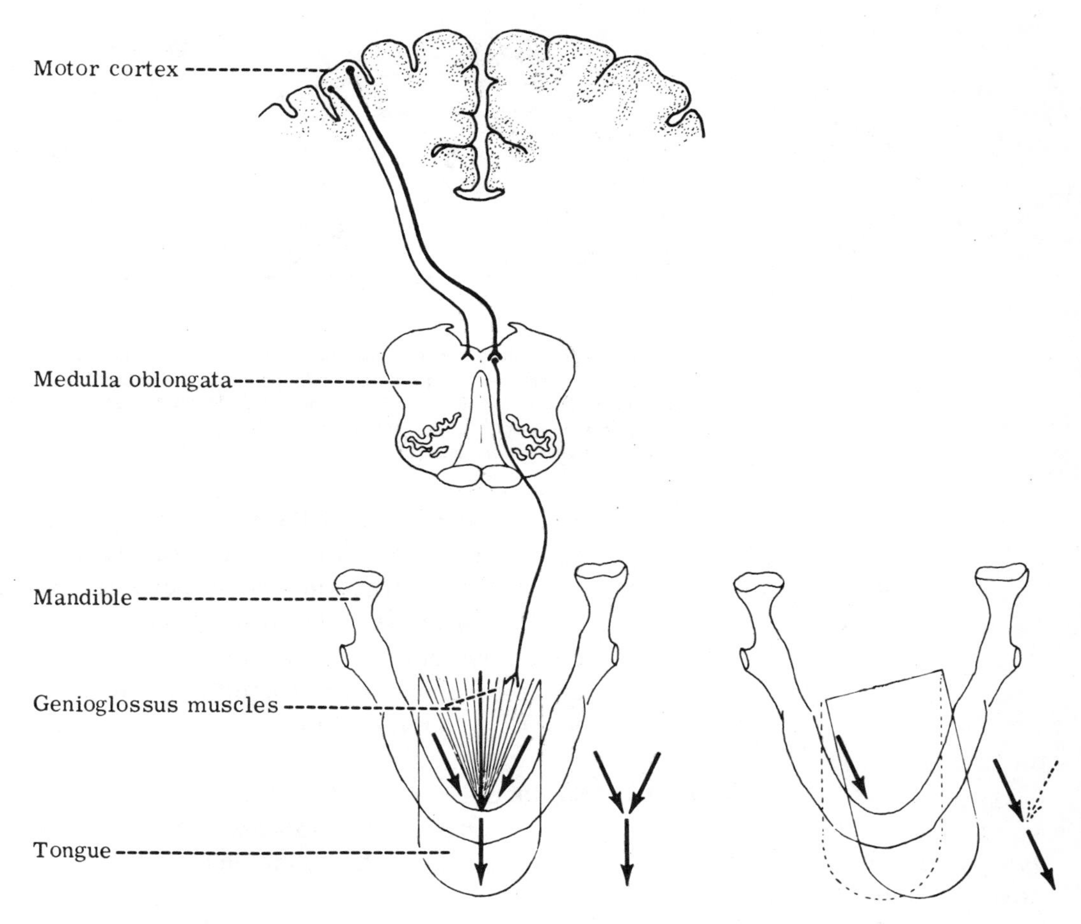

FIG. 6-11. Action and innervation of the genioglossus muscle. To the right is a diagram showing the deviation of the tongue when only the right genioglossus muscle contracts, pulling the *base* of the tongue forward on the right and protruding and deviating the *tip* of the tongue to the left.

Answers	Frames
disuse denervation	goes ______________ atrophy. A muscle deprived of its nerve supply undergoes ______________ atrophy.
disuse denervation myopathic	4. Muscular atrophy also occurs from primary diseases of muscle, which result in death of muscle fibers. This atrophy is called *myopathic* atrophy. List the three types of muscular atrophy: *a.* From prolonged inactivity, ______________ atrophy. *b.* From LMN lesions, ______________ atrophy. *c.* From primary diseases of muscle, ______________ atrophy.
	5. Each efferent axon of a peripheral nerve may innervate one or more muscle fibers. In some small muscles, such as the extraocular, each motor axon is thought to innervate only one muscle fiber. In large muscles, such as the gluteus maximus or quadriceps femoris, each motor axon branches to innervate as many as 150 muscle fibers. One LMN, its axon, and all muscle fibers innervated by it are called a *motor unit.* See Fig. 6-12.
all	6. If a normal LMN discharges a nerve impulse, ☐ some / ☐ all / ☐ none of the muscle fibers of the motor unit would be expected to contract.

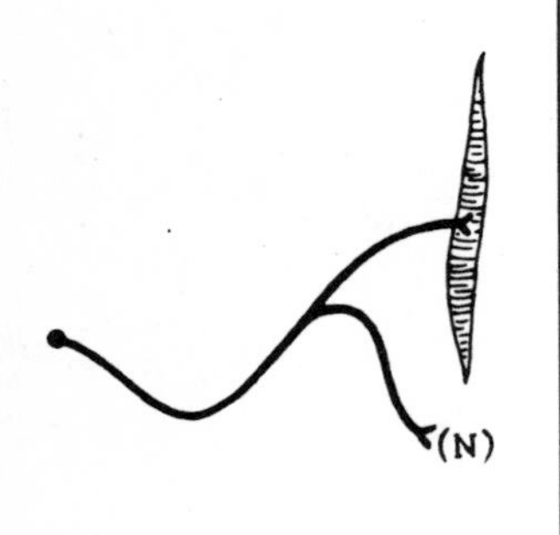

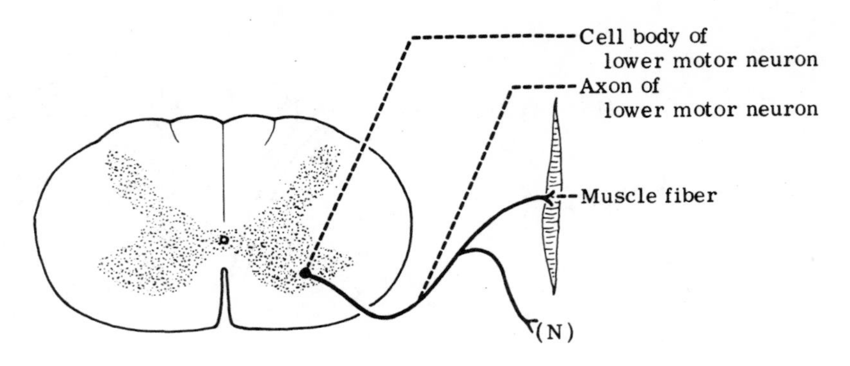

FIG. 6-12. Cross section of spinal cord and motor nerve to show the composition of a motor unit. It consists of the LMN (including the neuron body and its axons) and all muscle fibers innervated by the axon. *N* stands for any number of additional muscle fibers between 1 and 150. The larger muscles have larger values of N. Encircle the portion of the drawing which defines the motor unit and compare with the drawing in the answer column.

7. The muscle fibers of the motor unit are grouped together in a *fascicle.* In general, when the fascicle of muscle fibers of a motor unit contracts, the contraction can be seen clinically as a small ripple or twitch. Such a twitch is called a *fasciculation.* You have all probably experienced twitching of an eyelid: that is a fasciculation. Fasciculations are apparent to the observer and may be felt and seen by the patient.
   a. Define a motor unit: ______________________________

Ans: An LMN, its axon, and all its muscle fibers.

A small muscular twitch called a fasciculation

   b. If a single motor unit discharges, what would be seen clinically and what is the technical name for it? ______________________________

8. Normally, motor units discharge only when stimulated by UMNs or other afferent impulses. If a needle wired to an amplifier and oscilloscope is inserted into a normal resting muscle, no electrical activity is recorded. When the patient contracts the muscle, showers of electrical potentials are seen on the oscilloscope screen. The electrical potentials are caused by depolarization of muscle fibers as the motor units discharge. The recording of the electrical activity from muscle is called *electromyography* (EMG). See Fig. 6-13*A*.
9. When the LMN, either the cell body or axon, is diseased, its membrane loses stability. The neuron discharges impulses spontaneously, randomly, rather than only in response to appropriate stimuli. The resulting muscular twitches seen clinically are called ______________ .

fasciculations

10. As seen on an oscilloscope, fasciculations look like Fig. 6-13*B*.
11. The spontaneous discharge causing the fasciculation may arise distally in the axon or proximally in the cell body. If the impulse arises distally, it is still propagated into the branches of the axon as though it came down the axon from the cell body as usual. Hence, all muscle fibers of the fascicle contract.
12. If the neuron dies or the axon is completely severed from the cell body, the distal part of the axon degenerates, *Wallerian* (Augustus Waller, 1816–1870) degeneration. See Fig. 6-14.

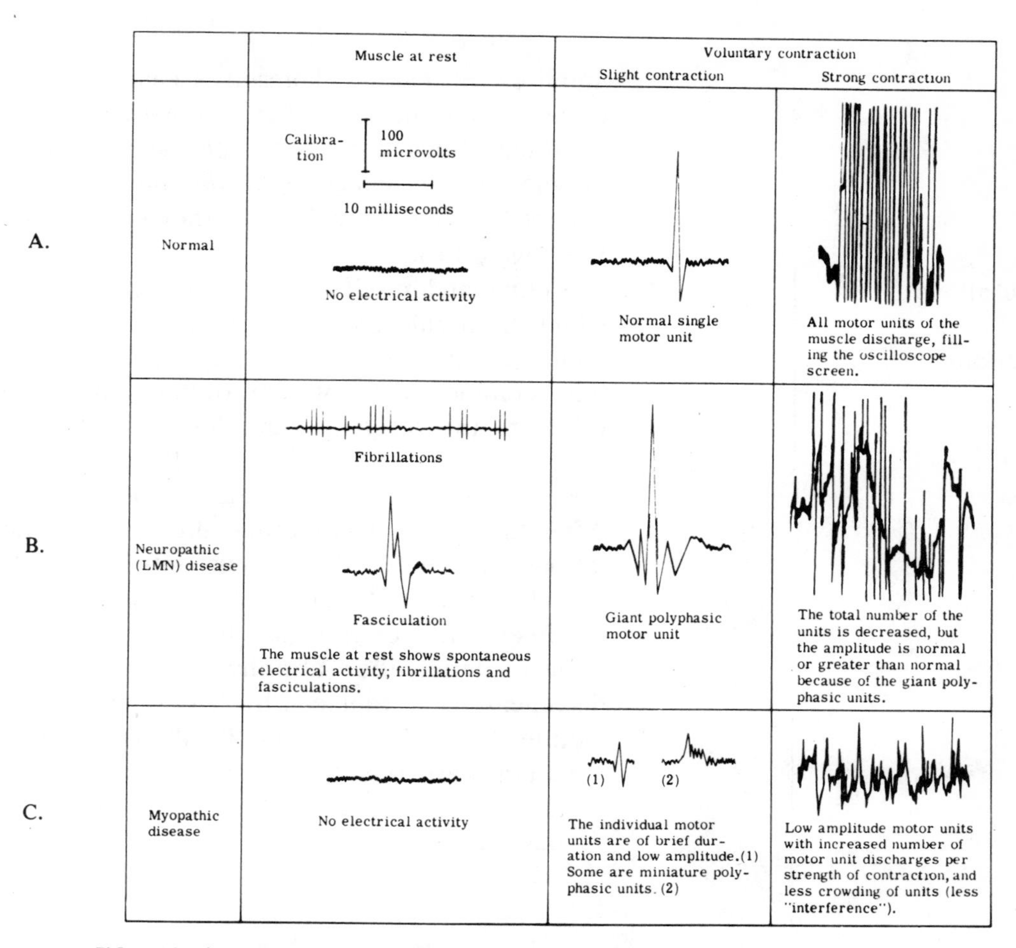

FIG. 6-13. Electromyographic (oscilloscopic) tracings of the electrical activity recorded from muscle. Only some of the common, typical findings are depicted here. *(Courtesy of Dr. Mark Dyken.)*

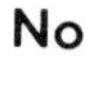

13. After Wallerian degeneration has taken place, would the muscle fibers contract in response to volitional effort or electrical stimulation of the peripheral nerve trunk? ☐ Yes / ☐ No.

14. After denervation by Wallerian degeneration of the motor axon, the muscle fiber undergoes a period of hyperexcitability, *Cannon's law of hyperexcitability of denervated structures.* It is as if the muscle fibers were trying to compensate for an insufficiency of nerve

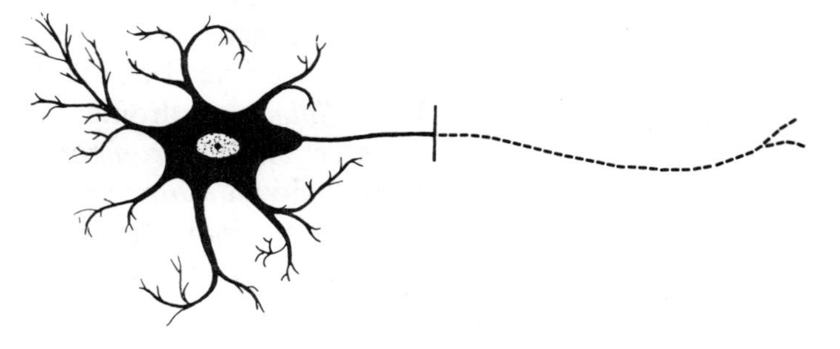

FIG. 6-14. Neuron to show Wallerian degeneration. The distal part of a severed neuronal process dies when deprived of the metabolites provided by the nucleus and organelles of the cell body. These substances move centrifugally from the cell body by axoplasmic flow to maintain the nutrition of the neuronal ramifications. Wallerian degeneration is only a specific example of the general rule that cytoplasm cannot survive when separated from its nucleus.

impulses by making themselves easier to discharge. Thus, the membrane of the muscle fiber depolarizes spontaneously and the fiber contracts. Such a random, spontaneous contraction of an individual muscle fiber is called a *fibrillation.* As a general rule, fibrillations cannot be seen clinically, but they can be "seen" by the oscilloscope. See Fig. 6-14*B*.

fasciculations

fibrillations

15. The clinician himself sees the twitches called __________________, while the oscilloscope is required to "see" the individual muscle fiber contractions called __________________.

nerve
muscle

16. The common denominator of fasciculations and fibrillations is that both are the result of pathologic instability of cell membranes, the __________________ cell in the case of fasciculations and the __________________ cell in the case of fibrillations.
17. After the death of nerve and muscle cells, no fasciculations or fibrillations can occur. They occur only during the period when the cells are abnormal, but not dead. The phase of hypersensitivity of muscle fibers after denervation lasts for months or years, until the final stage of denervation atrophy, in which the muscle dies and the cells disappear, to be replaced by fatty or fibrous tissue.
18. Define fasciculations and fibrillations. Include the operations by which they are detected and their pathophysiology: __________________

Ans: Fasciculations are contractions of muscle fascicles, detected by clinical inspection or by characteristic EMG waves. They indicate an abnormal depolarization of the cell membrane of the LMNs, causing contraction of all muscle fibers of the motor unit. Fibrillations are spontaneous contractions of individual muscle fibers, detected by characteristic EMG waves. They indicate a state of hyperexcitability of the muscle fibers following denervation.

19. Another electromyographic change of denervation is *giant polyphasic motor units.* These giant EMG waves are of greater amplitude and of more complex form than normal motor unit discharges. The pathophysiology of giant polyphasic units is disputed, but they signify LMN disease. See line B of Fig. 6-13.

fasciculations
fibrillations
giant polyphasic

20. The *clinical* syndrome of LMN lesions is paresis or paralysis and atrophy. The *electromyographic* syndrome of LMN lesions is spontaneous individual *motor unit discharges* called __________________, spontaneous individual *muscle fiber discharges* called __________________, and the appearance of __________________ motor units.

C. LMN lesion of XII

Notice from Fig. 6-11 that one XIIth nerve innervates one half of the tongue. With a unilateral XIIth nerve lesion, the atrophy and weakness thus affect only one side. Having given the general rules about fasciculations and fibrillations, I now regret to mention that the tongue may violate them. Otherwise, the rules hold firm. Authorities differ as to whether the rippling movements seen in the denervated tongue represent fibrillations or fasciculations, and, in fact, tiny ripples play across the surface of many normal tongues. Thus, you had best read tongue ripples cautiously, relying on the pattern of weakness and atrophy for diagnosis.

Bibliography

See Chapter 13 for EMG bibliography.

Patel, A. N., Razzak, Z. A., and Dastur, D. K.: Disuse atrophy of human skeletal muscles, *Arch, Neurol.,* 20:413-421, 1969.

D. *UMN innervation and lesions of XII*

1. In Fig. 6-11 notice that the hypoglossal nucleus receives crossed and uncrossed UMN fibers. Using a colored pencil, draw in the UMN and LMN innervation from the *left* motor cortex. Notice that the line representing crossed fibers is somewhat thicker.
2. The percentage of crossed UMNs varies from person to person. For the tongue, the number of crossed UMN fibers is intermediate, considerably more than 50 percent and considerably less than 100 percent. In this respect, the UMN innervation of the tongue most closely resembles the innervation of ☐ forehead elevation / ☐ eyelid closure / ☐ lip retraction.
3. After a unilateral lesion of the corticobulbar fibers for XII, the patient usually shows a ☐ moderate and transient / ☐ severe and permanent weakness of the tongue.
4. With a lesion of the *right* hemisphere, the tongue would deviate to the ☐ right / ☐ left when protruded; use Fig. 6-11 to reason out the answer.
5. With a lesion of the *right* XIIth nerve, the tongue would deviate to the ☐ right / ☐ left when protruded.

E. *Clinical testing of XII*

1. Inspection of the tongue at rest.
   a. Inspect the tongue for the most reliable sign of an LMN lesion, ______________.
   b. Rippling of a normal tongue frequently indicates incomplete relaxation. Ask the patient to make some tongue movements and then inspect it again after he again tries to relax it. Rippling of one half of the tongue, if that half is weak and atrophic, supports the diagnosis of an LMN.
   c. With a unilateral LMN lesion you would see ☐ bilateral atrophy / ☐ hemiatrophy.

eyelid closure

moderate and transient

left

right

atrophy

hemiatrophy

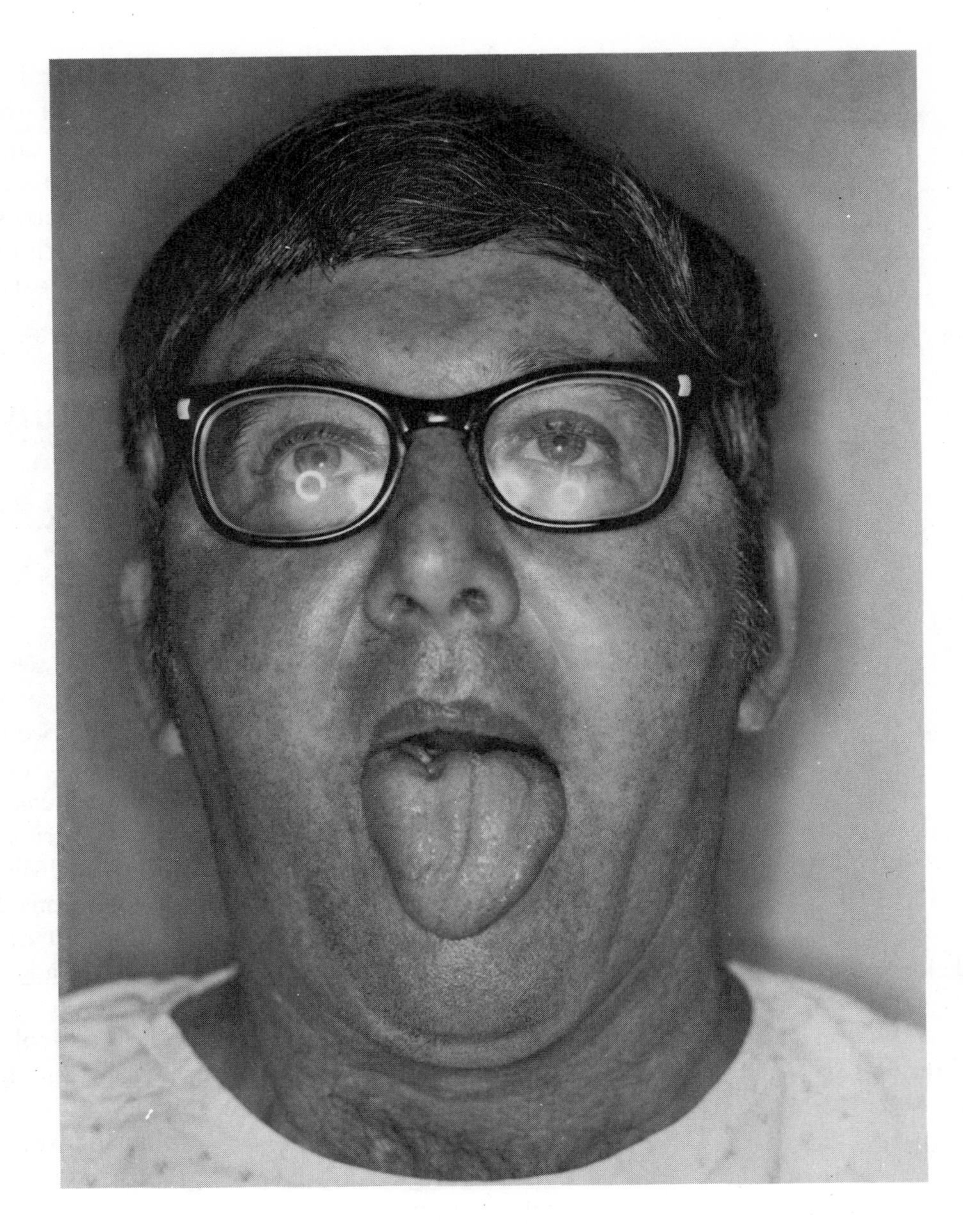

FIG. 6-15. This patient was asked to stick his tongue straight out.

d. Palpation may help resolve questionable hemiatrophy. Palpate each half of the tongue between your thumb and index finger.

2. Tongue motility is tested by having the patient protrude his tongue, pushing it to the right and left. Strength is difficult to evaluate. Have the patient press his tongue against his cheek while you press against it with your fingers. Keep your tongue-in-cheek while you evaluate this rather unreliable test.
3. How would you inspect for correct alignment of the tongue when it is protruded? ______________________________
____
____

Check alignment of median raphe with notch between medial incisors

right
moderate

4. If the tip of the tongue deviates, the patient has either a *UMN* or an *LMN lesion.* Suppose the tongue deviates to the *left.*
   a. If the lesion is UMN it involves the ☐ right / ☐ left hemisphere. The weakness is usually ☐ severe / ☐ moderate.
5. The clinical distinction between a UMN and an LMN lesion of the XIIth nerve rests on supporting evidence of other UMN signs in other movements or upon positive evidence of LMN involvement. The clinical and EMG signs of an LMN lesion of one XIIth nerve are: ____

Ans: hemiatrophy, unilateral fasciculation or fibrillation, and usually severe paralysis with obvious deviation to the paralytic side when the tongue is protruded.

6. Inspect the tongue of the patient in Fig. 6-15 and describe the abnormalities. The patient was instructed to stick out the tongue.

Ans: The tongue shows right-sided atrophy, and deviation of the tip to the right.

right XIIth
nerve

   a. These clinical findings indicate that a lesion has interrupted the ☐ right/ ☐ left ☐ XIIth nerve/ ☐ corticobulbar tract.
   b. The patient in Fig. 6-15 suffered from a glioma of the medulla oblongata.

Bibliography

Currier, R. D., Giles, C., and DeJong, R.: Some comments on Wallenberg's lateral medullary syndrome, *Neurology,* 11:778-791, 1961.

DeJong, R.: *The Neurologic Examination,* 3d ed., New York, Hoeber Medical Division, Harper & Row, 1967.

VI. Tests for pathologic fatiguability of the cranial nerve muscles

A. If a patient complains of diplopia, dysphagia, dysphonia, or dysarthria, particularly if these complaints are intermittent, or if you find an unexplained ocular, facial, or bulbar palsy, such as ptosis, strabismus, or mild hypernasal speech, suspect myasthenia gravis. Myasthenic patients may have little or no deficit when rested, as when first arising in the morning, but as the day wears on, or as they use their cranial nerve muscles to look, talk, swallow, or chew, the weakness becomes increasingly severe. This pathologic fatiguability of muscles, particularly of cranial nerve muscles, is virtually pathognomonic of myasthenia gravis. Myasthenic patients have a deficit in cholinergic transmission at the motor endplates of skeletal muscle. The diagnosis depends on demonstrating the pathologic fatiguability by clinical and electrical tests and proving that a cholinergic drug will restore strength.

The clinical tests chosen depend on the particular muscles implicated by the patient's history, and whether they display some evident weakness at the time of examination. If the patient complains of double vision or ptosis, select the eye muscles, or if the complaint involves dysphagia-dysarthria or dyspnea, select the oropharyngeal and breathing muscles. To bring out latent weakness of a muscle not overtly weak, require the patient to make repetitive or prolonged contractions. To test for ptosis or diplopia, carefully measure the height of the palpebral fissure and record the range of eye movements. Pay particular attention to the range of upward eye movement, the ocular movement which has the least range and is frequently weak in myasthenics. Then have the patient follow your finger up and down through a full range of movement 100 times. Then measure the height of the palpebral fissure and again record the range of eye movements. Test lateral eye movements by measuring the distance between limbus and lateral or medial canthi before and after the repetitive exercise test, or have the patient hold the eyes in a deviated position for a timed period. Test oropharyngeal function by actually timing the patient while reading aloud, swallowing a glass of water, waggling the tongue from side to side, counting to 100, or chewing gum or paraffin a given number of times. Test palatal function by timing how long the patient can sustain an "EEE . . .", and test breathing by measuring vital capacity before and after a timed period of hyperventilation. As another quick, quantitative, apparatus-less test for breathing sufficiency, useful in myasthenia or other neurologic disorders, ask the patient to take a full, deep breath and to count aloud from one upward. Control the rate of counting by tapping your finger at the rate of one per second. The average adult patient should reach at least 30. Try this test yourself. The point is that you must have some quantifiable or measurable end point to prove that repetitive use of the muscle causes pathologic fatiguability.

Electrical testing for myasthenia requires repetitive stimulation of a peripheral nerve while recording the amplitude of the action potentials generated in the muscle fibers (Jolly test). Myasthenic patients show a decrement in the amplitude of muscular contraction after repetitive electrical stimulation of the nerve. The repetitive nerve stimulation test provides entirely objective data. It eliminates the need for the patient's active, willful participation, required by the repetitive exercise tests.

Pharmacologic proof that the pathologic fatiguability results from a defect in cholinergic transmission requires restoration of strength by injecting a cholinergic drug. The most frequently used is intravenous edrophonium (Tensilon®), a short-acting anticholinesterase.

**B. *Procedure for an adult:*

1. Determine some measurable end point, as just discussed in Sec. A.
2. Have cardiopulmonary resuscitation equipment available, as when giving any intravenous medication, and provisions for relief of bladder or bowels.
3. Draw up 1 cc of 10 mg/cc edrophonium in a tuberculin syringe. Draw up 0.4 mg of atropine in another syringe to counteract any excessive reaction to the edrophonium.
4. Draw up 1 cc of sterile saline solution in another tuberculin syringe to serve as a placebo control.

5. Anchor an intravenous needle with flexible tubing to connect to the syringes.
6. Describe the procedures of the test to the patient, but do not state whether the injection will make the patient stronger or weaker. Forewarn the patient that some subjective responses may occur, consisting of symptoms and signs of cholinergic stimulation. The cholinergic effect on skeletal muscles consists of a feeling of tightness in previously weak muscles, such as the ocular muscles, and fasciculations. The sympathetic effect consists of sweating. The parasympathetic effects consist of blurred vision (pupilloconstrictor and ciliary muscles), salivation (salivary gland stimulation), bradycardia (vagomimetic), abdominal cramping and diarrhea (vagomimetic), and urinary urgency and urination (pelvic sympathomimetic). If you will review all of the cholinergic endings in the peripheral motor system—skeletal, sympathetic, and parasympathetic—you will have an organizing principle to remember all of these effects, rather than memorizing them as a list. Then invoke the rostrocaudal principle to "think through" the parasympathetic end organs of the eye and the oral, thoracic, and abdomino-pelvic cavities.
7. Have an assistant inject 0.1 cc of sterile saline every 30 sec for five injections. You measure whatever you have chosen to measure. Placebo-reacting patients may show very dramatic effects, including fainting, but the injection will produce no measurable improvement in motor function in a patient with organic disease.
8. Inject edrophonium at the rate of 0.1 cc (1 mg) every 30 sec either until you obtain some measurable improvement or the patient becomes uncomfortable. Thus you must proceed to one or the other of these two end points, or you may not have given sufficient edrophonium to adequately test the patient. Some myasthenic patients have an extreme tolerance for the medication. If you do not give enough to cause side effects, you may not have given enough for an adequate therapeutic trial.

VII. Summary of the motor examination of the cranial nerves

And now the crucial test: can you sit down with a patient and actually examine the cranial nerve motor function? If you did your job when taking the history, you have already observed the patient's eye movements and blinking, noted the degree and symmetry of other facial movements, inspected the relation of the lids to palpebral fissures, looked for en- or exophthalmos, listened to phonation, and the articulation of labials, linguals, and palatals, and noted the spontaneous swallowing of saliva. If these are all normal, the patient just can't have too much wrong with cranial nerve motor function, but you must do a formal examination anyhow.

The formal examination of cranial nerve motor function begins with the eyes. We test motility last in the ocular sequence for a reason. We can then flow smoothly through the entire cranial nerve motor examination, yes, III to XII, in just 45 sec in a normal cooperative patient. No, the 45 sec is not a misprint. Get a partner and rehearse Table 6-9 today, tomorrow, and every day until you meet the 45 sec criterion.

TABLE 6-9. Method for Rapid Sequential Screening of the Motor Function of the Cranial Nerves

Nerves	Commands to patient by examiner	Observations and tests by examiner
III, IV, VI	"Follow my finger."	Move finger through the ⊢——⊣ and watch for asymmetrical corneal light reflections, lid-limbus relations, nystagmus, and pupilloconstriction during convergence. Inquire about diplopia.
VII	"Look up at the ceiling."	Watch for asymmetry or absence of forehead wrinkling and eyebrow elevation.
	"Close your eyes tight and don't let me open them."	Look for asymmetry of wrinkles radiating from lateral canthi and try to force lids open with your fingers.
	"Draw back the corners of your mouth" or "Smile."	Look for asymmetry of the nasolabial folds. Have patient make labial sounds if speech sounded abnormal.
	"Draw down the corners of your mouth hard."	Look for asymmetry of movement and for wrinkling of skin on neck from platysma action.
V	"Bite your jaws together hard."	Palpate the masseter muscles.
	"Open your jaw as wide as possible."	Look for deviation of the tip by sighting on the notch between the medial two incisors.
	"Hold your jaw to one side."	Try to push it back. Repeat test to the opposite side.
XII	"Stick out your tongue as far as possible."	Look for deviation, atrophy, and fasciculations. Test for lingual articulations if speech sounded abnormal.
	"Move your tongue from side to side."	Look for weakness or slowness of movement.
X	"Say, Ah."	Look for asymmetrical palatal elevation. Test for palatal articulations and do gag reflex if speech or swallowing were abnormal.
XI	"Turn your head to one side and don't let me push it back."	Try to push head back to midline. Inspect and palpate SCM muscles. Repeat maneuver to opposite side.

7

Examination of the Somatic Motor System (Exclusive of Cranial Nerves)

But the expression of a well-made man appears not only in his face,
It is in his limbs and joints also, it is curiously in the joints of his hips and wrists.
It is in his walk, the carriage of his neck, the flex of his waist, and knees . . .
To see him pass conveys as much as the best poem, perhaps more.

— Walt Whitman

I. Inspection of the body contours, postures, and muscular actions

A. *Initial appraisal*

1. The motor examination begins as soon as you meet the patient. Study his every activity, how he sits, stands, walks and gestures, his postures, and his general level of activity. Unobtrusive observation of the patient's spontaneous activity often discloses more than formal tests, particularly in infants or mentally ill patients.
2. Next, undress the patient and stand him under an overhead light. Undergarments may remain in place, in deference to modesty, but you must, at some time during the examination, look under them. If you leave one-third of the body covered, you can do only two-thirds of an examination. Before the cock crows, one of you will violate this commandment that thou shalt undress every patient. Your own anxieties about viewing a nude patient may exceed those of the patient about being viewed nude. After all, the patient came to you expecting to be examined.
3. Next, ponder, yes *ponder,* the patient's somatotype—his body contours and proportions, his "build"—comparing it with the standard normal figure of a person of like age and sex. From abnormalities in the patient's *gestalt,* sometimes from just a glance at the silhouette, the clinician

can diagnose an immense number of syndromes, such as arachnodactyly, achondroplastic dwarfism, and Down's syndrome.

4. Next, scrutinize the size and contours of the patient's muscles, looking for atrophy or hypertrophy. Then, look for body asymmetry, joint malalignments, fasciculations, tremors, and involuntary movements. Proceed in an orderly, rostrocaudal, neck-to-toe sequence, and continually compare right and left sides.
5. Next, ask the patient to walk freely across the room. Watch for unsteadiness, a broad-based gait, and lack of arm swinging. Request the patient to walk on the toes, heels, and in tandem (heel-to-toe along a straight line). Request a deep knee bend. Request a child to hop on each foot and to run.
6. Now, to remember the preceding five steps in the preliminary appraisal of the motor system, turn to section VI, step A of the Summarized Neurologic Examination and rehearse them and recite them. Yes, I'll ask you to demonstrate them by and by.

B. *Significance of the preliminary appraisal*

These preliminaries provide an enormous amount of critical information. With normal muscle size and contours, with normal station and gait, with a normal deep-knee bend, and with no visible tremor or involuntary movements, the motor system is most likely normal (and, in all probability, not much is wrong with the sensory system or mentation). However, formal tests of fatiguability, coordination, muscle tone, reflexes, and muscle strength remain.

II. Principles of strength testing

A. *Introduction*

1. Even if an iron bar loses much of its strength, it may remain too strong for you to bend. Contrariwise, tissue paper offers too little resistance. You cannot accurately gauge the strength of movements that are too strong for you to overcome or too weak to provide a certain minimum resistance. Select for strength testing those movements in which the expected strength of the patient matches your own.
2. In the next section, the instructions assume that you will study with another student and do the strength tests on each other. How else can you learn to match your strength against another's? And something else: yes, you should strip down in order to see the muscles and tendons in action. First, after getting your partner, rehearse the steps of section VI, step A of the Summarized Neurologic Examination. Do you remember all of them? No? That's why you may need another rehearsal.

B. *Relation of length to strength of a muscle*

1. With your partner, work through Fig. 7-1*A* to *D* to test biceps and triceps strength. In all strength tests, the participants should exert maximum power, but they should reach a peak in a slow crescendo without jerking. The examiner does the tests by pulling or pushing on the patient's wrist with one hand while stabilizing the patient's elbow or shoulder with the other hand.

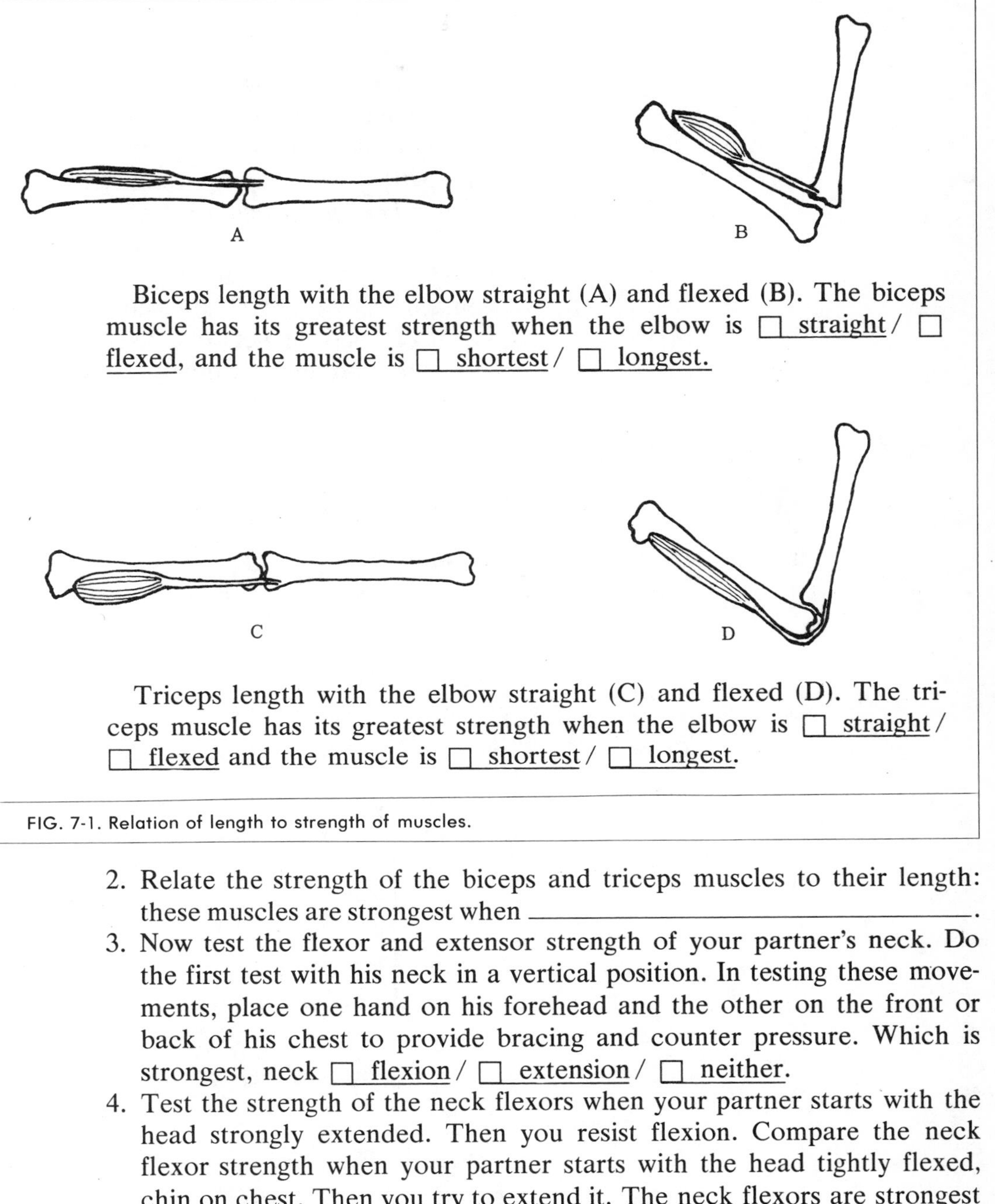

Biceps length with the elbow straight (A) and flexed (B). The biceps muscle has its greatest strength when the elbow is ☐ straight / ☐ flexed, and the muscle is ☐ shortest / ☐ longest.

flexed
shortest

Triceps length with the elbow straight (C) and flexed (D). The triceps muscle has its greatest strength when the elbow is ☐ straight / ☐ flexed and the muscle is ☐ shortest / ☐ longest.

straight
shortest

FIG. 7-1. Relation of length to strength of muscles.

2. Relate the strength of the biceps and triceps muscles to their length: these muscles are strongest when ______________________.

they are shortest

3. Now test the flexor and extensor strength of your partner's neck. Do the first test with his neck in a vertical position. In testing these movements, place one hand on his forehead and the other on the front or back of his chest to provide bracing and counter pressure. Which is strongest, neck ☐ flexion / ☐ extension / ☐ neither.

extension

4. Test the strength of the neck flexors when your partner starts with the head strongly extended. Then you resist flexion. Compare the neck flexor strength when your partner starts with the head tightly flexed, chin on chest. Then you try to extend it. The neck flexors are strongest with the neck ☐ flexed/ ☐ extended, when the flexor muscles are ☐ shortest/ ☐ longest.

flexed
shortest

5. To see whether we have discovered a general length-strength law, test the quadriceps femoris and hamstring muscles. With the knee extended, the quadriceps femoris muscle is ☐ strongest / ☐ weakest and ☐ shortest / ☐ longest.

strongest
shortest

6. Thus, we have confirmed the length-strength law that muscles are strongest when ______________________.

they act from their shortest position.

Note: The physiologists' length-strength law that contraction strength increases with resting length suggests the opposite conclusion.

bent

7. In general, you can test strength more accurately in muscles of weak or modest strength when the patient starts from a position of strength, e.g., neck flexed. However, in testing a very strong muscle, you place it at a disadvantage to bring it within your range of strength. Thus, to reduce the strength of the triceps muscle to bring it within the testing range, test the patient with his elbow ______________.

C. *How to remember the strongest of opposing sets of muscles*

1. We have shown that one set of opposing muscles excedes the other in strength, often by a considerable amount, e.g., neck extension versus flexion. Unless we can find a general law to recall automatically the strongest of opposing sets of muscles, we face the oppressive task of memorizing each set individually. If we look at a quadruped, or, better, a man in quadrupedal position, the solution leaps out at us. See Fig. 7-2.

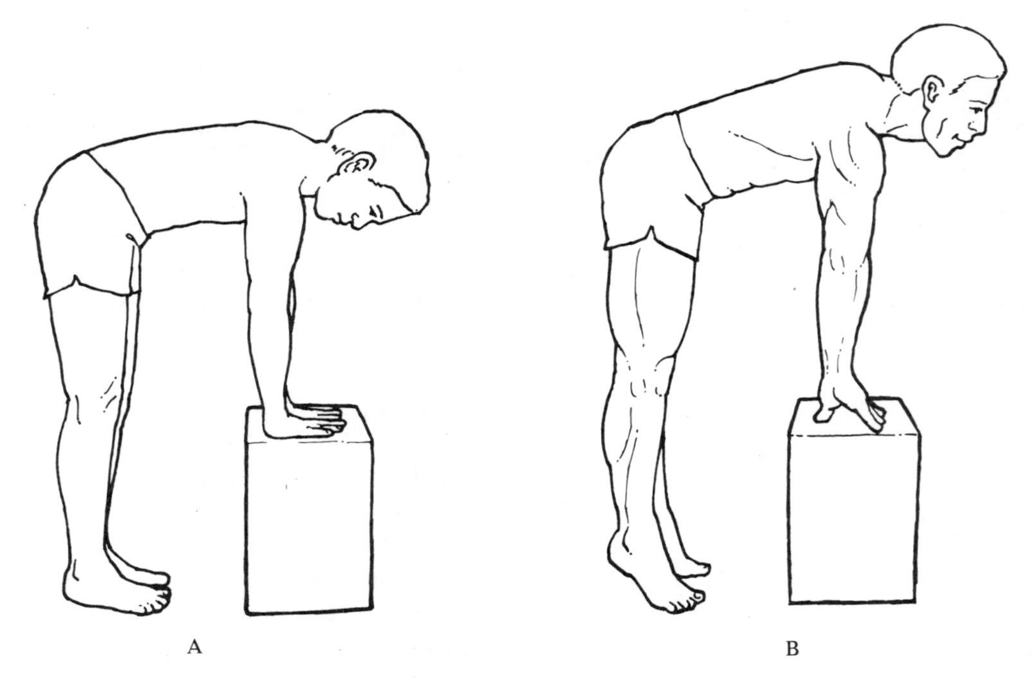

FIG. 7-2. Man in quadrupedal posture. *A.* Relaxed. *B.* Raising on fingers and toes.

2. Stand up and assume the posture of Fig. 7-2*A* and *B*. Of particular importance, assume posture *B*. Notice then how the triceps muscle locks the upper extremities against collapse from the pull of gravity and how the quadriceps femoris locks the lower. Buttocks and back extensors erect the trunk, holding it from collapse by gravity when the individual stands or, equally important, when he leaps or locomotes. When leaping or locomoting, the hands and feet flex downwards. The muscles which support the standing or locomoting posture against collapse by the pull of gravity constitute the antigravity muscle system. Invariably, the strength of these antigravity locking, locomoting, and leaping muscles exceeds the opposing set.
3. Using the principle of the superior strength of the antigravity locking,

flexion
trunk extension
plantar flexion
flexion

locomoting, and leaping muscles, predict the strongest of these opposing movements:

☐ Wrist extension / ☐ flexion
☐ Trunk extension / ☐ flexion
☐ Foot dorsiflexion / ☐ plantar flexion
☐ Toe extension / ☐ flexion

4. Confusion may arise in applying the antigravity theory to arm abduction. When abducting, the arm acts against the pull of gravity, but the abductor muscles do not support the skeletal posture against collapse by gravity when the animal stands or locomotes; hence, they are not postural antigravity muscles and, quite to the contrary, their opponents are. Consider as examples of postural antigravity muscles the pectoral and latissimuss dorsi muscles. The pectoral muscles prevent the forelimbs from straddling out when the animal stands (imagine the leverage acting to spread a giraffe's legs). The latissimus dorsi muscles pull the forelimbs backwards, thrusting the shoulders forward and upward, i.e., against gravity, when the quadruped locomotes. Consequently, the adductor and flexor muscles acting at the shoulder exceed their opponents, the abductor-extensor muscles. Applying this consideration to the hip, which would be stronger? ☐ hip abductors / ☐ hip adductors. Explain.
5. The antigravity theory predicts not only the strongest muscles, but also how much stronger they are. Your arm and hand strength cannot even begin to overcome the antigravity muscles when set in their strongest positions (head and trunk extended; jaw closed; arms and legs extended; wrists, fingers, feet, and toes flexed). But your arm and hand strength just about equals or barely overcomes the antagonistic muscles when set in their strongest position (head and trunk flexed; jaw open; arms and legs flexed; wrist and fingers extended; and feet and toes dorsiflexed).

adductors
Well, read the last paragraph again if you aren't sure.

III. The sequence of muscular testing

A. You have to have a routine for testing muscles. The simplest routine to remember? Test in rostrocaudal order.

B. After testing cranial nerve muscles, simply shift caudally to the neck.

C. Test neck flexor and extensors

1. Which is the weakest of these movements? ________________
2. In what position should the patient place his head to bring flexion strength up into the best range to test? ________________

flexion

head flexed

D. The shoulder girdle muscles

1. The trapezius has been tested with the cranial nerves.
2. Have the patient extend his arms forward, to the sides, and over his head. Inspect from front and back. Look for scapular movement, particularly winging of the dorsal border away from the rib cage.
3. After testing free movement of abduction and elevation of the arms, test the strength of these movements. Here is where you must build your own catalog of experience. Have your partner hold his arms straight out to the sides. Push down on them as he resists you. Where do you push? That depends on you. If you are a woman, push down on the forearms or wrists. If you are a strong man, push down just

proximal to the elbows to reduce your leverage. Select a point where your strength in pushing down about equals that of the standard average person of the height, weight, age, and sex of your patient.

4. Everything is going smoothly at this point. I could just continue to machinegun you with instruction, but how do *I* know what to do next? The answer is easy. Consider the *possible* movements and test those you have not tested. Table 7-1 summarizes the movements. Work through them with your partner.

TABLE 7-1. Method of Testing Shoulder Girdle Strength

Action	Commands and maneuvers
Arm elevation	Command patient to hold his arms straight out to the sides. Press down on both arms at a point where you expect your strength to approximate the patient's.
Arm adduction downward	With the patient's arms extended to the sides, he resists your efforts to elevate them.
Arm adduction across the chest	With the arms extended straight in front, the patient crosses his wrists. You try to pull them apart.
Scapular adduction	With the patient's hands on his hips, the patient forces his elbows backwards as hard as possible. Standing behind him, you try to push them forward.
Scapular winging	Have the patient try a pushup or lean forward against a wall, supporting himself with outstretched arms.

5. Arm abduction is complex, involving supraspinatus action to initiate the act, deltoid action to carry the arm to shoulder height, and scapular rotation to continue the elevation to the vertical position. The scapula is held in place against the chest wall by the serratus anterior and trapezius muscles.

E. *Upper arm muscles*

1. The major movements are flexion and extension of the elbow.
2. *Flexors* are tested by having the patient hold his arm tightly flexed as you attempt to straighten it by pulling at his wrist. When average man contests average man, the battle is a stalemate, therefore, just about proper. By grasping more proximally on the forearm, you can reduce your leverage for children or weak subjects.
3. *Extensors,* so you might think, are tested by having the patient hold his arm extended. But the triceps is tremendously strong, and average man against average man, the exten*dor* wins easily. If, however, you can overcome the patient's extended arm, he has significant weakness. A subtler test is to start with the patient's arm flexed as in testing the flexors, but this time you try to keep the arm flexed while he extends it. The triceps is put at a mechanical disadvantage by this maneuver, and average man against average man, the examiner will win, but barely. Since this test pits nearly equal strengths, it is better for discovering slight loss of power in the triceps than the arm extended position.

extension

arm extended

partially dorsi-
flexed

palm down

F. Forearm muscles

1. *Flexors* of the wrist are tested by asking the patient to make a fist and to hold his wrist flexed against your efforts to extend it.
2. *Extensors* of the wrist are tested by having the patient hold his wrist cocked-up (dorsiflexed) as you try to press it down. While wrist flexion is very strong, wrist extension pits approximately equal strength against the examiner. Therefore, in general, wrist ☐ extension / ☐ flexion is the better test.
3. Test pronation-supination of the forearm by twisting the patient's wrist after he assumes a posture of strength for the muscle under test. How do you position his arm to minimize supination by the biceps? __________ __________.

G. Finger movements

1. Inspect and palpate the thenar and hypothenar eminences carefully for size and asymmetry. Look for atrophy of interosseous muscles. Most old people show obvious interosseous atrophy.
2. *Finger flexion* is tested by having the patient squeeze your fingers. If he is strong, give him only two or three, putting his grip at a disadvantage, or you may rue it. To add an element of fun to the test, particularly with a child, and to keep the patient working at top strength, I frequently grasp the patient's wrist with one hand to steady his arm and place two fingers of my other hand in his hand. Then I instruct him, "Don't let me get away," as I try to pull my fingers from his grasp.
   a. Try this experiment: grip a pencil as tight as possible in your fist. Notice that your wrist automatically *dorsiflexes*. Have your partner try to pull the pencil out of your grip when your hand is in the normal position it automatically assumes when you tighten your grip. Then, hold your wrist *flexed* as strongly as possible and have him try to pull the pencil out of your grip. Finger flexion is strongest when the wrist is ☐ strongly flexed / ☐ partially dorsiflexed.
   b. This experiment shows that partial dorsiflexion of the wrist allows the strongest grip. Partial dorsiflexion is the functional position of the hand, the position chosen when putting a cast on the forearm or wrist to treat a fracture, or when splinting the wrist to maintain optimum hand position while the patient recovers from paralysis.
3. *Finger extension* is tested by having the patient hold out his hands with the fingers hyperextended. Simply turn your hand over so that the dorsum of your fingernail presses against the dorsum of his. Then you can carefully match his extensor strength against yours.
4. Test adduction-abduction of the fingers as usual by matching your strength against the patient's. But figure it out carefully. Assume that you want to test the first dorsal interosseous muscle of your partner's (or your own) left hand. This muscle abducts the index finger. To match the strength of the patient's finger, you should place the terminal phalanx of your index finger alongside the terminal phalanx of his. If he holds his hand palm down, should you hold your palm down or palm up to match muscle against muscle? ☐ palm down / ☐ palm up. Work through the fingers, learning how to match abductors and adductors. See Fig. 7-2.1.

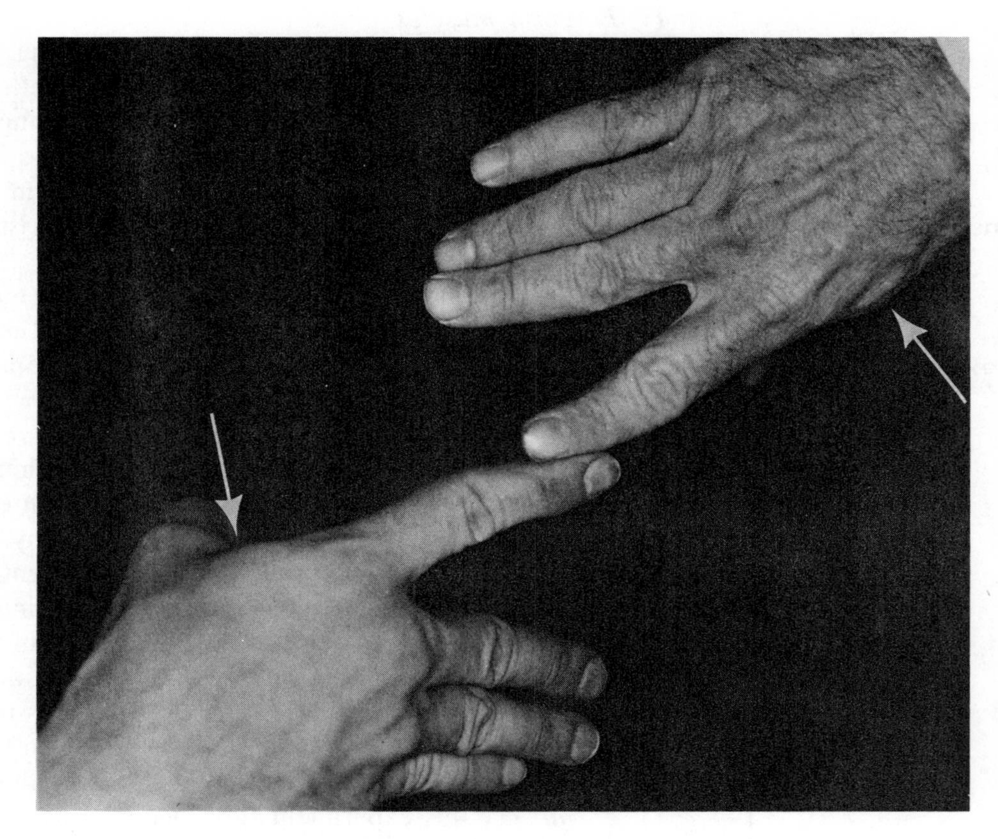

FIG. 7-2.1. Method of matching the examiner's finger strength against the patient's. Notice the bulging first dorsal interosseous muscle (arrows) of both examiner and patient.

H. *Abdominal muscles*

1. *Position.* Have the patient supine (on his back). Ask him to do a situp, or to elevate his legs or his head. At the same time watch the umbilicus as the abdominal muscles contract and palpate the muscle action. If he has equal strength in all four quadrants of the abdomen, the umbilicus will remain centered. But, if the *lower* abdominal muscles are weak, and the *upper* are intact, the umbilicus would migrate __________ *ward* when the patient contracts his abdominal muscles.

upward

   a. Suppose the *right* abdominal muscles were weak, the *left* normal. In which direction would the umbilicus migrate when the patient lifts his head or legs, contracting the abdominal muscles? ☐ up / ☐ down / ☐ right / ☐ left.

left

   b. In general, if some abdominal muscles are weak, the umbilicus will migrate ☐ toward / ☐ away from the pull of the intact muscles during strong abdominal contraction.

toward

   c. The umbilical migration test is invaluable for localizing the level of spinal cord lesions. The umbilicus is innervated by the 10th thoracic segment of the spinal cord. If the patient has a transverse spinal cord lesion at this level, all muscles caudal to T10 are paralyzed. The umbilicus migrates ☐ upward / ☐ downward when the patient contracts his abdomen.

upward

I. Large back muscles are so strong that they cannot be readily tested in the average patient. Two tests can be done:

1. *Position.* Have the patient prone (face down):
   a. Ask him to arch his back and rock on his stomach.
   b. Inspect and palpate the paraspinal muscles.
2. Have the patient bend forward at the waist and straighten up.

J. The hip girdle

1. *Position.* Patient supine.
   a. Have the patient hold his legs abducted as you try to press them together.
   b. Then have him try to hold them adducted as you try to pull them apart.
2. *Position.* Patient prone: have the patient lift his knee from the table surface to test the strength of his hip extensors.
3. *Position.* Patient supine.
   a. Have the patient lift his knee off the table surface.
   b. Try to push it back down to test the hip flexors.

K. The thigh muscles

1. The deep-knee bend has already tested the quadriceps, which ordinarily is too strong to test by opposition, but if you try to hold the leg flexed, the quadriceps is at a mechanical disadvantage in straightening the leg. Compare the strength of extension of both legs.
2. The knee flexors are tested by having the patient hold the knee at a 90° angle while you try to straighten it.

L. The leg muscles

1. *Position.* Patient sitting or reclining.
   a. Have the patient dorsiflex, invert, and evert his foot. Inspect, palpate the leg, and check for strength of these movements.
   b. These movements pit equal strength against equal strength and are very useful tests. Plantar flexion of the foot is ordinarily too strong for you to test by opposition. Have the patient raise himself up on his toes, supporting his entire weight, one foot at a time. If you had the patient walk on his toes, as requested under general inspection, this part of the exam is already done.
   c. Have the patient hold his toes flexed or extended, and you try to press them back to the neutral position.

M. The screening tests for muscle strength during the routine physical examination

1. To test the strength of every muscle in every patient would squander time. For the routine examination, the strength of a few selected movements serves as a sample of all. The history and preliminary appraisal permit you to tailor the muscle examination to the patient's problem by selecting the critical muscles for testing and the conditions under which the tests should be done. For example, if the patient complains of weak-

ness after exertion, have him climb stairs before testing him. If he says that his muscles "freeze up" when cold, put his arm in ice water before testing it. If his muscles cramp when he writes, have him write. So often, physicians fail to examine the patient under conditions which reproduce his symptoms.

2. The irreducible minimum routine strength examination of every patient for whom you claim to have done a physical examination consists of section VI, step C of the Summarized Neurologic Examination. Rehearse it.
3. In patients with neurologic symptoms and signs, you must go far beyond this minimum examination.

N. Detailed testing of individual muscles

The diagnosis of specific nerve injuries requires detailed testing of individual muscles. Of the many manuals available, the first one listed in the bibliography fits in your bag and can be carried around. This economical little pamphlet is a best buy for conciseness and quality.

O. Recording the muscle examination

1. Table 7-2 lists the clinically testable muscles or movements. For a normal patient who has no neuromuscular signs or symptoms, a simple statement on the medical record might suffice, but if you see the patient again in a month, and he now has some weakness, only a detailed record will prove that you actually tested the muscle and did not overlook something.
2. Several grading systems are used in recording muscular strength. The strength can be estimated on a scale from 0 to 5, 0 for complete paralysis, 5 for normal strength. Or, you can use a word system, such as *paralysis, severe weakness, moderate weakness, minimal weakness,* and *normal.*

Bibliography

Aids to the Examination of the Peripheral Nervous System. Medical Research Council (Great Britain) Memorandum no. 45, 1st ed., London, Her Majesty's Stationery Office, 1976.

D'Ambrosia, R. D. (ed.): *Musculoskeletal Disorders, Regional Examination and Differential Diagnosis,* Philadelphia, J. B. Lippincott Co., 1977.

Daniels, L., Williams, M., and Worthingham, C.: *Muscle Testing, Techniques of Manual Examination,* 3rd ed., Philadelphia, W. B. Saunders Co., 1972.

Hollinshead, W.: *Functional Anatomy of the Limbs and Back,* 3rd ed., Philadelphia, W. B. Saunders, 1969.

Kopell, H., and Thompson, W.: *Peripheral Entrapment Neuropathies,* Baltimore, The Williams & Wilkins Co., 1963; 2nd ed., 1976.

Paine, R.: Abnormal gaits in children, *Clin. Proc. Child. Hosp.,* 22:43-51, 1968.

Rosse, C., and Clawson, D.: *Introduction to the Musculoskeletal System,* New York, Harper & Row, 1970.

Sunderland, S.: *Nerves and Nerve Injuries,* 2nd ed., New York, Churchill Livingstone, 1979.

P. Direct percussion of muscle: It will come as no surprise to the cognoscente in physical diagnosis that after inspecting and palpating a muscle, it ought to be percussed.

TABLE 7 – 2. Chart for Recording Muscle Tests

Right side						Left side			
Fascicu-lations	Tone	Size	Strength	MUSCLES	LEVEL OF NEURAXIS	Strength	Size	Tone	Fascicu-lations
				Temporal	Cranial nerve V				
				Masseter	V				
				Pterygoid	V				
				Frontalis	VII				
				Orbicularis oculi	VII				
				Mouth	VII				
				Platysma	VII				
				Soft palate	X				
				Pharynx	X				
				Sternomastoid	XI				
				Trapezius	XI				
				Tongue	XII				
				Neck, flexors	C 1-6				
				Neck, extensors	C1-T1				
				Scapular	C 4-7				
				Pectoralis major	5-T1				
				Deltoid	C 56				
				Biceps	56				
				Triceps	678				
				Wrist, extensors	678				
				Wrist, flexors	678 T1				
				Digits, extensors	678				
				Digits, flexors	78 T1				
				Thenar	8 1				
				Hypothenar	8 1				
				Interossei	8 1				
				Back					
				Abdomen	T 6-L1				
				Iliopsoas	L1234				
				Adductors, thigh	234				
				Abductors, thigh	45 S1				
				Gluteus max.	5 S12				
				Quadriceps femoris	234				
				Hamstrings	45 S12				
				Tibialis anterior	45 S1				
				Toes, extensors	45 S1				
				Peronei	45 S1				
				Gastroc.-soleus	5 S12				
				Toes, flexors	5 S12				

1. *Percussion irritability of muscle.* Independent of reflex or volitional contraction, muscle fibers have the inherent property of contracting in response to direct percussion.
   a. Bare your biceps muscle and strike its belly a sharp blow with the *point* of your reflex hammer. You will see a faint dimple or ripple at the percussion site. Strike a crisp blow and get the hammer out of the way because the ripple is very transient. It results from contraction of the muscle fibers directly percussed. It demonstrates the intrinsic irritability of muscle and is not a reflex. In fact, in LMN lesions, when the muscle is denervated, percussion irritability of muscle is *increased* for a period of time.
   b. Percussion irritability of muscle is not a reflex. We will discuss muscle stretch reflexes in the next section. Because of percussion irritability, however, the muscle stretch reflex is not elicited by percussing the muscle directly, but by percussing its tendon.
2. *Percussion myoedema.* Sometimes muscle percussion causes a tiny hump at the percussion site. Its physiology is poorly understood. It is seen in some normal people and often in debilitation, uremia, and myxedema.
3. *Percussion myotonia*
   a. Place your hand on the table, palm up. Sharply percuss your thenar eminence with the point of your percussion hammer. If your thumb slowly rises up from your palm and holds up, you have got problems. You have *percussion myotonia.*
   b. Next place a tongue blade under your tongue and percuss your tongue as you watch it in the mirror. If your tongue mounds up, you have *percussion myotonia.*
   c. Myotonia can be demonstrated in another way. The patient is asked to make a tight fist and to flip his fingers open as quickly as possible on command. If he has myotonia, he cannot open his fingers rapidly, because of sustained "after contraction" or delayed relaxation of the flexors. Myotonia is seen in myopathies, mainly myotonia dystrophica and myotonia congenita, and also in paramyotonia congenita and some types of periodic muscular paralysis associated with a disturbance in potassium metabolism.

irritability
myoedema
myotonia

4. List the three muscular responses to direct percussion: percussion ______________, percussion ______________, and percussion ______________.

irritability

5. Of these responses, only percussion ______________ is normally found.

myoedema

6. Some normal people may show percussion ______________.

myotonia
muscle

7. No normal people have percussion ______________. It indicates a primary disease of the ______________, hence a myopathy.

Bibliography

Brody, I. A., and Rozear, M. P.: Contraction response to muscle percussion; physiology and clinical significance, *Arch. Neurol.,* 23:259-265, 1970.

Brooke, M. H.: *A Clinician's View of Neuromuscular Diseases,* Baltimore, The Williams & Wilkins Co., 1977.
Dyken, P.: Extraocular myotonia in families with dystrophia myotonica, *Neurology,* 16: 738-740, 1966.
Patel, A., and Swami, R.: Muscle percussion and neostigmine test in the clinical evaluation of neuromuscular disorders, *New Engl. J. Med.,* 281:523-526, 1969.
Walton, J. N. (ed.): *Disorders of Voluntary Muscle,* London, Churchill Livingstone, 1974.

IV. Examination of muscle stretch reflexes

A. Physiology of the muscle stretch reflexes

1. Study this classification of muscle:

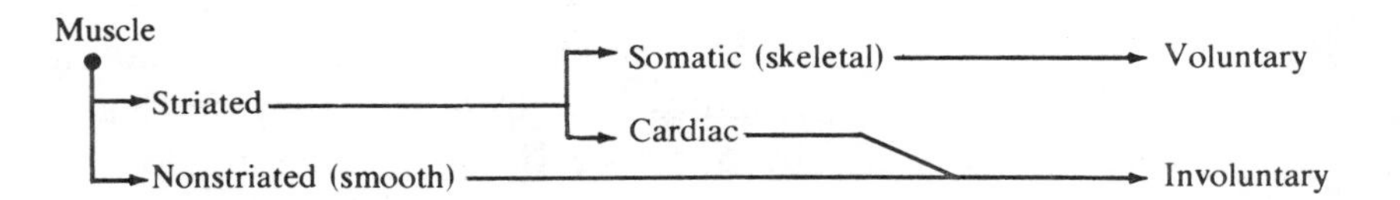

2. Evolution has perfected muscle fibers for precisely one thing: contractility. Whenever a muscle fiber is stimulated by a chemical agent, electricity, or mechanical stretching such as by percussion, the fiber contracts. Stretch is not only the basis of percussion irritability but also of a different phenomenon, reflex irritability. Somatic muscles have specialized stretch-sensitive receptors called *muscle spindles.* Study Fig. 7-3.

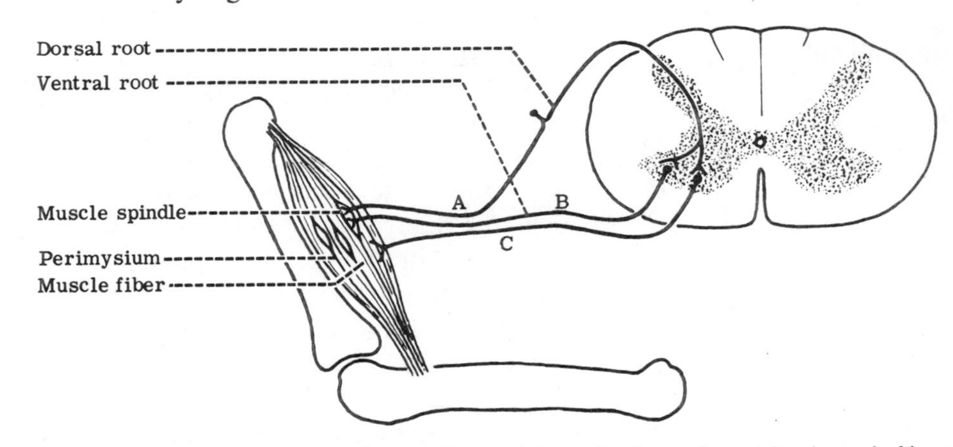

FIG. 7-3. Muscle spindle innervation. The muscle spindles are tiny bags of specialized muscle fibers, located in the equatorial plane of the muscle. They have an afferent and an efferent nerve supply, axons *A* and *B*. The regular muscle fibers have only an efferent axon, C.

3. The muscle fibers of the spindle originate and insert into the perimysial connective tissue which ultimately is continuous with the tendons. The muscle spindles can be regarded as "muscles within a muscle." If the joint in Fig. 7-3 *extends*, the tendon pulls on the perimysium and stretches the muscle spindles. If the joint is flexed, the muscle spindles are ☐ stretched / ☐ relaxed.

relaxed

4. The information that the spindle muscle fibers have changed length

relax

is relayed to the neuraxis by axon *A* in Fig. 7-3. In order that the muscle spindles remain sensitive to stretch throughout the entire range of muscle movement, they must readjust their length whenever the length of the muscle changes. If the part has been *flexed*, the muscle fibers of the spindle contract slightly to maintain their original tension. If the part has been extended, the spindles would □ relax / □ contract to maintain their original tension.

5. The resting length and the resting tension of the spindle fibers are reset for each change in muscle length. The readjustment of spindle tension is effected by axon *A*, afferent, and axon *B*, efferent, in Fig. 7-3.
6. Electromyography shows that the fibers of a resting muscle are electrically silent. If, however, the recording needle is inserted into a spindle fiber, they are found to chatter incessantly because they maintain some degree of stretch-detecting tension. Whenever the muscle spindles are stretched, they send an afferent volley into the neuraxis by axon *A*. If the stretch is slow, the spindles signal intermittently and asynchronously. The spindles quickly adapt to the new length and resume a baseline level of activity. If the stretch is rapid, essentially instantaneous, all spindles signal synchronously. A strong afferent volley enters the neuraxis over axon *A*.
7. The strong afferent volley stimulates the LMNs. The resultant discharge of motor units is seen clinically as a muscular contraction, the muscle stretch reflex (MSR). The efferent axon is axon *C*, of Fig. 7-3. This axon innervates the regular muscle fibers, while axon *B* innervates the spindle fibers.

muscle spindles

regular muscle fibers

reduced

8. The event which initiates the MSR is stretch of the □ muscle spindles / □ regular muscle fibers.
9. The resultant twitch of the muscle is the result of contraction of the □ muscle spindles / □ regular muscle fibers.
10. When the MSR acts, the muscular contraction pulls the ends of the tendons closer together. The tension on the muscle spindles momentarily is □ reduced / □ increased whenever the tendons approximate each other. Hence, the spindles cease firing abruptly, and the MSR ends abruptly.
11. When the muscle comes to rest at a new length, what adjustment takes place in the muscle spindles? ________________________

____

Ans: They reset their tension to the baseline level.

12. Explain why only a quick stretch elicits an MSR:

____

____

____

____

Ans: All spindles must fire rapidly and synchronously to discharge the LMNs. If the stretch is too slow, the spindles fire slowly and asynchronously, and they adapt to the new resting length without sending a sufficiently strong volley to discharge the LMNs.

13. Muscle fibers can be made to contract in response to stretch of the

percussion

muscle spindles

enhanced

reduced or abolished

muscle membrane by direct percussion of the fiber. This phenomenon is called ______________ irritability of muscle.

14. In contrast to percussion irritability, reflex irritability of muscle depends on a strong volley of afferent impulses initiated by the stretch of the ______________ ______________, which are specialized stretch receptors.
15. Percussion irritability is temporarily ☐ eliminated/ ☐ enhanced/ ☐ unchanged when the muscle is denervated (Cannon's law).
16. Reflex irritability is ☐ reduced or abolished/ ☐ enhanced/ ☐ unchanged by denervation.

Bibliography

Davson, H., and Segal, M. B.: *Introduction to Physiology, Vol. 4: Mechanisms of Motor Control,* London, Academic Press, 1978.

Granit, R.: *The Basis of Motor Control,* New York, Academic Press, 1970.

Yahr, M., and Purpura, D.: *Neurophysiological Basis of Normal and Abnormal Motor Activities,* Hewlett, N.Y., Raven Press, 1967.

B. Technique of eliciting an MSR (muscle stretch reflex)

1. *Holding the percussion hammer*

   a. A percussion hammer permits you to strike a rapid blow, producing the instantaneous stretch of muscle spindles necessary to elicit a MSR. You must use a loose wrist and hold the hammer loosely between the thumb and forefinger. Think of the hammer handle as a bird: hold it too tightly and you crush it to death. Hold it too loosely and it flies away. Fig. 7-4 shows how a loose wrist and grip permits a double whiplash effect, imparting the maximal terminal velocity to the hammer head.

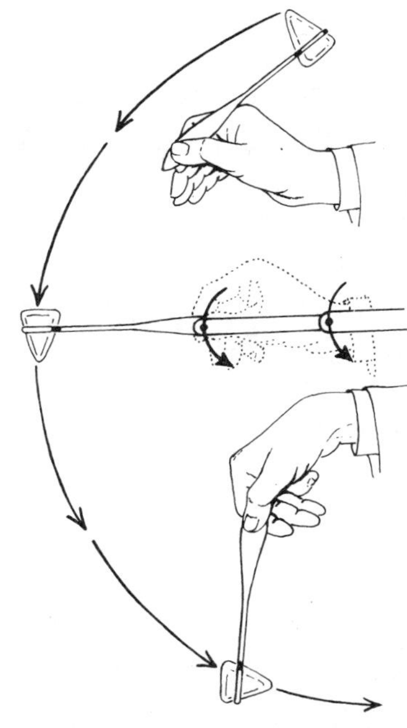

FIG. 7-4. Technique for striking a blow with a reflex hammer. Notice the loose, double pivot action at the wrist and fingers.

b. Practice by holding your wrist six inches above a hard table top. Strike the top a crisp blow. With the correct terminal velocity and looseness of wrist and grip, the hammer head bounces all of the way back up and falls backward across the crevice between thumb and forefinger.

2. *Position of the patient*
   The part to be tested should be at rest, with the muscle relaxed and the joint it moves placed so that the blow on the tendon deforms the tendon and transmits a stretch to the muscle spindles. Usually the best position is intermediate, between full extension and full flexion.
3. Although all somatic muscles will respond to a stretch stimulus by contracting, only a few muscles are sampled in the routine examination. The technique for eliciting these reflexes is shown in Figs. 7-5 to 7-17. Work through these figures, testing the reflexes on yourself where possible, and on another subject. Do the reflexes in pairs, directly comparing right and left sides (except for the jaw reflex).

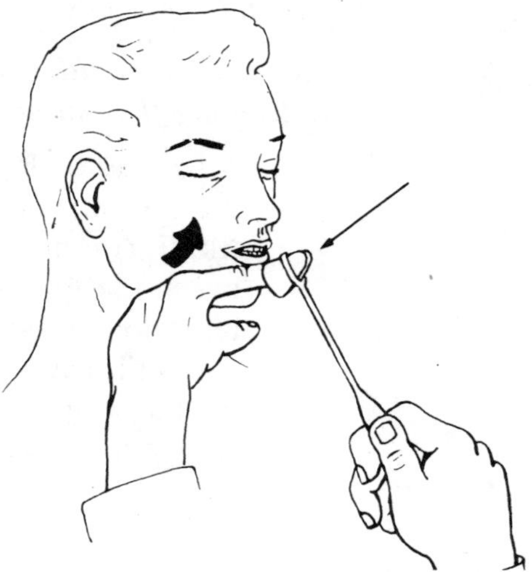

FIG. 7-5. *Jaw reflex.* The patient lets his jaw sag loosely open. The examiner rests his finger across the jaw and strikes it a crisp blow. In this and subsequent illustrations, the direction of the percussion hammer blow is shown by the thin arrow, the direction of the response by the thick arrow.

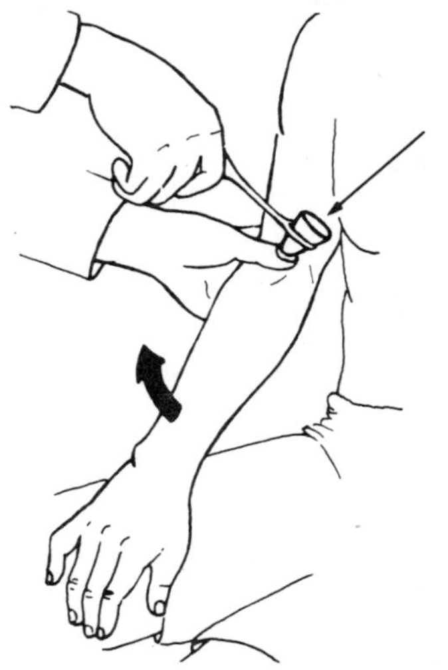

FIG. 7-6. *Biceps reflex.* The biceps tendon is placed under slight tension by the examiner's thumb. The examiner strikes his thumbnail a sharp blow.

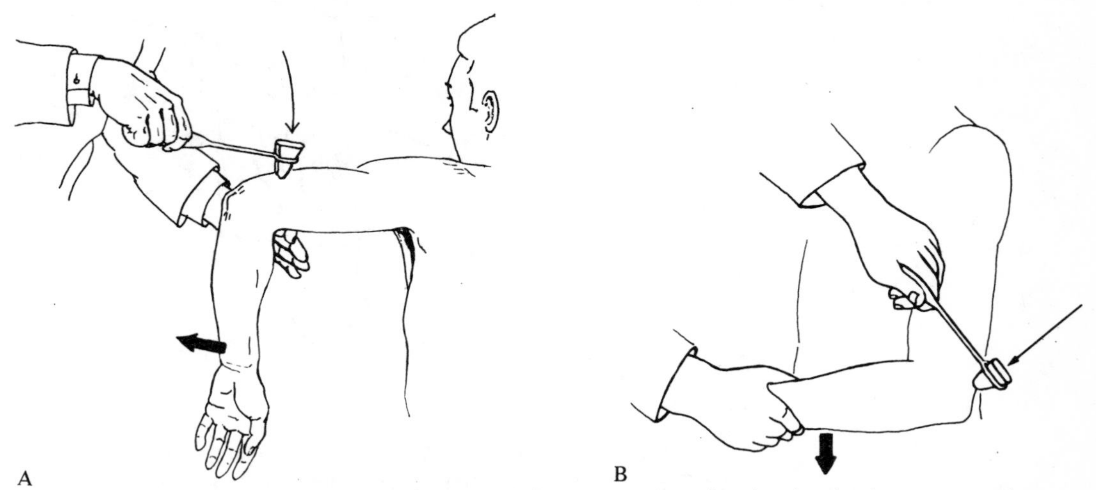

FIG. 7-7. *Triceps reflex. A.* Dangle the patient's forearm over your hand and strike the triceps tendon. *B.* Cradle the patient's forearm in your hand and strike the triceps tendon.

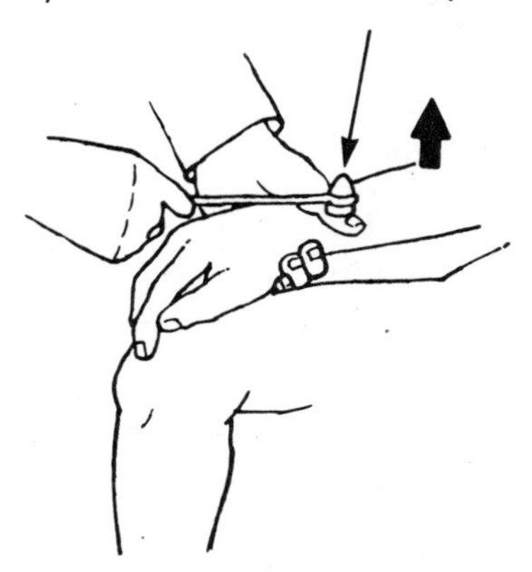

FIG. 7-8. *Brachioradialis reflex.* As in eliciting the triceps reflex, the examiner first tries with the patient's arm at rest on the thigh and then, if necessary to get a response, he lifts the forearm with his free hand. He may cradle both forearms simultaneously to compare more accurately the responses of the two sides. Notice the hammer striking the examiner's thumb rather than the patient's radius.

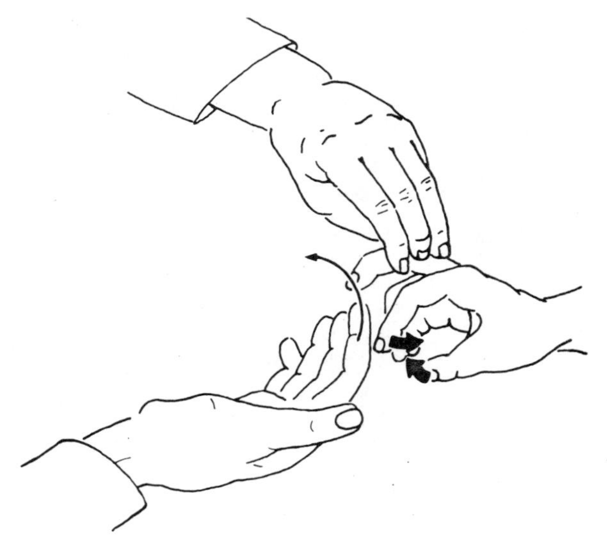

FIG. 7-9. *Finger flexion reflex* (Tromner's method). The patient's hand is relaxed, supported only by the examiner, who briskly flips the patient's distal phalanx upward, as though trying to flip a handful of water high into the air. The patient's fingers and thumb flex in response to the stretch of the finger flexor muscles.

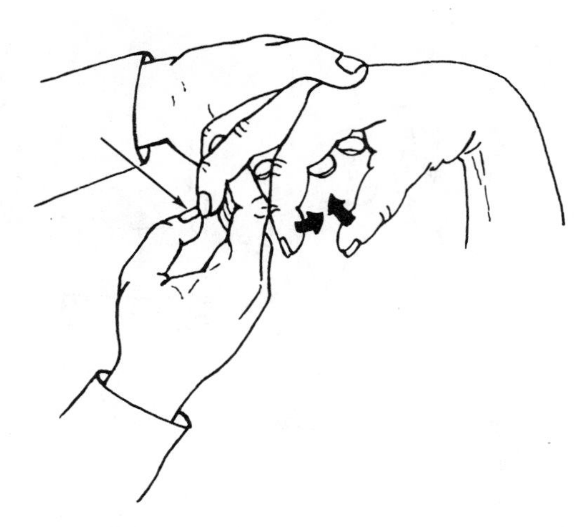

FIG. 7-10. *Finger flexion reflex* (Hoffman's method). The examiner depresses the distal phalanx and allows it to flip up sharply. The extension of the phalanx stretches the flexor muscles, causing the fingers and thumb to flex. This method is effective only when the patient's MSRs are very brisk.

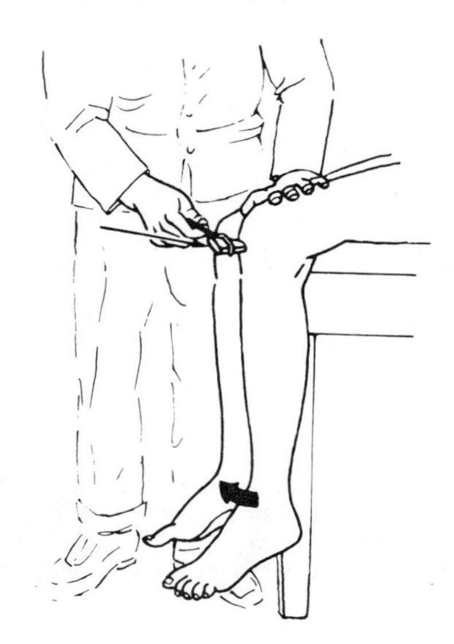

FIG. 7-11. *Quadriceps femoris reflex*, patient erect. The examiner strikes the patellar tendon a crisp blow. He places his hand on the knee to feel as well as to see the magnitude of the response.

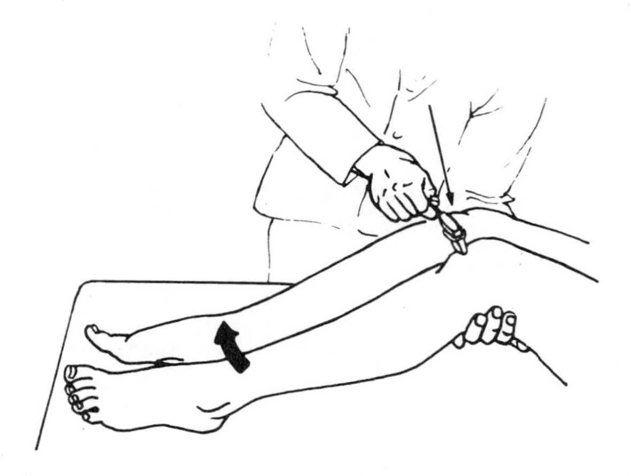

FIG. 7-12. *Quadriceps femoris reflex*, patient supine. The examiner bends the patient's legs to place slight tension on the patellar tendon. The blow then will deform the tendon and transmit a stretch to the muscle.

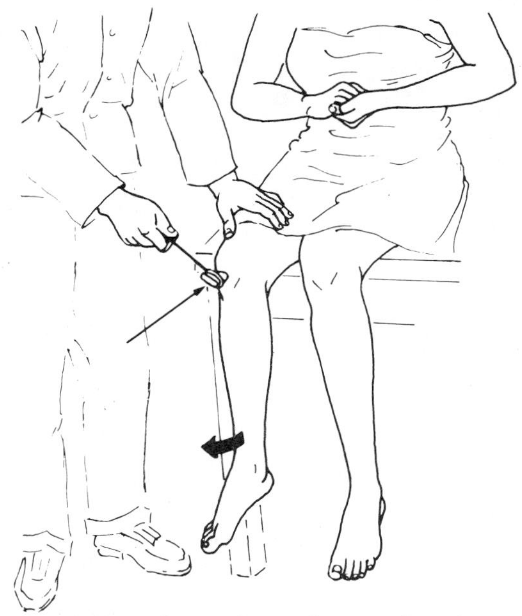

FIG. 7-13. *Pull method* of Jendrassik for reinforcing the quadriceps reflex. The patient grips his hands and pulls apart hard while the examiner strikes the tendon.

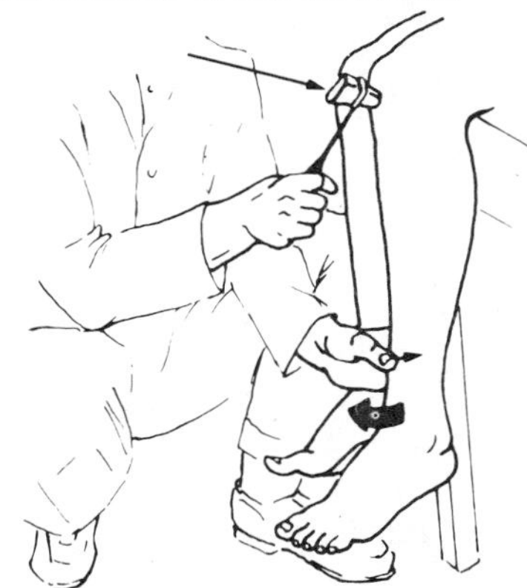

FIG. 7-14. *Counterpressure method* for reinforcing the quadriceps reflex. The examiner applies slight pressure with his thumb (small arrow) against the patient's tibia. The patient counteracts the thumb pressure by slightly tensing his quadriceps femoris muscle. Then the examiner strikes the quadriceps tendon.

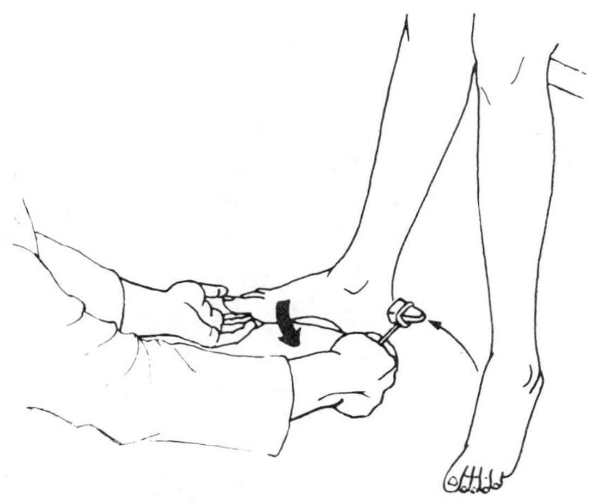

FIG. 7-15. *Triceps surae reflex*, patient sitting. The patient completely relaxes the leg. The examiner places slight tension on the Achilles tendon by dorsiflexing the foot. Reinforcement is tried if no reflex is obtained.

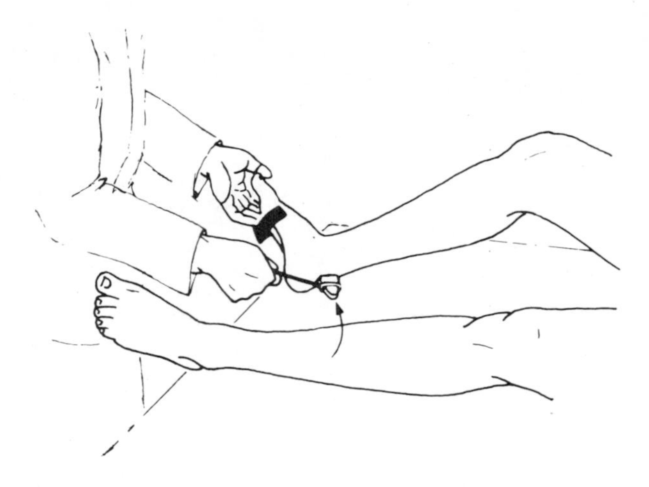

FIG. 7-16. *Triceps surae reflex,* patient supine. The knee is bent to relax the triceps surae muscle and the foot is dorsiflexed to allow the examiner to control the tension necessary to elicit the reflex. Reinforcement is tried if no reflex is obtained.

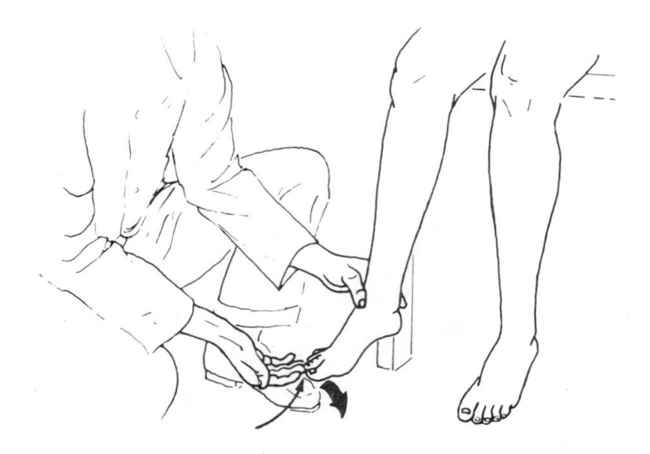

FIG. 7-17. *Toe flexion reflex* (Rossolimo's method). The maneuver is identical with the finger flexion method, Fig. 7-9.

C. *What to do if you get no response in your attempt to elicit an MSR*
   1. Make sure you have struck the blow crisply.
   2. Change the mechanical tension on the muscle by:
      a. Moving the part to a slightly different position.
      b. Compressing the tendon slightly more, or slightly less, with your finger.
   3. Try *reinforcement*
      a. Excitability of the MSR is enhanced by slight *voluntary* contraction of the muscle. This can be done by having the patient make a strong voluntary contraction of a muscle you are *not* testing. Thus, if you fail to get a quadriceps femoris reflex after several trials, have the patient lock his fingers together and pull hard, as shown in Fig. 7-13. The voluntary UMN innervation of the arm muscles "overflows" to increase the excitability of the LMN pool of the lower extremities.

b. If these maneuvers fail, the patient can be asked to tense slightly the muscle being tested. Request the patient to just counterbalance slight pressure you apply against the action of the muscle, as shown in Fig. 7-14.

4. If all maneuvers are ineffective, you conclude that the MSRs are absent, which always indicates a pathologic condition, with these exceptions:
   a. In infants, normal children, and young adults, the jaw reflex is difficult to elicit.
   b. In infants, the tendons are not well developed, and it is difficult to elicit the biceps, triceps, quadriceps, and triceps surae reflexes. The quadriceps is difficult to elicit because the patella is not developed, but by positioning the leg nearly straight, with the infant recumbent, the quadriceps reflex usually can be obtained.
   c. In young children, especially girls, the biceps reflex remains hard to elicit because the tendon is not prominent.

D. Analyze this clinical problem

partially bent across her thigh

1. Suppose you want to examine the biceps reflex of a 38-year-old conscious woman. She is seated and positioned with her arm ______________________________.

2. Although you have struck a crisp blow, you got no MSR. List the maneuvers you must try before concluding that the patient has no biceps MSR. ______________________________.

Ans: Place more or less tension on the tendon with thumb pressure. Re-position the elbow at a slightly different angle. Ask her to "tense" her leg muscles (extend her legs) for reinforcement. (The counterpressure method of reinforcement cannot be used conveniently for arm reflexes.)

3. In the same patient, you are unable to elicit the quadriceps reflex when the patient is sitting. What maneuvers do you try before concluding she has no quadriceps MSR? ______________________________

Ans: Request the patient to lock her hands and pull; ask the patient to counterbalance the slight pressure you apply against the tibia, the *pull* and *counterpressure* methods of reinforcement. If these fail, place her supine and try different positions of flexion of her legs. Above all make sure you strike the tendon a crisp blow.

E. Nomenclature of the MSRs

1. All the methods for eliciting MSRs involve stretching the muscle by tapping on its tendon, or by percussing the bone of insertion of the tendon, as in the brachioradialis (radial) reflex. The reflex should be named according to the muscles which respond or the part which moves. The common denominator of all the maneuvers which elicit a MSR, whether it is tapping a tendon, a bone, or flipping a digit, is that the muscle spindles are mechanically ______________.

stretched (stimulated)

2. The fact that the MSR was elicited by tendon percussion led to the archaic, misleading name of "deep tendon reflexes" for the MSRs. This name carries the connotation that the receptor for the reflex is in the tendons. In fact, most studies suggest that tendon receptors are inhibitory to the MSR. Here is what one author said: "It seems, therefore, most desirable to discard the term 'tendon reflex' altogether. The phenomena are, according to the explanation above given, dependent on a 'muscle reflex' irritability, which has nothing to do with the tendons. If we wish to describe them by a general term, it will be best to employ 'tendon-muscular phenomena,' but the intervention of tendons is not necessary for their production; the one condition which all have in common is that passive tension is essential for their occurrence, and they may more conveniently be termed myotatic contractions (myo = muscle; teinein = to stretch). The irritability, on which they depend, is due to and demonstrative of a muscle reflex action which depends on the spinal cord."
3. This conclusion was offered in 1885 by William Gowers (1845-1915). One section of Gowers' book (pages 222-230) stands as a great classic in reflexology, because he synthesized a complex body of knowledge into a single word, *myotatic*. But his plea for rational, informative terminology has fallen unheeded. Each generation of medical students is taught the "deep tendon reflexes" and almost universally fails to understand the spindle mechanism.

Bibliography

Gassel, M., and Diamantopoulos, E.: The Jendrassik maneuver. I. The pattern of reinforcement of monosynaptic reflexes in normal subjects and patients with spasticity or rigidity, *Neurology,* 14:555-560, 1964.

Gowers, W.: *Diagnosis of Diseases of the Brain and of the Spinal Cord,* New York, William Wood & Co., 1885.

Hagbarth, K-E., Wallin, G., Burke, D., and Lofstedt, L.: Effects of the Jendrassik manoeuvre on muscle spindle activity in man. *J. Neurol. Neurosurg. Psychiatry,* 38:1143-1153, 1975.

Wartenberg, R.: *The Examination of Reflexes,* Chicago, Year Book Medical Publishers, Inc., 1945.

F. Recording the MSRs by using a stick figure

1. The MSRs and, as we shall see later, other reflexes can be recorded for interpretation at a glance. The MSRs are graded on a scale from 0 to 4+. See Table 7-3.

TABLE 7-3. Grading of MSRs	
0	Areflexia
±	Hyporeflexia
1 to 3	Average
3+ to 4+	Hyperreflexia

2. Notice in Fig. 7-18*A*, a normal subject, that the finger and toe flexion MSRs may not be obtainable. The important feature of any reflex pattern is not the absolute value assigned, but the asymmetry or discrepancy between one part of the body and another.

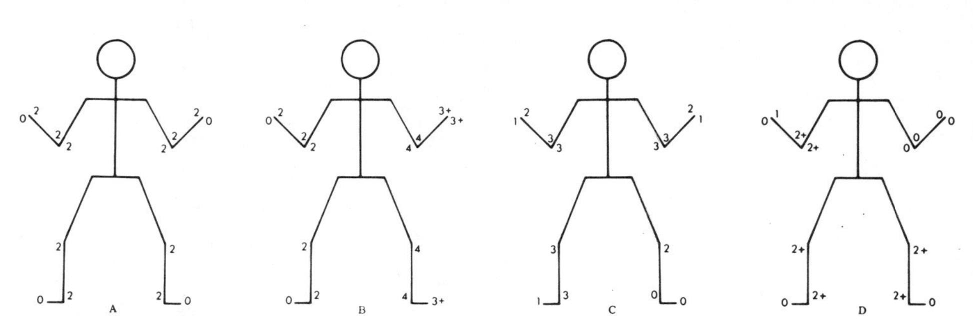

FIG. 7-18. Stick figure method of recording muscle stretch reflexes (MSRs).

b. hyperreflexia on the L.
c. quadriceps hyporeflexia, triceps surae, and toe areflexia on the L.
d. areflexia left arm.

3. How would you describe the reflex pattern of:
   a. Fig. 7-18*A:* This pattern is normal.
   b. Fig. 7-18*B:* ____________________
   c. Fig. 7-18*C:* ____________________
   d. Fig. 7-18*D:* ____________________

G. *Clinical analysis of the causes of areflexia or hyporeflexia.* Areflexia is pathologic, excepting toe and finger MSRs, and in some infants and children whose tendons are not yet strongly developed. Since the threshold for MSRs has a normal range of variability, some subjects with generalized hyporeflexia or hyperreflexia will not be pathologic, but will merely be at one end of the normal range. In deciphering the cause of areflexia or hyporeflexia, you must think through the reflex arc. See Fig. 7-19.

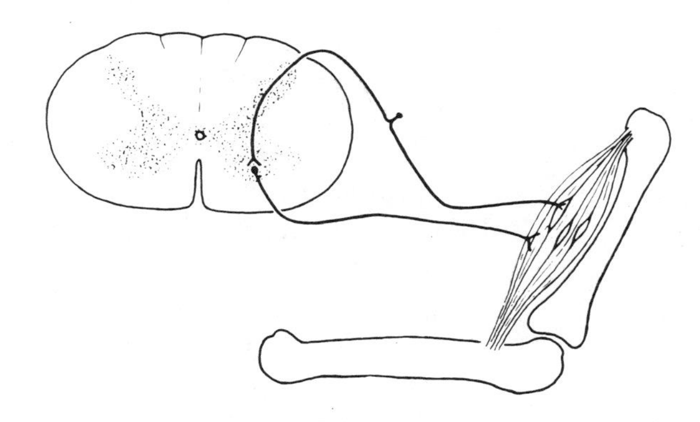

FIG. 7-19. Simplified diagram of the arc for the muscle stretch reflex. This reflex can be regarded as a closed ring, the muscle being both receptor and effector.

1. You may begin at any point since the muscle converts the arc into a circle, but let us establish the habit of starting with the *receptor.* The adequate stimulus is stretch of the muscle. If you get no response, then

Hit crisper blow, alter tendon tension by finger pressure or repositioning, try reinforcement.

ask this question: Was my stimulus adequate? Outline the clinical maneuvers to elicit a reflex when you fail on your first attempts: ____.

strongly

weakly

The two methods of reinforcement are:

a. To have the patient contract ☐ strongly / ☐ weakly a set of muscles *not* being tested.

b. To have the patient contract ☐ strongly / ☐ weakly the muscle being tested.

2. If you are certain that you have applied the stimulus for the MSR properly, the next step in thinking through the reflex arc is to consider the integrity of muscle spindles and afferent limb. We cannot directly check the integrity of the muscle spindle clinically, but we have a means to test the afferent limb.

No

a. Suppose you cut a dorsal root supplying afferent fibers to the cord from the muscle spindles, could you get an MSR? ☐ Yes / ☐ No.

b. If the dorsal root is cut, the patient loses sensation in the distribution of the root. Hence, if the lesion causing areflexia is in the afferent arc, the patient should also lose sensation.

No

c. Would you expect the muscle to be paralyzed if only the afferent limb of the reflex arc was interrupted? ☐ Yes / ☐ No. Explain ____

Ans: As long as UMN and LMN pathways are intact, the muscle fibers will contract and movement is possible. In tabes dorsalis, for example, the axons of the dorsal roots selectively degenerate and the spinal cord is partially deafferentiated. Since the afferent axons from the muscle spindles are lost, the patient is areflexic, but he is not paralyzed.

No

d. Would the patient whose areflexia was caused by a lesion confined to the afferent arc show muscular atrophy, fasciculations, and fibrillations? ☐ Yes / ☐ No. Explain ____

Ans: Atrophy, fasciculations, and fibrillations indicate interruption of the efferent arc, a lesion of the LMN.

3. Knowing that the stimulus is proper and the *af*ferent arc is intact, you consider next the LMN, the *ef*ferent side of the arc.

axon

a. The term *LMN* includes both the cell *body* of the neuron and its *axon.* Hence, an LMN lesion means any lesion affecting the body of the neuron or the ______________ running to the end organ.

No. The afferent neurons remain intact.

b. Many diseases attack bodies of LMNs. Poliomyelitis, one of the most specific, destroys LMNs, with little effect on the dorsal horns. A poliomyelitis patient is areflexic in the involved muscles because the LMNs which form the beginning of the efferent arc are destroyed. Would such a patient lose sensation? Explain.

4. After the LMN cell body, the next level to consider is the *efferent axon.* The efferent axon may be interrupted by mechanical lesions such as cuts or compression. Many toxic-metabolic disorders, such as lead poisoning, may predominantly affect efferent axons, causing a *motor neuropathy.* Other toxins, such as arsenic, regularly affect both afferent and efferent axons, causing a *sensorimotor neuropathy.* Irrespective of cause, irrespective of involvement of the afferent system, a lesion of the LMN cell body or axon has essentially the same effect on the muscle:

a. The reduction in muscle bulk of a LMN lesion is called ______________________________.

b. The reduction or loss of muscular power is called ______________________________.

c. The spontaneous twitches seen by the clinician are ______________________________.

d. The spontaneous muscle fiber contractions which, in general, can only be detected by EMG recording are called ______________ and the large complex wave forms are called ______________________________ units.

e. The MSRs are ☐ normal/ ☐ increased/ ☐ absent or decreased.

f. Read the answers to *a* through *e*: *They comprise the syndrome of LMN lesions.*

denervation atrophy

paresis, palsy, or paralysis (the three *p*'s)

fasciculations

fibrillations

giant polyphasic motor

absent or decreased

5. The next level of the efferent arc to consider is the *neuromyal junction.* We did not consider the synapse of the afferent axon on the ventral motoneuron because we do not know of any clinical disorders confined solely to this synapse.

a. The major disturbance of the neuromyal junction is *myasthenia gravis,* a defect in the transmission of the nerve impulse from nerve to muscle.

b. Myasthenia is a disease of fluctuating intensity. Complete areflexia is unusual unless the person is in a myasthenic "crisis."

6. The final level of the reflex arc is the *effector,* the *muscle.*

a. Many primary diseases of muscle cause areflexia, such as muscular dystrophy or myositis. They are all included in the term *myopathy.* The afferent and efferent limbs of the reflex arc are preserved in these patients, but the end organ is diseased.

b. In some myopathies, the muscle goes through a transitory phase of increased bulk, called *pseudohypertrophy,* but the final result of most myopathies is muscular atrophy, *myopathic* atrophy.

c. We may now summarize the types of muscular atrophy:

(1) Atrophy solely from lack of exercise, as a leg in a cast, is called ______________________________ atrophy.

(2) Atrophy from interruption of efferent axons is called ______________________________ atrophy.

(3) Atrophy from primary disease of muscle is called ______________________________ atrophy.

7. *Atrophy* must be distinguished from *aplasia* or *hypoplasia.*

a. A muscle which has lost bulk after previously having been normal is properly said to be ______________________________ *ic.*

disuse

denervation

myopathic

atrophic

aplastic

hypoplastic

Receptor
Afferent axons
LMN (including efferent axon)
Neuromyal junction
Effector

b. A muscle which is congenitally *absent* is called ______________ *ic*.

c. A muscle which is small because of lack of normal embryologic or postnatal development is called ______________ *ic*.

8. Summarize the clinically significant stations in the reflex arc, beginning with the stimulus: ______________

____

____

____

H. *Analyze this patient.* The patient is a 52-year-old man. Four weeks before hospital admission, he became violently ill with nausea, vomiting, and bloody diarrhea. Four days before admission, he began to have severe pain in his extremities. On the day of hospitalization, he also noticed weakness in his legs. His cranial nerves were normal. He had slight paresis of his hand muscles and severe leg weakness, most pronounced distally. He was hyporeflexic in the arms, areflexic in the lower extremities. He had difficulty distinguishing pinprick and light touch over his hands. His feet were almost anesthetic. He had no muscular atrophy on admission, but it became evident in 10 days. An EMG on admission disclosed no spontaneous activity indicative of fasciculations or fibrillations. Within 10 days the hand and leg muscles became atrophic. A second EMG, done 4 weeks after hospitalization, disclosed fasciculations and numerous fibrillations in the muscles which were clinically weak and areflexic.

A combined sensorimotor neuropathy

Symptom of severe pain, distal sensory loss; areflexia

weakness; areflexia; later atrophy, fasciculations and fibrillations.

1. This patient had ☐ only a motor / ☐ only a sensory / ☐ a combined sensorimotor neuropathy.
2. From the history and examination the evidence for sensory neuropathy was: (Review the case protocol to sift out the answers.)

   ____

   ____

   ____

3. The evidence for motor neuropathy was: ______________

   ____

   ____

4. The sensorimotor neuropathy coming on within weeks after a severe gastrointestinal disturbance suggested poisoning. Chemical tests of the patient's urine for lead, mercury, and arsenic showed high arsenic levels. Questioning of the patient disclosed domestic strife. The wife admitted trying to poison her husband with rat poison. The patient was treated with dimercaprol and made a satisfactory, but incomplete, recovery.
5. The onset of fasciculations and fibrillations about 4 weeks after the first signs of LMN disease indicates the approximate time required for these signs of denervation to appear. The full syndrome of LMN lesions takes time to develop. Even if a nerve is cut with a knife, fibrillations usually do not appear for 3 weeks or more. Some signs are early and persist for the duration of the disease. Other signs appear later. Rank the LMN signs as they evolved in the course of the patient's illness, and you will have the relative times that they occur in LMN disease in general:

☑ early

☑ intermediate

☑ late

	Relatively early	Intermediate	Late
Paresis, paralysis, and areflexia	☐	☐	☐
Atrophy	☐	☐	☐
Fibrillations and fasciculations	☐	☐	☐

Bibliography

Jenkins, R.: Inorganic arsenic and the nervous system, *Brain,* 89:479-498, 1966.

I. Clinical analysis of hyperreflexia

1. Some normal individuals have very brisk MSRs. They are at the opposite end of the range of normal variation from individuals whose MSRs are hypoactive. The commonest cause of pathologic hyperreflexia is interruption of UMN pathways between cerebrum and LMNs. If the hyperreflexia is indeed pathologic and caused by a UMN lesion, other signs will tie the hyperreflexia into a diagnostic pattern, a syndrome. If a patient has hyperreflexia on the left side, and it is the result of a UMN lesion, you would expect to find some degree of weakness when you test the strength of the left side.

UMN

2. A syndrome of hyperreflexia in the paretic or paralytic muscles would be strong evidence of ☐ a UMN / ☐ an LMN lesion.
3. To understand the full syndrome of UMN lesions, it is helpful to classify the signs into one of two groups. Those behaviors or normal activities the patient loses because of the UMN lesion are called *deficit phenomena*. Those behaviors which are exaggerated, unmasked, or released after the UMN lesion are called *release phenomena.*

release

deficit

   a. Hyperreflexia after a UMN lesion is classed as a ☐ release / ☐ deficit phenomenon.
   b. Paresis or paralysis after a UMN lesion is classed as a ________ phenomenon.
4. The deficit in strength after a UMN lesion is readily explained by the interruption of impulse conduction from the UMNs to the LMNs. Specification of the exact upper motoneurons whose interruption causes release phenomena leads to some difficulty. For many decades, neurologists have accepted the dictum that pyramidal tract interruption is responsible both for the deficit *and* the release phenomena. I am willing to accept the pyramidal tract theory, as are many others (see Walshe; Van Gijn). Dissenting opinions are summarized by Bucy. You may, if you wish, substitute the term *pyramidal tract* for *UMN,* or you may, if you wish, use only *UMN* to be noncommittal. Whatever theory the neurologist expounds, he will behave as if the pyramidal theory is true when he makes diagnoses.

5. Hyperreflexia has many causes. The dendrogram, Fig. 7-20, shows some. Again we illustrate the principle that a sign generates many diagnostic possibilities. The syndrome formed by integrating the sign with other evidence produces the diagnosis.

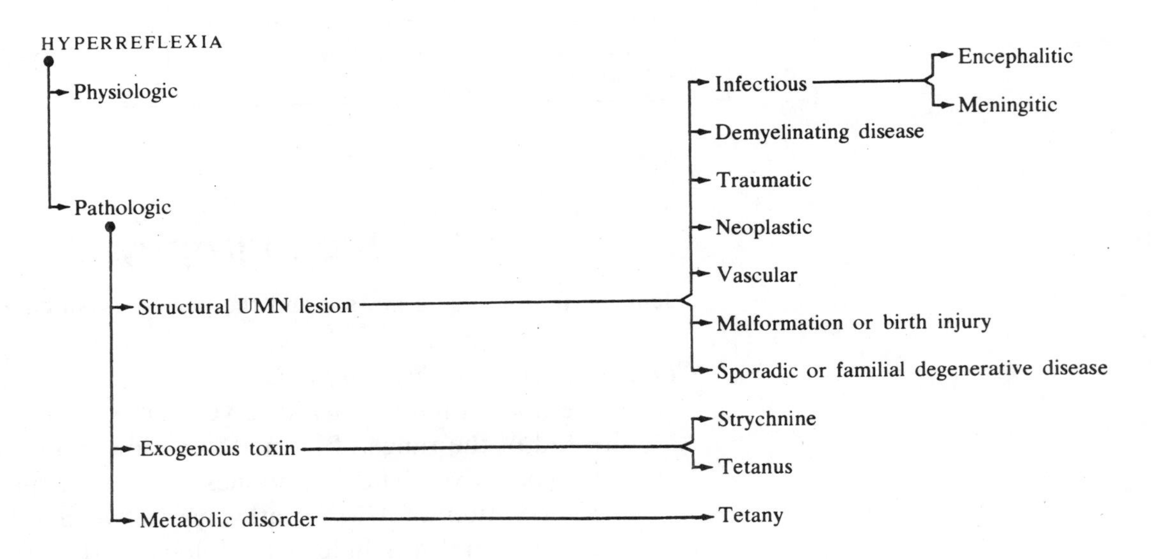

FIG. 7-20. Some causes of hyperreflexia. (Reference only.)

J. Clonus

1. The hypersensitivity of the MSRs is readily demonstrated by the percussion hammer, and it can also be demonstrated in another way, by eliciting *clonus.* See Fig 7-21. The knee is slightly flexed, relaxing the triceps surae muscle. The examiner briskly jerks the foot up and slightly outward. He continues to apply pressure with his fingers against the sole of the patient's foot. The foot oscillates between flexion and extension for as long as the pressure is applied.

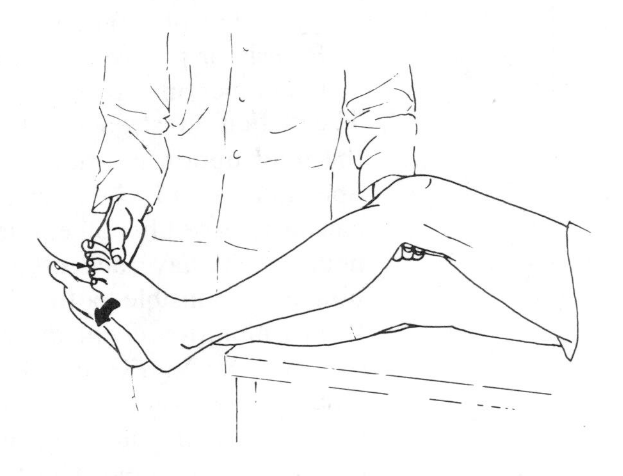

FIG. 7-21. Method for eliciting ankle clonus.

2. *The mechanism of clonus*
   a. The quick dorsiflexion of the patient's foot stretches triceps surae. See Fig. 7-22*A*, thin arrow. Triceps surae responds by contracting, and the foot plantar flexes, Fig. 7-22 *B*, thick arrow.
   b. The examiner continues to apply light pressure against the ball of the foot, opposing plantar flexion. When the MSR stops, the examiner's pressure immediately dorsiflexes the foot again, Fig. 7-22*C*, thin arrow. The restretching of triceps surae causes plantar flexion, Fig. 7-22*D*. As long as the examiner applies the proper pressure to elicit an MSR from triceps surae, the foot continues to oscillate.

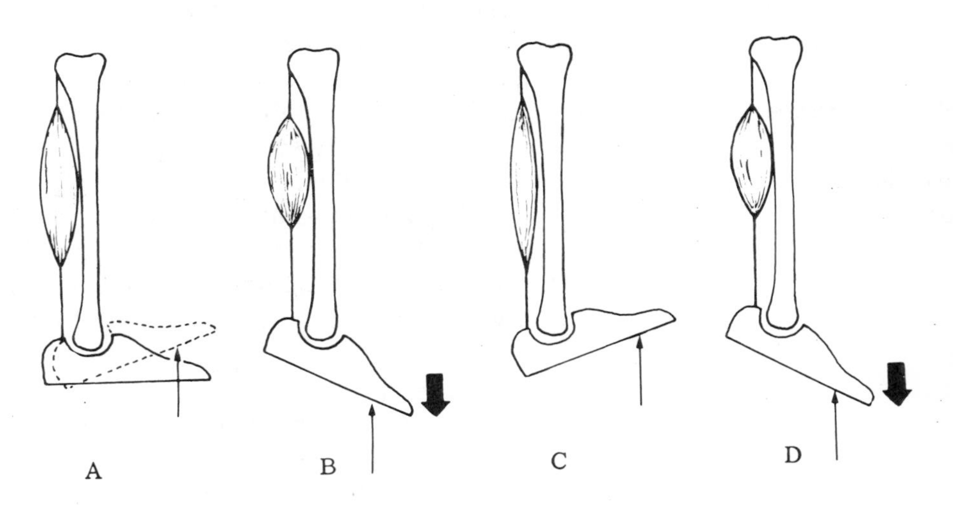

FIG. 7-22. Mechanism of ankle clonus. The thin arrow represents the light pressure applied by the examiner to the ball of the patient's foot.

leg extended

3. Wrist and patellar clonus are elicited by the same method as ankle clonus. To elicit patellar clonus, grasp the patella between your thumb and forefinger. Jerk *downward* briskly and maintain downward pressure. Try this test on your own patella. What position must your leg be in to grasp the patella and have the quadriceps muscle relaxed to initiate the stretch reflex? ☐ leg extended / ☐ leg flexed.
4. Some normal individuals with physiologic hyperreflexia will have a few clonic jerks, called *abortive clonus*. Only *sustained clonus* is pathologic.

a UMN lesion

release

5. Sustained clonus in a patient with hyperreflexia would give supportive evidence that the patient had ☐ a UMN lesion (pathologic hyperreflexia) / ☐ physiologic hyperreflexia.
6. Clonus is classed as a ☐ release / ☐ deficit phenomenon.
7. Why must the initial movement of the part be brisk to elicit clonus?
   ____
   ____
   ____

Ans: The movement must stretch the muscle spindles rapidly enough to initiate a muscle stretch reflex.

8. Give an *operational* definition of clonus. (Include the maneuvers and what response occurs.) ____
____
____

Ans: Clonus is a series of to-and-fro oscillations of a part initiated by a quick jerk and maintained by slight pressure.

9. What is the *pathophysiology* and *clinical interpretation* of clonus?
____
____
____
____

Ans: Clonus is a series of repetitive MSRs, a release phenomenon, indicating pathologic hyperreflexia, usually as a result of a UMN (pyramidal tract) lesion.

unilaterally independent
Hyperreflexia
clonus

10. To summarize the syndrome of UMN lesions, as developed to this point, we can state that the patient shows:
    a. Paresis or paralysis, most severe in those movements which are ☐ bilaterally synchronous / ☐ unilaterally independent.
    b. ☐ Hyperreflexia / ☐ hyporeflexia of the MSRs.
    c. Oscillatory to-and-fro movements called ______________, which are elicited by a quick stretch.
11. To understand another component of the UMN syndrome, *spasticity*, requires a general discussion of muscle tone.

K. Muscle tone

1. Place your forearm flat on a table top, with your wrist dangling over the table edge. Supinate your forearm so that your radius is on top, the ulna resting directly on the table edge. After relaxing this arm completely, grasp its hand with your other hand and flex and extend the wrist as fully as possible.
2. As your active hand moves your relaxed hand, the active hand will feel slight resistance. This slight resistance to passive movement is normal muscle tone. (The ultimate range of joint movement is set by the ligaments.)
3. Try now to relax your elbow and, with your other hand, flex and extend your forearm. The purpose of these exercises is to give you insight into how hard it is to relax a part completely. Do not become impatient if your patients are not any better at it than you are. Keep working patiently until the part is completely relaxed before judging tone.
4. Muscle tone is operationally defined as the *muscular* resistance (apart from gravity) the examiner feels when he moves a patient's resting joint.
5. Normally the resistance of the muscle to passive movement has two components:
    a. The *elasticity* of the muscle, which ordinarily is slight unless the muscle is fibrotic.
    b. The *number and rate of motor discharges*, which is the critical variable. The number and rate of motor unit discharges is a consequence of:

(1) The stimulation of LMNs by muscle spindles and other receptors in skin, tendons, joint, and bone.
(2) The stimulation of LMNs by pyramidal and extrapyramidal pathways.

6. The tone detected by the examiner is the algebraic sum of all influences on the LMNs, excitatory and inhibitory. Since the pathways affecting tone are numerous and the theories about it complex and conflicting, we will be content with the operational findings and their clinical implications, rather than attempting a detailed physiologic analysis. In this way, we will not err in giving explanation priority over the operational data to be learned.
7. It is easy to surmise that the two possible alterations of tone are too much tone, ***hypertonia***, and too little tone, ***hypotonia***.

L. Hypertonia

1. The two most common hypertonic states are *spasticity* and *rigidity*.
2. *Spasticity* is operationally defined as the increased muscular resistance the examiner feels when he moves a joint briskly, in which the initial resistance quickly fades away. It is like opening an ordinary pocket-knife blade. The initial resistance of the blade, as it is first opened, quickly yields as the blade straightens out. The similar phenomenon in muscle tone is called *clasp-knife* spasticity. See Fig. 7-23.

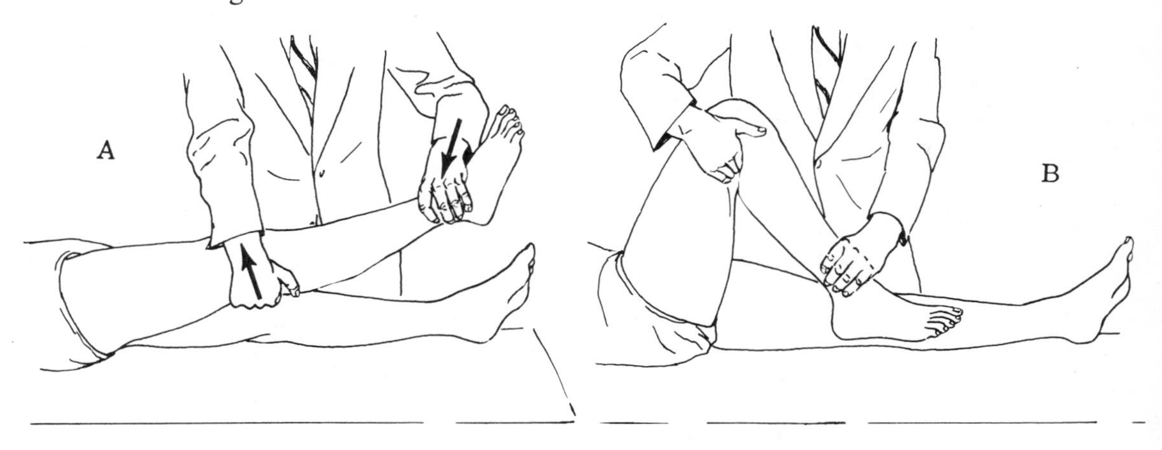

FIG. 7-23. Method for eliciting clasp-knife spasticity in the lower extremities. A. The examiner lifts the patient's leg with one hand, placing the other under the patient's knee. As briskly as possible, in fact with a jerk, he simultaneously pushes *down* with the ankle hand and *up* with the other. B. The spastic leg catches and then molds to the flexed position.

a. Since a brisk movement is necessary for eliciting clasp-knife spasticity, as in eliciting MSRs or clonus, we can infer that it represents increased sensitivity of the MSRs. The resistance felt is simply a muscle stretch reflex, according to this interpretation. While hyperreflexia, clonus, and clasp-knife spasticity usually parallel each other in intensity, occasionally one feature predominates, out of proportion to the others. Evidently something is lacking in our explanation, but that is the way we will have to leave it.

b. The three release phenomena, presented to this point, and indica-

hyperreflexia, clonus, clasp-knife spasticity

tive of a pyramidal tract lesion are ____________________

3. *Rigidity* is operationally defined as the increased muscular resistance the examiner feels when he moves a resting joint, in which the resistance persists throughout the entire range. Within certain limits, the resistance is the same, regardless of range or velocity of movement. It is like bending a piece of clay, solder, or a lead-pipe. Hence, it is called *lead-pipe rigidity.* The pathophysiology of lead-pipe rigidity is highly debated, but we will say, for purposes of clinical diagnosis, that its presence indicates a lesion of extrapyramidal pathways, in the circuitry of basal ganglia, diencephalon, and brainstem. Much evidence points also to a disturbance in the muscle spindle mechanism, determined perhaps in part by abnormal influences of extrapyramidal pathways on the LMNs, but a brisk stretch is unnecessary to elicit lead-pipe rigidity, in contrast to clasp-knife spasticity.
4. Lesions frequently affect both pyramidal and extrapyramidal pathways. Hence, mixtures of spasticity and rigidity are common.
5. Give an operational definition of clasp-knife spasticity:

____

See frame *L2*

6. Give an operational definition of lead-pipe rigidity:

____

See frame *L3*

pyramidal

extrapyramidal

7. Clasp-knife spasticity indicates a lesion of the ____________ pathway, while lead-pipe rigidity indicates a lesion of the ____________ pathways.
8. Check the signs which require a brisk stimulus to elicit:
   a. ☐ Clasp-knife spasticity.
   b. ☐ Lead-pipe rigidity.
   c. ☐ Muscle stretch reflex.
   d. ☐ Clonus.

a ☑
b
c ☑
d ☑

9. Why do the signs checked in frame 8 require a brisk stimulus to elicit?

____

To activate muscle spindles

Bibliography

Pyramidal Tract

Bucy, P.: Is there a pyramidal tract? *Brain,* 80: 376-392, 1957.

Chokroverty, S., Rubino, F., and Haller, C.: Pure motor hemiplegia due to pyramidal infarction. *Arch. Neurol.,* 32:647-648, 1975.

DeMyer, W.: Number of axons and myelin sheaths in adult human medullary pyramids, *Neurology,* 9:42-47, 1959.

DeMyer, W.: Ontogenesis of the rat corticospinal tract, *Arch. Neurol.,* 16:203-211, 1967.

Leestma, J. E., and Noronha, A.: Pure motor hemiplegia, medullary pyramid lesion, and olivary hypertrophy. *J. Neurol. Neurosurg. Psychiatry,* 39:877-884, 1976.

Levitt, L. P., Selkoe, D. F., Frankenfield, B., and Schoene, W.: Pure motor hemiplegia secondary to brainstem tumour. *J. Neurol. Neurosurg. Psychiatry,* 38:1240-1243, 1975.

Nyberg-Hansen, R., and Rinvik, E.: Some comments on the pyramidal tract, with special reference to its individual variations in man, *Acta Neurol., Scand.,* 39:1-30, 1963.

Ropper, A. H., Fisher, C. M., and Kleinman, G. M.: Pyramidal infarction in the medulla: A cause of pure motor hemiplegia sparing the face. *Neurology,* 29:91-95, 1979.

Walshe, F.: On the role of the pyramidal system in willed movements, *Brain,* 70: 329-354, 1947.

Hypertonia

Ashby, P., and Burke, D.: Stretch reflexes in the upper limb of spastic man, *J. Neurol. Neurosurg. Psychiat.,* 34:765-771, 1971.

Burke, D., Gillies, J., and Lance, J.: The quadriceps stretch reflex in human spasticity, *J. Neurol. Neurosurg. Psychiat.,* 33:216-223, 1970.

Clemente, C. D.: Neurophysiologic mechanisms and neuroanatomic substrates related to spasticity. *Neurology,* 28:(2)40-45, 1978.

Rushworth, G.: Spasticity and rigidity: an experimental study and review, *J. Neurol. Neurosurg. Psychiat.,* 23:99-118, 1960.

Thomas, J.: Muscle tone, spasticity, rigidity, *J. Nerv. Ment. Dis.,* 132:505-514, 1961.

Weisendanger, M.: *Pathophysiology of Muscle Tone,* Berlin, Springer, 1972.

M. Hypotonia (flaccidity)

1. Muscle tone depends on the activity of motor units as driven by the play of excitatory impulses on the LMNs. Pyramidal and extrapyramidal lesions apparently increase the sensitivity of LMNs to afferent impulses arriving via the dorsal roots. At least we find that section of dorsal roots in normal or hypertonic subjects abolishes muscle tone.
2. *Hypotonia from lesions at the level of the reflex arc.* Review Fig. 7-19.
   a. Section of *dorsal* roots, removing the excitatory impulses coming from the muscle spindles, would cause ☐ hypertonia / ☐ hypotonia / ☐ no change in tone.
   b. Section of *ventral* roots would cause ☐ hypertonia / ☐ hypotonia / ☐ no change in tone.
   c. *Primary myopathies,* causing death of muscle fibers, would cause ☐ hypotonia / ☐ hypertonia / ☐ no change in tone.
3. Paresis or paralysis would occur with ☐ dorsal root lesions / ☐ LMN lesions / ☐ myopathies.
4. Denervation atrophy occurs with ☐ dorsal root lesions / ☐ LMN lesions / ☐ myopathies.
5. Loss of sensation occurs with ☐ dorsal root lesions / ☐ LMN lesions / ☐ myopathies.

hypotonia

hypotonia

hypotonia

LMN lesions and myopathies

LMN lesions

dorsal root lesions

dorsal root, LMN lesions, and myopathies; all three.

6. **Absence of MSRs could occur with ☐ dorsal root lesions / ☐ LMN lesions / ☐ myopathies.**
7. The previous frames illustrate some of the combinations of signs found with lesions of the reflex arc. Complete Table 7-4 with check marks to summarize the various diagnostic patterns.

TABLE 7-4. Clinical Signs and Probable Diagnosis of Lesions at the Level of the Reflex Arc

Clinical signs	Probable diagnosis		
	Dorsal root lesion	LMN lesion	Myopathy
Areflexia, hypotonia, loss of sensation. No atrophy, weakness, or EMG abnormalities.	☐ 1	☐ 2	☐ 3
Weakness, areflexia, atrophy, hypotonia, fasciculations, and fibrillations. No sensory loss.	☐ 1	☐ 2	☐ 3
Weakness, areflexia, atrophy, hypotonia. No sensory loss fasciculations, or fibrillations.	☐ 1	☐ 2	☐ 3
Weakness, hyporeflexia, atrophy, hypotonia, percussion myotonia. No sensory loss, fasciculations, or fibrillations.	☐ 1	☐ 2	☐ 3
Weakness, areflexia, atrophy, hypotonia, loss of sensation, fasciculations, and fibrillations.	☐ 1	☐ 2	☐ 3

☑ 1

☑ 2

☑ 3

☑ 3 (myotonia dystrophica)

☑ 1 ☑ 2 (sensorimotor neuropathy)

8. **Although cerebral and brainstem lesions sometimes are associated with hypotonia, the anatomic substrate is unknown. Cerebellar lesions regularly cause hypotonia, as will be discussed later. Another important cause of hypotonia is cerebral or spinal shock.**

N. Cerebral or spinal (neural) shock

1. Immediately after acute, severe UMN lesions, such as a large cerebral infarct or spinal cord transection, the paralyzed limbs may be hypotonic and areflexic or hyporeflexic. We call the stage of hypotonic paralysis after an acute UMN lesion *neural* shock (diaschisis of Monakow), or more specifically *cerebral* or *spinal* shock, depending on the lesion level. The term *shock* in this context has nothing to do with blood pressure.
2. Neural shock implies that the lesion is ☐ small and evolved slowly / ☐ large and evolved slowly / ☐ large and evolved rapidly.

large and evolved rapidly

3. The paralyzed limbs of the patient with a slowly evolving UMN lesion usually show hypertonia and hyperreflexia, but after an acute, severe UMN lesion, the paralyzed limbs may initially show hypotonia and hyporeflexia.
4. Hypotonia and hyporeflexia would qualify as ☐ release / ☐ deficit phenomena.

deficit

5. If a patient originally in a stage of neural shock begins to recover movement, the recovery usually parallels the appearance of release phenomena, such as hyperreflexia. In the chronic stage of an acute UMN lesion as well as after any UMN lesion of slow onset, the patient shows both deficit and release phenomena. Thus, the clinical signs of a UMN lesion depend on the rapidity of onset and the size of the lesion. If the patient has only deficit signs, what do you assume about the size and rapidity of onset of the lesion? ______________________ ______________________.

large and acute in onset

V. Examination of the superficial reflexes

Note: Since you will do tests on your bare foot, do this part of the text in your own living quarters. Get a reflex hammer, a broken tongue blade, and a key to use as stimulating objects.

A. Introduction

To complete the UMN syndrome, we turn from the MSRs, clonus, and spasticity to a different set of phenomena, the superficial reflexes. The MSRs are elicited by stimulation of receptors deep to the skin. Hence, MSRs are classed as *deep* reflexes. Those skeletal muscular responses elicited by stimulation of surface receptors in skin and mucous membranes are called *superficial* reflexes.

B. Technique for eliciting superficial plantar reflexes

1. The toes can be made to move in response to *muscle stretch* or *deep stimuli,* and to *superficial* stimuli. Fig. 7-24 shows one method, the method of Babinski, for eliciting reflex toe movement by superficial plantar stimulation.

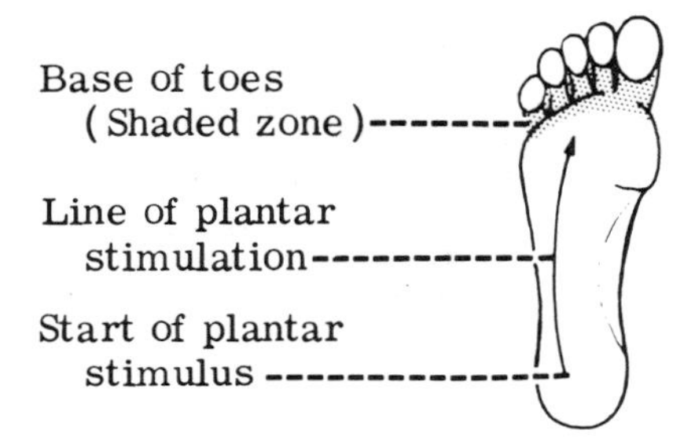

FIG. 7-24. Sole of the right foot. The arrow marks the plantar stroke. Notice that it stops short of the shaded zone, the base of the toes.

   a. A blunt object, such as a broken edge of a tongue blade, a key, or the butt of a reflex hammer is stroked along the lateral aspect of the sole. See the arrow in Fig. 7-24. Normally the large toe and frequently the others flex. The plantar stroke must have the correct dimensions of *length, velocity,* and *pressure* to elicit the response.

   b. Try the test on your own foot and if possible, another person's. Try different velocities and pressures, using the length shown in Fig. 7-24. Notice that the stroke stops short of the base of the toes.

2. When preparing to elicit the plantar reflexes, place the patient supine with the limbs symmetrical and extended, the legs straight out, and the arms at the sides.
3. In trying the plantar stimulus on yourself, what errors in positioning did you have to make? ______________________________
____
____

All of them! Your leg was flexed, your trunk was bent, and your posture was asymmetrical.

4. From experience, you know that a plantar stimulus may be uncomfortable. The patient, if senile, demented, or paranoid, may view the act of plantar stimulation as unnecessary, ludicrous, or even hostile, unless you prepare him for it. Check the best statement to insure the patient's relaxation and cooperation.
   - ☐ *a.* "Hold still while I tickle the bottom of your foot."
   - ☐ *b.* "I am going to scratch the bottom of your foot."
   - ☐ *c.* "Don't move your foot, I am going to stimulate your sole."
   - ☐ *d.* "I am going to press gently on your foot. If it's unpleasant tell me."

☑ *d.*

5. Next, hold the patient's ankle with one hand. Why would you do this?

   ____

   ______________________________.

Ans: To prevent the patient from pulling his foot away and to permit you to maintain the proper pressure of your stimulating object against the sole.

6. The stimulus object is placed at the *heel* and moved along the sole, as shown in Fig. 7-24. The object is moved along the ☐ medial margin / ☐ lateral margin / ☐ center of the foot.

lateral margin

7. Notice in Fig. 7-24 that the plantar stroke stops short of the base of the toes. Extending the stroke to the base of the toes produces unpredictable responses.
8. *Length* is only one of the significant variables of the plantar stimulus.
   - *a.* Another variable is the amount of ______________ you use to hold the object against the sole.

pressure

   - *b.* A third variable is the ______________ at which the object is moved.

velocity

9. Hence, the three important variables are the ______________, ______________, and ______________ of the stroke.

length, pressure, velocity

10. After practicing on your own feet, you will appreciate that the plantar stimulus should be made with slight pressure. Patients with sensory disorders may have extremely tender soles. Some are unable to tolerate the plantar stimulus. Thus, you should be careful to use slight pressure for your first attempt.

C. The criterion for success in eliciting a reflex

1. The goal in eliciting any reflex is to get a *constant* response. If you get no response or inconstant responses, you must vary your stimulus.
   - *a.* Consider *length* first: you have already started at the heel and cannot get much more length there. You must avoid the ______________ of the toes. What is left is to swing the stroke across the ball of the foot.

base

   - *b.* On Fig. 7-25, draw the usual length of the stroke in a solid line. Then draw the extension of the stroke in a dotted line and check against the drawing in the answer column.
2. If you get no response or variable responses using gentle pressure and different lengths, the next step is to increase the pressure. What consideration limits the amount of pressure you should apply?

   ____

the patient's comfort

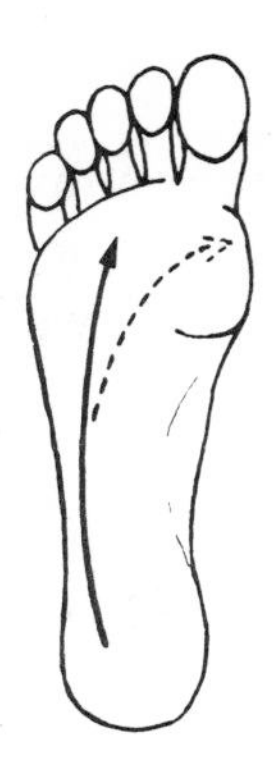

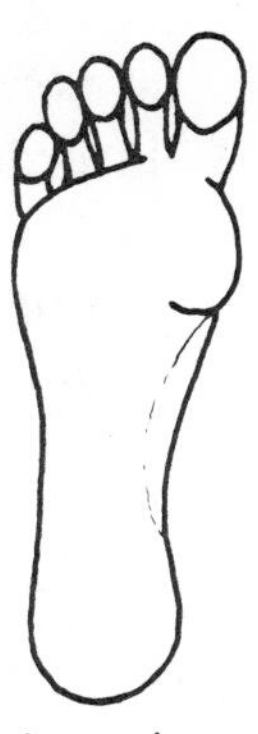

FIG. 7-25. Blank for drawing the stroke used for the plantar stimulus.

velocity

reproducibility of toe movement

3. If you still do not get a reproducible response after varying length and pressure, you would vary the ________________ of the stroke.
4. What is the criterion by which you know you have used the correct plantar stimulus? ________________

D. In summary:

Supine, legs extended, parts symmetrical.

It produces unpredictable toe movements.

The stimulus was improper in respect to length, velocity or pressure.

Well, would your statement put you at ease?

1. What is the correct position of the patient for the plantar stimulus? ________________.
2. Why stop short of the base of the toes with the plantar stroke? ________________.
3. If you obtain no response with your first plantar stimulus, what is the most likely explanation? ________________.
4. Write a soft statement to forewarn the patient for a plantar stimulus. ________________.

E. Anatomy of the plantar reflex arc

1. The zone from which a reflex can be elicited is called the *reflexogenous zone*. The reflexogenous zone for the normal plantar reflex is usually restricted to the first sacral dermatome (S_1). Notice in Fig. 7-26 the area of the S_1 dermatome and its relation to lumbar segments 4 and 5 (L_{4-5}).
2. Cover Fig. 7-26 and shade in the S_1 dermatome in Fig. 7-27.

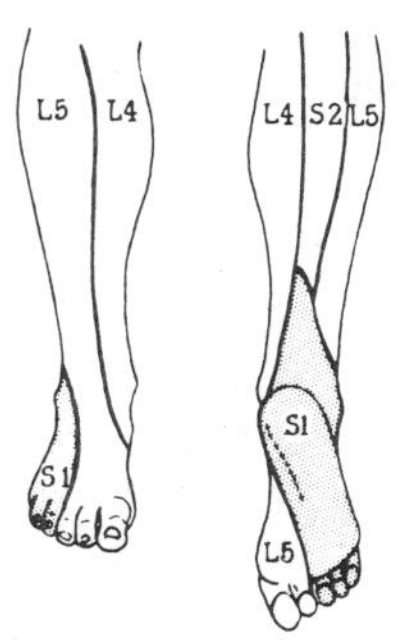

FIG. 7-26. Dermatomes of the foot.

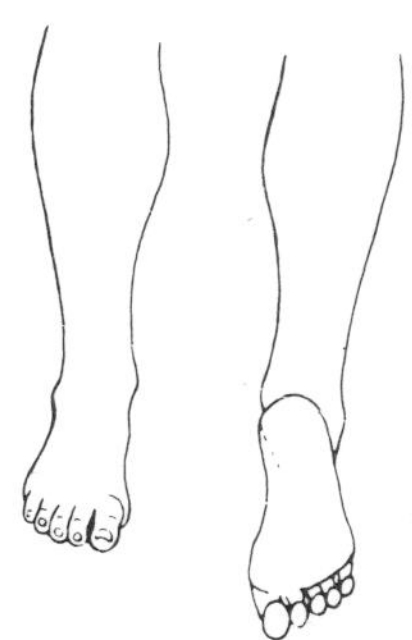

FIG. 7-27. Blank for shading the S_1 dermatome.

receptor	3. In order to analyze any reflex, you have to "think through" the reflex arc. Use Fig. 7-28 to answer the following frames. Notice that according to previous principles of thinking through a reflex arc, we begin at the ________________.
S_1	*a.* The reflexogenous zone for the plantar stimulus is the __________ dermatome.
skin	*b.* The receptor nerve endings are located in the ☐ skin / ☐ muscle / ☐ bone.

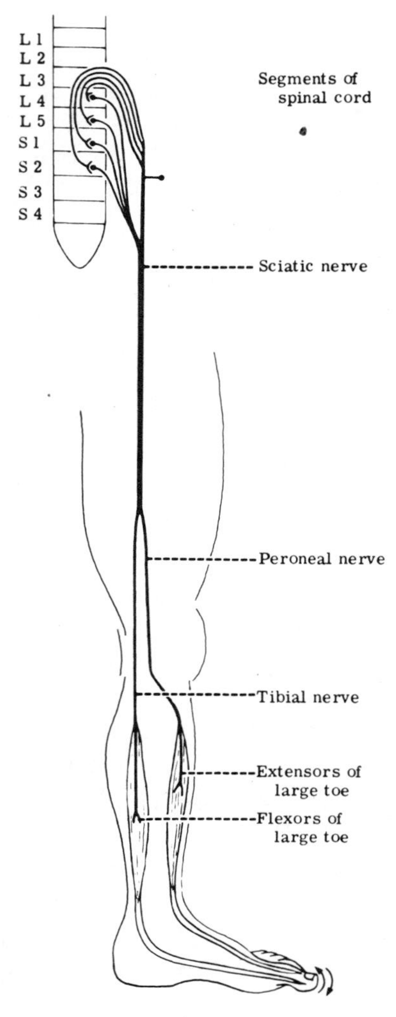

FIG. 7-28. Reflex arc for the plantar reflexes. For simplicity, the diagram shows the flexor hallucis brevis in the calf rather than in the foot. See Van Gijn, 1977.

superficial	*c.* Therefore the plantar reflex is classed as ☐ superficial / ☐ deep.
sciatic	*d.* The *afferent* nerve is the tibial nerve. It is a branch of the ________________ nerve.
lumbar (4 and 5) sacral (1 and 2)	*e.* The spinal cord segments involved in the plantar reflex are the 4th and 5th segments of the ________________ part of the cord and the 1st and 2nd segments of the ________________ part.

tibial
peroneal

f. The sciatic nerve has two large branches which separate just proximal to the knee. The branch to the toe *flexors* is the ______________ nerve, and the one to the extensors is the ______________ nerve.

sciatic

g. The major nerve which divides into tibial and peroneal branches is the ______________________ nerve.

No
The toe flexor muscles would be paralyzed.

h. Suppose a patient has a lesion of the tibial nerve, could you obtain a *flexor* plantar response? ☐ Yes/ ☐ No. Explain__________
____
____

tibial

i. What nerve would you cut to interrupt both the *afferent* and *efferent* arc of the normal plantar response, leaving the toe extensor muscle innervated? ______________________.

F. Physiology of the normal plantar response

1. *Introduction.* As long as the sensory pathways remain intact and the patient conscious, the patient perceives the plantar stimulus as uncomfortable. The subjective experience seems to consist of a mixture of tickling, pressure, and pain. The stimulus for the plantar reflexes is thought to act mainly through the *pain* receptors in the skin. However, one cannot safely infer from the subjective component of the reflex precisely which receptors do, in fact, cause the response, since the stimulus activates several types of afferent endings.

pain

2. On the basis of the noxious subjective experience of the patient, we would suspect that the major receptor for the plantar stimulus would be the nerve endings for ______________________ sensation.
3. Because the stimulus is noxious you have been instructed to inform the patient what is to be done and to carry out one other maneuver just prior to applying the stimulus, which is to grasp the patient's ankle.

pressure

4. This maneuver is necessary so that you have control of the only stroke variable which can stimulate pain endings. This variable is __________. Clinical interpretation of the plantar reflexes will require first a short detour into the physiology of summation.
   a. In Fig. 7-29 are the oscilloscopic patterns of electrical shocks. The shock in Fig. 7-29*A* did not elicit a response when applied to a patient's nerve. In Fig. 7-29*B*, in which only the *duration* of the shock was increased, the patient felt a sensation.

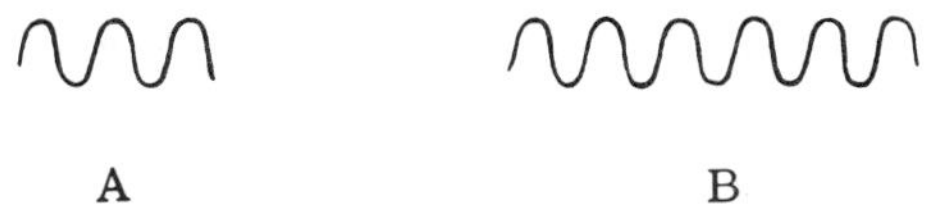

A B

FIG. 7-29. Oscilloscopic pattern of electrical stimuli.

summation

   b. A stimulus which changes as in Fig. 7-29*A* to *B* to elicit a response is said to *summate* or to undergo *summation*. In this example, the stimulus accumulates over time. We say that temporal __________ ______________ has occurred.

spatial

temporal
spatial

summation

temporal

spatial

temporal
spatial

c. Suppose you move an object a distance of 500 micra across a patient's skin, and he feels no movement. Then if you move it 1,000 micra, using the same time and pressure, he feels movement. The response occurs because the object acts on an increased area of skin. This would be an example of □ spatial/ □ temporal summation.

d. In performing the sensory and reflex examinations, you use the two types of summation, ______________ and ______________, repeatedly.

5. When the plantar stimulus is applied, the toe will not move until the object has reached the instep or ball of the foot. This delay in the response after initiating the stimulus indicates that to increase the excitability of the LMN pool, ______________ has to occur.
6. The fact that a finite period of time is required for the object to get from the heel to the instep suggests that ______________ summation is necessary.
7. Because your object successively stimulated more receptors as it moved along, you could also infer that ______________ summation may have occurred.
8. Thus, to get the flexors of the toes to contract, the central excitatory state of the motoneurons of the toe flexors was increased both by ______________ and ______________ summation.
9. *Normal variations and additional movements in response to a plantar stimulus.*

   a. Some normal persons will show little or no toe or leg movement after a plantar stimulus, but most normal persons tend to withdraw their foot from a plantar stimulus, as well as flexing the great toe. The withdrawal movement consists of dorsiflexion of the ankle, and flexion of the knee and hip, a *flexion synergy,* like your response to stepping on a tack. The tensor fascia lata, hamstrings, and tibialis anterior muscles visibly and palpably contract as part of this flexion synergy. Watch for and check these actions as you apply the plantar stimulus.

   b. The small toes may fan, but this does not constitute a consistent or clinically important part of the plantar reflex (Van Gijn, 1977).

****G. *The role of agonist-antagonist contraction in the plantar reflex***

1. Reflexes differ greatly in the adequate stimulus and in the complexity and number of muscles acting. The MSR is a relatively simple reflex involving the contraction of only one muscle or even only one part of one muscle. In some reflexes, the action of the prime mover, the *agonist,* is opposed by simultaneous contraction of the *antagonist*. In other reflexes, the antagonist contraction is inhibited.
2. In the normal plantar reflex, we know that the toe flexors contract because we can see the toe flex. The question is whether the toe extensor muscles contract in opposition to the flexors and are simply overpowered by the flexors, or whether the toe extensors contract

at all. This question is crucial for clinical interpretation of plantar responses. What pathologic conditions or laboratory experiments would provide conclusive evidence that the toe extensor muscles contract simultaneously with the flexors in the plantar reflex? Work out your answer on scrap paper. If you cannot think of a way to solve the problem try one of the hints below.

Hints:

a. Begin by "thinking through" the reflex arc, Fig. 7-28. Would a lesion at a particular site help answer the question?

b. How would you detect extensor muscle contractions even if the toe moved in the direction of the flexors?

c. Could you use electromyography?

3. *Answers to frame 2*

   a. The clinically minded investigator would look for patients in whom the flexor muscles of the toe were inactivated by disease, leaving the afferent impulses from the sole intact. Such a situation might be realized by a lesion of the nerve to the flexor muscles, a muscle injury, or by a disease such as anterior poliomyelitis which might happen to destroy the LMNs supplying the flexors, leaving all *afferent* axons from the sole and *efferent* axons to the extensors intact.

   b. The laboratory minded investigator would make simultaneous electromyographic recordings from the flexors and extensors as he applied the plantar stimulus.

   c. Landau and Clare concluded that both flexors and extensors of the toe contract simultaneously in response to a plantar stimulus, with the outcome a mechanical competition between these muscles, but Van Gijn disagrees. At the spinal cord level, however, some integrative mechanism must fight out whether flexion or extension will occur.

H. Pathologic variations in the plantar reflexes

1. After interruption of the UMN pathways to the lumbosacral reflex centers, a plantar stimulus causes the great toe to dorsiflex (extend) rather than plantar flexing. We call this a *dorsiflexor* or *extensor* plantar response, or *Babinski* sign (Joseph Babinski, 1857–1932). See Fig. 7-30*A*.
2. The flexor synergy which withdraws the leg of a normal person after a plantar stimulus usually becomes more prominent and stereotyped after pyramidal tract interruption. See Fig. 7-30*B*. You detect this withdrawal by visual inspection and by the tug of the patient's ankle against your grasp.
3. Some patients voluntarily extend their large toe after a plantar stimulus, contaminating the reflex-induced response. In addition, a struggling child or some patients with involuntary movement disorders may inadvertently dorsiflex the great toe. To best identify an extensor toe sign, carefully notice the relation of toe extension and leg withdrawal to the plantar stimulus. With a true extensor toe sign, the toe usually begins to extend only after the plantar stroke has moved some distance along the sole to produce spatial and temporal summation. The toe remains tonically extended as the stroke continues, and then promptly returns

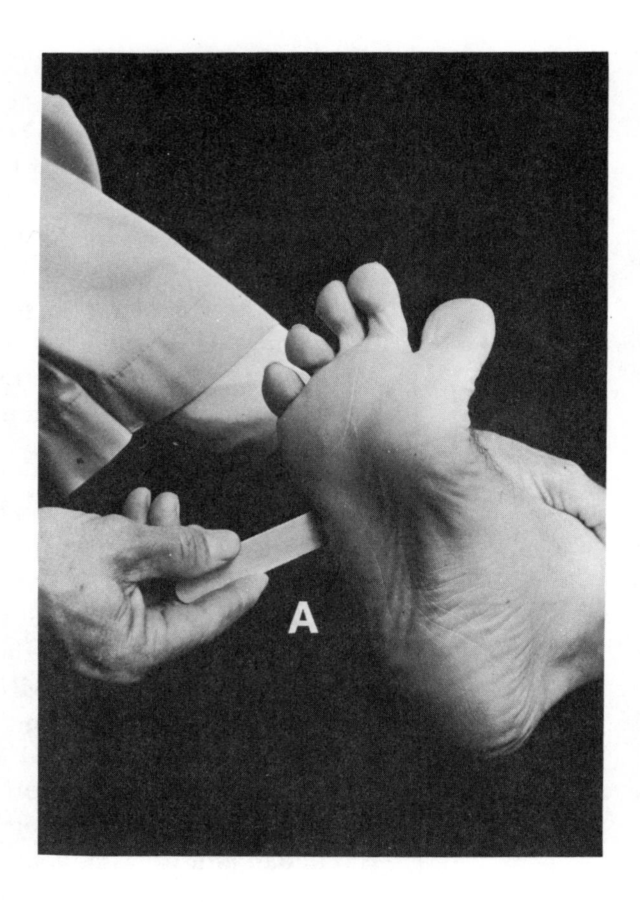

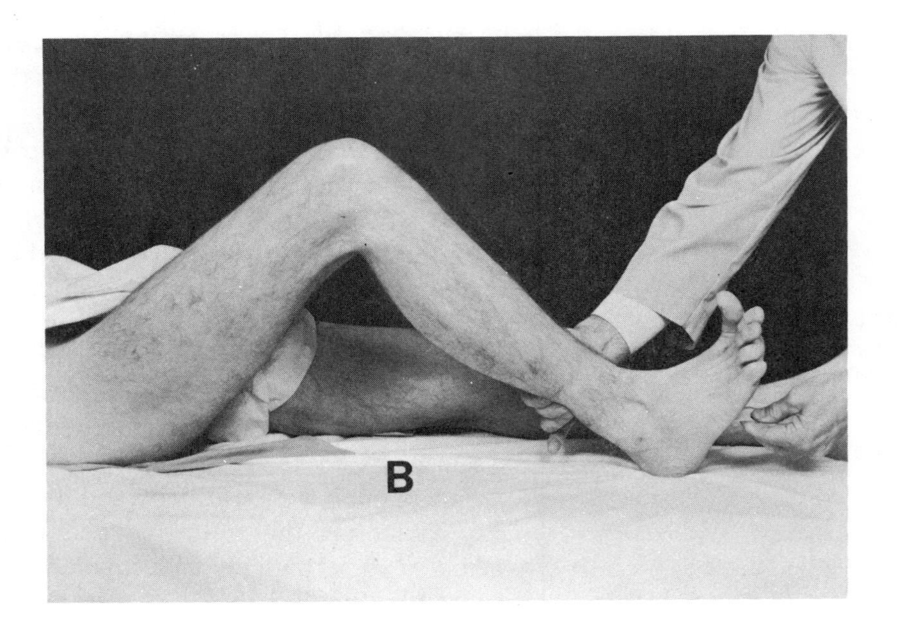

FIG. 7-30. Responses to a plantar stimulus. (A) Extension (dorsiflexion) of the great toe in response to a plantar stimulus in a patient with an upper motor neuron lesion. (B) Flexor withdrawal reflex (triple flexion reflex) consisting of dorsiflexion of the ankle, and flexion of the knee and hip in response to plantar stimulus.

to the neutral position after release of the stroke. Thus, you must confirm that the toe movement is indeed related to, provoked by, and dependent on the plantar stimulus, and that any flexion of the leg displays a similar correlation. To establish it as a reflex, the response should show a "machine-like fatality," to use Sherrington's words. Any other relation of the toe or leg movement to the plantar stimulus, or an inconstant relation, falls under suspicion of a false response.

release

4. The extensor toe sign would be classed as a ☐ deficit/ ☐ release phenomenon because ____
____.

Ans: It is a new behavior or response which the patient did not display before the UMN lesion and which is unmasked by the UMN lesion.

5. Clinicians regard the extensor toe response as a sign of anatomical or pathophysiological interruption of the pyramidal tract (Van Gijn; Walshe). No other hypothesis fits the facts as well. However, as with other features of the UMN syndrome, such as spasticity, some uncertainty exists about the exact UMN pathway that is responsible (Nathan and Smith). Pathophysiological conditions that result in extensor toe signs, with or without the other features of the UMN syndrome, include toxic-metabolic coma, epileptic seizures, trauma, transient ischemic attacks, and hemiplegic migraine. The patient's prompt and full recovery provides the proof of a transient pathophysiological state rather than anatomic interruption of UMN pathways.

I. Explanations for the otherwise puzzling absence of extensor toe signs in patients who have UMN lesions, or, How to avoid being fooled

1. *Consider this patient.* He was a 24-year-old man who struck his head on the bottom of a swimming pool when he dived in. His neck was forced sharply backward. He immediately became paralyzed and anesthetic from the neck down. When examined shortly after his neck injury, all movement except diaphragm contractions, all sensation, and all reflexes were absent caudal to the lower cervical region.

spinal shock

   a. Such a phase of complete paralysis, hypotonia, and areflexia after an acute, severe spinal cord injury is called ______________.
   b. Within 8 days, his MSRs returned and became very hyperactive. Extensor toe signs appeared and sensation started to return. Within 15 days after injury, all release phenomena were present and he began to have active movement. Eight weeks after the injury he was able to move all extremities. Six months after the injury, he had slight hyperreflexia of the left leg and a suggestive extensor toe sign on the left, but otherwise he seemed normal.
   c. The patient had suffered a contusion of the spinal cord which had temporarily interrupted all impulse transmission through the lesion site. After recovery, he still had residual signs indicating that some UMN axons on the left side of the cord had been permanently destroyed.
   d. After an acute neurologic lesion, the extensor toe sign may be absent during the stage known as spinal or cerebral (neural) shock,

and this is one explanation for absence of an extensor toe sign when the patient has a UMN lesion.

2. In other patients, absence of the extensor toe sign may have a simple mechanical explanation: compression damage to the common peroneal nerve blocks efferent impulses to the extensor muscles of the toe. The usual site of compression of the common peroneal nerve is where it crosses the fibula. Feel the head of your fibula. Move your fingertip a half a centimeter or so distally. Pressing fairly hard, move your fingertip back and forth across the fibula. You should be able to feel the nerve slip back and forth under your finger. See Fig. 7-31.

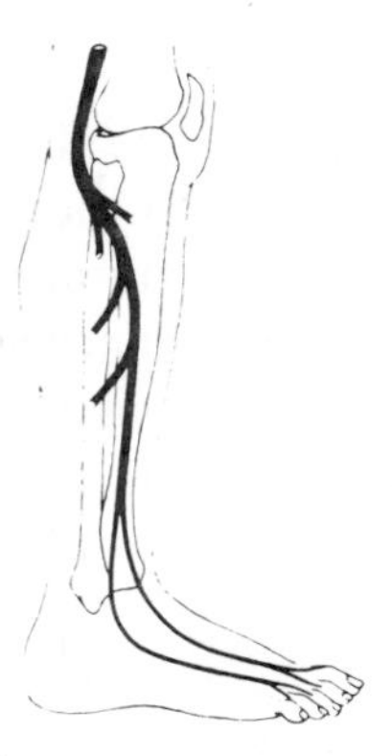

FIG. 7-31. Distribution of the common peroneal nerve. Notice how it courses superficial to the fibula, where it is exposed to injury.

3. In patients paralyzed from any cause, the common peroneal nerve is frequently damaged because the paralyzed leg may rest in outward rotation, in the same position, for long periods of time, compressing the nerve between the fibula and the bed or other surface. This mechanism accounts for many instances in which the extensor toe sign is unexpectedly absent when the patient undoubtedly has a UMN lesion.
4. Since the common peroneal nerve supplies all foot and toe extensors, damage to it causes a foot drop. The patient cannot dorsiflex his foot. It will drop, and he will drag his toes when he walks. When the patient's UMN paralysis improves, it is tragic if the major disability remaining is the peroneal palsy, which precludes a satisfactory gait. The peroneal nerve, ulnar nerve, and other nerves have to be protected by proper positioning and nursing care during the paralytic phase of UMN lesions and when applying casts for fractures.
5. The superficial position of the nerve accounts for a common cause of foot drop, the so-called "crossed knee palsy" in which the nerve is compressed when a person sits with one knee crossed over the other. Cross your legs and notice how the peroneal nerve may be entrapped between the fibula and the lateral condyle and patella of the opposite knee.

6. Give two basically different reasons why an extensor toe sign may be absent in a patient who undoubtedly has a UMN lesion.

____

____

Ans: (1) Spinal or cerebral shock. (2) A lesion of the reflex arc, such as peroneal nerve injury, loss of afferent impulses, etc.

7. Even when all the foregoing alternative explanations are excluded, some patients with UMN lesions will fail to show one or more of the deficit or release phenomena. We can only hide behind the mask of "biologic variability." But don't use that disguise as a substitute for careful analysis of all the possible pathogenic factors.

J. Changes in the stimulus dimensions and reflexogenous zone for the plantar reflexes after a UMN lesion

S_1

1. To get a plantar response in some patients requires a fairly selective combination of site, length, velocity, and pressure of the stimulus. The usual reflexogenous zone for the plantar reflexes, either normal or pathologic, is the ______________ dermatome. Shade this dermatome in Fig. 7-32.

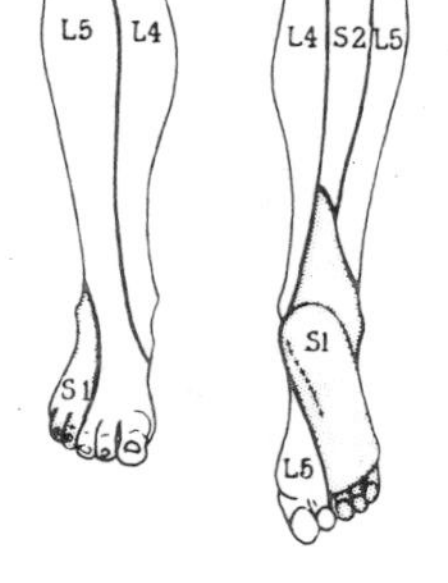

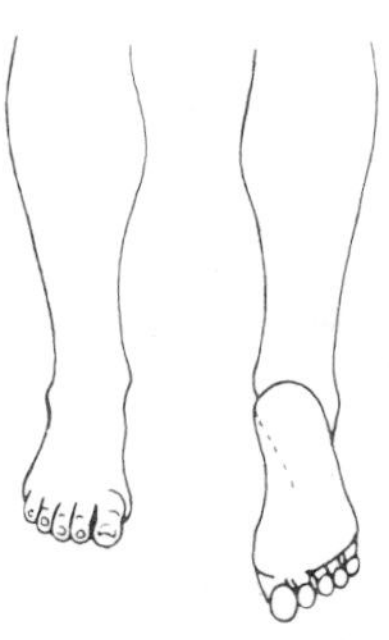

FIG. 7-32. Blank for shading the S_1 dermatome.

2. In some patients the extensor toe sign and leg withdrawal lose all local signature or local specificity. Almost any stimulus of any part of the skin caudal to the level of UMN interruption results in toe extension, with a strong flexor synergy or flexion spasms. Such patients usually have severe structural lesions, often complete spinal cord transection.
3. *Additional methods of eliciting superficial toe reflexes*

lateral

   a. Babinski's method is stimulation of the ☐ medial/ ☐ lateral margin of the sole.

   b. Other eponymic maneuvers to elicit toe movement from superficial stimuli are given in Fig. 7-33. The importance of Fig. 7-33 is not the eponyms, but the behavior you go through in the various maneuvers. Having different eponyms, these maneuvers are frequently referred to as if they were separate signs. But when considered physiologically, as stimuli, the maneuvers betray a beguiling simplicity which unifies them. Since many of the maneuvers apply the stimulus outside of S_1, the usual reflexogenous zone, they are in general less effective than stimuli within the S_1 dermatome. In the normal person they do not usually cause toe flexion, but with UMN lesions, they tend to elicit toe extension just as with the Babinski maneuver.

c. Do the maneuvers of Fig. 7-33 on yourself and another subject, paying attention to the stimulus properties of each maneuver.

4. If you can divine the common properties of the stimuli used in the maneuvers of Table 7-33, you will find a beguiling simplicity. What are the common features of the stimuli? ______________________________
____
____
______________________________________.

Descriptive Name	Eponym	Maneuver
A. Plantar toe reflex	Babinski	Move an object along the lateral aspect of the sole. 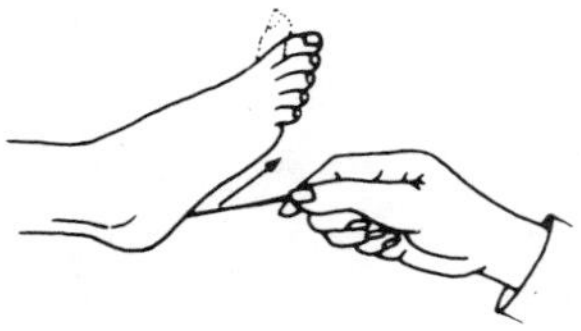
B. None	Chaddock	Move an object along the lateral side of the foot. 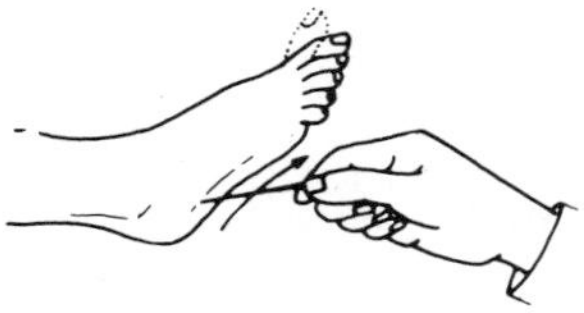
C. Achilles-toe reflex	Schaeffer	Squeeze hard on the Achilles tendon. 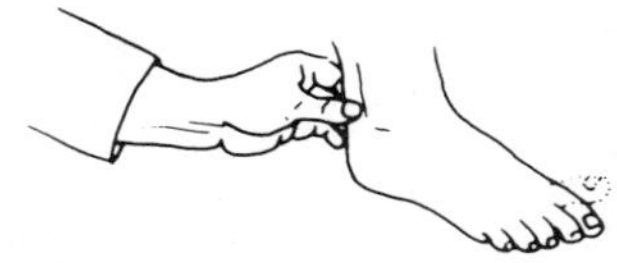
D. Shin-toe reflex	Oppenheim	Press your knuckles on the patient's shin and move them down. 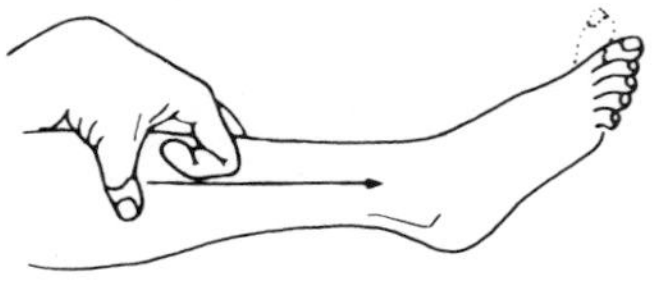
E. Calf-toe reflex	Gordon	Squeeze the calf muscles momentarily. 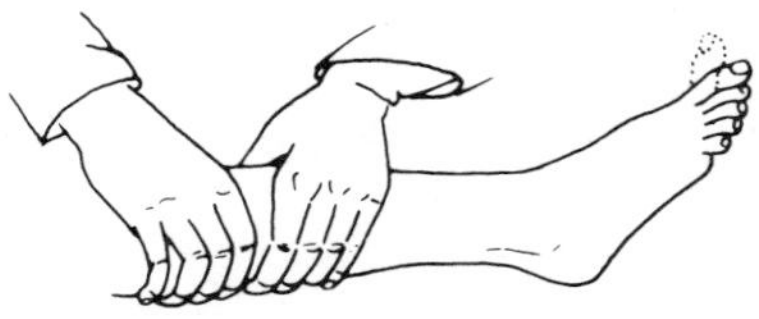
F. Pinprick-toe reflex	Bing	Make multiple light pinpricks on the dorsolateral surface of the foot. 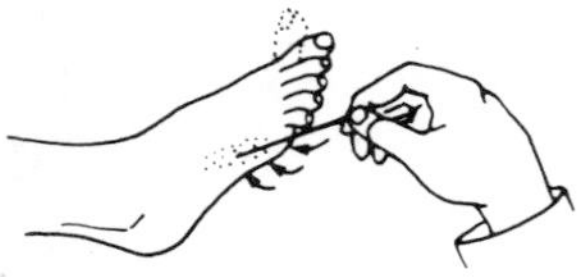
G. Toe pull reflex	Gonda, Stransky	Pull the 4th toe outward and downward for a brief time and release suddenly. 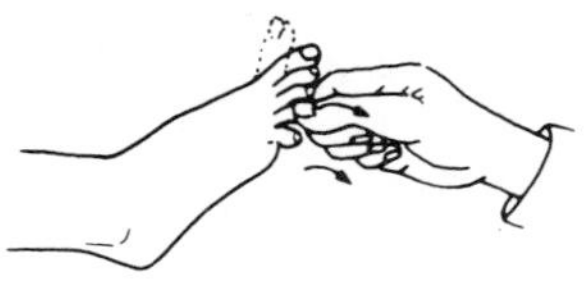

FIG. 7-33. Methods for eliciting the extensor toe sign.

Ans: In each maneuver, the stimulus acts over a similar interval of time, stimulates more than one point of skin, and causes a noxious or uncomfortable sensation. We can infer that it is a spatially and temporally summated, noxious superficial stimulus which elicits the response. That's what this business of toe signs is all about.

5. Armed with this information you are now capable of "discovering" a dozen new signs yourself. Run your thumbnail down the shin and you have ______________________*'s* sign. Squeeze on a corn (a very effective way to get an extensor toe response) and you have another sign, and so on. Thus, it is simply ludicrous to separate the Babinski sign from the Chaddock sign, as if they were different entities, when all you have done operationally is to stimulate slightly different areas of the S_1 dermatome. The response from the S_1 dermatome is the most constant and useful. If a convincing, reproducible response is obtained from the S_1 dermatome, the other maneuvers are superfluous.

Insert your own name

6. *Coming to terms*
   a. The best terminology is to say that the patient has a *flexor plantar response* or an *extensor plantar response*, whichever is found. If you use an eponym and speak of a "Babinski sign" or "Chaddock sign," it is infelicitous, redundant, to say the patient has a positive Babinski sign. There is no negative Babinski sign. The sign is either present or not. However, you may find either a *flexor* or an *extensor* plantar response. A generic term used to describe the result when *any* maneuver causes extension of the large toe instead of flexion is an *extensor toe sign.*
   b. If you feel that your education is deficient unless you are well equipped with eponyms, try this mnemonic: B is for Babinski, stimulate the *bottom* of the foot. C is for Chaddock, stimulate the *side*. G is for Gordon, *grip* the calf. O is for Oppenheim's, *on* the shin maneuver. S is for Schaeffer, *squeeze* the Achilles tendon.

K. The plantar responses in infants

1. In normal infants an extensor plantar response is frequently obtained, especially if the pressure used is slight. Strong plantar pressure may elicit a plantar grasp reflex which competes with toe extension.
2. The characteristic of the plantar response in normal infants is *variability*, extension on one occasion, flexion on the next. Hence, the extensor toe sign, while always to be viewed as pathologic in older patients if the reflex arc is intact, does not convict the infant of a UMN lesion. In general, the older the patient and the more constant the extensor response, the more likely the patient has a UMN lesion.
3. Contrast the clinical significance of an extensor toe response in infants and older subjects. ______________________________
____
____
____

Ans: Normal infants show variability, with extensor and flexor toe responses. In older subjects, extensor responses indicate a UMN lesion.

L. Technique of eliciting the superficial abdominal and cremasteric reflexes

1. The superficial abdominal and cremasteric reflexes are elicited by stroking the skin of the abdominal quadrants or thighs, as shown in Fig. 7-34.

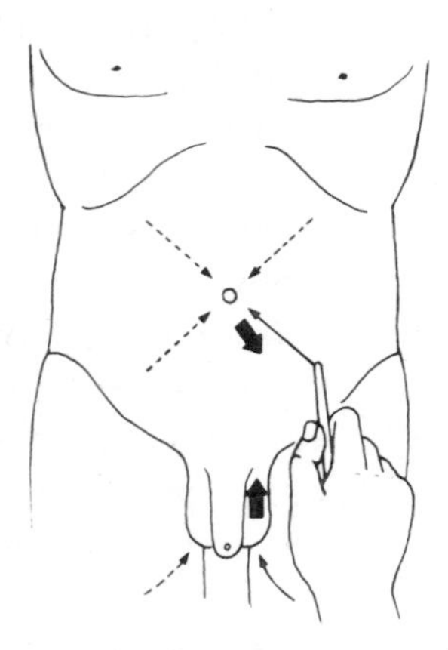

FIG. 7-34. Method for eliciting the superficial abdominal and cremasteric reflexes. The thin arrows are the direction of the examiner's stroke, and the thick solid arrows are the direction of the response.

2. Using a broken tongue blade, the blunt end of a reflex hammer, or a pin, practice obtaining the superficial abdominal reflexes on yourself and another subject. The subject should be sitting or reclining. You may be unable to obtain the reflex on yourself, but by trying, you will learn two important things:
   a. The stimulus is unpleasant to the patient.
   b. The response is difficult to obtain if the abdominal muscles are too tense. Since you will have to flex or raise your head, you may tense your muscles too much. On the other hand, a slight degree of abdominal tension may facilitate the response.
3. The normal response to abdominal skin stimulation is twitching of the umbilicus ☐ toward / ☐ away from the quadrant stimulated.
4. The normal response to thigh stimulation is ☐ elevation / ☐ depression of the ☐ ipsilateral / ☐ contralateral / ☐ both testicles. (No counterpart of this reflex can be obtained in females.)
5. From your previous experience, you will recognize immediately that the abdominal stimulus has the same properties as the plantar stimulus. That is, the stimulus, if perceived by the patient, is ______________, and it undergoes ______________ and ______________ summation.
6. Therefore you use the same consideration for the patient's comfort as in eliciting plantar reflexes: the first stimulus is applied ______________.

toward
elevation
ipsilateral

unpleasant
spatial
temporal

gently!

M. Effect of UMN lesions on the abdominal and cremasteric reflexes. These superficial reflexes are absent or diminished after UMN lesions. No substitute movement, such as dorsiflexion of the toe, occurs. Thus the effect of UMN lesions would be classed as a ☐ deficit / ☐ release phenomenon.

deficit

N. Natural history of the abdominal and cremasteric reflexes

1. You will find it difficult to elicit abdominal reflexes in young infants. The patient, adult or infant, must be relaxed and able to sustain the somewhat uncomfortable or tickling sensation produced. If his abdomen is tense, no response will be observed. As the infant matures, the abdominal reflexes can be elicited.
2. In normal old or obese patients, or in multiparous women whose abdominal muscles have been stretched, the abdominal reflex is often absent.
3. During the acute phase of a UMN lesion, the abdominal and cremasteric reflexes are usually absent. Later they may recover. If the brain lesion is inflicted early in life, these reflexes regularly return. Thus, in the acute phase of a UMN lesion, abdominal and cremasteric reflexes would be absent, but in the ________ phase of the lesion they may have recovered.
4. What 2 features of the superficial reflexes in young infants would indicate a UMN lesion in a more mature patient? ________

chronic

extensor toe signs, and absence of abdominal reflexes

O. Summarize the full syndrome of the chronic phase of UMN lesions (apart from spinal or cerebral shock) with respect to the effect on:

1. Movements: (Give the general rule as to whether proximal or distal parts are most severely affected.) ________.
2. MSRs: ________.
3. Muscle tone: ________.
4. Plantar reflexes: ________.
5. Abdominal-cremasteric reflexes: ________.

Paresis or paralysis most severe in unilaterally independent or distal parts
Hyperreflexia
Clasp-knife spasticity
Extensor toe sign
Absent at first but may recover

P. Recording the superficial reflexes

1. In the stick figure used to record the MSRs, the toe response is recorded by an arrow in the appropriate direction. The abdominal and cremasteric reflexes are recorded as 0 if absent, ± if equivocal or barely present, and + if normally active. See Fig. 7-35.

Ans. to frame 4:

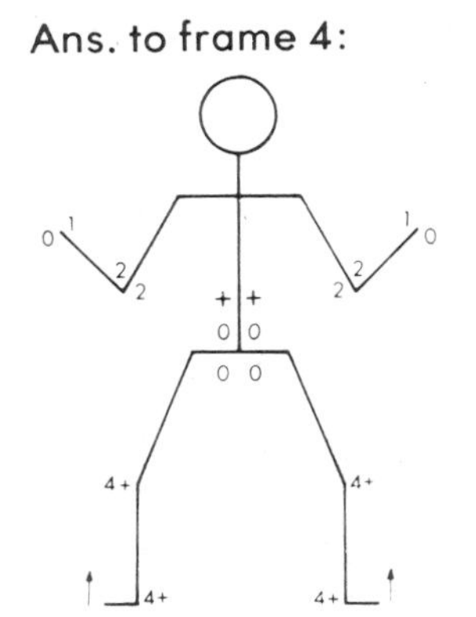

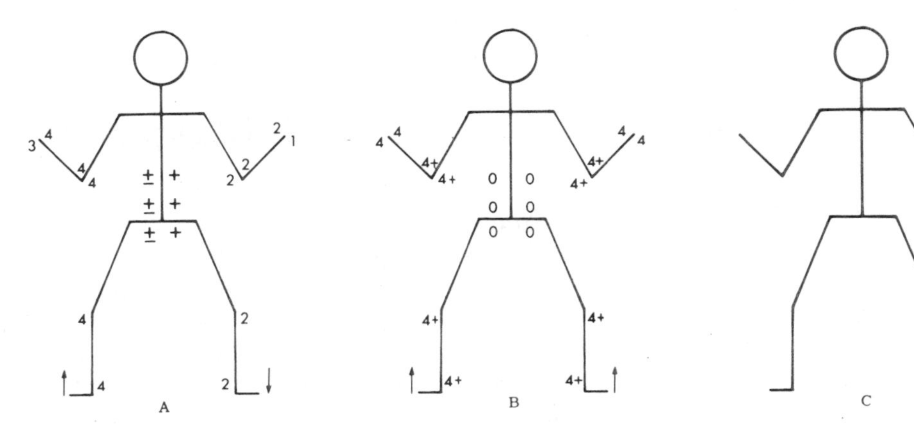

FIG. 7-35. Recording of reflex changes after UMN lesions.

hemiplegia

quadriplegia

See figure above.

migrate upward

2. In Fig. 7-35*A*, the result would be consistent with ☐ hemiplegia / ☐ quadriplegia / ☐ paraplegia?
3. Fig. 7-35*B* records ☐ hemiplegia / ☐ quadriplegia / ☐ paraplegia.
4. The next patient is paraplegic with a chronic lesion at the 10th thoracic level. The 9th and 10th thoracic segments innervate the upper half of the abdomen, the 11th and 12th the lower. Thus, his UMN signs appear only distal to T10. Fill in Fig. 7-35*C* to show the reflex pattern expected.
5. What would happen to the patient's umbilicus in Fig. 7-35*C* if he were supine and attempted to elevate his head and shoulders? ________ ________.

Q. Summary of the syndromes of UMN and LMN lesions

1. Complete Table 7-5. Assume the patient does not have neural shock and answer in terms of general principles, not in terms of the possibility of exceptions.
2. When a patient has a severe, acute UMN lesion, he may show no ☐ release / ☐ deficit phenomena, but he will always show ☐ release / ☐ deficit phenomena.

release
deficit

UMN	LMN
✓	
	✓
✓	
	✓
	✓
✓	
	✓
✓	
✓	
	✓
✓	*
✓	

TABLE 7-5. Clinical Syndrome of UMN and LMN Lesions

1 UMN	2 LMN	3 Characteristic
		Paralyzes movements in hemiplegic, quadriplegic, or paraplegic distribution, not individual muscles
		Paralyzes individual muscles or sets of muscles in root or peripheral nerve distributions
		Atrophy of disuse only (late and slight)
		Atrophy of denervation (early and severe)
		Fasciculations and fibrillations
		Hyperactive MSRs
		Hypoactive or absent MSRs
		Clonus
		Clasp-knife spasticity
		Hypotonia
	*	Absent abdominal-cremasteric reflexes
		Extensor toe sign

***Note:** Direct disease of the LMNs to the effector muscles abolishes these reflexes, but disease confined to other LMNs does not.

Bibliography

Gijn, J. Van: *The Plantar Reflex: A Historical, Clinical, and Electromyographic Study,* Meppel (The Netherlands), Krips Repro, 1977.

Landau, W., and Clare, M.: The plantar reflex in man, with special reference to some conditions where the extensor response is unexpectedly absent, *Brain,* 82:321-355, 1959.

Nathan, P., and Smith, M.: The Babinski response: a review and new observations, *J. Neurol. Neurosurg. Psychiat.,* 18:250-259, 1955.

Walshe, F.: The Babinski plantar response, its forms and its physiological and pathological significance, *Brain,* 79:529-556, 1956.

VI. Involuntary movements and nonparalytic disorders of movement

A. *Introduction*

We experience ourselves as having free will. This experience leads us to classify movements as voluntary and involuntary. Then we must puzzle over behaviors like breathing, sphincter constriction, and postural reflexes which are both voluntary and involuntary. Puzzlement leads to bewilderment when we try to classify the bizarre behavior of mental patients which they experience as involuntary.

It can be argued that all behavior is the outcome of laws as binding as those governing reflexes. In fact we can almost state that if we understand the neurophysiology of a behavior, such as a muscle stretch reflex or tonic neck reflex, we regard it as involuntary, and if we do not understand the neurophysiology of a behavior, such as a man rioting, we regard it as voluntary. If we could translate motivation into neuronal properties, we could see why your free will directs you to turn left instead of right as you go out the door. The experience of having a free will, then, would become an artifact of consciousness, rather than a mystical energizing force within the personality.

Interesting discussions of determinism versus free will are found in Tolstoy's *War and Peace* and Clarence Darrow's defense plea in the Leopold-Loeb murder trial. Although the free will theory of behavior is a metaphysical doctrine of unprovable validity, physicians get on the witness stand every day to testify that some outcast who has dismembered a child or murdered a President acted in possession of his faculties, of his own free will. Yet the very act he committed is the clearest kind of evidence that he could not control his impulses. Is it worthwhile, then, to argue that by force of free will he could have acted otherwise? If we could only understand how the neurons act when a man commits a crime, or when mired in poverty, or when caught in a neurotic web . . . if we could only understand the surge of electrical currents through the brain's circuits, the ebb and flow across synaptic clefts of the excitatory and inhibitory neurohumors which trip the delicate balance between repose and aggression.

All right, I will not dwell on this point forever. I am trying to state that the notion of willed movement can be accepted for the limited purposes of clinical diagnosis, but I personally do not wish to generalize it to encompass criminology, sociology, and the questions of blame and responsibility for behavior. The stark clinical facts are these:

1. Patients will come to see you because they do, indeed, have movements they cannot willfully control.
2. We can utilize operational definitions to guide clinical analysis.

B. *The operations for identifying voluntary and involuntary movements*

1. *Identifying normal voluntary and involuntary movements*
   - *a.* A voluntary movement is one that the standard normal man can start or stop at his own or an observer's command.
   - *b.* An involuntary movement is one that the standard normal man cannot stop at his own or an observer's command.
2. *Identifying syndromes of abnormal involuntary movements.* As the neurologist conceives involuntary movements, he means those movements

caused by structural or biochemical lesions of the nervous system. Disease-induced involuntary movements fall into patterns allowing recognition without recourse to the patient's testimony, in most cases. Here is the pivotal point, the art of inspection again. To see is to diagnose. If the physical evidence is inconclusive, the psychiatric history usually leads to the diagnosis. The operations for making a clinical decision are these:

a. Find out when the movements started, under what conditions they appear and disappear, and their evolution over time. In other words, what is the history?

b. Describe the pattern of the movements, their distribution, rate, amplitude, and force. In other words, what are the physical findings?

c. Compare the clinical data with a standard catalog of involuntary movement syndromes.

3. *Effects of pyramidal and extrapyramidal lesions on movements*

a. Pyramidal tract lesions paralyze voluntary movements.

b. Extrapyramidal lesions, which interrupt the complex motor circuitry between the cortex, basal ganglia, thalamus, brainstem, cerebellum, and LMNs, have a variable effect on movements. The patient may show a reduction in voluntary movements, usually because of rigidity, or may show excessive involuntary movements, with relatively intact voluntary movements. In a patient with extrapyramidal movements, a second lesion, inflicted by disease or surgery, in the extrapyramidal circuits may paralyze the abnormal involuntary movements, while still sparing voluntary movements. However, in a patient with extrapyramidal involuntary movements, interruption of the pyramidal tract causes not only the expected paralysis of voluntary movements, but also paralyzes the abnormal involuntary movements. Thus no simple equation of pyramidal tract = voluntary movements, extrapyramidal tracts = involuntary movements applies.

C. *Some normal involuntary movements*

1. *Physiologic tremor*

a. Place a large sheet of paper between your index finger and the adjacent finger, and hold your arm straight out in front of you. The rustling of the paper is *physiologic tremor.* The tremor has a frequency of about 10 cps.

b. We do not know the full basis for physiologic tremor. It comes from a composite of neurally mediated oscillations and the ballistic effects of respiratory and cardiac actions (ballistocardiogram). Thus, it has neurologic and mechanical components.

2. *Physiologic synkinesias:* (syn = with; kinesia = moving). A synkinesia is an involuntary or automatic movement that accompanies a voluntary movement. Close your eyes and your eyeballs automatically roll up (Bell's phenomenon). Walk and your arms swing. Cough and your latissimus dorsi muscles contract. Look up and your frontalis muscle contracts. Use these examples to identify other synkinesias. The degree

of volition in the synkinesias varies. You can't stop Bell's phenomenon, but you can stop your arms from swinging when walking.

3. *Myoclonic jerks*
   a. You have at some time felt your head jerk upright when just falling asleep (in a lecture hall or while doing a programmed text). The jerk and the sudden restoration of consciousness are the result of a sudden discharge in the reticular activating system of the brainstem. It is essentially a startle reaction, an alerting response.
   b. You may have felt a twitch of your whole biceps muscle, perhaps after doing some unaccustomed work. This too is a myoclonic jerk, confined in this instance to a single muscle.
   c. Myoclonic jerks may occur as a sign of epilepsy or other nervous system diseases. What is *physiologic* under one circumstance is *pathologic* under another.
   d. Myoclonic jerks are to be distinguished from fasciculations. Define a fasciculation. ______________________________
   ____
   ____

Ans: A twitch of part of a muscle due to random discharge of an LMN and its fascicle of muscle fibers.

myoclonic
fasciculation

   e. A twitch of a whole muscle or groups of muscles is called a ______________ jerk, while a twitch of a single fascicle of muscle is a ______________.

4. *Benign fasciculations*
   a. Normal subjects may have fasciculations, particularly after exercise. When fasciculations are unusually numerous or persistent, they are given the diagnostic label *benign fasciculations,* if the subject has no weakness or other signs of LMN disease. Twitching of an eyelid is a benign fasciculation.
   b. What clinical and electromyographic signs enable you to distinguish benign from pathologic fasciculations? ______________
   ____
   ____
   ____

Ans: If pathologic, fasciculations implicate LMN disease. Therefore, you look for other evidence of LMN disease: weakness, hypo- or areflexia, hypotonia, and denervation atrophy as supported by EMG evidence of fibrillations and giant polyphasic motor units along with the fasciculations.

D. *The dyskinesias*

1. Broadly defined, dyskinesias could include any difficulty with movement, whether too much movement, *hyper*kinesia, or too little, *hypo*kinesia. In use, the terms have some restrictions.
2. Hypokinesia refers to a reduction in the amount of movement or the activity level of the patient. The causes range from depression to extrapyramidal syndromes. By custom, neurologists generally do not apply the term hypokinesia to various types of paralysis such as hemiplegia or even quadriplegia.

3. Hyperkinesia refers to an increase in the amount of movement or the activity level of the patient. Some neurologists would restrict the term to extrapyramidal hyperkinesias. Others might include any excessive movements, from fasciculations to the hyperkinesis of children. (Considering my colleagues' peculiarities, I won't belabor strict definitions.) For description we can recognize tremorous and nontremorous hyperkinesias.

E. *Tremorous hyperkinesias*

1. *Rest tremors* occur when the part is at rest.

   a. *Emotional tremor* is present at rest, but it worsens during volitional movement: witness the quavering knees and voice of the novice orator. From your own experience you know that emotional tremor, like physiologic tremor, is ☐ rapid / ☐ very slow and of ☐ very great / ☐ low amplitude.

   rapid
   low

   b. *Familial tremor* is a tremor of similar frequency as physiologic tremor, about 10 cps, but of greater amplitude. Apparently it is of neural origin, although its pathophysiology is poorly understood. It affects the hands predominantly and follows an autosomal dominant hereditary pattern.

   c. *Senile tremor* has a frequency of about 6 to 10 cps and occurs in the older patient. Senile and familial tremor merge in their clinical manifestations, but senile tremor while frequently familial, may result from non-familial lesions of aging. See Critchley for a more complete discussion of these commonplace tremors.

   d. *Parkinsonian tremor* is rhythmic with low amplitude and a frequency of about 5 cps. Drum your fingertips on the table, making 25 beats per 5 sec, and you will observe two characteristics of this tremor: moderate frequency and low-to-moderate amplitude. In contrast to emotional tremor, it disappears or dampens during intentional movement. Parkinsonian tremor, like virtually all involuntary movement disorders, is accentuated during emotional stress. The uninitiated observer is apt to think the patient is feigning to attract attention, but it is an organic disease caused by a lesion of the ☐ pyramidal / ☐ extrapyramidal system.

   extrapyramidal

      (1) Parkinsonian tremor differs from emotional tremor by ☐ increasing / ☐ decreasing in amplitude during volitional movement, and resembles every other type of tremor by ☐ increasing / ☐ decreasing during emotional stress.

      decreasing
      increasing

      (2) Although it seems paradoxical, the resting tremor of Parkinsonism, a hyperkinesia, is regularly associated with a hypokinetic feature, ☐ clasp-knife spasticity / ☐ lead-pipe rigidity.

      lead-pipe rigidity

2. *Intention* tremor appears during intentional movements. The patient's hand, while resting on his lap, shows no tremor, but upon movement, a fairly rhythmic tremor commences which increases in amplitude as the hand approaches an end point. It implies a lesion of the cerebellar efferent system as does postural tremor with which it merges.

3. *Postural* tremor occurs during the maintenance of an intentional posture, such as holding the hands outstretched. As the patient holds

his hands outstretched, he has a regular, rhythmic tremor of several cps. As he brings his finger in to touch his nose the tremor disappears or decreases. When he holds his fingertip on his nose, the tremor reappears, and it is often exaggerated temporarily. When the patient places his hands in his lap, at rest, he has no tremor. Before answering the next frames, review the tremorous hyperkinesias and organize your own list of them or make your own dendrogram.

parkinsonian

disappearing

a. Since it disappears or decreases during movement, postural tremor is like ______________________ tremor.

b. Postural tremor differs from Parkinsonian tremor in ☐ disappearing / ☐ appearing when the patient is completely at rest.

c. Postural tremor results from a lesion of the efferent cerebellar pathway through the rostral part of the brainstem, of which more later.

4. Review frames *E*1*b*, *E*2, and *E*3 and act out the tremors described.
5. Give the clinical characteristics of Parkinsonian tremor: ______________
____
____

Ans: Parkinsonian tremor appears at rest, has a low amplitude and a regular frequency of 5 cps, disappears during intentional movement, and exacerbates during emotional stress.

cerebellar or cerebellofugal

6. Intention and postural tremors indicate a lesion of the ☐ cerebellar or cerebellofugal/ ☐ basal ganglia pathways.

F. The kymographic records of tremors

1. From these kymographic recordings, identify the type of tremor and the pathophysiologic basis:

a. The patient is sitting quietly in a chair. The tremor looks like this:

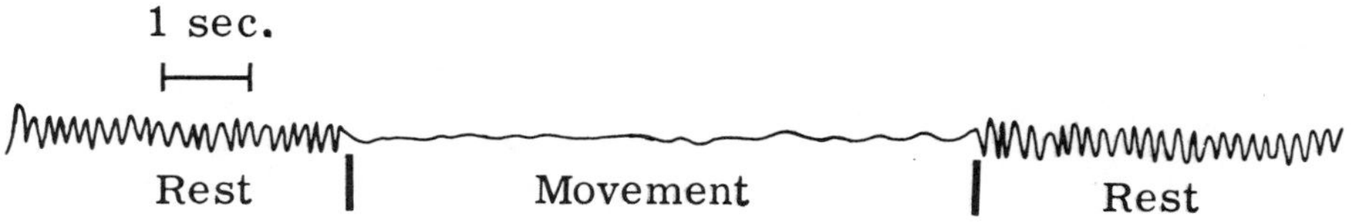

FIG. 7-36. Kymographic record of tremor. See text.

5 or 6

rest

extrapyramidal

Parkinsonism

b. The rate of the tremor is about ____________ cps.

c. Since the tremor is absent during intentional movement and present at rest, it is classified as a ☐ rest / ☐ intention / ☐ postural tremor.

d. This type of tremor signifies a lesion of the ______________ pathways and is characteristic of the disorder called ______________ __________ (eponym).

2. This patient was sitting quietly in a chair. He was asked to extend his arms. When he held his arms outstretched, no tremor was seen. When asked to touch his index finger tip to his nose, he showed a tremor like this:

1 sec.
Arms out-stretched
Moving finger in to touch nose
At rest on nose

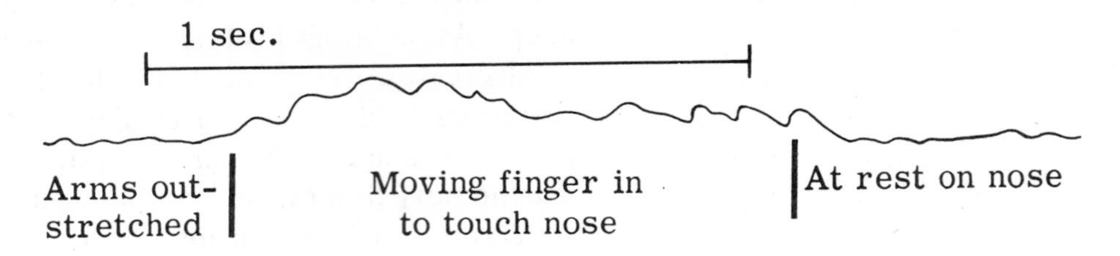

FIG. 7-37. Kymographic record of tremor. See text.

intention

cerebellar

a. After he reached his nose, he showed very little tremor. This tremor is called ______________ tremor.

b. It signifies a lesion of the □ pyramidal/ □ basal ganglia/ □ cerebellar pathways.

3. This patient, while reclining quietly in bed, had no tremor. When asked to hold out his arms, he showed this tremor:

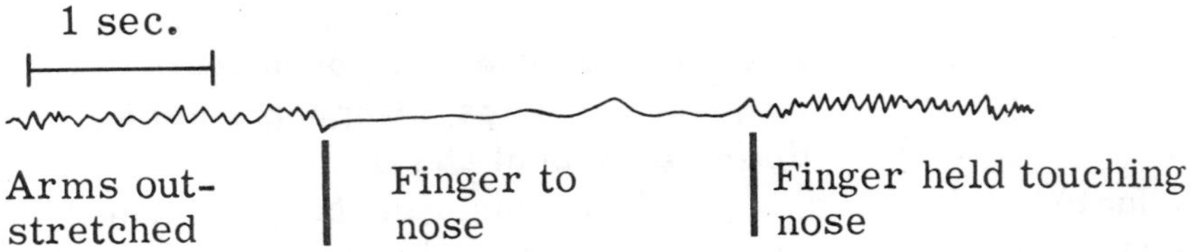

1 sec.
Arms out-stretched
Finger to nose
Finger held touching nose

FIG. 7-38. Kymographic record of tremor. See text.

postural

cerebellum

a. After he reached his nose, the tremor was accentuated. This tremor is called ______________ tremor.

b. It signifies a lesion of the efferent pathway from the ______________ ______________.

G. Types of nontremorous hyperkinesias

1. *Chorea:* random, quick movements, simulating fragments of normal movements — a grimace, elevation of a finger or arm, a misstep when walking, a grunt when speaking. Extremity, speech, facial, and respiratory actions are all affected. At one time or another, you have started to make a movement (perhaps reaching up to pick your nose) and then suddenly decided it was inappropriate and arrested it midway. Or after starting such a movement, you may have diverted it to brushing back your hair. Nevertheless, anyone watching would see the deviation from the usual smooth movement. When such quick fragments of movement occur randomly and involuntarily, they are called ______________. Perhaps this hyperkinesia is best remembered as the fidgets.

chorea

2. *Athetosis:* slow, writhing movements of the fingers and extremities. If severe, athetosis affects speech and respiration. These movements come and go and do not hold the part in a fixed posture for long periods. They are usually seen in patients who also have pyramidal tract signs, and mixtures of athetosis with hemiplegia, spastic quadriplegia, or diplegia are common, especially in cerebral palsy. The quick ran-

chorea
athetosis

dom fidgety movements called ______________ are in contrast to the slow writhing distal movements called ______________.

3. *Dystonia:* very slow, alternating contraction-relaxation of agonists and antagonists. When one movement predominates, holding the part in one position for long periods of time, a fixed contracture of the joint occurs. The muscular pull leads to severe, pretzel-like positions, resulting in fixed scoliosis (axial) and limb (appendicular) deformities.

chorea
athetosis

dystonia

a. The sustained postural deviations of dystonia differ from the quick fragments of movement called ______________, and the slow, writhing movements called ______________.

b. The patient with very slow, sustained contractions of axial or appendicular muscles, has the movement disorder called ______________.

c. You might best regard dystonia, athetosis, and chorea as way stations along a continuum of involuntary movements, not as discrete entities. They differ perhaps more in their speed than in any other way. Chorea ranks fastest, each individual movement measured in a second or even less, a little faster than myoclonic jerks (but sometimes hard to distinguish from them). Next comes athetosis measured just a little longer. Then comes dystonia, which lasts many seconds to minutes, or even longer as in spasmodic torticollis, a form of dystonia in which the head remains deviated for long periods of time. If you like an oversimplified 1,2,3 mnemonic, think of chorea as lasting 1 second or less, athetosis as 1-2 seconds, and dystonia as 3 or more seconds.

d. Although dystonia is traditionally classed as an extrapyramidal movement disorder, the lesion site and pathophysiology are unknown.

4. *Hemiballismus:* violent flinging movements of one half of the body. The root *ballista* means to throw, as in ballistics. The patient acts as if he were trying to fling away a handful of snakes. Hemiballismus usually comes on acutely in elderly, hypertensive patients. The lesion is predictable for most cases. A peculiar, sharply delimited hemmorhage destroys the subthalamic nucleus of Luys. This almond-sized and almond-shaped diencephalic nucleus is a way station in the extrapyramidal system.

chorea

greater

half

rest
lead-pipe
oculogyric

a. Being very fast, hemiballismus is most similar to ☐ chorea / ☐ athetosis / ☐ dystonia.

b. Hemiballismus differs from chorea in having much ☐ greater / ☐ smaller amplitude of movements and in usually being limited to one- ______________ of the body.

5. *Oculogyric crises:* spasms of upward deviation of the eyes and head. These spasms are common in Parkinsonism. Some motor disturbances in Parkinsonism are ______________ tremor, ______________ rigidity, and ______________ crises.

6. *Tics:* quick, stereotyped movements of face, tongue, or extremities. In contrast to the preceding hyperkinesias, the sequence of movements is always identical. All of us have minor tics or tic-like tendencies: wrinkling of the forehead, followed by blinking the eyes, or hitching up the trousers, or a shrug of shoulder. You see a number

of tic-like maneuvers when a basketball player prepares to shoot a free throw, or a tennis player prepares to serve. The tic somehow relieves anxiety and is seen most prominently in moments of stress, in patients with obsessive-compulsive personality traits. Tics are regarded as psychogenic, but there is a syndrome of multiple tics and the utterance of four letter words, which is of unknown origin, but probably organic (syndrome of Gilles de la Tourette). Of the movement disorders discussed, tics are most like ________________ in being quick, brief, and of moderate amplitude, but they differ from the other hyperkinesias in being ☐ purely random / ☐ rigidly stereotyped in pattern.

chorea

rigidly stereotyped

7. *Restless legs syndrome (Ekbom's syndrome):* When attempting to rest or sleep, these patients feel an irresistible urge, often described as an actual sensation in the legs, to keep their legs continuously in motion. No force of will can hold them still. You may have noticed a similar restlessness after exhaustive exercise, or some drugs induce it.
8. *Drug-induced extrapyramidal syndromes and the tardive dyskinesias:* Psychotropic medications (tranquilizers, antipsychotic, and antidepressant drugs) alter the balance of neurotransmitters in the motor circuits. These chemical lesions imitate the effect of anatomic lesions, producing similar hypo- and hyperkinesias, ranging from parkinsonism to dystonia. The movement disorder may appear at any time after starting medication.

   Tardive dyskinesia refers to a hyperkinetic syndrome appearing during chronic psychotropic medication, usually manifested most prominently by face, lip, tongue, and jaw movements, but which may include other types of hyperkinesias or hypertonias in other parts of the body. Tardive dyskinesia resists therapy and may be permanent.
9. *The hyperkinetic child:* Hyperkinetic children display an excessive amount of rapidly changing motor activity. Their inappropriate and usually annoying activity consists of fidgeting, pushing, pulling, banging, rummaging, scattering, clamoring, whining, and running. Rather than a standard, stereotype like athetosis or dystonia, the movement disorder consists of the sheer quantity of activity which continues with little regard for other people, or danger, and responds but little to reward and punishment. No specific known brain lesion underlies this hyperkinesia. Some hyperkinetic children have subtle or overt brain damage with mental retardation. Others may have superior intelligence.
10. *Akathisia:* Akathisia refers to a condition (generally in an adult), in which there is displayed motor unrest manifested by continual shifting of postures or continual moving around. When questioned, these patients often complain of an actual feeling in their muscles of a need to move. Akathisia appears as part of Parkinson's disease and as a result of psychotropic medications. It merges with a variety of cursive states such as compulsive walking or running. We might think of restless legs as a localized type of akathisia or of childhood hyperkinesis as its generalized childhood counterpart. We do not know what critical differences might separate these various syndromes of motor unrest, nor what similarities of pathogenesis they might share.

11. *Epilepsy:* tonic or clonic spasms of all or part of the body represent one manifestation of epilepsy which presents differential diagnostic problems with involuntary movement syndromes. Myoclonic jerks merge imperceptibly with the epilepsies.

H. A summary of involuntary movements (hyperkinesias), by operational definition

1. For clinical diagnosis, we will define hyperkinesias as *any* extra muscular activity caused by a lesion of the nervous system.
2. For the clinical characteristics in *a* to *q*, write down the proper descriptive diagnosis in the blank to the right. Where possible, act out the motility disorder described:

Answer	Clinical characteristic	Blank
a. Fibrillations	*a.* Spontaneous random individual contractions of denervated muscle fibers, detected by EMG.	*a.* __________
b. Fasciculations	*b.* Spontaneous random twitches of small parts of muscles, detected by clinical inspection and EMG.	*b.* __________
c. Myoclonic jerks	*c.* Sudden spontaneous contraction of a muscle or group of muscles, which may simulate a startle reaction.	*c.* __________
d. Tics	*d.* Spontaneous, stereotyped sequence of muscular contractions, seen most prominently in facial muscles in patients with obsessive-compulsive personality traits.	*d.* __________
e. Epilepsy	*e.* Spontaneous tonic or clonic jerking of the body, often accompanied by loss of consciousness.	*e.* __________
f. Chorea	*f.* Spontaneous, quick movements, simulating fragments of normal movements, usually most prominent in extremities.	*f.* __________
g. Athetosis	*g.* Spontaneous, slow writhing movements of fingers and extremities, sometimes involving face and axial muscles.	*g.* __________
h. Dystonia	*h.* Spontaneous, long-sustained deviations of appendicular and axial parts, with alternating agonist-antagonist contractions, ultimately leading to fixed deformities.	*h.* __________
i. Hemiballismus	*i.* More or less incessant (during waking hours) wild, flinging movements of one-half of the body, seen usually in elderly hypertensive patients.	*i.* __________

j. Oculogyric crises

k. Restless legs syndrome

l. Hyperkinetic child syndrome

m. Parkinsonian tremor

n. Intention tremor

o. Postural tremor tremor

p. Familial tremor

q. Senile tremor

r. Tardive dyskinesia

s. Akathisia

j. Spontaneous upward deviation of the eyes and head, seen usually with rest tremor and lead-pipe rigidity. *j.* ______

k. Irresistible wandering of the legs when the patient tries to rest. *k.* ______

l. Incessant, driven, usually assaultive or aggressive behavior in a child. *l.* ______

m. A tremor at rest of 6 cps which dampens or disappears on intentional movement. *m.* ______

n. Irregular tremor of a movement in progress, but no tremor at rest. *n.* ______

o. Rapid tremor of an outstretched hand, which dampens when a movement is in progress and reappears when a new posture is held. *o.* ______

p. A 10 cps tremor of the hands which has an autosomal dominant hereditary pattern. *p.* ______

q. An 8 cps tremor of the head or head and hands, occurring in an elderly patient. *q.* ______

r. A therapy-resistant hyperkinesia usually with predominant face, lip, and tongue movements that appear after prolonged ingestion of psychotropic medications. *r.* ______

s. A state of motor unrest in an adult, characterized by irresistible shifting of postures and moving around. *s.* ______

athetosis

I. Identify the involuntary movements shown in Fig. 7-39A and B. The patient is a 47-year-old woman who was born with a motor system disorder which has persisted with little change over the years. For the photographs, the patient was requested to extend her arms out in front of her and hold them there. Similar movements appear when she is at rest or walking. The movements have a slow rate and low to moderate force and amplitude. They would best be classified as ______________.

J. Avoiding pitfalls (pratfalls) in distinguishing psychogenic and organic motility disturbances

1. Hysterical movement disorders may imitate organic disease. The diagnosis of a *psychogenic* movement disorder must be based on a positive history of mental illness, in which the movement disorder

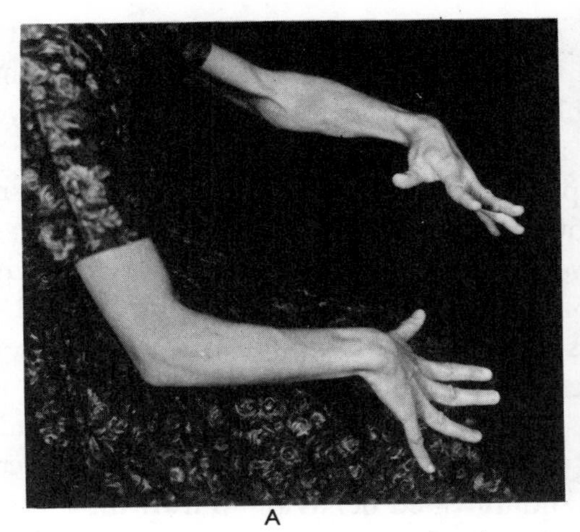
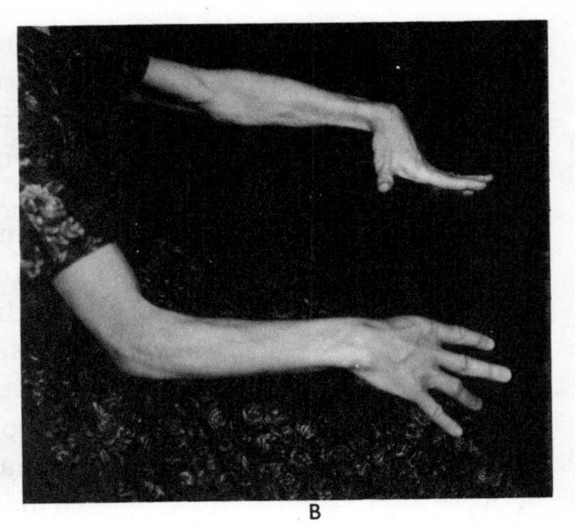

A B

FIG. 7-39. Action sequence of involuntary movements.

is only one shadow in a pattern of maladjustment. The diagnosis of an *organic* movement disorder rests on signs of organic disease and a positive history compatible with organic disease. And then, of course, the patient may have both lice and fleas, a psychogenic and an organic disorder in combination.

2. All, yes *all*, of the involuntary movements and tonic disturbances we have discussed are worse when the patient is under emotional tension. The tremor at rest of the Parkinsonian patient may be accentuated when you simply walk up to the bedside. The patient, previously at rest, with little or no tremor, may begin to rattle the bed. The novice usually interprets this as evidence that the patient has a psychogenic disorder and is putting on a show.
3. Just as all motility disorders discussed here are made worse by emotional tension, they are made better by tranquility and repose. Hence, when the patient is asleep, the hyperkinesias disappear. The postural deformity of the dystonic patient may not relent completely, but most muscular contractions and tremors cease.
4. The various hyperkinesias are not mutually exclusive. Transitions between all the categories occur, and the same patient, over the evolution of his illness, may show one or more motility disturbances. Hence, what starts as athetosis may end as dystonia.
5. The commonest cause today of hypokinetic or hyperkinetic motility disturbances is tranquilizer drugs. These drugs cause astonishing motility disturbances and should be the first thought in the differential diagnosis of a motility disturbance. This is another paradox; tranquility quiets involuntary movements and tranquilizing drugs may cause them.
6. Mothers of hyperkinetic children invariably appear distraught, depressed, and defeated by their inability to cope with their child. If, however, the child appears calm during the period of examination, as some will, the doctor may mistakenly conclude that the mother does not have a justifiable complaint. Thus the immediate inspection of the patient, that serves so well to recognize the standard hyperkinesias of extrapyramidal

origin, may fail in recognizing the hyperkinetic child if the observation period is too brief. On the next visit, make the child remain for a considerable period in the waiting room before you keep the appointment. Then, after the child has demolished your decor, exasperated your other patients, and driven your receptionist mad, you will understand the mother's plight.

7. *Editorial note:* Not too long ago patients with involuntary movement syndromes such as chorea were imprisoned in stocks or executed as possessed of demons and devils. Our understanding of disease has advanced us beyond that barbaric stage, yet we still punish or execute people whose behavior we do not understand. Let us, then, revisit the theme with which I introduced this chapter: can we distinguish between willed and unwilled behavior? Surely the twitch of a muscle in response to stretch is an inexorable, unwilled behavior. But once we admit that restless legs might also result from an inexorable pathophysiological force, where do we place similar compulsions like drug-seeking, stealing, fire-setting, or murder? When do these behaviors become inexorable, in the sense that they have escaped the control of the person's will? Can we ever enter another person's mind and testify as to the quantitative balance between willed and unwilled vectors? You can sit in your armchair debating free will forever, like judges and lawyers. Or you can ask whether the anatomy of the patient's brain differs from normal, what subtle alterations might exist in the neurohumoral balances, how the life experiences of the brain shaped its synapses and circuitry, and how such factors alter the brain's perceptions and responses. These are the operational questions that impel you to get out of your chair to investigate, to make studies, and to devise experiments.

Bibliography

Aigner, B., and Mulder, D.: Myoclonus. Clinical significance and an approach to classification, *Arch. Neurol.,* 2:600-615, 1960.

Aron, A. M., and Carter, S.: Sydenham's chorea, in *Scientific Approaches to Clinical Neurology,* Goldensohn, E. S., and Appel, S. H. (eds.), Philadelphia, Lea & Febiger, 1977.

Chase, T. N., and Kopin, I. J.: Drug-induced disorders of movement in *Scientific Approaches to Clinical Neurology,* Goldensohn, E. S., and Appel, S. H. (eds.), Philadelphia, Lea & Febiger, 1977.

Cooper, I.: *Involuntary Movement Disorders,* New York, Hoeber Medical Division, Harper & Row, 1969.

Critchley, E.: Clinical manifestations of essential tremor, *J. Neurol, Neurosurg. Psychiat.,* 35:365-372, 1972.

Darrow, C.: *Attorney for the Damned,* Arthur Weinberg (ed.), New York, Simon and Schuster, 1957.

DeMyer, W.: Spasmodic torticollis, status marmoratus and status dysmyelinatus in *Scientific Approaches to Clinical Neurology,* Goldensohn, E. S., and Appel, S. H. (eds.), Philadelphia, Lea & Febiger, 1977.

Ekbom, K.: Restless legs syndrome, *Neurology,* 10:868-873, 1960.

Fahn, S., and Duffy, P.: Parkinson's disease, in *Scientific Approaches to Clinical Neurology,* Goldensohn, E. S., and Appel, S. H. (eds.), Philadelphia, Lea & Febiger, 1977.

Harrington, R., et al.: Ictal tremor, *Arch. Neurol.,* 14:184-189, 1966.

Klawans, H. L., Moses, H., III, Nausieda, P. A., Bergen, D., and Weiner, W. J.: Treatment and prognosis of hemiballismus, *N. Engl. J. Med.,* 295:1348-1350, 1976.

Lippold, O.: Physiological tremor, *Sc. Amer.,* 65-74, 1971.

Molina-Negro, P., and Hardt, J.: Semiology of tremors, *Can. J. of Neurol. Sci.,* 2:23-30, 1975.

Onuaguluchi, G.: Crises in post-encephalitic Parkinsonism, *Brain,* 84:394-414, 1961.

Putnam, T. (ed.): *The Diseases of the Basal Ganglia,* vol. XXI, *Res. Publ. Assoc. Res. Nervous Mental Disease,* Baltimore, The Williams & Wilkins Co., 1942.

Shapiro, A. K., Shapiro, E. S., Bruun, R. D., and Sweet, R. D.: *Gilles de la Tourette Syndrome,* New York, Raven Press, 1977.

Stevens, H.: Paroxysmal choreo-athetosis, *Arch. Neurol.,* 14:415-420, 1966.

Yahr, M: Involuntary Movements, from *Scientific Foundations of Neurology,* Critchley, M. (ed.), Philadelphia, F. A. Davis Co., 1972.

Zeman, W., and Dyken, P.: Dystonia musculorum deformans, in *Handbook of Clinical Neurology,* Amsterdam, Elsevier Pub. Co., vol. 6, 1968.

Zeman, W., and Whitlock, C.: Symptomatic dystonias, in *Handbook of Clinical Neurology,* Amsterdam, Elsevier Pub. Co., vol. 6, 1968.

V. Summary of the somatic motor system examination

With another student rehearse Section VI, A-H, of the Summarized Neurological Examination, until you attain proficiency.

8

Examination for Cerebellar Dysfunction

But how great was his apprehension, when he farther understood, that [the force of parturition] acting upon the very vertex of the head, not only injured the brain itself, or cerebrum, — but that it necessarily squeezed and propelled the cerebrum towards the cerebellum, which was the immediate seat of the understanding! — Angels and ministers of grace defend us! cried my father, — can any soul withstand this shock? — No wonder the intellectual web is so rent and tattered as we see it; and that so many of our best heads are no better than a puzzled skein of silk, — all perplexity, — all confusion within-side.

— *The Life and Opinions of Tristam Shandy Gentleman*
Laurence Sterne (1713 - 1768)

I. Introduction

A. *What the cerebellum does not do.* Since cerebellar destruction causes only motor deficits, Laurence Sterne correctly satirized the speculative neurophysiology of his time. The cerebellum is not "the immediate seat of the understanding" nor is any other fragment of the brain.

1. The cerebellum has no clinically evident role in consciousness, emotion, intellect, homeostasis, or autonomic functions.
2. The cerebellum has no clinically evident role in the conscious appreciation of sensation, despite massive sensory connections.
3. The cerebellum has no clinically evident role in willing movements to occur, despite massive motor connections. (See Evarts.)

B. *What the cerebellum does do.* To the clinician, the major role of the cerebellum is to coordinate willfully directed muscular contractions.

1. You would err, however, if you attributed all coordination to the cerebellum or all incoordination to cerebellar lesions. As Hughlings Jackson (1834-1911) stated, "It will not suffice . . . to speak of coordination as a separate 'faculty.' Coordination is the function of the whole and every part of the nervous system." Visual, tactile, auditory, pyramidal, and extrapyramidal circuits all contribute, but intrinsic to coordination is proprioceptive input (proprioceptors transmit positional information from muscles, joints, and vestibular system).

2. Proprioceptors inform the cerebellum about joint position and the length of and tension on muscles; that is to say, what the muscles are doing. The brain decides where to move the body parts, that is to say, what the muscles are to do. From this information, the cerebellum aids in coordinating the range, velocity, or strength of contractions to produce steady volitional movements and steady volitional postures. Thus as the crucial test for cerebellar dysfunction, examine the patient for unsteady volitional movements and for unsteady volitional postures.

3. Now, if you understand the role of the cerebellum, you can correctly answer this question: Could cerebellar function be tested in a paralyzed or comatose patient? ☐ Yes/ ☐ No. Explain: ______________________________ ____ ____.

No. He makes no willed movements or willed postures.

C. *Cerebellar phylogenesis*

1. You will understand the clinical syndromes of the cerebellum best if we start where the cerebellum started, with its phylogenesis.
2. The cerebellum evolved out of the vestibular nuclei. It is condemned by its origin to straddle forever the vestibular nerves and nuclei at the pontomedullary junction and to retain forever its connections with the vestibular system—the law of original innervation.
3. Vestibular proprioceptors provide information about the movement of the head and its position in relation to the pull of gravity. Having no limbs, primitive animals evolve only a small nubbin of cerebellum to coordinate the axial muscles which position the head, trunk, and eyes. This nubbin of cerebellum is called the *flocculonodular* lobe.
4. In all higher animals, the cerebellum retains its flocculonodular lobe-vestibular connections and their axial functions, but the budding limbs and expanding cerebrum impress new roles. The cerebellum must now coordinate axial (trunk) and appendicular (limb) muscles. The emergence of bipedal posture places particular demands on gait coordination. The newer portion of the cerebellum which evolves to receive most of the proprioceptive input from limbs and trunk is the *anterior* lobe.
5. The latest part of the cerebellum develops in equal measure with the cerebrum. Its most conspicuous input comes from the corticopontocerebellar pathways, and it is called the *posterior* lobe. (See Larsell.)
6. To recapitulate: we recognize three lobes of the cerebellum, the *anterior, posterior* and *flocculonodular,* based on phylogenesis and the major source of afferent connections. Complete Table 8-1.

TABLE 8-1. Some Major Afferent Pathways to the Lobes of the Cerebellum

Major afferent source	Lobe
Vestibular system	________ lobe (archicerebellum)
Spinocerebellar tracts (from trunk and extremities)	________ lobe (paleocerebellum)
Corticopontocerebellar tracts	________ lobe (neocerebellum)

flocculonodular
anterior
posterior

7. Since distinct clinical syndromes result from lesions of each of the lobes, and the syndromes predict the location and type of lesion, we have to look closer at the anatomy and connections of the cerebellum.

II. Anatomy of the cerebellum

A. *The three cerebellar lobes*

1. The cerebellum is subdivided *transversely* into three lobes and *longitudinally* into three parts, one midline vermis uniting two hemispheres. Learn these structures in Fig. 8-1.

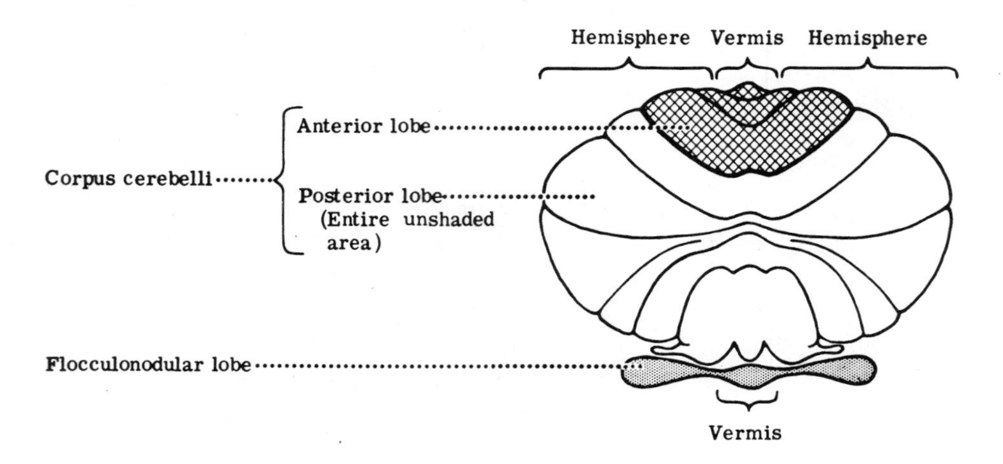

FIG. 8-1. Schematic dorsal view of the cerebellum (Larsell's nomenclature). In reality, the flocculonodular lobe is rolled under, out of sight, when the cerebellum is viewed dorsally.

Note: In the cerebellum, bump and crevice anatomy has reached the height of unreality. Angevine et al. list 24 different nomenclatures. The clinician can get along with Fig. 8-1, based on Larsell. You will have to realize that authors use the same names for different subdivisions. If the author is thoughtful, he tells you the scheme he is using; if not, you won't be the only confused reader.

2. Fig. 8-2, is a drawing of an actual cerebellum. In contrast to the schematic representation of lobes in Fig. 8-1, the flocculonodular lobe is rolled under in proper position. Label the lobes.

A. Anterior

B. Posterior

C. Flocculonodular

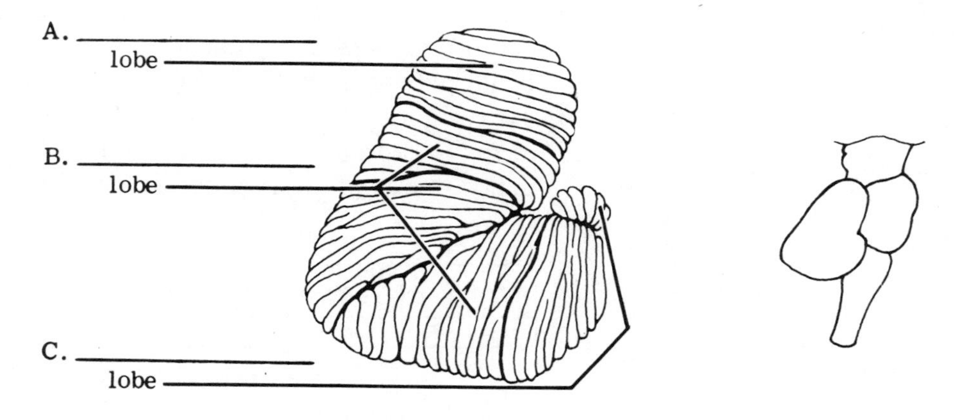

FIG. 8-2. Right lateral view of the cerebellum. The insert at the right shows the relation of the cerebellum to the brainstem. Label the lobes at A to C.

B. The three pairs of cerebellar peduncles

1. The fiber pathways in and out of the cerebellum form three pairs of peduncles. These thick stalks anchor the cerebellum to the pons. Learn Fig. 8-3, where the cut surfaces of the peduncles are exposed after the cerebellum has been sliced off.

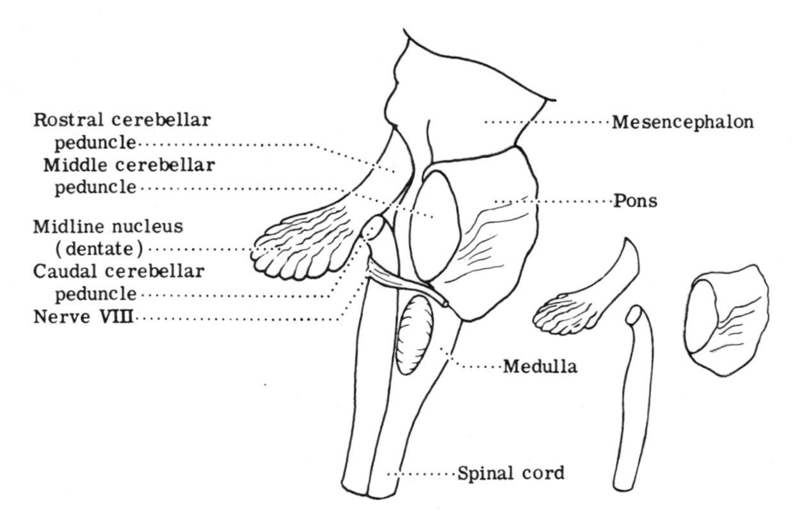

FIG. 8-3. Right lateral view of the brainstem to show the cerebellar peduncles. The insert at the right is an exploded view of the peduncles.

pons

2. The three pairs of peduncles anchor the cerebellum to only one division of the brainstem, the ☐ mesencephalon / ☐ pons / ☐ medulla.

posterior

3. Therefore, all afferent and efferent cerebellar fibers pass through the pons and through one of the peduncles. The simplest peduncle, the middle peduncle, conveys the pontocerebellar fibers and, indeed, mostly corticopontocerebellar fibers. It is made memorable by the lilting mnemonic of the L's: largest, lateralest, and latest. It is the *l*argest by far of the cerebellar peduncles, conveys the *l*argest pathway to the cerebellum (from the cerebrum, the largest part of the brain), contributes to the *l*ateral aspect of the pons (the largest division of the brainstem), is the *l*atest to develop phylogenetically, and ends in the largest lobe of the cerebellum, the ______________ lobe.
4. The inferior peduncle, as you might expect from its neighbors, the spinal cord, medulla, and VIIIth nerve, conveys spinocerebellar, medullocerebellar, and vestibular fibers.
5. The superior peduncle conveys most of the efferent fibers which leave the cerebellum. From its direction and angulation in Fig. 8-3, you can see it diving rostrally into the pons, aimed towards the mesencephalon and cerebrum.

middle

superior (rostral)

inferior (caudal)

   a. The peduncle of the corticopontocerebellar pathway is the ______________.
   b. The major efferent peduncle is the ______________.
   c. Medullary, vestibular, and many spinocerebellar afferents enter the cerebellum via the ______________ peduncle.

C. The major afferent connections of the cerebellar lobes

1. For the purist in neuroanatomy, we will recall and profess that the dorsal spinocerebellar tract enters the cerebellum via the inferior peduncle, whereas the ventral spinocerebellar curves rostralward to enter via the superior peduncle—but we can make no particular clinical use of these facts. What you should know is that both tracts end in the anterior lobe, mainly in the vermis. These tracts provide proprioceptive input to the anterior lobe from the muscles of the trunk and extremities.
2. When activating muscles for voluntary movements, the cerebrum informs the cerebellum via the corticopontocerebellar pathway, which ends mainly in the ______________ lobe.

posterior

3. Recall that the lobe which arose out of the vestibular system and retains strong vestibular connections throughout its phylogenetic history is the ______________ lobe.

flocculonodular

   a. Of the 3 nerves attached to the pontomedullary sulcus, the VIIIth is the most ☐ dorsal / ☐ ventral. The other two, in ventrodorsal order, are ______________ and ______________.

dorsal
VI, VII
(Review Fig. 3-10 if you missed.)

   b. Notice in Fig. 8-2 that the flocculonodular lobe rests on the pontomedullary junction, convenient to the entrance zone of the VIIIth nerve, its source of afferent impulses.

D. Circuitry of the cerebellum

1. All incoming afferent impulses ascend through the white matter of the cerebellum ultimately to influence large Purkinje neurons of the cerebellar cortex. Axons from the Purkinje neurons descend through the white matter of the cerebellum to synapse on the midline nuclei of the cerebellum. These nuclei sit in the roof of the 4th ventricle. Learn the flow of impulses in Fig. 8-4.

Afferent pathway
Purkinje neurons in cerebellar cortex
Midline nucleus
Efferent pathway

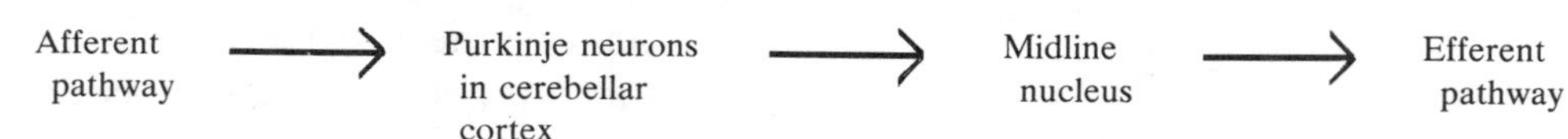

FIG. 8-4. Flow of impulses through the cerebellum.

2. *The cortico-ponto-cerebello-rubro-thalamo-cortico-spinal circuit*
   a. Well, yes, instead of using a word like that I could just say that cerebral hemisphere lesions cause ☐ contralateral / ☐ ipsilateral signs, whereas and in direct contrast, cerebellar hemisphere lesions cause ☐ contralateral / ☐ ipsilateral signs if that's all you want to know. But with the more elegant if more demanding way to do it, you learn the actual circuit which underlies the correlation between lesion side and clinical signs. To learn it won't reduce you to a basket case, and you will know a great deal more clinical neurology. Anyway, as you can verify at your next opportunity, thinking through this circuit, a cerebral act, delays impending orgasm, a reflex act, and prolongs copulation.

contralateral

ipsilateral

   b. Study Fig. 8-5 this way:
      (1) Learn the labeled structures.

(2) Start at the frontal motor cortex and trace a motor impulse down from the motor cortex to the cerebellar cortex, back to the motor cortex, and down the pyramidal tract.

(3) Using a colored pencil, draw the circuit on the other half of Fig. 8-5.

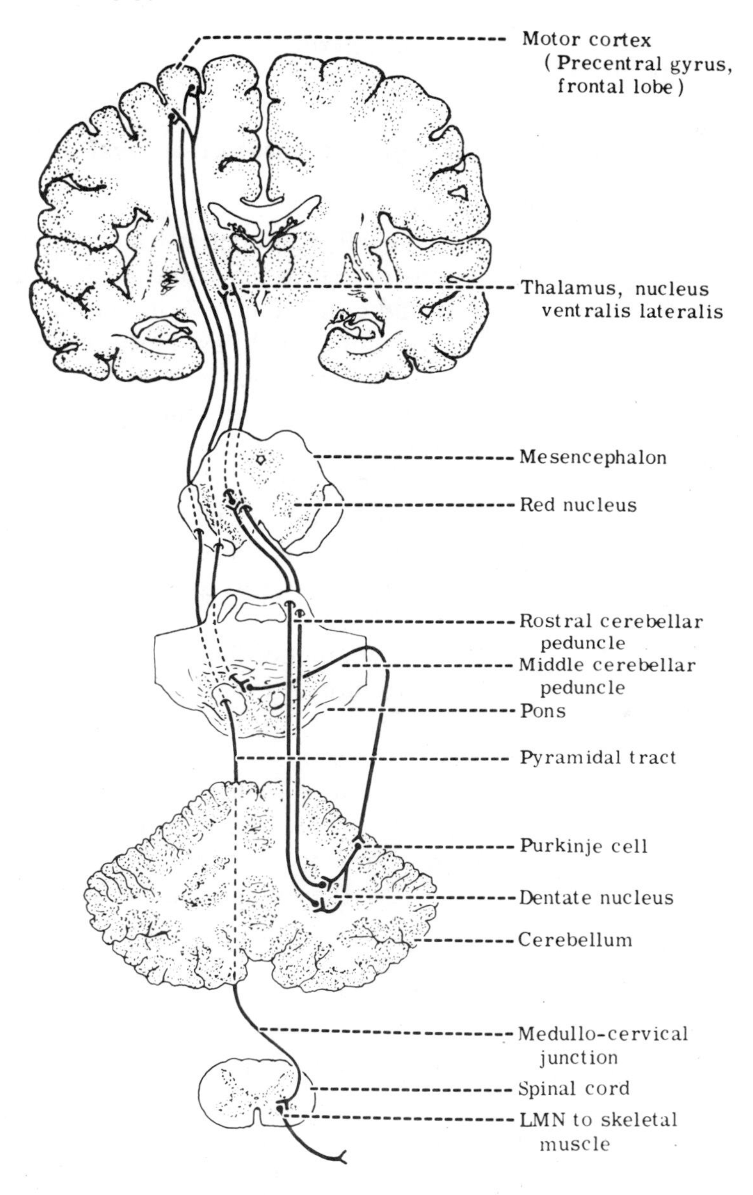

FIG. 8-5. Diagram of the cerebro-cerebello-cerebral circuit. By this pathway, the cerebellum feeds back information to the cerebral motor cortex to influence its commands to the LMNs via the pyramidal tract. Thus, the circuit functions in the equilibration of muscular contractions during volitional movement. Start at the cortex and trace through the circuit. Notice that the cerebro-cerebello-cerebral circuit double crosses the midline and that the pyramidal crossing brings the influence of one cerebellar hemisphere back to the same side.

contralateral

3. By means of the single pyramidal decussation, a cerebral hemisphere controls volitional movements on the ☐ ipsilateral / ☐ contralateral side of the body.

ipsilateral

cerebral

cerebellar

4. By means of double crossing pathways in conjunction with the pyramidal tract, a cerebellar hemisphere ultimately coordinates movements on the ☐ contralateral / ☐ ipsilateral side of the body.
5. Thus, one-sided UMN signs implicate a lesion of the contralateral ______________ hemisphere, whereas one-sided incoordination implicates a lesion of the ipsilateral ______________ hemisphere.

III. Clinical signs of cerebellar dysfunction

A. Introduction

1. Clinically, cerebellar lesions manifest as incoordination of a volitional movement or of a volitionally maintained posture. As a model to understand cerebellar deficits, consider drunkenness. Alcohol and other depressants, such as barbiturates, poison vestibulocerebellar neurons effectively, albeit not exclusively. If you have ever been or seen an inebriated person, the syndrome will crystalize for you immediately.
2. A drunken person incoordinates whenever he contracts any of his muscles. Thus, he sways when he stands, reels when he walks, slurs when he talks, and has jerky eye movements when he looks. He experiences his limbs as loose and floppy. If we apply technical terms to these features, as is the habit of physicians, the cerebellar syndrome is defined.
   a. The incoordination of volitional movements is called intention tremor or *dystaxia* (ataxia, taxis—ordering or arranging in rank and file).
   b. The slurred speech, like any neurogenic disturbance of voice articulation, is called *dys* ______________.
   c. The jerky, oscillatory eye movements are called ______________.
   d. The floppiness of the extremities is called ______________.
   e. List the 4 major clinical signs of the cerebellar syndrome: ______________, ______________, ______________, and ______________.
3. The exact relation of nystagmus to pure cerebellar lesions remains in some dispute. Cerebellar lesions often also affect the vestibular pathways and brainstem (Hood et al., 1973; Carlow and Bicknell, 1978).

dysarthria
nystagmus
hypotonia

dystaxia, dysarthria, nystagmus, hypotonia

B. Clinical tests for dystaxia of station (stance) and gait

1. Inspect the patient for swaying when standing, which is a volitional posture, and for dystaxia of gait, which is a volitional movement. The unsteady stance and reeling gait of the drunken person need no wordy description. To compensate for his unsteadiness, the cerebellar patient assumes a broad-based stance and broad-based gait, just as a toddler does before he gains coordination, or an elderly patient does after he loses some of his. To challenge the patient's coordination, we overcome his broad-base by asking him to stand with his feet together. Similarly to expose gait incoordination, use a test known to every policeman: ask the patient to step along a straight line, placing the heel of one foot

directly in front of the toe of the other, so-called *tandem* walking. Now stand up and try this test yourself. You will see that to balance on a narrow base takes no little ability.

3. To judge broad-based gaits, you must know where the heels fall in relation to the midline when a normal person walks. You will remember this point forever if you try this test, but first, just for fun, guess where the medial margins of the heels fall in relation to the midline: ☐ on/ ☐ 2.5 cm off/ ☐ 3-5 cm off/ ☐ more than 5 cm off.
   a. Now stand up, and walk at normal pace in a straight line. Hitch up your garments so that you can note the exact placement of your heels. Where do they fall in relation to the midline? ______________________________________

   see next frame

   b. Unless you are huge-thighed, your heels fell *upon* the line. Verify this the next time you are girl (boy) watching, or just as instructive, note the neat and precise tightrope placement of a dog's hind feet.
4. To the original four signs of cerebellar dysfunction, ____________, ____________, ____________, and ____________, we can add a swaying, broad-based stance and gait. Review these signs until you know them.

dystaxia
dysarthria
hypotonia
nystagmus

C. Clinical tests for arm dystaxia

1. *Finger-to-nose test*
   a. The patient starts by holding his hands straight out in front. The examiner inspects for tremor during this volitionally maintained posture. The patient then is instructed to place his index finger on the tip of his nose. The examiner inspects for intention tremor (dystaxia) of the movement in progress and how precisely the patient can touch the tip of his nose.
   b. If the patient has a tremor of his outstretched hands which disappears during movement and reappears when he holds his finger at his nose, it is called a ____________ tremor.
   c. This tremor indicates a lesion of the ____________ cerebellar peduncle (brachium conjunctivum) which runs to red nucleus, thalamus, and to the ____________ area of the cerebral cortex.
   d. If the patient maintains the posture of his outstretched arms well but has tremor during the finger-to-nose movement, it is called ____________ tremor.
   e. Dystaxia of the right hand implicates a lesion of the ☐ ipsilateral/ ☐ contralateral cerebellar hemisphere.

   postural
   superior
   motor
   intention
   ipsilateral

   f. When the dystaxic patient has to reach a specific end point, such as finger-to-nose, he frequently undershoots or overshoots the mark. He has metered the distance wrong; hence, we say this error indicates *dysmetria*. It is not a qualitatively different phenomenon from dystaxia. It is again dysequilibrium of muscular contraction, in this case of the agonist-antagonist contractions which arrest movement.
2. *The rapid-alternating movements tests for dystaxia-dysmetria*

a. The patient holds out his hands and pronates and supinates them as rapidly as possible. The hands are tested separately and together. The dystaxic hand overshoots one time, undershoots the next, and is slower than normal. See Fig. 8-6.

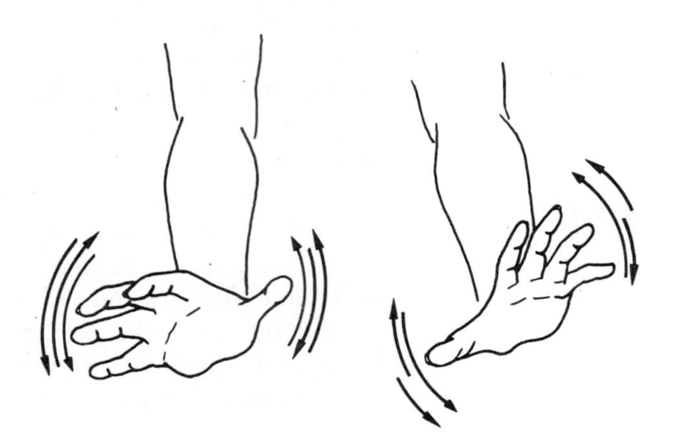

FIG. 8-6. *Pronation-supination test* for dystaxia-dysmetria of the hands.

b. An alternative method is the *thigh-slapping test.* The patient slaps his thigh, first with the palm and then with the back of his hand, as rapidly as possible. See Fig. 8-7.

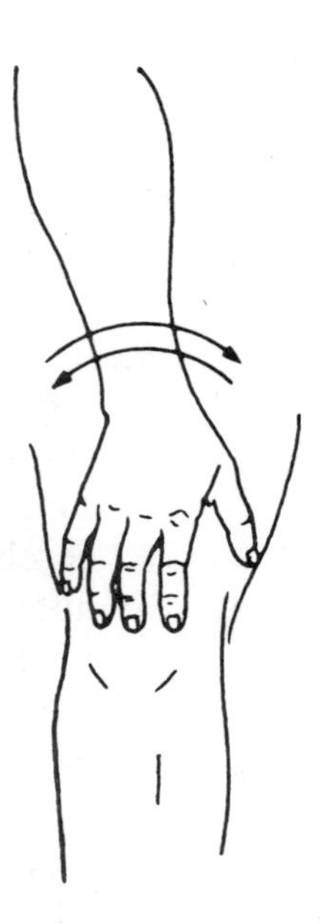

FIG. 8-7. *Thigh-slapping test* for dystaxia-dysmetria. The cerebellar patient slaps irregularly, and he frequently turns his hand too much or too little in alternately slapping the front and the back of his hand on his thigh.

You can see *and* hear the difference if one hand is dystaxic. If both are slightly dystaxic, you have to conjure up the image of the standard normal person.

c. Try the two rapid-alternating movement tests on yourself.

d. The technical term for dystaxia-dysmetria of rapid alternating movements is *dysdiadokokinesia*, a lovely dactylic trimeter. This ĭs thĕ fórĕst prĭmévăl: dýs dĭ ă dó kŏ kĭ né sĭ ă. This term describes nothing qualitatively different. It means only incoordination of muscular contractions during rapid alternating movements.

D. *Clinical tests for leg dystaxia*

1. In addition to gait testing, a highly useful, specific test for leg dystaxia is the heel-to-shin test. The patient is supine or sitting. He is instructed to place one heel precisely on the opposite knee and run the heel down his shin.
2. Try this test yourself. Again you may be surprised that such a simple task offers a considerable challenge. Does your leg waver any as you do the test?

E. *Clinical demonstration of hypotonia*

1. Muscle tone is operationally defined as ________________________________
____
____

Ans: the muscular resistance felt by the examiner when he moves the patient's resting extremity.

2. *Inspection for hypotonia*
   a. In a normal person, muscle tone helps to limit joint excursions. When the muscles are flaccid, the patient assumes postures uncomfortable to a normal subject — rag doll postures.
   b. When walking, the hypotonic patient gives a floppy, loose-jointed appearance. His arms fail to swing properly, his knees may bend backward slightly, his head and trunk bob — rag doll gait.
3. *MSRs.* The MSRs can be elicited in the cerebellar patient, but once elicited, fail to check normally. The phenomenon is best seen with the quadriceps femoris reflex. The patient sits with his legs swinging freely over the edge of a table. After the reflex is elicited, the leg normally stops swinging in one to two excursions. The legs of the cerebellar patient swing like a pendulum, without the normal checking of excursion by muscle tone. Pendular reflexes are also seen after pyramidal tract lesions, which usually cause some degree of spasticity and hyperreflexia. The apparently paradoxical fact that pendular reflexes are seen both with cerebellar lesions and hypotonia and pyramidal tract lesions and hypertonia serves to illustrate some of the complexities of the relationship between clinical signs and muscle tone.
4. Three methods for detecting hypotonia are ________________________________
____
____

inspection for rag doll postures and gait, passive movement, and pendular reflexes

F. *Overshooting and checking tests*

1. A dysequilibrium in postural stability can be brought out by testing the ability of the patient to maintain a posture or position against a sudden, unexpected displacement.

2. The patient stands with outstretched arms, eyes closed. See Fig. 8-8.
3. The patient is instructed, "I am going to bump your arms. Hold them still. Don't let me move them." The examiner strikes the back of the patient's wrist with a sharp blow, strong enough to displace the arm. The normal subject's arm returns quickly to its initial position. The cerebellar patient's arm oscillates back and forth; it *overshoots* several times.
4. A second overshooting test, the *arm-pulling* test, is shown in Fig. 8-9.

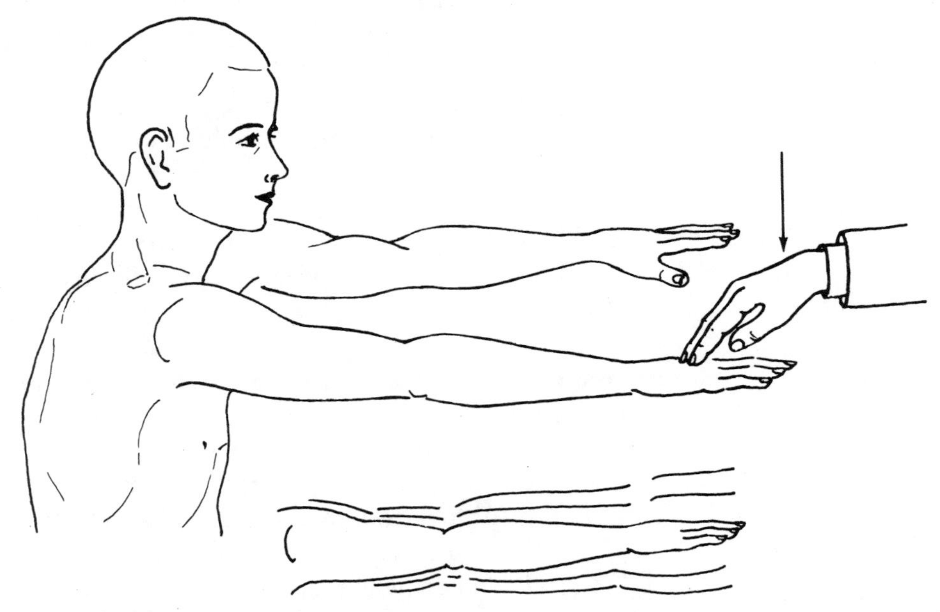

FIG. 8-8. *Wrist-slapping test* for abnormal overshooting oscillations after sudden displacement of a part that is maintaining a volitional posture. The thin arrow shows the direction of the examiner's blow, which displaces the part.

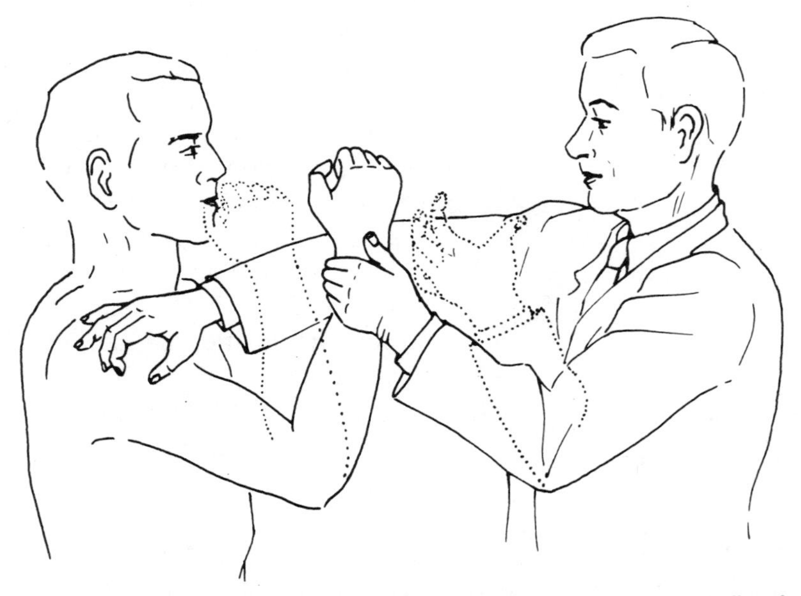

FIG. 8-9. *The arm-pulling test* for overshooting. It is a test of how well the cerebellum functions to check movement and to maintain a given posture after sudden release of tension on a muscle which is voluntarily contracting.

a. For this test the patient flexes his arm and the examiner pulls hard against it. Then the examiner suddenly releases his grip. The cerebellar patient fails to check the flight of his arm.

b. Precaution: notice how you put your own arm between the patient's arm and face. In this way you keep him from hitting himself in the face if he has a cerebellar lesion.

c. Angel points out that neurologists have erroneously called the overshooting phenomenon the rebound sign of Gordon Holmes.

G. *The effect of cerebellar lesions on eye movements*

1. Nystagmus results from lesions of the eye, cerebellum, vestibular system, or their brainstem pathways. The close anatomic relation of brainstem structures means that several of them may be affected by the same lesion. One type of nystagmus regularly occurs after acute lesions of one cerebellar hemisphere. It is described in the nystagmus dendrogram. See Figs. 5-10 and 5-11. Note this:

   a. The nystagmus from each source, ocular, cerebellar, vestibular, and brainstem, has different clinical characteristics.

   b. It is futile for the average physician to try to memorize the differential features. Consult a dendrogram when you need the information.

H. *Additional features of cerebellar deficits*

1. The possible ways to demonstrate the basic cerebellar deficits of dystaxia, hypotonia, and overshooting can be proliferated endlessly. One interesting feature is *decomposition of movement*, although it is difficult to assess clinically. The patient performs a movement as though it were decomposed into its component parts. It is like learning an activity "by the numbers." If the patient is asked to touch his nose when his arms are at his side, he will do it in two stages. He will lift the arms to the level of his nose (movement 1) and then bring the fingertip to his nose (movement 2). The normal person performs both movements simultaneously. This and other cerebellar tests are discussed by Gordon Holmes (1876-1965). Holmes was one of the founders of modern clinical neurology. I think you would enjoy his classic article, a summation written near the end of his career.
2. *Effect of cerebellar lesions on strength and endurance.* The cerebellar patient may complain of mild weakness and fatiguability. Testing of strength by dynamometry shows some decrease in the maximum force of contraction. The pathway which connects the cerebellar cortex with the cerebral motor cortex is the probable explanation. Review this circuit in Fig. 8-5. When the cerebellar cortex is electrically stimulated in the experimental animal, the cerebral motor cortex becomes more sensitive to stimulation. When the cerebello-cerebral pathway is sectioned, the motor cortex becomes less sensitive to stimulation. Apparently cerebellar impulses facilitate discharge of the cerebral motor cortex. The cerebellar patient lacks this facilitation and is unable to muster full discharge of his UMNs.

I. Summary of clinical tests for cerebellar dysfunction

1. Complete Table 8-2.
2. Find a normal subject and practice the cerebellar tests in the order listed in Table 8-2.

Free walking for broad-based gait and tandem walking.

Inspect and have patient follow your finger through fields of gaze.

Finger-to-nose; pronation-supination test, thigh-slapping test.

Wrist-slapping test and arm-pulling test.

Heel-to-knee test

Inspection for rag doll postures and rag doll gait.

Passive movement of extremities.

Pendular quadriceps reflexes.

TABLE 8-2. Tests for Cerebellar Dysfunction

Abnormality	Method of examination
Gait dystaxia	
Nystagmus	
Arm dystaxia and disturbance of alternating movement	
Overshooting	
Leg dystaxia (other than gait)	
Hypotonia	

J. As a review, before learning some specific cerebellar syndromes, draw the cerebro-ponto-cerebello-dentato-rubro-thalamo-cortico-spinal circuit in Fig. 8-10. Compare your drawing with Fig. 8-5.

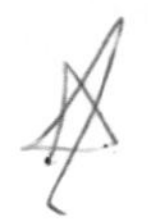

IV. Analysis of patients

A. Patient 1

1. *Medical history.* This 53-year-old man awakened one morning and upon arising, fell to his left side. He became dizzy and vomited and struggled back into bed. When he called to his wife, he noticed that his speech was slurred. He had been hypertensive many years and had had a myocardial infarct at the age of 50.
2. *Physical findings.* The patient was conscious, cooperative, and intact mentally. He was dysarthric. He had a bidirectional nystagmus, with the quick movement to the side of gaze. The nystagmus was of higher amplitude on looking to the left. No nystagmus was apparent when he looked slightly to the right of center. He had slight weakness of abduction of the left eye and complained of diplopia on looking to the left. Cranial nerve examination was otherwise normal. He was unable to walk unless supported. He had severe dystaxia on

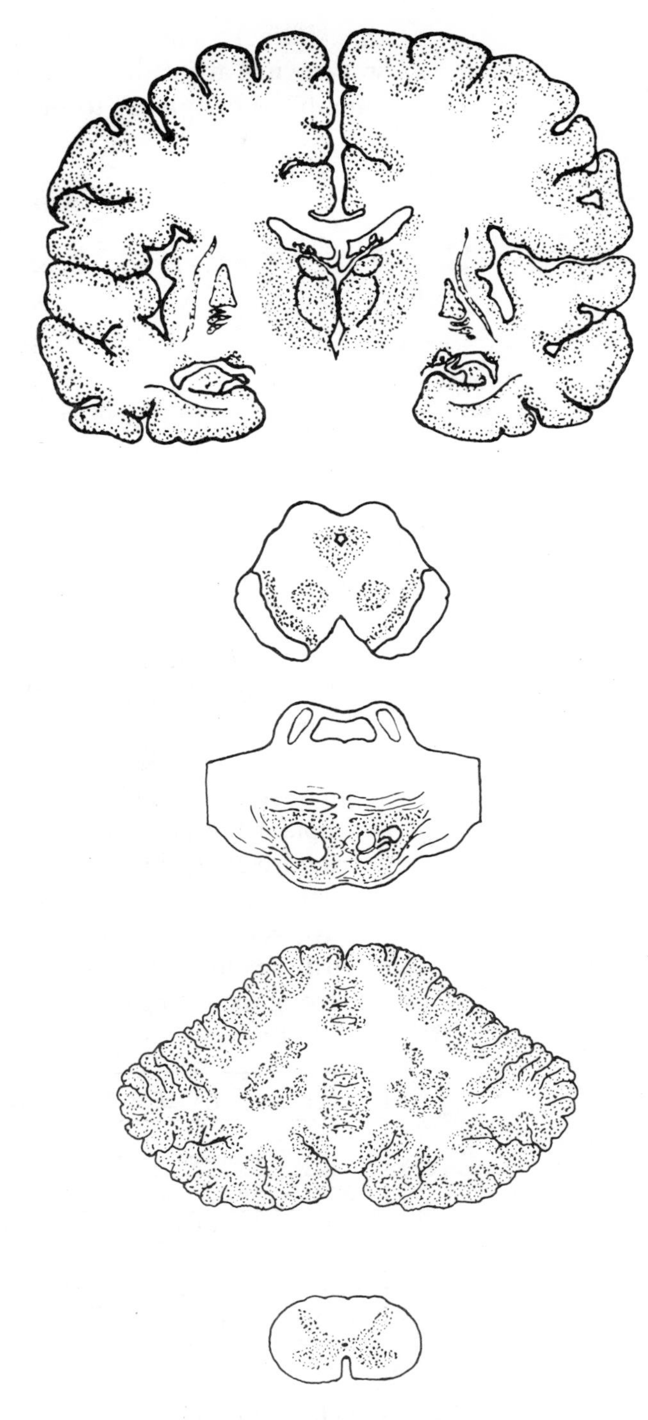

Check with Fig. 8-5.

FIG. 8-10. Blank for drawing the cerebro-cerebello-cerebro-pyramidal pathway.

finger-to-nose and heel-to-knee testing on the left side only. Alternating movements were poorly performed on the left. The left arm overshot. The left quadriceps femoris reflex was pendular. Muscle tone was reduced on the left. Strength of all movements was somewhat impaired, but the right extremities and lower facial muscles were weaker than the left. Fig. 8-11 shows the reflex examination: Body sensation was normal to testing, but the patient reported that his right side felt "numb" as compared to the left. Study Fig. 8-11.

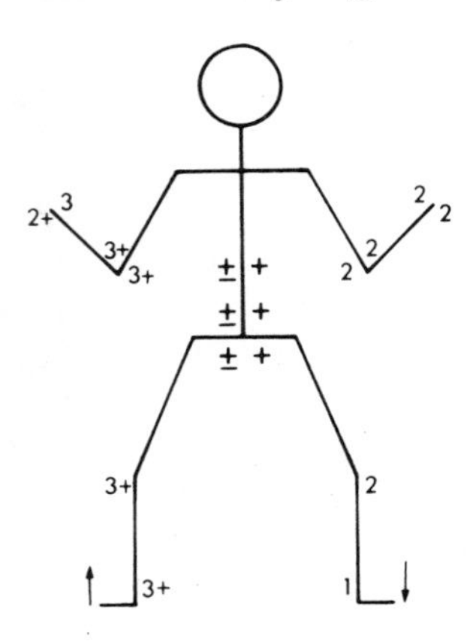

FIG. 8-11. Reflex figurine of patient 1.

3. *Lesion localization in patient 1*
   a. Before continuing with the text, you may want to try to reach your own conclusions as to where and what the lesion is. Review of brainstem cross sections, Figs. 3-14 to 3-17, page 92, may be helpful.
   b. In seeking a single lesion or at least a single pathologic process to explain the patient's findings, we first of all assemble the data that require explanation. We then sort out the specific findings to focus on them. Our patient had both pyramidal and cerebellar system signs; involvement of either or both systems might account for his dysarthria and inability to walk. Thus, these latter two features are not of strong localizing value. Complete Table 8-3.

R	L
	VI
✓	
	✓
✓	
	✓

TABLE 8-3. Localizing Findings in Patient 1

Clinical sign or symptom	Found on patient's Right	Left
Cranial nerve palsy (specify which nerve)		
UMN (pyramidal tract) signs, face spared		
Cerebellar signs		
Sensory complaint		
Nystagmus, bidirectional, with null point		

pons

basis

left

   c. The diplopia and weakness of ocular abduction implicate a VIth nerve lesion, but it might be at any site from the nucleus to the muscle. However, the pyramidal tract, sensory, and cerebellar findings require a central lesion. The association of a LMN VIth nerve palsy on the *left* and pyramidal signs in the *right* extremities suggests a lesion in the ☐ mesencephalon / ☐ pons / ☐ medulla, and it would be in the ☐ tectum / ☐ tegmentum / ☐ basis on the ☐ right / ☐ left side.

d. At the brainstem level, the pathway for somatic sensation via the medial lemniscus has already crossed the midline. Review Fig. 3-15, page 92, to see how a single pontine lesion could explain the left VIth nerve palsy, right-sided pyramidal tract signs, and right-sided sensory complaint.

left cerebellar

e. The left-sided dystaxia implicates a lesion of the □ vermis / □ right / □ left cerebellar hemisphere.

Yes. Left cerebellar hemisphere

f. Review the nystagmus dendrograms, Fig. 5-10 and 5-11, pages 142 and 143, and state whether the patient's nystagmus has any localizing value: ______________________.

Normal facial movements and no MLF syndrome.

g. What normal findings in our patient would indicate that the dorsal part of the pontine tegmentum is intact? (**Hint:** Review Fig. 3-15, page 92, to see what structures would have caused clinical signs if they had been destroyed. For example, does he show a medial longitudinal fasciculus (MLF) syndrome?) ______________________.

They had left the pyramidal bundle to migrate into the tegmentum caudal to the lesion site.

h. Since the patient's hemiparesis included his face, the lesion destroyed the corticobulbar axons to the VIIth nerve nucleus. What does this fact tell you about the course of the corticobulbar fibers to the VIIth nucleus? ______________________.

4. *Subsequent course of the patient*

After two weeks the patient began to improve steadily. His speech became nearly normal and the nystagmus virtually disappeared. His right-sided pyramidal signs became much less obvious and his diplopia disappeared. He remained with some residual left-sided cerebellar signs. Fourteen months later he returned to the hospital and died from a second myocardial infarct.

5. *Clinicopathologic correlation*

a. Autopsy examination disclosed severe cerebral arteriosclerosis, with two lesions in the brain: a large, old infarct of the ventral part of the left cerebellar hemisphere and a small, old infarct of the left basis pontis, just rostral to the VIth nerve and encroaching slightly into the pyramidal tract.

VII (Review Fig. 6-4 if you erred.)

b. The cerebellar features are classic for acute destructive lesions of a cerebellar hemisphere: infarct, abscess, or trauma. The additional lesion in the left basis pontis, accounting for the right-sided pyramidal tract signs and VIth nerve palsy, was not continuous with the cerebellar infarct. If the lesion had been continuous, from the left basis pontis dorsally into the cerebellar hemisphere, a second motor cranial nerve, nerve ____________ would have been affected along with VI.

c. Both infarcts occurred at the same time and were caused by occlusion of the left vertebral artery which supplies the medulla and cerebellum with blood and along with the right vertebral artery forms the basilar artery to supply the pons and rostral brainstem.

Hence, if we set aside the right-sided pyramidal syndrome and left VIth nerve palsy caused by the pontine lesion, this patient had typical manifestations of the *syndrome of the cerebellar hemisphere:* ipsilateral cerebellar signs, a particular type of bidirectional nystagmus, and dysarthria.

B. Patient 2

1. *History.* The patient was a 48-year-old alcoholic, with a history of severe drinking for 13 years and numerous previous hospitalizations for drunkenness, convulsions, and delirium tremens. He had difficulty walking for 3 years, so much that his family thought he had been drinking, even when he was sober. He had been drinking heavily for 10 days before admission, but had stopped 3 days before hospitalization.
2. *Physical examination.* The patient was malnourished and unkempt. He was uncertain of the time and date. Cranial nerves were normal. He had no nystagmus or dysarthria. Finger-to-nose and overshoot tests of the arms were normal bilaterally, although he was generally somewhat tremulous. He had an unsteady, broad-based gait and was unable to tandem walk. He had truncal unsteadiness when sitting or standing. The heel-to-shin movements were strikingly dystaxic. His quadriceps femoris reflexes were pendular. See Fig. 8-12.

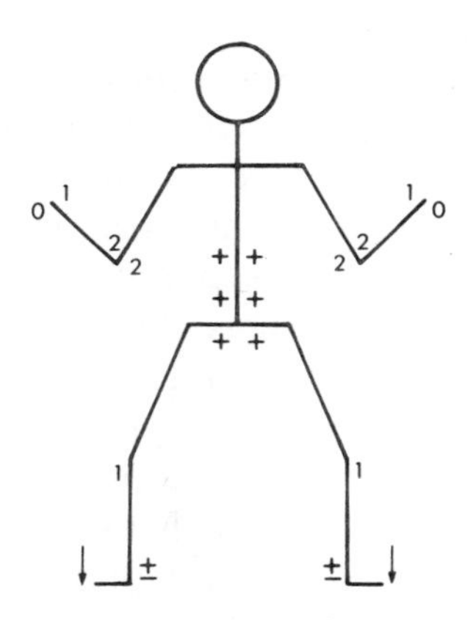

FIG. 8-12. Reflex figurine of Patient 2.

3. *Course.* Five days after hospitalization, the patient began to have severe delirium tremens with hyperpyrexia, and convulsions. The hyperpyrexia became irreversible and the patient died. At autopsy, the cerebellum was examined by making a sagittal cut through the vermis. All the folia of the rostral part of the vermis were severely atropic. Microscopically the rostral vermis and adjacent anterior lobe cortex proved to be badly damaged.
4. *Clinicopathologic correlation*
   a. Which figure of 8-13 best shows the distribution of cerebellar signs this patient had? ☐ A/ ☐ B/ ☐ C.

☑ B

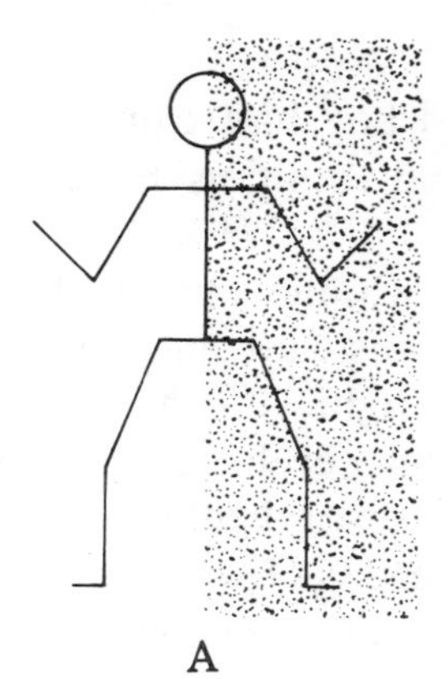
A

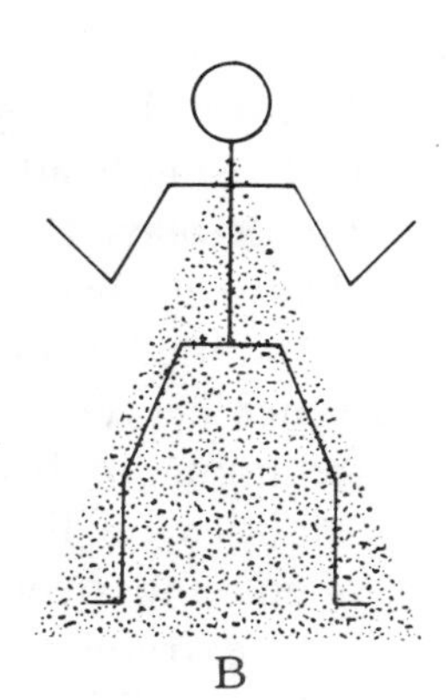
B

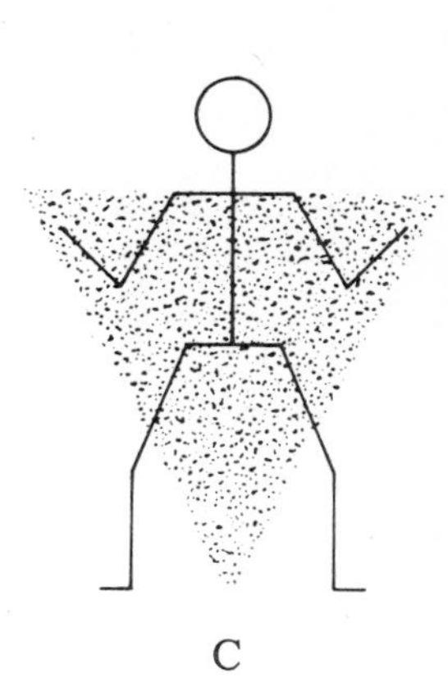
C

FIG. 8-13. Distribution of cerebellar signs. See text for description.

☒ A
anterior

spinocerebellar

cranial nerve
musculature
legs

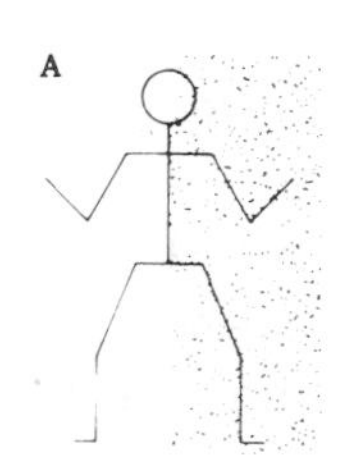

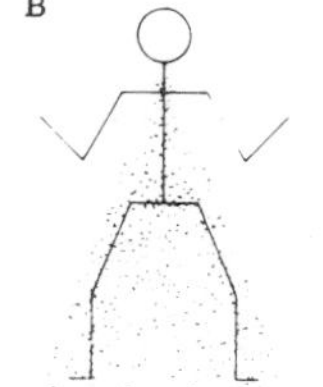

b. Which figure shows the distribution of cerebellar signs in the first patient? ☐ A / ☐ B / ☐ C.

c. The rostral vermis and adjacent cortex is part of the ________ lobe of the cerebellum.

d. The rostral part of the vermis receives proprioceptive information from the legs and trunk via the ________ tracts.

e. The clinical picture of classical cerebellar signs in the legs, mild truncal dystaxia, minimal or no arm dystaxia, and absence of dysarthria or nystagmus predicts a rostral vermis lesion, as was found in this patient. Most common in severe alcoholism and malnutrition, it presents the closest approximation to an *anterior cerebellar lobe syndrome* found in human disease. The feature which permits antemortem prediction of the lesion is the gradient of cerebellar signs. The cerebellar signs are *least* severe in the ☐ cranial nerve musculature / ☐ arms / ☐ trunk / ☐ legs and *most* severe in ☐ cranial nerve musculature / ☐ arms / ☐ trunk / ☐ legs.

5. Shade the stick figures of Fig. 8-14 to contrast the distribution of cerebellar signs:

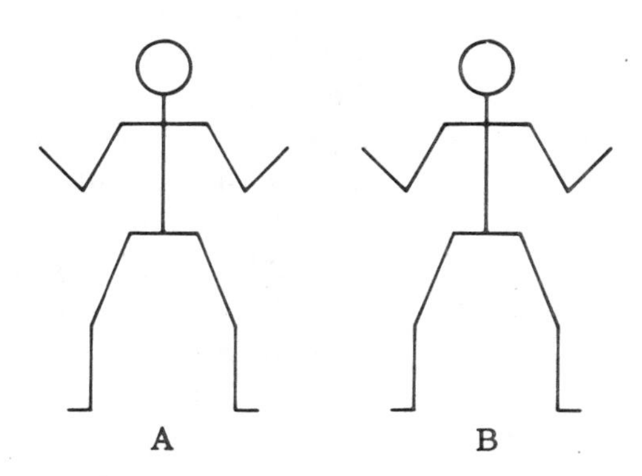

FIG. 8-14. Blanks to be filled in to show the distribution of cerebellar signs. A. Distribution of cerebellar signs in syndrome of the left cerebellar hemisphere. B. Distribution of signs in syndrome of the rostral vermis.

C. *Patient 3*

1. *History.* This 6-year-old boy had trouble walking for 3 months, with increasing headaches and vomiting. Formerly very active, he no longer ran or played.
2. *Physical examination.* Cranial nerve function was normal. When he walked, his gait was unsteady and he could not tandem walk. Sometimes he veered to the right, at others to the left. When the boy was reclining in bed, formal cerebellar tests showed no definite abnormalities on finger-to-nose or heel-to-knee testing or on rapid movement and overshoot testing. However, each time he got upright, he was extremely unsteady of trunk when sitting, and of trunk and legs when walking. He had faint nystagmus in the extreme field of gaze to each side, with a quick component in the direction of gaze. When his eyes were allowed to return slightly toward the midline, the nystagmus disappeared. The reflex pattern is shown in Fig. 8-15.

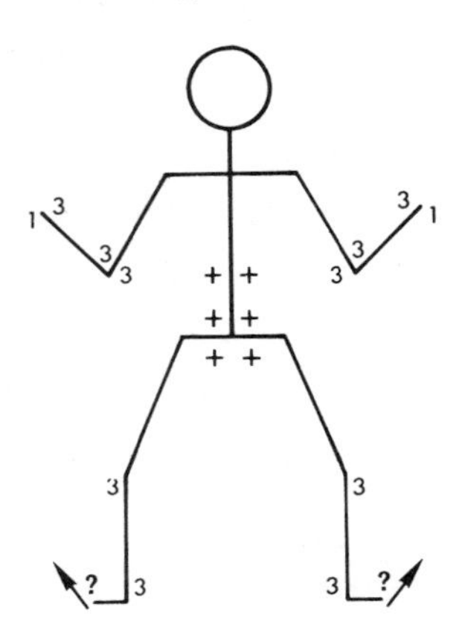

FIG. 8-15. Reflexes of Patient 3.

The sensory examination was normal. Skull radiographs showed split sutures. Subsequent diagnostic procedures led to a posterior fossa craniotomy. Arising from the caudal part of the vermis, the nodule of the flocculonodular lobe, was a medulloblastoma. It filled the fourth ventricle.

pseudonystagmus

3. *Clinicopathologic correlation.* From the nystagmus dendrograms, Figs. 5-10 and 5-11, identify the type of nystagmus: ____________
   a. The nystagmus was not clearly related to the neoplasm. It was a type called *pseudonystagmus*, which usually has no pathologic significance. The equivocal extensor toe signs and vomiting probably reflect compression of the medulla. Since the boy's sutures had split, he had no papilledema, as would be expected with an obstructed fourth ventricle.
   b. The critical clinical feature in this 6-year-old boy was a nearly pure syndrome of *postural disequilibrium* whenever he had to maintain an erect posture. On the other hand, formal cerebellar tests with the patient reclining were very nearly normal. It is tempt-

ing to suggest that the postural disturbance was caused by disruption of vestibulocerebellar and cerebellovestibular connections, that he had a *flocculonodular lobe syndrome.* But we schematize too much. "The facile gates of hell are too slightly barred." — Milton. The large size of the neoplasm and distorted posterior fossa anatomy silence further speculation.

c. Since the nodule of the flocculonodular lobe is in the caudal part of the vermis, we can contrast the *caudal vermis syndrome* of the present patient with the *rostral vermis syndrome* of patient 2, and the *cerebellar hemisphere syndrome* of patient 1. Then if we recognize a *pancerebellar syndrome* caused by any agent acting bilaterally, we see that the first stage in the diagnosis of cerebellar lesions is to classify, if possible, the patient's deficits into one of the four types of cerebellar syndromes. The four cerebellar syndromes are:

(1) Dystaxia predominantly in the legs, sparing the cranial nerve musculature, is the ______________________________ syndrome.

(2) Disequilibrium of stance and gait (axial disequilibrium) with little or no extremity dystaxia is the ______________________________ syndrome.

(3) Lateralized cerebellar signs limited to one half of the body is the cerebellar ______________________________ syndrome.

(4) Cerebellar signs bilaterally in all musculature, cranial, axial, and appendicular, is the ______________________________ syndrome.

rostral vermis (anterior lobe)

caudal vermis (flocculonodular lobe)

hemisphere (posterior lobe)

pancerebellar

D. Table 8-4 summarizes the four cerebellar syndromes. Study the clinical characteristics given in columns A and B, and from these characteristics complete columns C and D. Answers are given after the table.

1. Run down each of the subcolumns under B in Table 8-4 to see an important fallout from displaying the data in tabular form. The only column with a strong plus for each of the four cerebellar syndromes is the gait dystaxia column.
2. Gait disequilibrium is the one ubiquitous cerebellar sign, common to all four cerebellar syndromes. The upright posture and gait must be under cerebral control, for they eloquently bespeak, they reek, of goal and volition; you stand or walk for some purpose. Hence, gait testing is a most efficient clinical test for cerebellar dysfunction, as well as for many other motor deficits.
3. If the patient's signs fit into one of the four cerebellar syndromes, the probable causes immediately become delimited, and the proper diagnostic procedures can be completed. The pancerebellar syndrome is most difficult, because the causative agents span the ocean of possibility from heredofamilial diseases to the toxic effects of antiepileptic drugs.

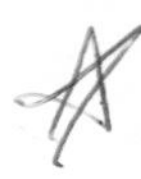

TABLE 8-4. Cerebellar Syndromes

A	B							C	D
Distribution of deficits	Dysarthria	Arm overshoot	Hypotonia	Dystaxia of: Arms	Dystaxia of: Gait and trunk	Dystaxia of: Legs	Nystagmus	Clincal syndrome of:	Lobe(s) most affected:
1. 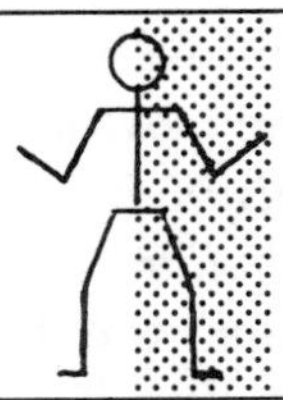	+	+	+	+	+	+	Bidirectional, coarser to side of lesion. Fast component to sides of gaze.		
2. 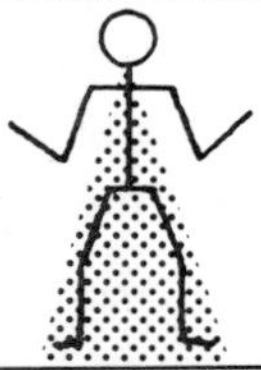	0	±	+	±	+	+	0		
3. 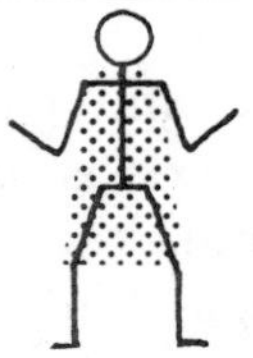	0	0	±	0	+	±	variable		
4. 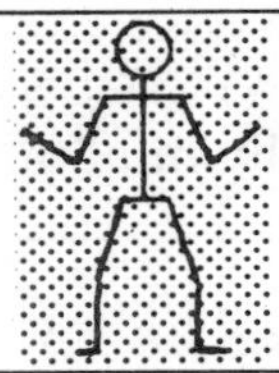	+	+	+	+	+	+	+(variable type)		

Answers to Table 8-4.

C	D
1. Cerebellar hemisphere syndrome	Mainly posterior, variably anterior lobe
2. Rostral vermis syndrome	Anterior lobe
3. Caudal vermis syndrome	Flocculonodular and posterior lobe
4. Pancerebellar syndrome	All lobes

E. *Etiologic implications of the four cerebellar syndromes.* Earlier in this chapter I gave a promissory note when I said that from knowledge of the cerebellar lobes and their syndromes you could predict or at least delimit the cause or lesion type. The rostral vermis syndrome results from alcoholism-nutritional deficiency. The caudal vermis syndrome implies a neoplasm, more often a medulloblastoma or ependymoma. The cerebellar hemisphere syndrome comes from an acute destructive lesion, most likely an infarct, neoplasm, or abscess. The pancerebellar syndrome requires a lesion which affects the entire cerebellum and, therefore, usually results from toxic-metabolic, demyelinating, or heredofamilial degenerative diseases. Thus, by correctly identifying the cerebellar syndrome, you come close to diagnosing the cause for the patient's illness, or at least you know which disorders head the list of diagnostic possibilities.

F. *Summary of the clinical examination for cerebellar dysfunction.* Rehearsal time: let's see whether you can do it. Give the commands, make the observations, and do the tests for cerebellar dysfunction. Start with gait testing and do section VI, step H, of the Summarized Neurologic Examination. Remember that you have already tested muscle tone and elicited the muscle stretch reflexes, which would have disclosed pendular reflexes and hypotonia.

(p. xviii)

Bibliography

Angel, R. W.: The rebound phenomenon of Gordon Holmes, *Arch. Neurol.,* 34:250, 1977.

Angevine, J., Jr., Mancall, E., and Yakovlev, P.: *The Human Cerebellum.* An Atlas of Gross Topography in Serial Sections, Boston, Little, Brown and Company, 1961.

Carlow, T. J., and Bicknell, J. M.: Abnormal ocular motility with brainstem and cerebellar disorders, in *International Ophthalmology Clinics: The Efferent Visual System and the Orbit,* Burde, R. M., and Karp, J. S. (eds.), 18:(1)37-56, 1978.

Evarts, E.: Brain mechanisms in movement, *Sci. Amer.,* 229:96-103, 1973.

Fields, W., and Willis, W.: *The Cerebellum in Health and Disease,* St. Louis, Warren H. Green, Inc., 1970.

Greenfield, J. G.: *The Spino-cerebellar Degenerations,* Oxford, Blackwell Scientific Publications, 1954.

Holmes, G.: The Cerebellum of Man, *Brain,* 62:1-30, 1939.

Hood, J. D., Kayan, A., and Leech, J.: Rebound nystagmus, *Brain,* 96:507-526, 1973.

Kark, R. A. P., Rosenberg, R. N., and Schut, L. J. (eds.): The Inherited Ataxias: Biochemical, Viral and Pathological Studies, in *Advances in Neurology, Vol. 21,* 1978.

Larsell, O., and Jansen, J.: *The Comparative Anatomy and Histology of the Cerebellum. The Human Cerebellum, Cerebellar Connections, and Cerebellar Cortex,* Minneapolis, University of Minnesota Press, 1972.

Victor, M., Adams, R., and Mancall, E.: A restricted form of cerebellar degeneration occurring in alcoholic patients, *Arch. Neurol.,* 1:579-688, 1959.

9

Examination of Cranial Nerve Sensation

"And there I stood, a man grown, shaking in the sunshine with that old boyish emotion brought back to me by an odour! Often and often have I known this strange rekindling of dead fires. And I have thought how, if our senses were really perfect, we might lose nothing out of our lives: neither sights, nor sounds, nor emotions . . ."

— Ray Stannard Baker

I. The senses

A. Classification

1. Like the concept of voluntary and involuntary movements, the classification of sensation is intuitive. Aristotle recognized five primary senses:
   a. Sight
   b. Sound
   c. Smell
   d. Taste
   e. Touch
2. Most modern classifications of sensation adopt the views of Charles Sherrington (1857 - 1952). Sherrington recognized *exteroceptors,* which mediate sight, sound, smell, and cutaneous sensation; *proprioceptors,* which mediate sensations of position and movement; and *interoceptors,* which mediate visceral sensations.
   a. The cutaneous *exteroceptors* mediate superficial skin sensation:
      (1) Touch
      (2) Superficial pain
      (3) Temperature
      (4) Itching and tickling
   b. The *proprioceptors* mediate deep somatic sensations from receptors beneath the skin, in muscles, joints, or internal ear. The senses of:
      (1) Position
      (2) Movement
      (3) Vibration
      (4) Pressure
      (5) Deep pain
      (6) Equilibrium (vestibular sensation)
   c. The *interoceptors* mediate sensations from receptors in the viscera:
      (1) Visceral pain
      (2) Pressure or distension
3. "Higher" sensations
   a. Form, size, and texture
   b. Weight
   c. Two-point discrimination

4. Looked at in another way, sensation can be classed as *general* or *special*. The special senses are sight, sound, taste, smell, and equilibrium. The general sensations are the rest.
5. You need not memorize sensory classifications if you remember the principle of systematization. Simply sort through your own senses starting at the nose, eyes, ear, skin, and so on over the exteroceptors of the body. Then visualize the body 3D, and you will encounter first the deep sensations of proprioception, and second, deep sensations of interoception.

B. *Sensory modalities*

1. Does anyone ever confuse the stench of carrion with a taste of honey, or a pinprick with a sound? Each different, each *unique* sensation not resolvable into elementary components is called a *sensory modality*. Ay, but there is the rub, in defining "unique," "resolve," and "elementary." We would have to accept the modality concept on faith alone, except that we can do these operations: stick yourself with a pin: there, that is one modality. Stroke yourself with a piece of cotton: there, that is another modality. We can, I think, agree that sight does not resolve into elementary modalities of sound and taste, but the sense of form — the perception of a cube in your hand — can be resolved at least in part, into touch and position sense. Thus, we can understand how elementary modalities might conglomerate into a sense of form and that the sense of form, which is a multimodal sensation, is more complex than pain, which is a unimodal sensation, a modality.
2. The neurologist could leave the problem of modalities to the philosopher if it were not for one thing. The wiring plan of the nervous system provides for modality separation. In fact, we might even suggest defining a modality as any sensation for which the nervous system has a unique pathway, but then we would be forced into negative definitions. What is sight? It is that sensation lost when both optic nerves are cut. We are back to relying on the private experience of the individual. It is customary then to define modalities by everyday intuitive experience.

C. *Basic principles of sensory physiology.* Summarized from the doctrine of specific nerve energies of Johannes Muller (1801 - 1858).

1. Sensation is an awareness of the states of the sensory neural pathways. All we know of the external world is that changes occur in the state of impulses in our receptor pathways.
2. No matter what the nature of the stimulus, stimulation of a sensory nerve causes the type of sensory experiences ordinarily mediated by the nerve. A blow on the eye causes a sensation of light; not taste, but light.
3. The same stimulus applied to different sensory organs causes sensation appropriate to the organ. Put a stimulating electrode on an auditory nerve and you *hear*. Put the same electrode on a somatic sensory nerve and you *feel*.

D. Implications of the theory of modality specificity

1. Since special senses have unique receptors, investigators have sought unique receptors for all modalities. Carried to its extreme, the theory of modality specific pathways requires unique receptors, unique peripheral axons, unique pathways through cord, brainstem, and thalamus, and unique cortical receptive areas. Recent studies have disputed the theory of modality specific skin receptors, but apart from this controversy, the theory of modality specific pathways is very nearly true, true enough for the clinician to use it to diagnose lesions.
2. When you test all sensations, you test the integrity of a large volume of nervous tissue. Add the volume of tissue assayed by testing motor pathways, and you have tested the integrity of the spinal cord, the brainstem, the cerebellum, and much of the diencephalon and cerebral hemispheres. The more pathways you sort through and find normal, the more certain you can be that the patient has no neurologic lesion. The more pathways you find affected, the closer you can predict the size, location, type, and cause of the lesion.

II. Smell (olfaction), the first cranial nerve

A. Olfactory receptor and nerve

1. Study Figures 9-1 and 9-2.
2. Mucus coats the olfactory nerve endings. Any odiferous agent must first dissolve in the mucus, which acts as the first censor for olfactory acuity. Colds or allergic rhinitis impair olfaction by mechanical reduction of air flow and by abnormal mucus secretion.
3. Olfactory impulses travel centrally past the ganglion cells. The ganglion cells are ☐ external to / ☐ within / ☐ internal to the cribriform plate.

external to

4. Axons from the olfactory ganglion cells form the olfactory nerve. The nerve perforates the ______________ plate.

cribriform

5. These perforations weaken the already wafer-thin cribriform plate, predisposing it to fracture during head trauma. The meninges may rupture initially or later when the patient coughs, causing cerebrospinal fluid to gush into the nose. During physiologic fluctuations in intracranial pressure, fluid refluxes into the subarachnoid space, introducing nasal bacteria and causing meningitis. Therefore, consider a cerebrospinal fluid fistula in the differential diagnosis of a runny nose (rhinorrhea). Neurosurgeons can close such a fistula if you can recognize it and refer the patient. How do you recognize it? Whenever a patient, usually one with a history of head injury and a runny nose, has loss of smell but does not have a cold or allergic rhinitis.
6. The olfactory axons cross the subarachnoid space to synapse on the olfactory bulbs. They shear off during head injuries, with or without cribriform plate fracture. The patient loses his sense of smell, a condition called *anosmia*. Some complications of a head injury are:
   a. The formation of a fistula between the nasal cavity and the ______________ space.

subarachnoid

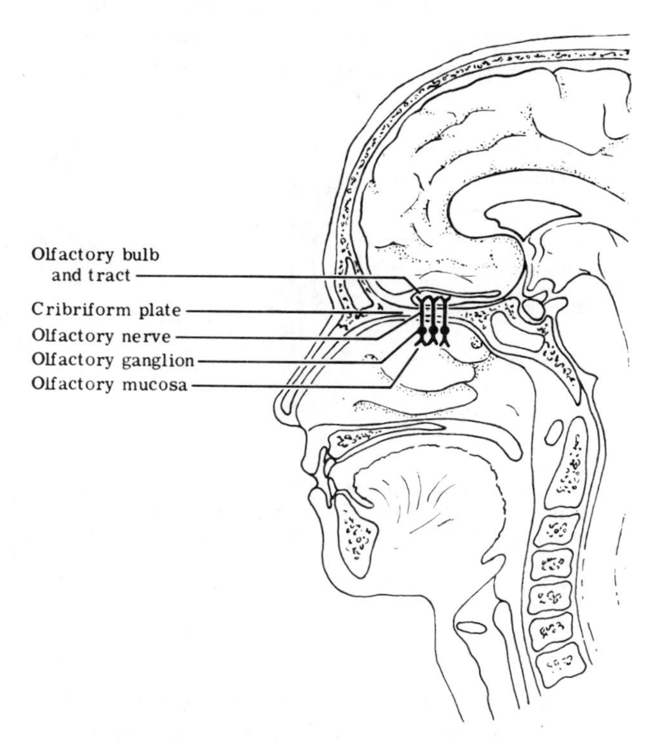

FIG. 9-1. Sagittal section of head to show olfactory nerve, bulb, and tract.

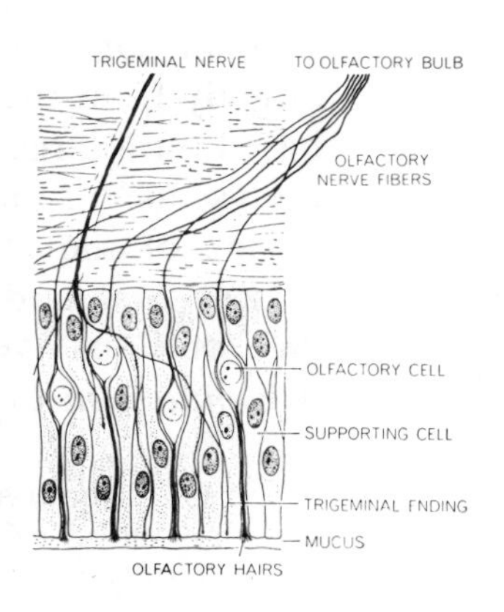

FIG. 9-2. Microscopic section of olfactory mucosa. (*From Amoore, et al., Sci. Amer.*, **210:42, 1964.**)

meningitis

anosmia

b. A potentially lethal complication of such a fistula is ________________ ____________.

c. Loss of smell, a condition called ____________________________.

B. Central pathways of olfaction and the concept of a rhinencephalon

1. After olfactory axons synapse on the olfactory bulbs, the further pathways lead to the adjacent fronto-temporal cortex and diencephalon, and through a bewildering array of circuits whose integrity we cannot test clinically. The term *rhinencephalon* encompasses the olfactory and olfactory-related central structures. Fig. 9-3 provides a concept of the

rhinencephalon and of its evolutionary significance. At one evolutionary stage, cerebrum and rhinencephalon were virtually synonymous. Thus, the rinencephalon has left its imprint forever on the human brain.

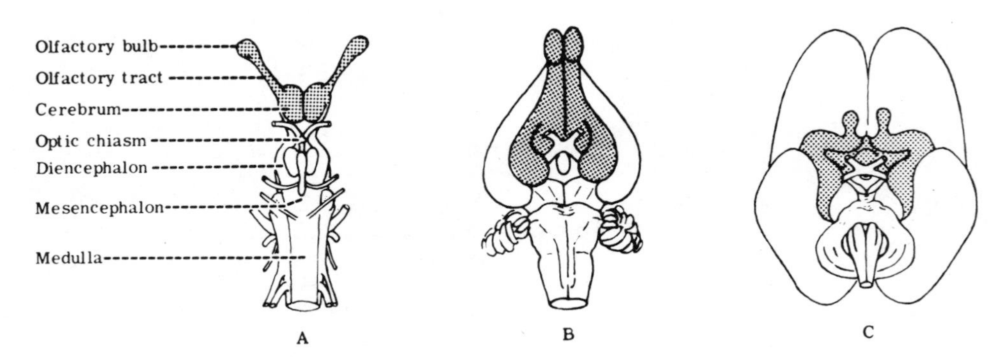

FIG. 9-3. Ventral view of shark (A), rabbit (B), and human fetal brain (C). The rhinencephalon is shaded. The cerebrum of the shark brain is mostly rhinencephalon. Notice, however, that in the rabbit and human brain, the non-rhinencephalic cortex (unshaded) which began as patches on the cerebral wall of primitive animals, has overgrown to dwarf the rhinencephalon. Nevertheless, the rhinencephalon set its imprint forever on the form and function of the brain.

2. The sense of smell originally served the two fundamental functions of *feeding* and *mating*. The human female no longer exudes the scent of the moth, but she assiduously replaces it with perfumes. The original importance of smell in these visceral drives located the visceral emotions in the parts of the diencephalon and cortex that evolved most directly from the olfactory ground plan. According to present theory, based on a large amount of research, these parts of the brain remain the "seats" of emotion and affective experience. In any event, smell is one of the most evocative of sensations. Here are the thoughts of Ray Stannard Baker again, as he set out on his farm one morning, some sixty years ago, to dig a ditch (David Grayson [pseudonym]: *Adventures in Contentment,* New York, Grosset, 1907):

> Of all hours of the day there is none like the early morning for downright good odours — the morning before eating. Fresh from sleep and unclogged with food a man's senses cut like knives. The whole world comes in upon him. A still morning is best, for the mists and moisture seem to retain the odours which they have distilled through the night. Upon a breezy morning one is likely to get a single predominant odour as of clover when the wind blows across a hay field or of apple blossoms when the wind comes through the orchard, but upon a perfectly still morning, it is wonderful how the odours arrange themselves in upright strata, so that one walking passes through them as from room to room in a marvellous temple of fragrance. . . .
>
> So it was this morning. As I walked along the margin of my field I was conscious, at first, coming within the shadows of the wood, of the cool, heavy aroma which one associates with the night: as of moist woods and earth mould. The penetrating scent of the night remains long after the sights and sounds of it have disappeared. In sunny spots I had the fragrance of the open cornfield, the aromatic breath of the brown earth, giving curiously the sense of fecundity — a warm, generous odour of daylight and sunshine. Down the field, toward the cor-

ner, cutting in sharply as though a door opened (or a page turned to another lyric), came the cloying, sweet fragrance of wild crab-apple blossoms, almost tropical in their richness, and below that, as I came to my work, the thin acrid smell of the marsh, the place of the rushes and the flags and the frogs. . . .

So I walked this morning, not hearing nor seeing, but smelling. Without desiring to stir up strife among the peaceful senses, there is this further marvel of the sense of smell. No other possesses such an after-call. Sight preserves pictures: the complete view of the aspect of objects, but it is photographic and external. Hearing deals in echoes, but the sense of smell, while saving no vision of a place or a person, will re-create in a way almost miraculous the inner *emotion* of a particular time or place. I know of nothing that will so "create an appetite under the ribs of death."

Only a short time ago I passed an open doorway in the town. I was busy with errands, my mind fully engaged, but suddenly I caught an odour from somewhere within the building I was passing. I stopped! It was as if in that moment I lost twenty years of my life. I was a boy again, living and feeling a particular instant at the time of my father's death. Every emotion of that occasion, not recalled in years, returned to me sharply and clearly as though I experienced it for the first time. . . .

And there I stood, a man grown, shaking in the sunshine with that old boyish emotion brought back to me by an odour! And I have thought how, if our senses were really perfect, we might lose nothing out of our lives: neither sights, nor sounds, nor emotions. . . .

— Ray Stannard Baker

3. *Déjà vu and déjà pensée*

One of the cortical receptive areas for smell is located in the uncus, a medial margin of the temporal lobe. Lesions of the uncus may cause the patient to have hallucinations of odor, usually very disagreeable odors. I recall one patient who tore down the walls of his room. Although otherwise rational he was convinced that he smelled a dead animal entrapped within them. Each time the odor came powerfully to him, he also had a peculiar feeling of familiarity, as if it had all happened before (just as Baker described). At autopsy the patient had a metastatic bronchogenic carcinoma in his uncus. The feeling of familiarity, as if a sensation was a recapitulation of a previous experience, is called *déjà vu* (previously or already seen) or *déjà pensée* (previously or already thought). Although we all have this experience from time to time, when the patient recounts it prominently, the clinician should suspect the patient's temporal lobe. If déjà pensée occurs with an olfactory hallucination, the probability of an anterior temporal lobe lesion is raised almost to a certainty.

C. *Clinical testing of olfaction*

1. *Stimulus*

a. From Fig. 9-2 we observe that two cranial nerves supply sensory fibers to the olfactory epithelium, cranial nerves number ______ and ______. Only cranial nerve ______ serves olfaction.

I V

I

b. In testing any sensation, the modality to be tested must be isolated from other modalities. Otherwise you do not know which sensory pathway you are testing. Which would be best to test the sense of smell, an irritating substance like ammonia or an aromatic substance like coffee? ☐ ammonia / ☐ coffee.

coffee

c. Ammonia irritates all receptors of a mucus membrane. Even the conjunctiva "smells" ammonia. To test smell, use a vial of coffee grounds. The vial should be opaque. Why? ________________

Ans: the principle of isolation of the function to be tested. You do not want the patient to see what you will use for a stimulus. You do not want to test how well he sees, but how well he can smell.

2. *Communication to the patient of what he is to do*
   a. Successful sensory testing depends on communication between you and your patient. Say to the patient, "Close your eyes and try to identify this odor."
   b. Compress *one* of the patient's nostrils and hold the vial in front of the *other.* Allow the patient a moment to respond.
   c. For the second trial, compress the opposite nostril and this time do *not* present the stimulus. By withholding the stimulus, you test the patient's suggestibility and attention to the test. In every sensory test you must build in safeguards of this type.
   d. The third time, present the stimulus to the untested nostril.
   e. If the patient cannot smell, he is said to have ________________

anosmia

D. Clinical interpretation of anosmia

1. To systematize analysis of anosmia, we will start at the receptor. What is the first barrier that any aromatic agent in the nasal cavity must dissolve in before it stimulates olfactory nerve receptors? ________________

mucus coating of the olfactory nerve endings

2. The most common causes of anosmia are the common cold and allergic rhinitis.
3. It is a saturnine fact that the sensitivity of all sensation decrements with aging. Sight, hearing, vibration sense; they all diminish. Hence, *aging*, the decay of the metabolic machinery of the neurons, is another common cause of anosmia in the elderly.
4. With head injuries, the delicate olfactory axons are easily sheared off as they cross the subarachnoid space. Lesions of the olfactory bulbs and tracts are next in order, and, while rare, the most significant lesions are meningeal neoplasms which obstruct the olfactory pathways by compression.
   a. Moving centrally from olfactory bulbs and tracts to olfactory cortex, we find that lesions here rarely if ever cause anosmia, but if they irritate the cortex which elaborates olfactory impulses into conscious appreciation, mainly the ________________ of the temporal lobe, the patient may experience hallucinations of disagreeable ________________.
   b. These olfactory hallucinations are likely to be accompanied by a peculiar mental experience, characterized by ________________

uncus

odors

familiarity, as if the event had all happened before (déjà vu or déjà pensée)

5. Anosmia must be integrated with the remainder of the history and physical examination in order to assess its significance as a signal of disease. The rubric for the differential diagnosis of anosmia leads through the dendrogram in Fig. 9-4:

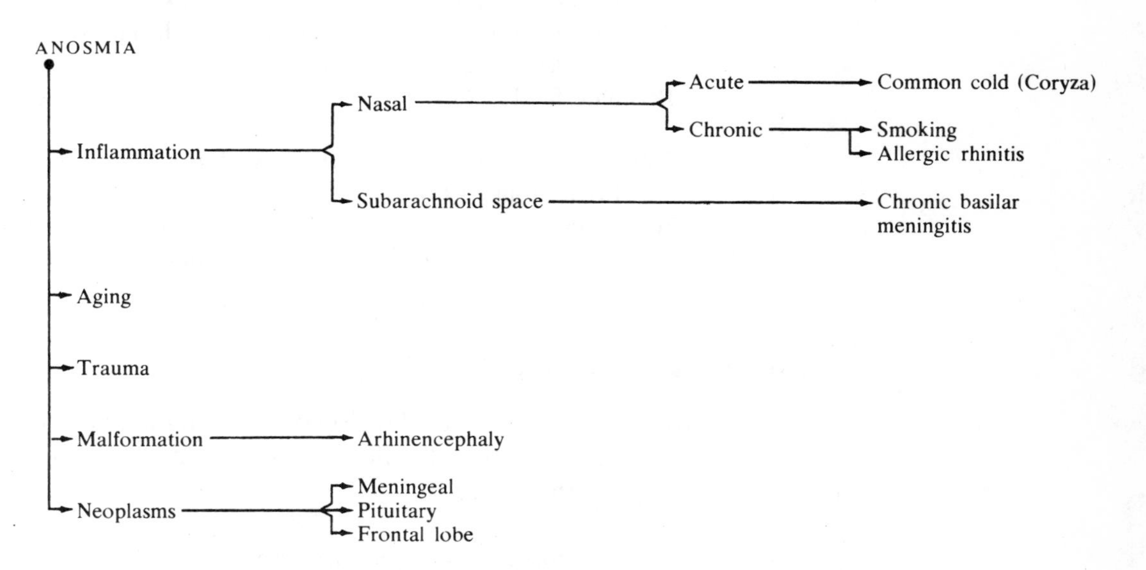

FIG. 9-4. Differential diagnosis of common causes of anosmia. (Reference only.)

6. The dendrogram for nasal drip is simple but important. Stain a nasal smear and place a drop of fluid on a glucose test tape (as used for urinalysis). CSF has free glucose, whereas mucus does not. See Fig. 9-5:

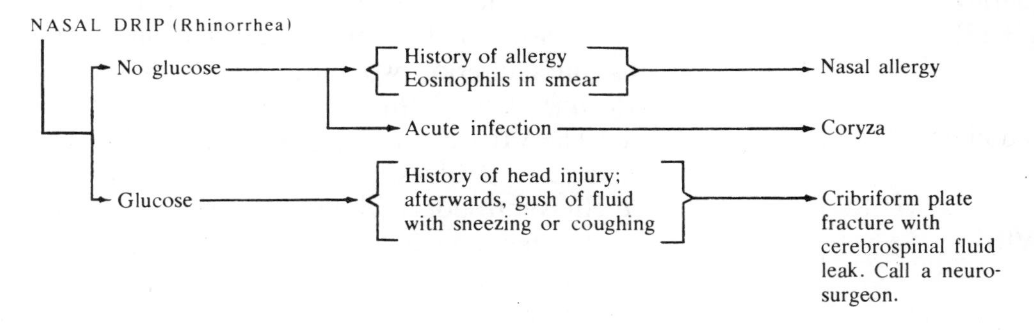

FIG. 9-5. Microdendrogram for nasal drip. (Reference only.)

7. Why does sneezing or coughing cause a discharge of cerebrospinal fluid from a cribriform plate fistula? ______________________

____

____

Ans: Increased intrathoracic pressure caused by coughing or sneezing is transmitted intracranially by the venous system, forcing fluid out of the cribriform plate fistula.

Bibliography

Allen, M., Jr., Gammal, T., Ihnen, M., and Cowan, M.: Fistula detection in cerebrospinal fluid leakage, *J. Neurol. Neurosurg, Psychiat.,* 35:664-668, 1972.

Amoore, J., Johnston, J., Jr., and Rubin, M.: The stereochemical theory of odor, *Sci. Amer.,* 210:42-49, 1964.

Brisman, R., Hughes, J. E. O., and Mount, L. A.: Cerebrospinal fluid rhinorrhea, *Arch, Neurol.,* 22:245-252, 1970.

Douek, E.: *The Sense of Smell and Its Abnormalities,* Edinburgh, Churchill Livingstone, 1974.

Schechter, P. J., and Henkin, R. I.: Abnormalities of taste and smell after head trauma, *J. Neurol. Neurosurg. Psychiatry,* 37:802-810, 1974.

III. Taste (or gustation)

A. *Receptors:* taste buds develop on the tongue and around the tonsillar pillars. Like olfaction, the chemical agents that stimulate taste must first dissolve in a liquid, the saliva.

B. *Neuroanatomy of peripheral connections*

1. The taste buds of the anterior two-thirds of the tongue are supplied by the. . . . What cranial nerve was it? Well, if you have forgotten, start at number I and sort through them:
   ________ smells, ________ sees.
   ________, ________, and ________ rotate the eye.
   ________ chews and feels front of head.
   ________ moves facial muscles, tears, salivates and ________.

   I, II
   III, IV, VI
   V
   VII, tastes (Should you review Table 3-2?)

2. Nerves IX and X innervate taste buds of the posterior third of the tongue and tonsillar pillars, areas inconvenient to test. Thus we only test the tongue's anterior two-thirds, VII's area. Learn Fig. 9-6.
3. *Review of the VIIth cranial nerve*
   a. The VIIth nerve attaches to the brainstem at the ________ sulcus.
   b. In ventrodorsal order, the nerves attaching to the brainstem at the pontomedullary sulcus are ________.
   c. VII passes into the internal auditory meatus in company with nerve ________.
   d. Since VII has only one ganglion, it holds the *primary* neuron for taste. This ganglion is the ________ ganglion.
   e. Ganglia always contain the ☐ primary/ ☐ secondary/ ☐ tertiary neuron of a sensory pathway.
   f. The geniculate ganglion receives its name from the knee-like downward bend of the VIIth nerve after it clears the ganglion and heads for the stylomastoid foramen.

   pontomedullary
   VI, VII, VIII
   VIII
   geniculate
   primary

C. *Central pathways for taste*

1. The neuroanatomy of the central connections for taste is not well enough known to be of use in clinical diagnosis.

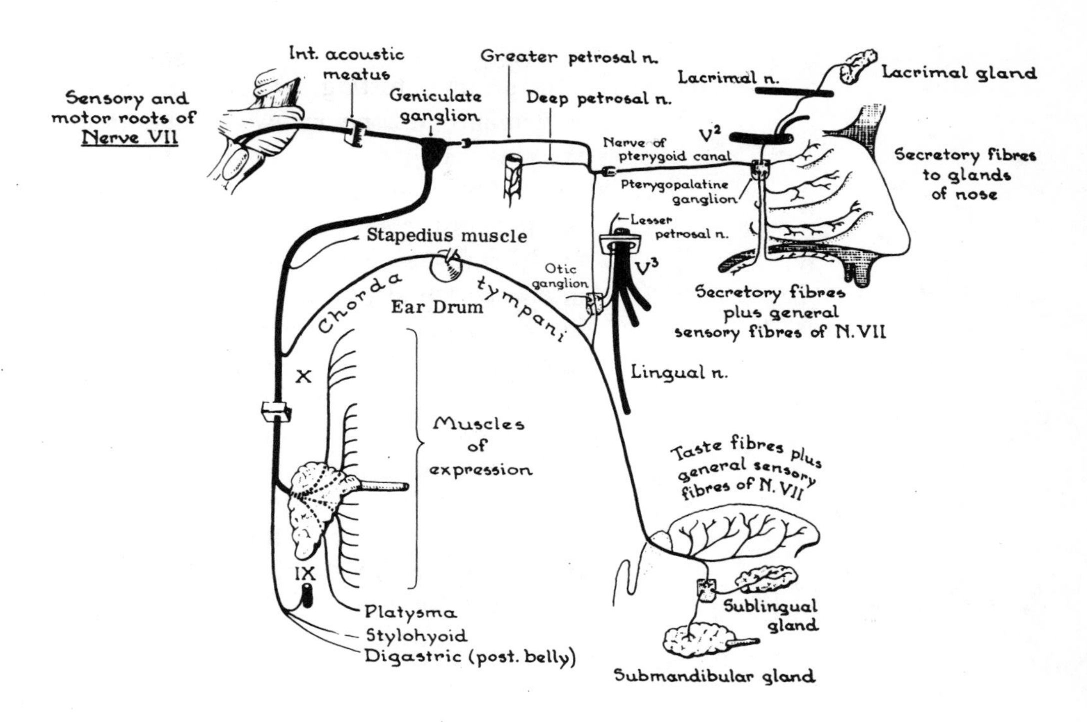

FIG. 9-6. Peripheral course of the VIIth cranial nerve. (*Modified from J. C. B. Grant: An Atlas of Anatomy, 5th ed., Baltimore, Williams and Wilkins Company, 1962.*)

2. Gustatory sensation is probably represented in the cerebral cortex, in the insular region (Island of Reil) of the frontal lobe. Occasionally, an irritative lesion in this part of the frontal lobe causes gustatory hallucinations.
3. If the patient has olfactory hallucinations, where is the lesion likely to be? ______________________.

uncus of temporal lobe

D. Clinical testing of taste

1. The stimulus is any salty, sweet, sour, or bitter substance. Salt, sugar, or quinine are suitable.
2. If you use salt or sugar keep them concealed from view. The patient who sees a white crystalline substance will almost automatically guess either salt or sugar.
3. *Communication with the patient*
   a. Tell the patient, "I want to place something on your tongue for you to taste. Stick out your tongue and keep it out. When you know what the taste is, hold up your hand."
   b. Place a few crystals of your test material on one half of the tongue and massage them around with a tongue blade. Test each half of the tongue separately.
   c. Allow a moment for the substance to dissolve.
   d. Have him rinse his mouth and then test the opposite side.
   e. For routine clinical purposes you need try only one substance.
   f. Test your own sense of taste.

E. Interpretation

1. This patient shows how the testing of taste aids in clinical diagnosis: A 26-year-old woman awoke one morning with her face "drawn to the side." Examination disclosed that on the right side she could not wrinkle her forehead, close her eye, pull back the corner of her mouth, or wrinkle the skin of her neck. The left side of her face moved normally, and her complaint of "drawing" of her face was due to the unopposed pull of the normal left-sided facial muscles, which pulled her lips to the left when she spoke. The remainder of the examination was completely normal, including taste sensation.
2. Let us work through the data to see how they lead us to conclude *where* and *what* the lesion is.
   a. In analyzing a motor deficit, the most important consideration is its distribution. Does it follow a *central* (pyramidal tract or UMN) distribution? Does it follow a *root* or peripheral *nerve* distribution?
   b. Which type of distribution does the motor deficit of the present patient follow? ☐ UMN / ☐ peripheral nerve.
   c. The paralysis involves the muscles of a single nerve, cranial nerve ______________.
   d. The distribution of the paralysis in the field of a single nerve excludes a neuromyal junction disorder or myopathy, which are widespread metabolic disorders, not limited to a single nerve.
   e. Since the paralysis can be explained by a single nerve lesion, we know it is a ☐ mononeuropathy / ☐ polyneuropathy / ☐ myopathy.
3. It is insufficient to say that the patient has an LMN facial palsy. We still have to specify where the lesion is along the course of the nerve. In analyzing a sensory disturbance or a reflex arc, we have established the principle of starting at the ______________________ because in this way we trace along the entire pathway of the nerve impulses.
4. In the present case, sensation of the VIIth nerve was normal. We have to analyze a motor mononeuropathy. Where should you start in order to utilize the principle of thinking along the course of impulse flow of a motor nerve? ______________________________
   ____
5. The VIIth nerve nucleus is located in the ☐ tectum / ☐ tegmentum / ☐ basis of the ______________________.
6. Since central lesions are rarely so discrete as to affect only one cranial nerve nucleus, we would expect neighborhood signs if the lesion were in the brainstem. Neighborhood signs, implicating the brainstem as the site of the lesion, would result from:
   a. Interruption of sensory, cerebellar, or corticospinal pathways.
   b. Involvement of adjacent nuclei or nerves. In addition to VII, the cranial nerve motor nuclei in the pons are ____________.
7. Since the patient had no neighborhood signs, the lesion is most likely ☐ inside / ☐ outside the brainstem.
8. Upon its exit from the brainstem, the VIIth nerve must cross the ______________ space, before entering the internal auditory meatus.
9. The region between the cerebellum and the brainstem is called the

Answers (margin): peripheral nerve; VII; mononeuropathy; receptor; at the nucleus or cell body of the LMN; tegmentum; pons; V, VI; outside; subarachnoid

VIII	*cerebellopontine angle.* A lesion here, such as a neoplasm, would involve not only cranial nerve VII, but also cranial nerve ________.
V and VI (and possibly IX, X, and XII)	10. As the neoplasm enlarged, it would involve more cranial nerves, both rostrally and caudally. Hence, it would affect in addition to cranial nerves VII and VIII, cranial nerves ________.
VIII	11. If the lesion is in the internal auditory meatus, what other cranial nerve should be affected besides VII? ________.
taste, ipsilateral anterior two-thirds	12. With any lesion of the VIIth nerve trunk from the point of exit from the brainstem to the geniculate ganglion, we would expect loss of ________ sensation on the ________ ________ of the tongue. The patient did *not* have this feature.
stapedius	13. In the middle ear, VII innervates one muscle, the ________ muscle. Contraction of this muscle dampens the vibration of the ossicles, protecting the inner ear from damage by loud sounds. With the stapedius muscle paralyzed, the patient experiences sounds as uncomfortably loud, a symptom called *hyperacusis.*
distal to (Should you review Fig. 9-6?)	14. Since these two abnormalities, loss of taste and hyperacusis were not found, the patient's lesion must be ☐ distal to / ☐ proximal to / ☐ within the middle ear.
	15. If distal to the middle ear, the lesion might be in the facial canal, but the deep location of the canal in the temporal bone bars clinical examination. If a lesion interrupted the VIIth nerve after its exit from the stylomastoid foramen, we would expect to find pain or swelling in the parotid region, as from an inflammatory or neoplastic mass, but no such abnormalities occurred.
neuromyal	16. The next link in a motor nerve comes at the terminal tips of its axons, where the axons contact their effector muscles, a region called the ________ junction.
	17. Explain why the patient's lesion is not at the neuromyal junction or muscle. ________________________________.

Ans: Neuromyal junction lesions or myopathies are diffuse metabolic disorders. The patient's paralysis is confined to a single nerve distribution.

18. Make a line across Fig. 9-6 at the most likely site of the patient's lesion. ________________________________.

Ans: Your line should cross the facial canal distal to the chorda tympani and proximal to the stylomastoid foramen.

19. The patient had "idiopathic facial paralysis" (Bell's palsy), a common mononeuropathy of the VIIth nerve. The lesion is a swelling of the nerve, in this patient, within the facial canal. It compresses and sometimes completely transects the axons and may occur at various sites along the facial nerve. The patient recovered good facial function by six weeks after onset.

20. This case shows that the major clinical value of testing taste is to localize lesions along the course of the VIIth nerve. Unless the patient has signs and symptoms implicating taste or smell of the VIIth nerve,

you do not have to test taste. This is one test you can frequently omit, but let it be an omission by discretion, not carelessness.

Bibliography

Adour, K. K., and Wingerd, J.: Idiopathic facial paralysis (Bell's palsy): Factors affecting severity and outcome in 446 patients, *Neurology,* 24:1112-1116, 1974.

Blatt, I.: Bell's palsy: Diagnosis and prognosis of idiopathic paralysis by submaxillary salivary gland flow and chorda tympani nerve testing, *Laryngoscope,* 75:1081-1091, 1965.

Börnstein, W.: Cortical representation of taste in man and monkey: I. Functional and anatomical relations of taste, olfaction, and somatic sensibility, *Yale J. Biol. & Med.,* 12:719-736, 1940. II. The localization of the cortical taste area in man and a method of measuring impairment of taste in man, *Ibid.,* 13:133-156, 1940.

Esslen, E.: *The Acute Facial Palsies,* New York, Springer-Verlag, 1977.

Sumner, D.: Post-traumatic ageusia, *Brain,* 90:187-202, 1967.

IV. Hearing

The specialist told him: "Fine let's leave it at that.
The treatment is done: you're deaf. That's how
It is you have quite lost your hearing."
And he understood only too well, not having heard.

— Tristan Corbiere

A. Anatomy of the cochlear division of VIII

1. *Receptor.* The organ of Corti is located in the cochlea. It is innervated by the cochlear (spiral) ganglion which also is in the cochlea. It contains the ☐ primary / ☐ secondary neuron for hearing.

   primary

2. Study Fig. 9-7 until you can trace an auditory impulse from cochlea to temporal lobe cortex. Begin by labeling the subdivisions of the brainstem on the left.
3. *Peripheral course.* The cochlear division of VIII, after combining with the vestibular division, runs through the internal auditory canal in company with cranial nerve ______. These two cranial nerves attach to the brainstem at the ______ sulcus.

   VII
   pontomedullary

4. *Central connections.* The cochlear axons synapse at the ______ nuclei.

   cochlear

   a. These nuclei drape around the ______ cerebellar peduncle.

   caudal (inferior)

   b. The cochlear nuclei contain the ☐ primary / ☐ secondary / ☐ tertiary neuron of the auditory pathway.

   secondary

   c. From the cochlear nuclei, the auditory pathway becomes about equally dispersed ipsilaterally and bilaterally. Therefore, you

A. Mesencephalon
B. Pons
C. Pontomedullary junction

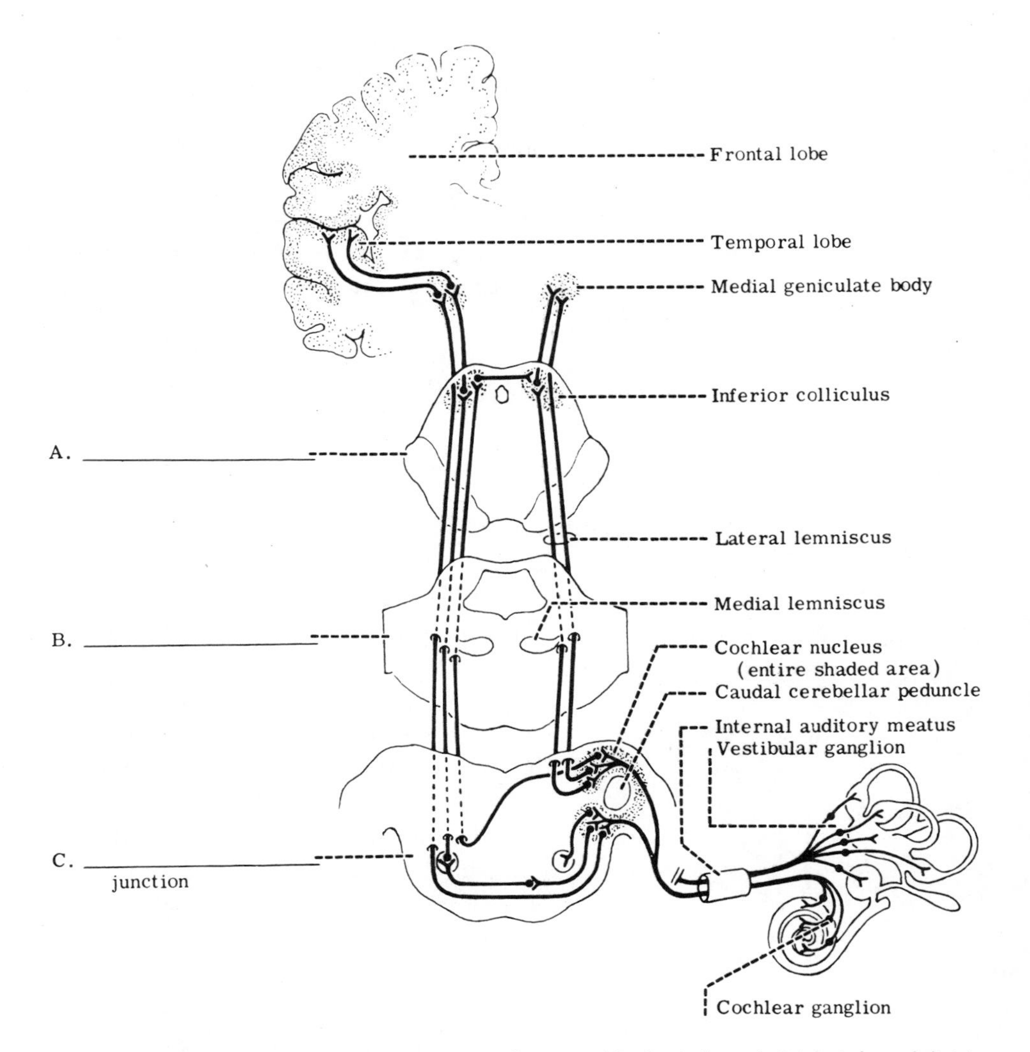

FIG. 9-7. Diagram of the cochlear (auditory) pathway. At blanks A through C label the subdivisions of the brainstem.

Answers	
would not	☐ would/ ☐ would not expect to find a profound unilateral hearing loss from a unilateral lesion of a central pathway.
ipsilateral	*d.* Complete transection of VIII would cause complete ☐ ipsilateral/ ☐ contralateral deafness.
medial	*e.* Axons from the cochlear nuclei ultimately reach the ______________ geniculate body, a thalamic nucleus. Some go directly, some synapse along the way.
lateral lemniscus medial	*f.* The name of the auditory pathway through the brainstem is the ______________ ______________, through which axons run to the ______________ geniculate body.
temporal	*g.* Neurons of the medial geniculate body relay to the superior surface of the ______________ lobe.
tertiary	*h.* The medial geniculate body contains ☐ primary/ ☐ secondary/ ☐ tertiary neurons of the auditory pathway.

No

i. Would you expect a temporal lobe lesion to cause complete deafness in either ear? ☐ Yes / ☐ No. Explain.

____

____

____

Ans: The central pathways have such extensive bilateral connections that unilateral deafness never occurs from a unilateral central lesion. Therefore, complete deafness in one ear must be due to a lesion in the peripheral apparatus of hearing.

j. Whenever you test hearing in a patient, "think through" the auditory pathway, naming the structures en route.

B. Clinical testing of hearing

1. *Introduction*

a. In the formal testing of hearing, a new concept of sensory function must be considered. In testing olfaction and taste, we did not concern ourselves particularly with the strength of the stimulus. We were mainly interested in a *yes* or *no* answer since smell and taste are difficult to quantify. When testing other sensations, we must consider the range of sensation, particularly *threshold.*

b. In testing muscle power, we required the muscle to display its full strength, and if it was too strong, we put it at a mechanical disadvantage to bring it within testing range. The severest test of a muscle is how strong it is. On the other hand, the severest test of a sensory system is not how strong a stimulus it can withstand, but how weak a stimulus it can detect. Hence, to put a sensory system to the severest test, use a ☐ minimal / ☐ maximal stimulus.

minimal

2. Test auditory threshold by presenting minimal stimuli.

a. Rub your fingers together beside each ear, or use a ticking watch or tuning fork (256 or 512 cps). Hold the fork prongs parallel to the ear, not perpendicular; try both positions to see why. The fork sound may reach the opposite ear. Mask the opposite ear by rubbing a piece of paper over it.

b. To semiquantitate the tests, compare the distance at which you hear the sound with the distance at which the patient hears it.

3. The *air-bone conduction test* of *Rinne* is for the relative efficiency of bone and air conduction of the sound vibrations.

a. Hold a faintly vibrating tuning fork on your mastoid process. When you can no longer hear the sound, hold the fork beside your ear. Can you again hear the sound? ☐ Yes / ☐ No. With this test you can decide which is the most efficient in the patient. Normally air conduction is ☐ more / ☐ less efficient than bone.

Do the test!

more

b. If you hold the tuning fork by your ear and put your finger in your ear, you know you won't hear its sound, but try this: place the fork against your mastoid and as you listen to the sound, press your finger hard into your ear. What happens to the sound? ______________________.

gets louder

increase
decrease

c. This test shows that a mechanical impediment in the auditory canal may cause an apparent □ increase / □ decrease in bone conduction and □ an increase / □ a decrease in air conduction.

d. Deafness or decreased hearing may be caused by a mechanical impediment to conduction of sound vibrations from the external ear through the auditory canal and ossicles of the middle ear. This type of hearing loss is called a *conduction* loss.

neurosensory

e. If the lesion is in the organ of Corti or the auditory nerve, it is called a *neurosensory* loss. Notice that when we say a patient has a conduction loss of hearing, we refer to conduction of sound vibrations through the auditory channels to stimulate the organ of Corti. We do not refer to conduction of nerve impulses through the VIIIth nerve. Loss of hearing from an VIIIth nerve lesion is called a □ conduction / □ neurosensory loss.

f. The reason for applying the tuning fork to the mastoid bone is that the bone mechanically transmits vibration to the inner ear to excite auditory impulses, bypassing the conduction channels of the external and the middle ear. In this way, integrity of the nerve can be tested even though a lesion blocks conduction of sound vibration through the normal channels.

g. Interpretation of the air-bone conduction test of Rinne.

(1) You have tested a patient and find that he hears better when the fork is applied to his mastoid process than when it is in the air beside his ear. The best inference is:

☑ (c)

□ (a) The patient is normal.
□ (b) The patient must have a lesion of the organ of Corti.
□ (c) The patient has a conduction lesion: a mechanical impediment such as wax in his auditory canal, a damaged drum, or immobility of the ossicles.
□ (d) The patient has a neurosensory lesion in the organ of Corti or of the auditory nerve.

☑ (d)

(2) If the test had shown reduced hearing for air and bone conduction of sound, the best inference is: □ (a) / □ (b) / □ (c) / □ (d).

center (If you are normal)
Yes (If you are normal)

4. *The sound-lateralizing test of Weber.* Place a vibrating tuning fork on the middle of your forehead or the vertex of your skull. Where does the sound seem to come from? __________________.
Is it equally loud in both ears? □ Yes / □ No.

Lateralizes to the occluded side

a. With the vibrating fork in place on the vertex of your head, press your fingertip in one ear and then the other. What happens to the sound? __________________

the same

b. Normally you hear the vertex vibration equally in both ears. If there is a mechanical impediment to sound conduction in one ear, the sound localizes to □ the same / □ the opposite / □ neither side.

opposite

c. If the patient has an auditory nerve lesion on one side, the vertex vibration sounds loudest on the □ same / □ opposite / □ neither side.

d. Only a consistent lateralization to one side is considered significant.

5. *Testing for a startle response to sound.* Sometimes you have to test auditory function in a noncooperative, hysterical, or malingering patient or an infant. You can gain a crude estimate of hearing by use of the *auditory-palpebral* reflex. If a person hears a loud sound, he involuntarily blinks. An assistant standing behind the patient, out of his line of sight, can clap hands or pop a bag. Observe the patient for blinking or a startle response. If the patient has a response, you are certain he hears something. If he does not respond, the significance of the test is doubtful.
6. *Interpretation of test results.* The critical point in analyzing hearing deficits is to decide whether the patient has a mechanical impediment to conduction of sound through the middle ear or has a nerve lesion. To interpret any test result, you must exclude obvious mechanical impediments such as damaged eardrums, wax, or foreign bodies in the external auditory canal. Therefore, you must look at the canal and drum with an otoscope as an integral part of every exam. Although you can exclude some mechanical impediments by otoscopy, you cannot exclude others, such as immobility of the ossicles.

a. A patient showed an increased auditory threshold to a ticking watch on the left; the vertex test lateralized to the left, and bone transmission was better than air transmission. These findings most likely indicate:

☐ (1) A normal patient.
☐ (2) A mechanical impediment, a *conduction* lesion.
☐ (3) Insufficient data to reach a conclusion.
☐ (4) Temporal lobe lesion.
☐ (5) An auditory nerve or cochlear lesion, a *neurosensory* lesion.

☑ (2)

b. Another patient showed an increased auditory threshold to the tuning fork on the left; bone and air transmission of sound were reduced on the left, and the vertex test lateralized to the right. Which inference in the preceding case best applies to this one?

☐ 1/ ☐ 2/ ☐ 3/ ☐ 4/ ☐ 5

☑ (5)

7. In testing visual fields we found that some patients are unable to detect stimuli from both sides. This test is called ________________ stimulation.

simultaneous (double, bilateral)

a. The same principle can be used for testing hearing. If the auditory pathways are shown to be intact by the previous tests, try simultaneous stimulation. Hold both of your hands up by the patient's ears. Gently rub your fingers together first on one side then the other, and have the patient point to the side from which the stimulus comes. Then rub the fingers of both hands to see whether he identifies the simultaneous stimuli. You may also snap your fingers, if you can make the sound equally loud on both sides.

b. Only a consistent inattention to sound from one side is significant. Repeat the test several times, using single and simultaneous stimuli.

C. Laboratory tests of auditory function

Among the otologist's vast array of tests, two, the *audiogram* and *BAER* test, have special value in distinguishing the type of hearing loss and site of the lesion. An *audiogram* consists of a curve which shows the patient's responses to electrically controlled sound of varying intensity and frequency. The *brainstem auditory evoked response,* or BAER test, produces waves which show the electrical responses of the auditory nerve and brainstem to sound, as discussed under Electroneurodiagnosis, page 430, Chapter 13.

D. Rehearse the clinical hearing tests, Section V, C, 3 of the Summarized Neurological Examination.

Bibliography

Arbit, E.: A sensitive bedside hearing test, *Ann. Neurol.,* 2:250, 1977.

Bierman, Pierson, W., and Donaldson, J.: The evaluation of middle ear functions in children, *Amer. J. Dis Child.,* 120:233-236, 1970.

Edwards, C. H.: *Neurology of Ear, Nose, and Throat Disease,* Toronto, Butterworths, 1973.

Heilman, K., et al: Auditory inattention, *Arch. Neurol.,* 24:323-325, 1971.

Jaffe, B. F. (ed.): *Hearing Loss in Children: A Comprehensive Text,* Baltimore, University Park Press, 1977.

Klingon, G., and Bontecou, D.: Localization in auditory space, *Neurology,* 16: 879-886, 1966.

Kohler, L., and Holst, H.: Auditory screening of four-year-old children, *Acta Paediat. Scand.,* 61:555-560, 1972.

Urmura, T., Suzuki, J-I., Hozawa, J., and Highstein, S.: *Neuro-otological Examination,* Baltimore, University Park Press, 1976.

V. Vestibular system

A. Introduction

1. If you were to ask me what are the most common symptoms, I would say, "Headaches, backaches, dizziness, fatigability, and blackout spells." If you were to ask what are the most difficult symptoms to diagnose, I would answer, "Headaches, backaches, dizziness, fatigability, and blackout spells."
2. In the patient's vernacular, dizziness encompasses a multitude. He may mean giddiness, light headedness, unsteadiness, "swimminess," vertigo, and so on. The patient usually does not deliver his symptom neatly packaged and labeled. Vertigo, if strictly defined, is not just a synonym for all complaints encompassed by dizziness. It means a sensation as though the person or the world were spinning around or undergoing movement.

B. Pathophysiology of the vestibular system

1. Lesions of the vestibular receptors, their nerves, or central connections cause vertigo and sometimes other sensations of movement. To

appreciate what the patient with vestibular disease experiences, try this experiment, but prepare yourself to fall during it. Follow the instructions carefully.

a. Place a penny on the floor about 40 to 50 cm from a bed or a fully cushioned easy chair (to serve as a receptacle in case you fall).

b. Stand directly over the penny, with it between your feet and with the receptacle to your *right*.

c. Bend your head forward to stare at the penny, and while staring at the penny, turn around to your right five complete turns, stopping with your right side toward the receptacle. At the end of the five turns, try to stand erect, look straight ahead, and hold your arms straight out. Record these observations:

(1) In which direction do you experience an illusion of movement? ☐ To the right / ☐ To the left.

Most persons feel as if they were spinning to the left.

(2) Which way do you tend to fall? ☐ To the right / ☐ To the left?

right

(3) Which way do your outstretched arms tend to deviate? ☐ To the right / ☐ To the left.

right

2. *The signs and symptoms of vestibular stimulation*

a. You will feel an illusion of movement immediately after you stop turning around the penny. For most of us, the illusion will be of rotation to the left, but it may be of some other type of movement. This experience is *vertigo.* With the vertigo, most of us will experience some *nausea,* and a few of us will vomit. The combination of vertigo and nausea will cause you to feel *anxiety.* If you have spun around enough to induce nystagmus, you will also experience *oscillopsia.* All in all it is a terribly uncomfortable experience. Summarize the symptoms of labyrinthine dysfunction: __________, __________, __________, and __________.

vertigo, nausea, anxiety, oscillopsia

b. The signs of labyrinthine disease are less spectacular than the symptoms. Most outstanding is falling, next is nystagmus. The remainder of the signs reflect autonomic dysfunction: pallor, sweating, vomiting, and hypotension. Motion sickness, which you have just sampled in the experiment, exemplifies a labyrinthine disorder with all the signs and symptoms.

c. Try the rotation experiment again, this time reversing directions and rotating to the left. The experience of vertigo is to the ☐ right / ☐ left and the direction of falling and arm deviation is to the ☐ right / ☐ left.

right
left

d. We can generalize that when the vertigo is in one direction, the falling and arm deviation are in the ☐ same / ☐ opposite direction.

opposite

C. *Peripheral anatomy of the vestibular system*

1. The end organs of the vestibular system are specialized nerve endings in the membranous labyrinth. For the detection of motion, the end organ is in the semicircular canals. The orientation of the canals is shown in Fig. 9-8.

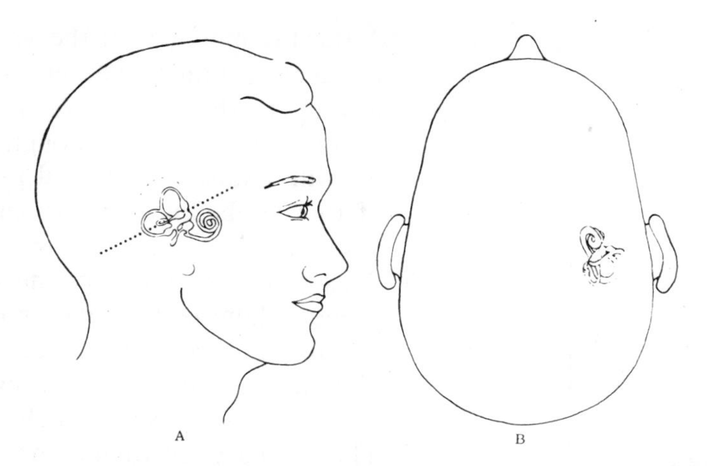

FIG. 9-8. Orientation of the labyrinth. The size of the labyrinth relative to the head is exaggerated for clarity of the drawing. *A*. Lateral view of right labyrinth. Notice that the plane (dotted line) of the "horizontal" semicircular canal is inclined upward 30° from the horizontal. B. Superior view of the head.

2. Fig. 9-9 emphasizes that the so-called horizontal canal is inclined upwards 30° from the horizontal plane.

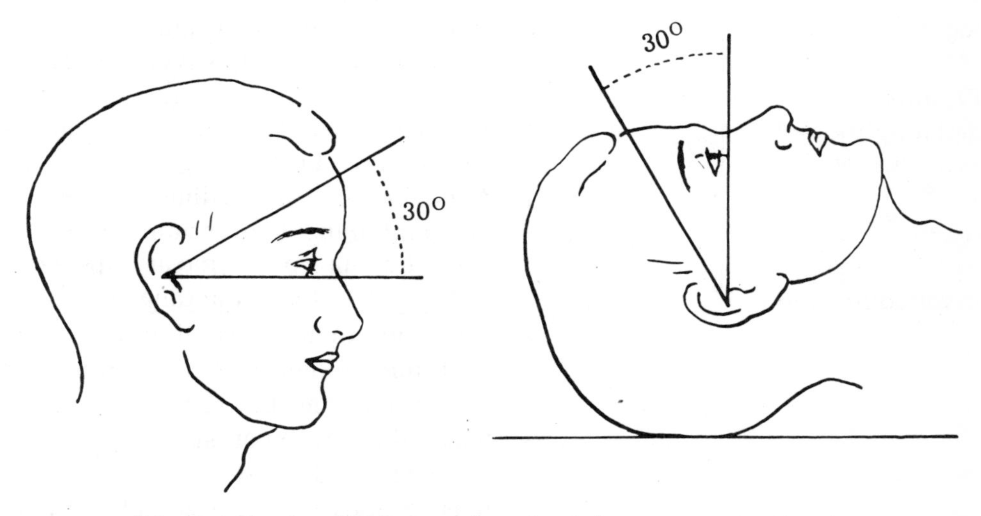

FIG. 9-9. Inclination of the horizontal canal with the patient erect and supine.

horizontal

3. When you tilted your head downward spinning around the penny, you placed the horizontal canal more nearly ☐ horizontal / ☐ vertical.
4. When you spun around with your head tilted down, the horizontal canal was in the plane of rotation. The canals are filled with fluid. As you turned, the fluid began to turn. When you stopped, the fluid continued to turn in the same plane, and you had the illusion of movement. The normal stimulus for the semicircular canals is rotation or movement of the fluid within them.
5. The semicircular canals of the vestibular apparatus detect turning. A second component, the utricle, is a gravity-operated receptor which responds to tilting. It can be thought of as an "out-of-position" receptor.

A third component of the vestibular apparatus, the saccule, responds to acceleration. The utricle-saccule system provides information leading to the correct vertical postures of the person when he sits, stands, and walks. Although this point is by no means established, we will assume for clinical purposes that the caudal vermis syndrome of the cerebellum reflects an interruption in the connections of this system.

6. All sensory receptors for the vestibular system are located in the membranous labyrinth of the internal ear. The vestibular ganglion is in the internal auditory canal. Hence, the primary vestibular neurons, like the primary cochlear neurons of VIII, are very close to their place of duty. So is the ganglion of sensory cranial nerve ________.

   I

7. The primary vestibular neurons synapse at the vestibular nuclei, located at the ________________ junction. Review Figs. 3-10 and 3-11.

   pontomedullary (Review Fig. 3-11 if necessary.)

8. The vestibular nuclei contain the ☐ primary/ ☐ secondary/ ☐ tertiary neurons in the vestibular pathway.

   secondary

D. Central pathways underlying vestibular signs and symptoms.

1. *The pathways for the signs of vestibular stimulation*
   - *a.* Since the major ocular sign of vestibular stimulation is ________, strong vestibular pathways run to cranial nerve nuclei ________, ________, ________, which innervate the eye muscles.

     nystagmus

     III, IV, and VI
   - *b.* The pathway linking the vestibular system with cranial nerve nuclei III, IV, and VI is the ________________________.

     medial longitudinal fasciculus (MLF)
   - *c.* A major sign of vestibulocerebellar dysfunction is a disturbance in maintaining equilibrium of the trunk. The cerebellar subdivision thought to be most important is the ☐ vermis/ ☐ hemispheres/ ☐ flocculonodular lobe.

     flocculonodular lobe
   - *d.* The autonomic signs of vestibular dysfunction (as well as direct anatomic studies) indicate strong connections between the vestibular system and the reticular formation.
   - *e.* Since the vestibular system provides positional information about the head and correlates head and eye movements with somatic muscle activity, the vestibular nuclei have strong descending systems to the spinal cord via the MLF and vestibulospinal tracts. These tracts along with reticulospinal tracts mediate postural reflexes, such as head and neck righting and tonic neck reflexes.
2. *The pathways for the symptoms of vestibular stimulation.* The fact that vestibular impulses influence consciousness implies a pathway to a thalamic nucleus and a cortical receptive area. These pathways to consciousness have not yet been convincingly established, but they undoubtedly exist. *A priori*, the vestibular center should associate with the auditory center in the superior temporal gyrus. Attempts to locate such a vertiginous center by electrical stimulation of the brain in conscious patients have not been decisive. Many epileptic patients complain of dizziness before their attacks, but few describe true vertigo. The symptom of dizziness has no localizing value,

while the symptom of vertigo suggests a lesion of the vestibular system or its brainstem connections.

vestibulospinal
flocculonodular
caudal (inferior)

MLF

3. *To summarize:* let us turn a vestibular impulse loose at the pontomedullary junction, at the site of the vestibular nuclei. If it goes caudally to the spinal cord, it can travel the ______ tract and the MLF. If it goes dorsally to the ______ lobe of the cerebellum, it travels via the ______ cerebellar peduncle. If the impulse goes into the reticular formation it goes via many short circuits of bewildering complexity. It it goes to the nuclei of the ocular muscles it travels via the ______. If it goes to the thalamus and cortex, we do not know how to write the ticket, but we can direct it in the general direction.

   In other words, the impulse can box the compass and go by vestibular pathways to every major subdivision of the nervous system: the cerebrum, the brainstem, the cerebellum, and the spinal cord.

E. *Preparation for testing of the vestibular system by caloric irrigation of the auditory canals*

1. Movement of the fluid within the semicircular canals from head rotation provides the normal vestibular stimulus.
2. Syringing the external auditory canal with warm or cold water artificially circulates semicircular canal fluid by inducing convection currents: the caloric test of vestibular function.
3. In preparation for the test, the patient's auditory canal must be inspected with an otoscope, for two reasons.
   a. A large wax plug may preclude adequate heat conduction. It should be removed before the test is done.
   b. If the patient's eardrum is perforated, you might instill water into the middle ear and cause pain and an infection.

vertigo,
nausea, anxiety,
and oscillopsia
nystagmus, falling or
postural deviation,
sweating, pallor,
vomiting, and
hypotension
sitting or reclining

4. Recall that the response to vestibular stimulation is subjective and objective. The subjective responses, the *symptoms,* are ______, ______, ______, ______.
5. The objective responses, the *signs,* are ______, ______, ______, ______, ______, ______.
6. Since the patient may experience vertigo and fall, how should you position him to prevent an accident? ______
7. The horizontal canal, being the most lateral, is most affected by temperature changes in the auditory canal. Even so, the weak convection currents set up in the semicircular canal by temperature changes require some assistance from gravity to cause sufficient fluid movement to stimulate the vestibular nerve endings. Cooling makes fluid heavier and to fall, heating makes it lighter and to rise. To add the effect of gravity to the convection currents, the horizontal canal should be *vertical.* Refer back to Fig. 9-9 to answer these questions:

30°
60°
backward

a. If the patient is reclining on his back, his head should be tilted ______ degrees forward to get his horizontal canal vertical.

b. If the patient is sitting, his head should be tilted ______ degrees ☐ forward / ☐ backward to get his horizontal canal vertical.

8. Because caloric testing makes the patient uncomfortable, the only sporting thing is to warn him. If you tell him the signs and symptoms to expect, you lose some of the objectivity and validity of the test. Therefore, say this, "I am going to rinse out your ear. It may be uncomfortable for you, but you'll manage all right."

F. Procedure for caloric irrigation

auditory canal (eardrum)

vertical

1. You will have a profound and enduring sympathy for your vertiginous patients if you have caloric irrigation done on yourself. Get a partner: Before you squirt in the water you must inspect the ______.
2. Since you are aware of what will happen, you can have the test done while sitting up. You will need to put the horizontal canal in the ______ plane.
3. How do you position the head to get the *horizontal* canal *vertical* when the patient is sitting up? ______

Ans: tilt it back 60°: 60 and 30 make 90. See Fig. 9-9.

4. When doing caloric irrigation on a patient, fit him with glasses having strong positive lenses (Frenzel glasses), which you can buy cheaply in a dime store. Glasses serve two purposes. They magnify the patient's eyes, making the nystagmus easier to see, and they blur his vision and interrupt fixation. Fixation inhibits induced nystagmus. Thus, the glasses increase the likelihood of nystagmus occurring and make it easier to study if it occurs.

44°
30°

vomits

5. Fill a 100-cc syringe with water which is at a temperature of 7° above or below the normal 37° C of body temperature. If warm water is used it should be at ______ degrees; cold water should be at ______ degrees. Gently instill the 100 cc of water into the external auditory canal over a period of 40 sec. Hold an emesis basin next to the ear to prevent wetting the patient (and also for emergency service if the patient ______).

   An alternative method of caloric stimulation, preferred by many, is to irrigate with 5 cc of ice water instead of the larger quantity of water at 30°.

6. Instruct the patient that at the end of the irrigation he is to try to sit erect, to try to look straight ahead, and to hold his arms straight out in front of him.

Get the answers for a-g from your own observations.

7. Get a partner and do caloric irrigation. Before irrigating, read *a-g* to learn what observations to make. To make all of them you may have to irrigate more than once. After irrigating, watch the eyes at least a minute before concluding that you will get no response. After nystagmus starts, make the other observations. Use the right ear and ice water.

   a. When his eyes are closed and his arms are straight out, the patient tends to deviate to the ☐ right / ☐ left.

b. When the patient's eyes are open, they deviate to the ☐ right/ ☐ left.
c. The fast component of the nystagmus is to the ☐ right / ☐ left.
d. Have the patient follow your finger to the sides. The nystagmus increases in amplitude when the patient looks ☐ to/ ☐ away from the direction of the fast component.
e. To test for past-pointing, have the patient elevate his right arm and try to bring it down on your fingertip, which you hold directly in front of him. He past-points to the ☐ right / ☐ left.
f. Ask about the direction of vertigo: ☐ to the right / ☐ to the left.
g. Record the duration of signs and symptoms: ______________________
____.

G. *Results of caloric irrigation test.* The results are to be analyzed, assuming that the *right* ear was irrigated with cool water.

jerk

1. The nystagmus has a fast and a slow phase. It is therefore a ☐ jerk / ☐ pendular nystagmus.

left

2. Nystagmus is conventionally named according to the direction of the fast or jerk movement. The nystagmus obtained on irrigation of the right ear with cold water is directed to the ☐ right / ☐ left.
3. The naming of nystagmus direction has always been a problem. The slow deviation of the eyes in vestibular nystagmus is the vestibular-induced phase. The quick jerk back is regarded as compensatory and may be abolished by cerebral lesions. If you want to name the nystagmus in terms of the slow component well and good, but again, you must understand that the terminology will differ from author to author.

right
left

4. Postural deviation and past-pointing were to the ☐ right / ☐ left.
5. The direction of the vertigo was ☐ right / ☐ left.

right

6. Here is what the subject should look like at the height of a strong vestibular response. In Fig. 9-10 which ear was irrigated with cold water? ☐ right / ☐ left.

30°
60°
horizontal
vertical

7. *To summarize:* when the right ear is irrigated with cold water the head is to be tilted ____________ degrees forward if the patient is reclining, or ____________ degrees backward if the patient is upright. The object of the position is to orient the ______________________ semicircular canal in the ______________________ plane.

right

a. The slow phase of the nystagmus, the deviation of the eyes, the truncal and arm deviation, and past-pointing were to the ☐ right/ ☐ left.

left

b. The vertigo was to the ☐ right/ ☐ left.

opposite

8. Since the vertigo was to the *left*, the postural deviations can all be regarded as reflex overcompensation for the erroneous information coming from circulation of fluid in the right horizontal canal. The patient compensates by a postural deviation in the ☐ same / ☐ opposite direction to the vertigo. In other words he feels as though he is moving to the left and compensates by leaning to the right.

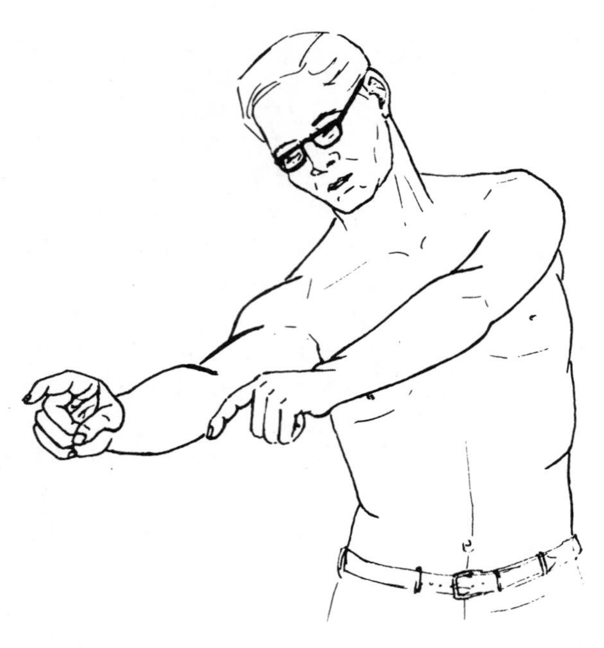

FIG. 9-10. Postural deviation in patient after one ear was irrigated with cold water. He was sitting upright with his head tilted backwards 60° during the irrigation.

H. Results, clinical interpretation, and use of caloric tests

1. After irrigating the auditory canal, look for nystagmus, recording its time of appearance, duration, and form. Normally, the nystagmus consists of conjugate horizontal eye movement with slow deviation of the eyes toward the side of the cold caloric stimulus and a quick jerk toward the opposite side. In section G, we reviewed the postural effects to provide an understanding of the mechanisms involved and to simulate the experience of the patient suffering from a vestibular disorder, but in actual clinical use we observe only the nystagmus.
2. Normal individuals respond variably to caloric irrigation. Some show little or no response from either ear. Determine whether irrigation of the two ears produces any consistent difference. Thus, a strong normal response from the right ear with little or no response from the left indicates a lesion of the vestibular end organ, nerve, or immediate central connections on the left.
3. *To summarize:*
   a. The signs of labyrinthine disease are ______________________________ ______________________________.
   b. The symptoms are ______________________________ ______________________________.
   c. What precautions are taken before doing the caloric irrigation test? ______________________________ ______________________________
   d. Describe the nystagmus expected after irrigating the left ear of a normal person with cold water: ______________________________ ______________________________ ______________________________ ______________________________.

nystagmus, postural deviation and falling, vomiting, hypotension, pallor, sweating

vertigo, nausea, anxiety, oscillopsia

Counsel the patient, do otoscopy, place the patient sitting or reclining

Horizontal with slow phase to the left and rapid phase to the right

4. Indications for caloric irrigation: do caloric irrigation if the history indicates dizziness, vertigo, or a hearing disorder, or if the examination discloses auditory dysfunction. Chapter 12 discusses caloric irrigation in coma, and Chapter 13 discusses objective recording of caloric or induced nystagmus by electronystagmography.

Bibliography

Barber, H. O.: Diagnostic techniques in vertigo, *Excerpta Medica, Journal of Vertigo,* 1:1-16, 1974.

Bender, M.: Oscillopsia, *Arch. Neurol.,* 13:204-213, 1965.

Bernstein, L.: Simplification of clinical caloric test, *Arch. Otolaryng.,* 81:347-349, 1965.

Carmichael, E., Dix, M., and Hallpike, C.: Observations upon the neurological mechanism of directional preponderance of caloric nystagmus resulting from vascular lesions of the brain-stem, *Brain,* 88: 51-74, 1965.

Doig, J.: Auditory and vestibular function and dysfunction, from *Scientific Foundations of Neurology,* Critchley, M. (ed.), Philadelphia, F. A. Davis Co., 1972.

Drachman, A., and Hart, C.: An approach to the dizzy patient, *Neurology,* 22:323-334, 1972.

Elia, J.: *The Dizzy Patient,* Springfield, Charles C Thomas, 1968.

Hood, J. D. (ed.): *Vestibular Mechanisms in Health and Disease,* New York, Academic Press, 1978.

Hughes, J. R., and Drachman, D. A.: Dizziness, epilepsy, and the EEG, *Dis. Nerv. Syst.,* 38:431-435, 1977.

Nelson, J.: The minimal ice water caloric test, *Neurology,* 19:577-585, 1969.

Tschang, H., and Harrison, M.: Note on the value of Frenzel's glasses for the recognition and qualitative evaluation of spontaneous nystagmus, *J. Neurol. Neurosurg. Psychiat.,* 34:362-366, 1971.

Wolfson, R. (ed.): *The Vestibular System and Its Diseases,* Philadelphia, University of Pennsylvania Press, 1966.

Zilstorff-Pederson, K., and Peitersen, E.: Vestibulospinal reflexes, *Arch. Otolaryng.,* 77: 237-242, 1963.

I. Positional nystagmus

1. *Introduction:* whenever a patient complains of dizziness, the physician should ask about the effect of changes in posture. Dizziness when first standing up, a phenomenon you have all experienced, suggests orthostatic hypotension. However, disease of the labyrinth or its central connections may produce sensory misinformation which may lead to dizziness. In these cases, you are apt to find positional nystagmus as an objective sign of the organicity of the patient's complaint and as a flag signaling that the labyrinthine system causes the mischief.
2. *Technique:* with Frenzel lenses in place, have the patient seated so that his head can be laid back over the edge of a table, as in Fig. 9-11. Test the patient by laying his head straight back, then erect him and lay him down with head turned to the right and repeat to the left. After laying the patient's head back, observe his eyes for nystagmus for one

minute before considering the test negative. At the end of the test, inquire whether the maneuver reproduced the patient's sensation of dizziness, but do not suggest that it should have.

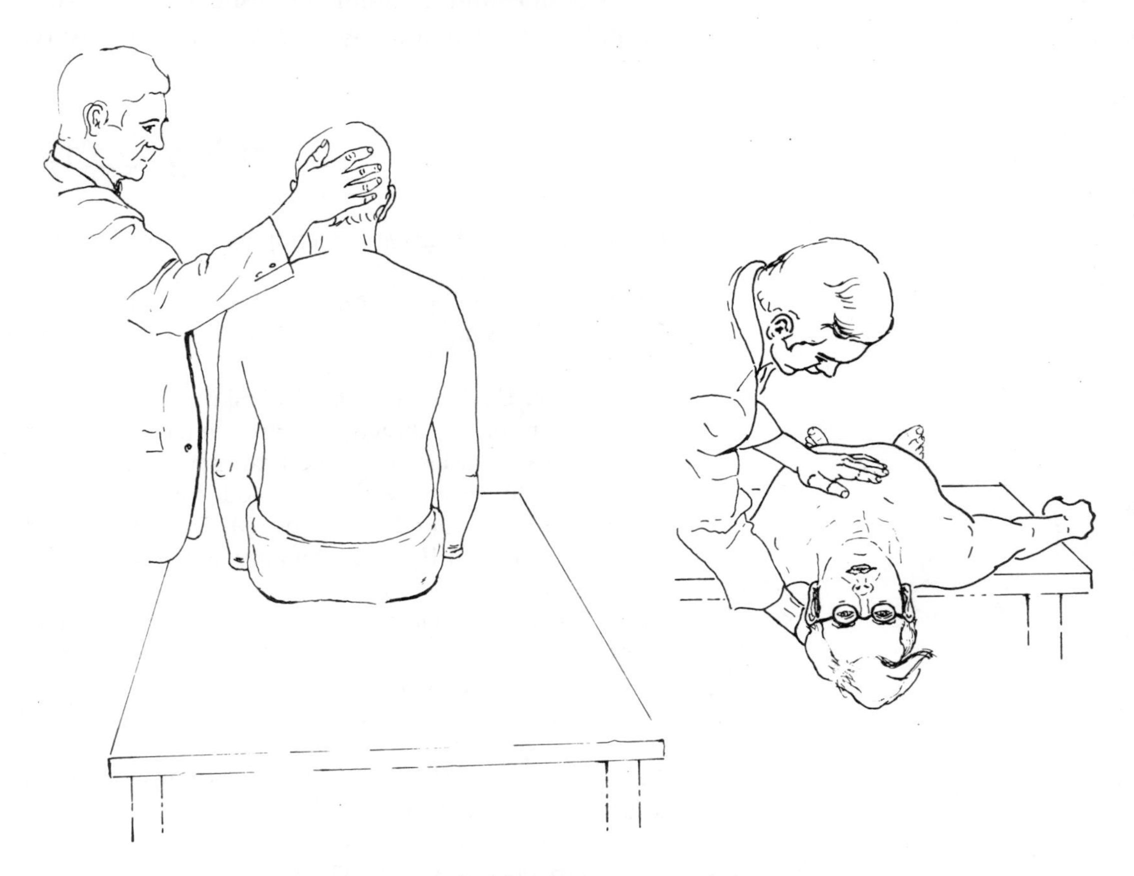

FIG. 9-11. Method for eliciting positional nystagmus.

Bibliography

Harrison, M., and Ozsahinoglu, C.: Positional vertigo: Aetiology and clinical significance, *Brain,* 75:369-372, 1972.

Schiller, F., and Hedberg, W.: An appraisal of positional nystagmus, *Arch. Neurol.,* 2:309-316, 1960.

J. *Hyperventilation*

Hyperventilation causes dizziness. Hyperventilation attacks occur commonly in an emotionally disturbed patient. Ask the patient to breathe as deep and fast as he can for 3 minutes. Time him and keep encouraging him to breathe hard during the entire test. At the end, ask whether hyperventilation reproduced his sensation of dizziness. Try this test yourself.

Some patients faint during this test, so-called *hyperventilation syncope;* therefore, place the patient in a chair or semireclining position before he hyperventilates.

VI. Somatic sensation from the face and mucous membranes of eyes, nose, mouth, and sinuses

A. Introduction

1. The modalities of sight, smell, taste, hearing, and equilibrium are the *special* senses. The modalities of touch, pain, temperature, pressure, and itching-tickling are the *general* senses.
2. The special senses all have special, unique receptors, and unique pathways. The theory of modality specific receptors and pathways for general sensory modalities, although once widely accepted, is presently disputed. Hence, no attempt will be made to describe the receptors. Apparently several of the general modalities share the same receptors and pathways.

B. Anatomy of facial and mucosal sensation

temporal, medial and lateral pterygoid, and masseter

1. The Vth cranial nerve mediates all general sensory modalities for the face and mucous membranes of the nose, cheeks, tongue, and sinuses. It has *no* special sensory fibers. It supplies branchiomotor fibers to all four of the masticator muscles, the ______________________ ______________________ muscles.
2. *Sensory domain of V.* Let us slice off the face, with a single scimitar blow, along the line shown in Fig. 9-12.

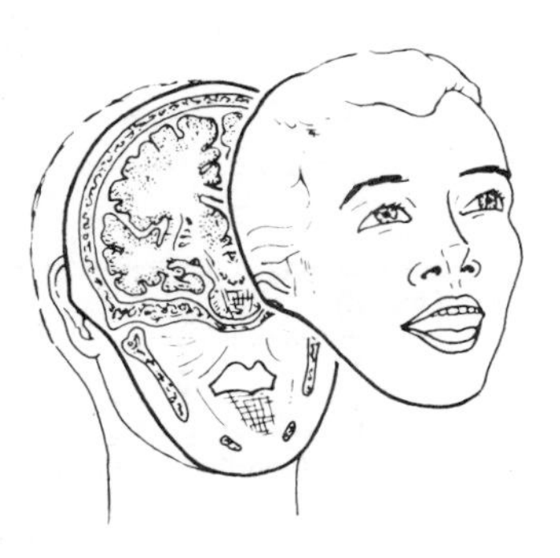

FIG. 9-12. The mask of Trigeminus. It is obtained by a single slice through the head with a scimitar. The mask that falls away is no ordinary Halloween mask. It is three dimensional. It contains all of the territory, both motor and sensory, innervated by the Vth nerve: skin, chewing muscles and their proprioceptors, mucous membranes, and the dura mater. Only the cerebrum itself has no nerve supply. Notice that the angle of the mandible is spared, left behind with the head: see also the face in Fig. 9-13 to fix this fact permanently in your mind.

3. Study Fig. 9-13 until you know the three divisions of the *tri*geminal nerve, their facial skin areas, and central connections. The mesencephalic nucleus of V does not conform to the other nuclei and will be discussed later.

C. Peripheral distribution of V

ophthalmic, maxillary, and mandibular

1. The three sensory divisions of V, the ______________________, ______________________, ______________________ branches, are the reason for naming V the *trigeminal nerve.*

primary

2. The ganglion of the trigeminal nerve is the trigeminal (semilunar, Gasserian) ganglion. It contains the ☐ primary / ☐ secondary / ☐ tertiary neuron of the sensory pathway from the face.

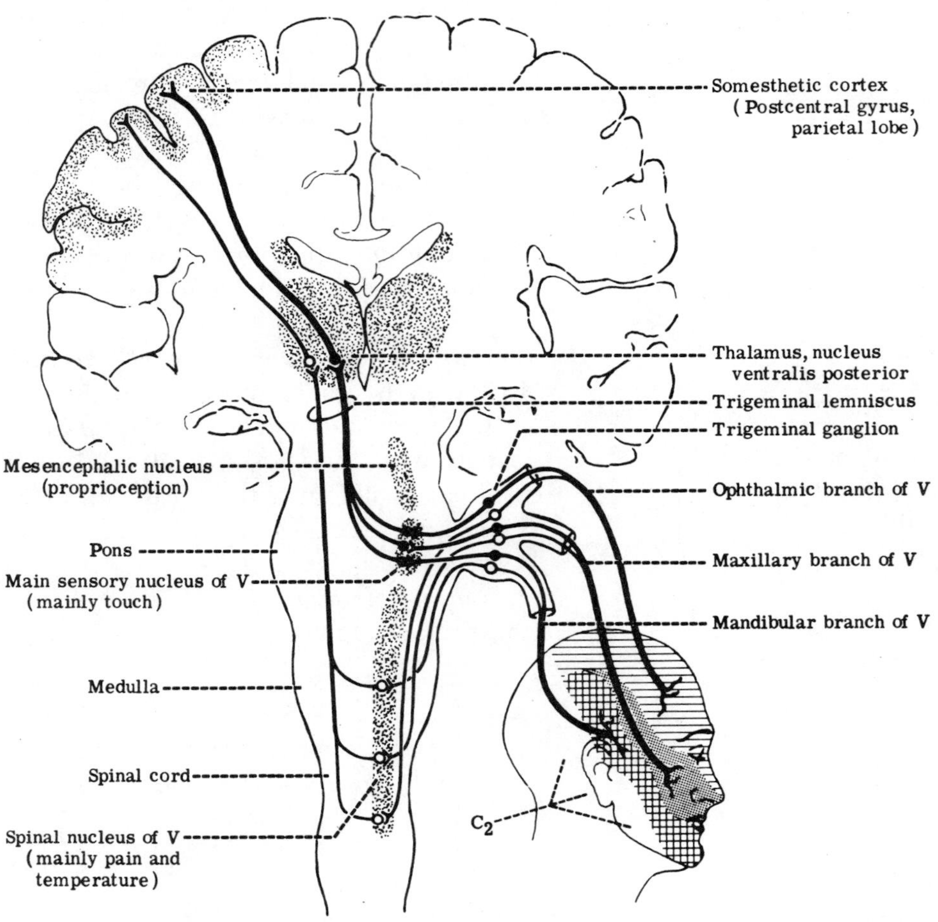

FIG. 9-13. Peripheral and central connections of the trigeminal nerve. Notice the pain and temperature pathway descending to the spinal cord. Compare the posterior margin of the line of facial innervation with Fig. 9-12.

dorsal root

3. The trigeminal ganglion corresponds to the ________________ ________________ ganglia of the spinal nerves.

pons

4. The trigeminal ganglion with its three sensory branches is attached by a single root to the ☐ mesencephalon / ☐ pons / ☐ medulla.

Note: to answer the optional frames,** you should have completed the previous optional sections.

I and VIII

**5. The ganglia of the primary neurons for the special senses mediated by cranial nerves ________________ are very near to, or in their end, organs. (If you don't recall the answer readily, what is the best way to systematize your approach?) ________________ ________________

Ans: Start at cranial nerve I and sort through them one by one.

secondary
thalamus
(diencephalon)

6. The trigeminal *nuclei* (*nuclei,* not ganglia) contain the ☐ primary / ☐ secondary / ☐ tertiary neuron of the trigeminal pathway.

7. Where is the tertiary neuron? ________________

Review Fig. 9-13 if you missed this one.

8. The mesencephalic portion of V forms an exception to the rule that the primary neuron of a sensory pathway is outside of the central nervous system. The retina is the other exception. The mesencephalic nucleus is a primary neuron within the neuraxis — a unique nucleus, but a fact of no clinical use. The mesencephalic portion of V is thought **to mediate *proprioceptive* function; the pontine and upper medullary portion mediates *touch,* and the spinal nucleus mediates *pain* and *temperature*. Thus, in rostrocaudal order, the functions mediated by the three portions of the sensory nucleus of V are: ____________, ____________, ____________, ____________.

proprioception, touch, pain, and temperature

9. Taken all together, trigeminal sensory fibers and nuclei extend from the rostral part of the cervical region of the spinal cord to the rostral part of the mesencephalon.

D. *Central connections of V*

1. The secondary neurons of V, like those of the cochlear pathway, synapse in the thalamus.
2. The trigeminal nuclei send axons to the thalamus by the ____________ lemniscus.

trigeminal

3. The cochlear pathway runs to the thalamus via the ☐ medial / ☐ lateral lemniscus.

lateral

4. Somatic sensory impulses from the remainder of the body, exclusive of the face, connect with the thalamus via the ☐ lateral / ☐ medial / ☐ trigeminal lemniscus.

medial (or combined spinal and medial)

5. We can generalize that a pathway that relays somatic sensory impulses to the thalamus is called a ____________.

lemniscus

6. The three lemnisci named thus far are the ____________ for facial sensation, the ____________ for hearing, and the ____________ for general somatic sensation exclusive of the face.

trigeminal
lateral
medial

7. In general the lemnisci contain axons from ☐ primary / ☐ secondary / ☐ tertiary neurons which have ____________ the midline. The ____________ lemniscus is a partial exception to this rule since it has many uncrossed axons.

secondary
crossed
lateral

8. *The domain of the lemnisci.* The tectum contains no long pathways, only a cerebellar pathway cutting through. The only long pathways in the basis are the corticofugal tracts. The lemnisci therefore must run through the ☐ tectum / ☐ tegmentum / ☐ basis of the brainstem. Trace the medial lemniscus through Figs. 3-14 to 3-17, page 92.

tegmentum

E. *Clinical testing of Vth nerve sensation: Touch, pain, temperature, and the corneal reflex*

1. Although the touch, pain, and temperature components of V can be tested separately, the proprioceptive function of the masticator muscles is not testable clinically.
2. *Touch* is tested by using a wisp of cotton. If the test object is too rigid, you will test not only the sense of touch, but also the sense of ________.

pressure

Principle of testing a single modality at a time

What principle of sensory testing would you have violated? ______________________________

a. The patient is requested to close his eyes. The cotton is touched lightly to each area of the three divisions of the nerve, alternating areas and sides of the face randomly. The patient is instructed to say "Yes" when he feels the touch stimulus.

b. Suppose you have touched several places and the patient has responded, "Yes." What would you do to test the patient's reliability and attentiveness? ______________________________

Ans: Occasionally withhold the stimulus and ask him whether he feels something. Recall that in testing the sense of smell we sometimes withheld the stimulus the patient was expecting.

3. Pain is tested by an ordinary straight pin, which has one blunt end and one sharp end. Why would you want an instrument with sharp and blunt ends? ______________________________

Ans: So that the ends can be alternated to monitor the reliability of the patient's responses.

a. In using a mechanical pain stimulus, such as a pin, you will cause a sensation of touch as well as of pain. This violates the rule of testing only one modality at a time. By presenting alternate touch and pain stimuli by using both ends of the pin, you overcome this objection.

b. The patient is instructed to respond by saying "Sharp" or "Dull," whichever sensation he feels. Since the patient will be somewhat apprehensive about being stuck with a pin, show him with his eyes open what you are going to do. Prick him lightly on the arm until he just feels the pain.

c. If you suspect from the history that the patient will have numb areas, start with a *normal* area to establish communication so that he knows what to expect. Have him shut his eyes to isolate the perception of pain from visual cues.

close his eyes

4. *Temperature* is tested by using two tubes, one filled with warm water and one with cold. Always test them on yourself first to make sure that they will not be uncomfortable. Avoid extremes of temperature. You want to test temperature *discrimination* near threshold, not maximal responses. Try the tubes on a normal part of the patient's body and have him respond by saying "Hot" or "Cold." Once he understands the test, he is instructed to ______________________________ to avoid visual cues.

a. Because pain *and* temperature run in the spinal root of V, they tend to be affected together by medullary lesions. When you test one you test both to some degree. Nevertheless, temperature should always be tested, not only on the face, but on the rest of the body, because you may get clear-cut abnormalities when pain testing is indecisive.

b. It has been said that the function of the internist or the surgical consultant is to do the rectal exam (and discover that the patient's baffling weight loss and back pain are from a metastatic prostatic carcinoma). Physicians habitually slight the same parts of the examination. Temperature testing is one of the most neglected parts of the neurologic examination. As a neurologist, I frequently find that my function is to do the temperature testing, and it frequently pays off.

5. *Testing the corneal reflex*
   a. The cornea is said to be able to detect only pain and temperature stimuli because it has none of the specialized receptors of the general cutaneous surface. Recent studies indicate that it can detect touch and other sensations.
   b. The corneal reflex consists of closure of the eyelid in response to touching the cornea. The afferent arc of the reflex is carried over the ______________ division of V.
   c. The eyelid is closed by the ______________ ______________ muscle which is innervated by the ______________ cranial nerve.
   d. The corneal reflex thus tests the integrity of two cranial nerves, ______________ and ______________.
   e. Instruct the patient to look to one side. With a wisp of cotton, touch the cornea of the *adducted* eye. Hold his lids apart to keep from stimulating the eyelashes, and bring the cotton directly in from the side to avoid entering the field of vision. In Fig. 9-14, make an X on the correct spot on the cornea to stimulate it without entering the patient's field of vision.

ophthalmic
orbicularis oculi
VIIth

V, VII

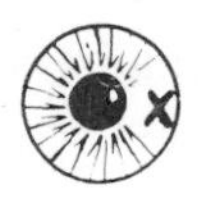

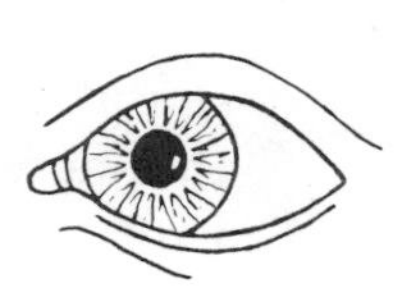

FIG. 9-14. Blank to mark the site for stimulation of the cornea to elicit the corneal reflex.

F. Practice testing Vth nerve sensation on a normal subject. First list the sensory functions to be tested: ______________ ______________ and the ______________ reflex.

Touch, pain, temperature, corneal

G. Clinical interpretation

1. Draw a line across the head of Fig. 9-15 to show the exact dividing line between the part of the head innervated by V and the cervical dermatomes. Compare with Fig. 9-13 to see how exact your line is.
2. Now shade and label the parts of the face supplied by each of the three major sensory branches of V. Check with Fig. 9-13.
3. Does V innervate the skin over the angle of the mandible? ☐ Yes/ ☐ No.
   a. If you included it in your drawing above, check again with Fig.

No

9-13: You missed a point of considerable clinical importance. Organic sensory loss of facial sensation from trigeminal nerve lesions spares the angle of the mandible, while hysterical loss of facial sensation includes it. Review Fig. 3-7A, page 78, and Fig. 9-13 to recall that cranial nerve V abuts on spinal nerve root C_2. This happens because the dorsal root of C_1 disappeared in the evolutionary rearrangement of the occipital dermatomes. Comparison

* Compare your drawing with Fig. 9-13.

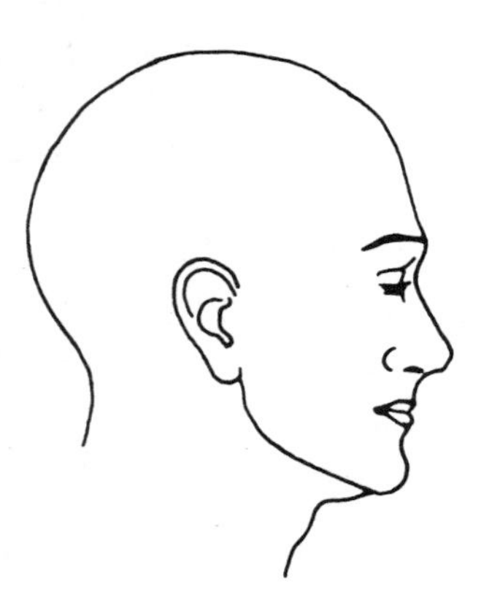

FIG. 9-15. Blank to draw in the sensory innervation field of the trigeminal nerve.

of hysterical and organic sensory losses leads to a profoundly useful general principle: hysterical patients lose sensation in accordance with their body image of a part; organic patients lose sensation in accordance with the wiring diagram of the nervous system. As a further example, we find that patients with hysterical loss of arm sensation usually have a sharp boundary at the shoulder because that agrees with the body image of the arm, but it does not agree with the actual anatomic distribution of peripheral nerves, nerve roots, or their central pathways.

affected

spared

b. Therefore in hysterical sensory loss of facial sensation, the angle of the mandible is ☐ spared/ ☐ affected whereas in organic loss of facial sensation due to a Vth nerve lesion, the angle of the mandible is ☐ spared/ ☐ affected.

H. Analyze this patient

1. A 76-year-old patient complains of severe pain in his face. His symptoms started 4 months ago and gradually worsened. He has become irascible and impossible to live with according to his wife. He has very brief, shocklike episodes of unbearable pain which run from the side of his cheek down to the tip of his jaw, on the right side only. Examination shows that all motor and sensory functions of the cranial nerves are normal except that it is difficult to test sensation over the right lower jaw because the patient is fearful of pain. Touching the right lower lip triggers excruciating shocks of pain into his right jaw. Because of it, he has been unable to eat and has lost 18 lb.

☑ c.

Mandibular division of right V

2. In differentiating organic from psychogenic sensory complaints one of the most important features is the distribution of the complaint. Is its distribution compatible with the anatomic organization of the sensory system, or does it conform to the person's mental image of his body? Is the distribution of the complaint compatible with a lesion of a *peripheral nerve, nerve root (dermatome),* or *central pathway?* Check the most probable explanation for the present patient:
   - ☐ *a.* In distribution of central pathway.
   - ☐ *b.* In distribution of a dermatome.
   - ☐ *c.* In distribution of a peripheral nerve or nerve branch.
   - ☐ *d.* The nonanatomic distribution, in combination with the patient's obvious personality change, indicate a psychogenic disorder.
3. What peripheral nerve area does the pain correspond to?

   ______________________________.
4. This patient had no other abnormalities on general physical examination or radiographic examination of his skull with a basilar view to show the foramina of exit of V. He had *trigeminal neuralgia,* a very typical idiopathic mononeuropathy which causes excruciating shock-like pain in one or more of the branches of the trigeminal nerve. The pain appears spontaneously, but is also set off by touching a "trigger point" on the cheek or inside the mouth.

I. Summary of the tests for the sensory functions of the cranial nerves. Rehearse sections V, steps C and D, of the Summarized Neurological Examination.

Bibliography

Bohm, E., and Strang, R.: Glossopharyngeal neuralgia, *Brain,* 85:371-388, 1962.

Darian-Smith, I.: Neural mechanisms of facial sensation, *Int. Rev. Neurobiol.,* 9:301-395, 1966.

Gordon, R., and Bender, M.: The corneomandibular reflex, *J. Neurol. Neurosurg. Psychiat.,* 34:236-242, 1971.

Humphrey, T.: "The central relations of the trigeminal nerve," in *Correlative Neurosurgery* (2nd ed.), Kahn, E. A., Crosby, E. A., Schneider, R. C., and Taren, J. A. (eds.), Springfield, Ill., Charles C Thomas, 1969.

Kerr, F.: The divisional organization of afferent fibres of the trigeminal nerve, *Brain,* 86:721-732, 1963.

Ross, R.: Corneal reflex in hemisphere disease, *J. Neurol. Neurosurg. Psychiat.,* 35:877-880, 1972.

Stookey, B., and Ransohoff, J.: *Trigeminal Neuralgia: its History and Treatment,* Springfield, Ill., Charles C Thomas, Publisher, 1959.

10

Examination of Somatic Sensation (Excluding the Face)

"Nature, indeed, has had a triple end in view in the distribution of nerves: she wished to give sensibility to organs of perception, movement to organs of locomotion, and to all the others the faculty of recognising the experience of injury."

— Galen (130 - 200 A.D.)

I. Introduction: The organization of general somatic sensation

A. Once you understand the Vth nerve, you understand the principles of the entire somatic sensory system.

1. There is a three-neuron path from periphery to cerebral cortex.
2. There is a variation within the three-neuron plan for the modalities of touch, pain and temperature, and proprioception. See Fig. 10-1 for the basic three-neuron plan and learn the names.
3. The primary neurons for any given spinal nerve collect on the dorsal root into a mass called a ____________________. (ganglion)
4. The primary ganglionic neuron sends a process peripherally to innervate sensory receptors each of which may detect one or more kinds of stimuli.
5. The primary neuron sends a process centrally to the central nervous system via the dorsal root to synapse on the ☐ secondary / ☐ tertiary neuron of the sensory pathway. (secondary)
6. The secondary neuron then ________________ the midline to synapse on a ☐ primary / ☐ tertiary / ☐ cortical neuron. (crosses; tertiary)
7. The tertiary neuron is located in the ________________, which relays impulses to the cerebral cortex. (thalamus)
8. A general term for a tract formed by the axons of secondary neurons as they ascend to the thalamus is ____________________. (lemniscus)
9. All somatic sensations and all special sensation, except smell, are thought to relay through a specific thalamic nucleus. With the exception of the special senses of taste and equilibrium, the relay nucleus has been identified. Thus, one of the major functions of the thala-

postcentral
parietal

mus is to relay sensory information to the somesthetic cortex located in the ______________ gyrus of the ______________ lobe.

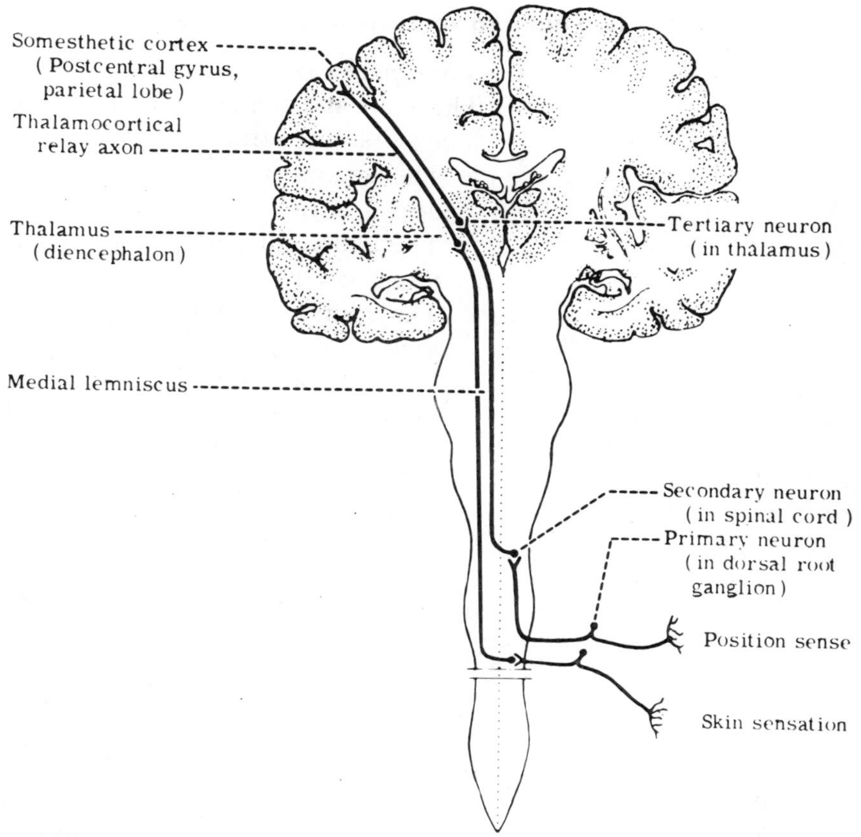

FIG. 10-1. The three-neuron plan for all somatic sensation. Start at the receptor and trace the pathway to the cerebral cortex.

contralateral

lateral geniculate

medial geniculate

ventralis posterior

ganglia
thalamus

10. Since pathways for all somatic modalities cross and then relay in the thalamus, a severe destructive lesion of the thalamus could cause loss of somatic sensation on the ☐ ipsilateral / ☐ contralateral side of the body. The thalamic nucleus which relays general somatic sensation is nucleus *ventralis posterior.*
11. The thalamic relay nucleus for sight is called the ______________ ______________ body.
    a. For hearing, a special somatic sensation, it is the ______________ ______________ body.
    b. For general somatic sensation it is the nucleus ______________.
12. All *primary* neurons for somatic sensation are located in ______________ ______________. The *tertiary* neurons are located in the ______________.
13. Therefore, to learn a sensory pathway, you only have to memorize the location of the secondary neuron. When you do so, you get this bonus: the axons from the secondary neurons decussate, and the decussation occurs just rostral to the nucleus. Hence, by knowing where the second-order neuron is you know where the lemnisci begin.

14. All general sensory impulses are relayed from the thalamus to the somesthetic cortex in the postcentral gyrus of the parietal lobe. Locate the parietal lobe in Fig. 10-1.

II. Pain and temperature sensation

A. Anatomic pathways

1. The pain and temperature pathway is given in Fig. 10-2. Learn the labels first, then trace the pathway to the cortex, noting these things.
   a. The secondary pain and temperature neuron is located in the dorsal horn.
   b. The course of pain and temperature impulses from *foot* to somesthetic cortex.
   c. The course of pain and temperature impulses from *hand* to somesthetic cortex.
   d. The pain and temperature axons from the foot and hand synapse on secondary neurons at, or within one or two segments of, their level of entry into the spinal cord, but the axons from the face descend through the brainstem to reach the secondary neuron. Review Fig. 9-13.

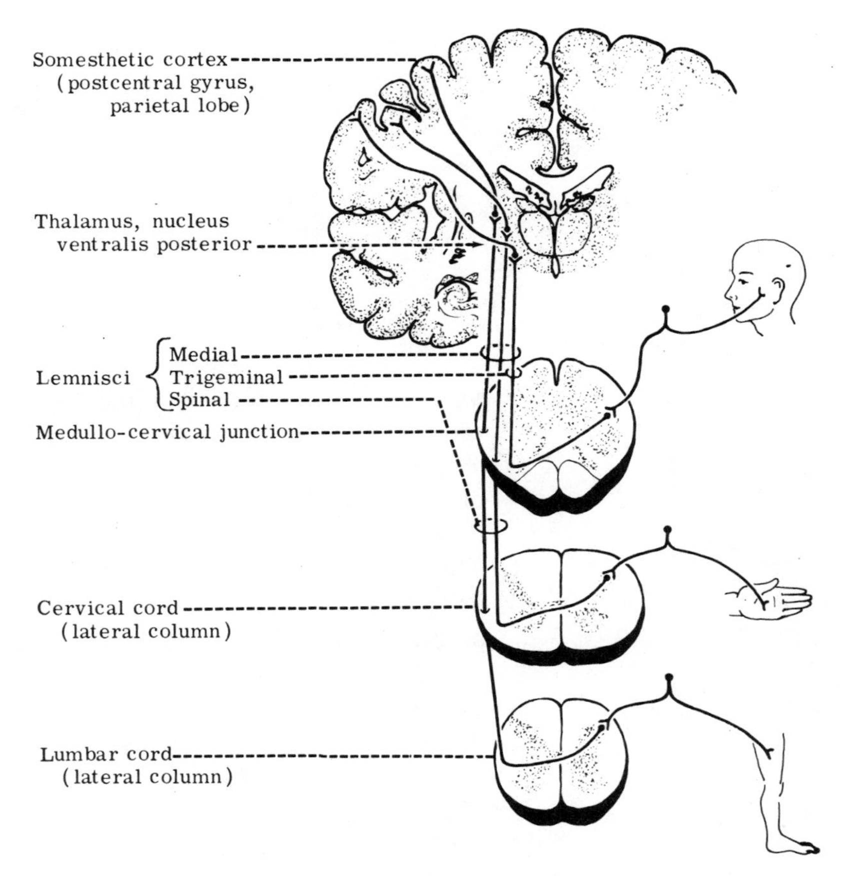

FIG. 10-2. Pathway for pain and temperature sensation from periphery to cerebral cortex.

2. The descent of the axons from the face permits the secondary nucleus to be continuous from the medulla to the last sacral segment. The

order of representation of parts in this continuous long columnar nucleus is face, neck, arm, trunk, lower extremity, and sacral region. The technical name for this nucleus is the *substantia gelatinosa of Rolando,* but you need remember only where it is and what it does.

3. The crossed axons of the secondary pain and temperature tract ascend the spinal cord in the ☐ ventral / ☐ lateral / ☐ dorsal column.

lateral

4. These ascending secondary pain and temperature axons form the lateral spinothalamic tract, which qualifies by definition as a lemniscus. Joined by the ventral spinothalamic touch pathway, the two together form the *spinal lemniscus*. Thus some of the lemnisci are:
   a. ______________________ lemniscus, which mediates facial sensation.
   b. ______________________ lemniscus, which mediates auditory sensation.
   c. ______________________ lemniscus, which mediates pain and temperature sensation through the spinal cord and brainstem.

trigeminal

lateral

spinal

5. Label the spinal lemniscus in Fig. 10-3.

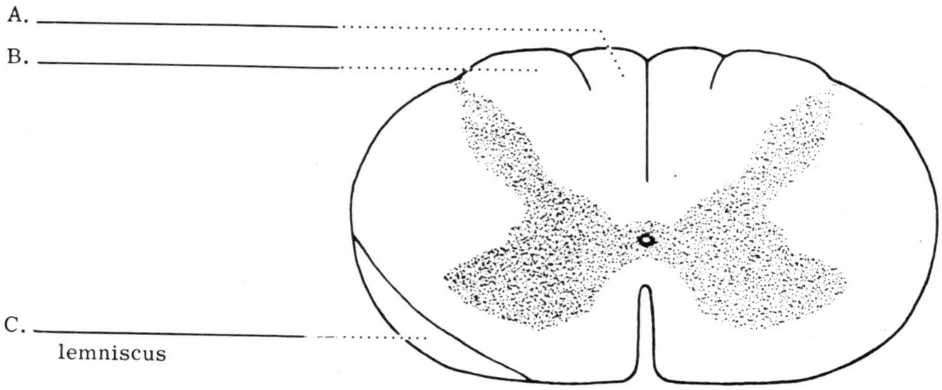

A. ______________________

B. ______________________

C. ______________________
lemniscus

FIG. 10-3. Cross section of spinal cord at fourth cervical segment. For the present, label only the spinal lemniscus.

A. Leg dorsal column (fasc. gracilis)
B. Arm dorsal column (fasc. cuneatus)
C. Spinal

6. What is the difference in the intraaxial course of the primary pain and temperature axons from the face and the rest of the body? ______________________ ______________________.

Ans: From the face, the pain and temperature axons descend through the brainstem, while from the body, the axons synapse within one or two segments of the level of entry.

7. Trace a nerve impulse for pain and temperature sensation from the skin on the lateral side of the foot to the cerebral cortex. Start by naming the dermatome: ______________________ ______________________ ______________________ ______________________.

Ans: S_1 dermatome *receptor* **to** *peripheral* **branch of dorsal root axon to** *central* **branch to** *secondary neuron* **in dorsal horn. Secondary axon crosses, ascends in**

spinal lemniscus **to** *tertiary neuron* **in n. ventralis posterior of** *thalamus.* **N. ventralis posterior relays to** *somesthetic cortex* **in postcentral gyrus of** *parietal* **lobe.**

B. Test pain and temperature on the rest of the body as described previously for the face. But now try this further experiment.

1. Make single pricks with an ordinary straight pin to compare your sensitivity on the face, dorsum of the hands and feet, and palms and soles. Does every single prick elicit pain? ________________.
2. Not every prick elicits pain. Therefore, make multiple, rapid (gentle) pricks at each test site before asking the patient to respond.
3. Discard each pin after use. I don't know how many angels can stand on the point of a pin, but at least one disease, infectious hepatitis, can.

No—and because of this the patient may give variable responses.

Bibliography

Beecher, H.: *Measurement of Subjective Responses:* Quantitative Effects of Drugs, New York, Oxford University Press, 1959.

Bonica, J. J. (ed.): International Symposium on Pain, in *Advances in Neurology, vol. 4,* New York, Raven Press, 1974.

Finneson, B.: *Diagnosis and Management of Pain Syndromes,* 2nd ed., Philadelphia, W. B. Saunders, 1969.

Fisher, C. M.: Thalamic pure sensory stroke: A pathologic study, *Neurology,* 28:1141-1144, 1978.

Hockaday, J., and Whitty, C.: Patterns of referred pain in the normal subject, *Brain,* 90:481-496, 1967.

Judovich, B., and Bates, W.: *Segmental Neuralgia in Painful Syndromes,* Philadelphia, F. A. Davis Co., 1944.

Keele, K.: *Anatomies of Pain,* Springfield, Ill., Charles C Thomas, Publisher, 1957.

Krayenbuhl, H., Maspers, P. E., and Sweet, W. H. (eds.): Pain—Its Neurosurgical Management, Part I: Procedures on Primary Afferent Neurons, in *Progress in Neurological Surgery, vol. 7,* New York, S. Karger, 1976.

Melzack, R.: Mechanisms of Pathological Pain, in *Scientific Foundations of Neurology,* Critchley, M. (ed.), Philadelphia, F. A. Davis Co., 1972.

Notermans, S.: Measurement of the pain threshhold determined by electrical stimulation and its clinical application: Part II. Clinical application in neurological and neurosurgical patients, *Neurology,* 17:58-73, 1967.

White, J., and Sweet, W.: *Pain, its Mechanisims and Neurosurgical Control,* Springfield, Ill., Charles C Thomas, Publisher, 1955.

C. Pain in the leg: nerve root compression and the leg raising (nerve root stretching) tests

1. Now consider this characteristic patient with the commonest leg pain of neurologic origin. For some time, in fact off and on for several years, this 34-year-old man has suffered from lumbosacral backache. A few weeks ago when straightening up, he felt a pop in his back, and since then he has had severe, sharp radiating pain into his foot along its lateral aspect. He sits rigidly in his chair, his trunk slightly tilted forward. When arising, he pushes himself erect with his arms. He stands with most of his weight on his unaffected leg, holding the knee of the affected leg slightly bent. The uneven weight distribution can be con-

firmed by placing your hand around his ankle with your thumb on his Achilles tendon. By squeezing firmly with your thumb, the tendon on the non-weight bearing leg yields. The Achilles reflex on that side is reduced. He has weakness of foot dorsiflexion on that side. His calf measures 1.8 cm less than the other. While such a clinical picture already points to the diagnosis of a nerve root syndrome, the leg raising tests help to confirm it. Two in number, the tests consist of the straight-knee leg raising test (Laseague's sign) and the bent-knee leg raising test (Kernig's sign).

2. *Technique of the straight-knee leg raising test (Laseague's sign):* The patient lies supine with his legs relaxed. Grasp the calf or heel of the affected limb and elevate it gently as far as possible, flexing the hip. See Fig. 10-4.

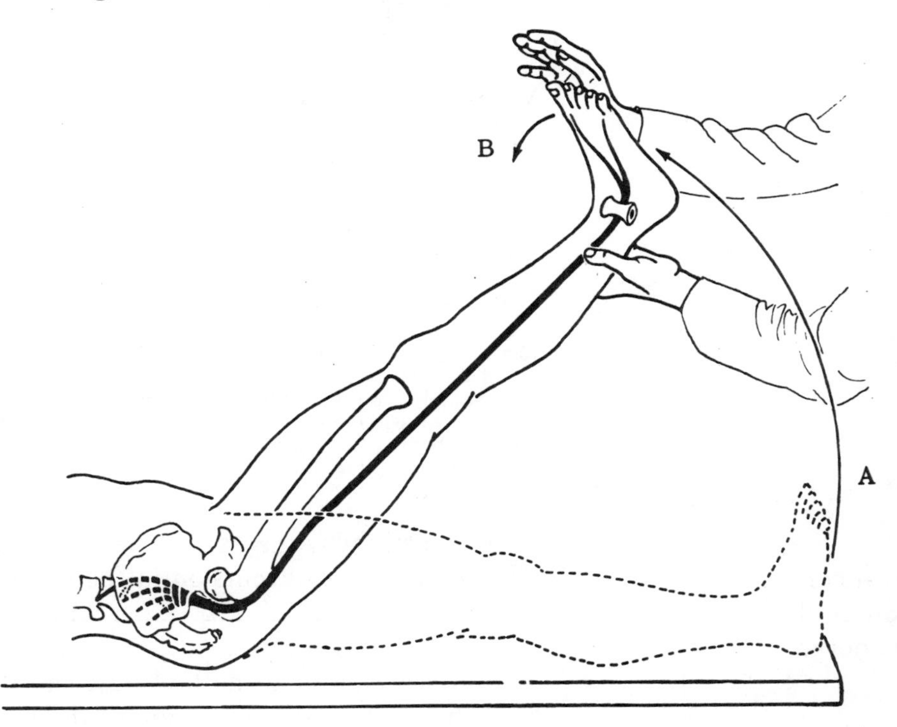

FIG. 10-4. Straight knee leg raising test. A. The examiner elevates the leg. B. He then dorsiflexes the foot. Both maneuvers stretch the sciatic nerve and elicit pain if the nerve roots are inflammed, compressed, or imprisoned by a mechanical lesion.

When you reached about 60° of elevation of the lower extremity, the patient winced with pain and flexed his knee. Then, holding the leg just short of the position of pain, gently dorsiflexing the foot brought another twinge of pain, the pain, as before, shooting into the lateral aspect of the foot. The same maneuvers on the unaffected limb produced nearly a normal range of movement, without pain.

3. *Explanation of the pain and limitation of leg elevation*

   a. Elevation of the lower extremity with the knee straight stretches the sciatic nerve. We might appropriately call it the *sciatic nerve stretching test.* As the nerve stretches, it pulls against any impediment to free movement. The resultant pain causes hamstring muscle spasm, flexing the knee and splinting against further extension, stretch, and pain. The commonest impediment by far is a ruptured intervertebral disc. See Fig. 10-5.

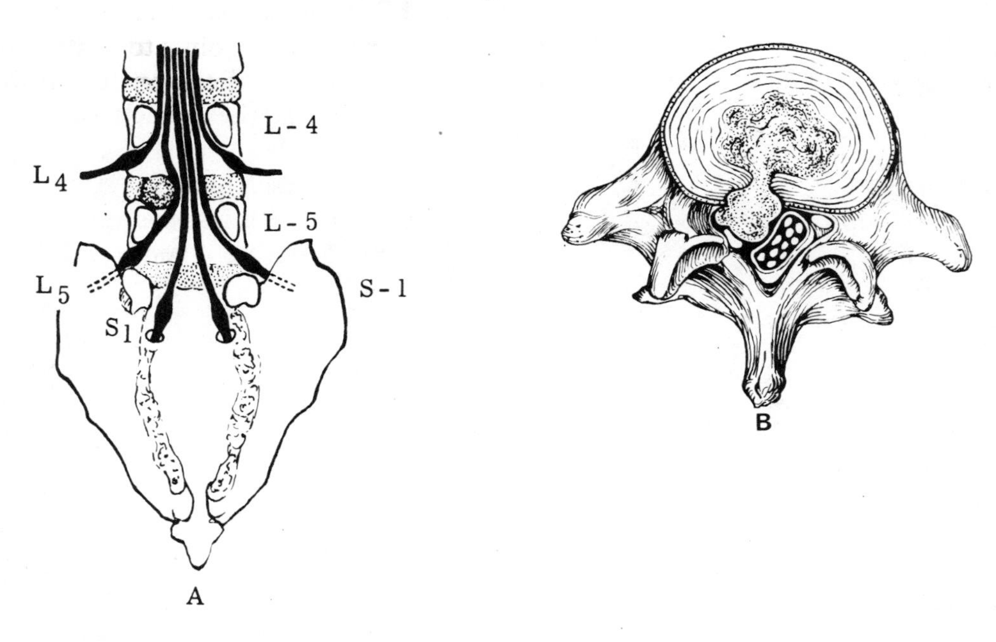

FIG. 10-5. Intervertebral disc herniation. A. Dorsal aspect of lumbosacral spine with the neural arches of the vertebrae and dura mater removed. Nerve roots labeled on the left side, vertebral bodies on the right. Notice how the nerve roots relate to the intervertebral discs and to their point of exit from the vertebral canal. The L_{4-5} disc has herniated, impinging on nerve root L_5. B. Transverse section of vertebrae L_5, as seen from above, showing disc herniation. The dural sac containing the cauda equina remains intact.

flexion relaxes tension on the sciatic nerve

b. Explain why the patient tended to flex his knee as you reached the end point of excursion in the straight-knee leg raising test? ______
____
______________________.

placed tension on the sciatic nerve

c. When you held the limb just short of maximum permissible elevation, why did dorsiflexion of the foot elicit a twinge of pain? ______
____
______________________.

flex it

d. In fact, we can interpret all the postural and movement limitations in the nerve root compression syndrome as pain protective. The splinting of the back by paravertebral muscle spasm, the flexed knee which relaxes tension on the sciatic nerve, and the limitation of straight leg raising. To prove this theory, we can do this: with the patient supine, set him up, leaving his legs flat against the bed. This action again stretches the sciatic nerve. What do you predict that the patient will do with the affected lower extremity to avoid pain? ______________________.

4. *The bent-knee leg raising test (Kernig's sign):* With the patient supine as for the straight-knee leg raising test, flex the limb at the hip while keeping the knee flexed. When the thigh reaches the vertical position, gently, *gently* straighten the knee. The patient will wince with pain,

and reflex hamstring spasm will prevent further straightening of the knee.

5. An accurate description of where the pain radiates often identifies the affected nerve root in a nerve root compression syndrome.
   a. If the patient complains that the pain radiates into his little toe or along the *lateral* side of his foot you would suspect the ____________________________ nerve root.
   b. If it radiates along the medial side of the foot or into the great toe, you would suspect the ____________________________ nerve root.

S_1 (review Fig. 7-26 if you erred.)

L_5. (Review Fig. 7-26 if you erred.)

Bibliography

DePalma, A. F., and Rothman, R. H.: *The Intervertebral Disc,* Philadelphia, W. B. Saunders Co., 1970.

Love, J.: Protruded intervertebral discs, Chapter 33 in Baker, A. and Baker, L., (eds.) *Clinical Neurology,* New York, Harper and Row, 1973.

III. Proprioception and vibration sense

A. The term *proprioception* comes from *proprius* = one's own, and *capio* = to take or capture; therefore, literally to take or capture one's own. The term refers to the capturing by receptors within the depth of one's own body the movements of one's own body parts. The body parts which move, and which movements its proprioceptive system captures, consist of one's own muscles and joints, i.e., the skeletomuscular apparatus, and one's otoliths and semicircular canal fluid, i.e., the contents of one's vestibular apparatus. Formally defined, *proprioception is the sense of movement, of position, and of skeletomuscular tension provided by deep mechanical receptors in muscles, joints, connective tissue, and the vestibular system.* And, we might add, is the system from which we obtain a sense of equilibrium. Charles Sherrington (1859-1952), to whom we owe the concept, put it this way:

> We arrived earlier at the notion that the field of reception which extends through the depth of each segment is differentiated from the surface field by two main characters. One of these was that while many agents which act on the body surface are excluded from the deep field as stimuli, an agency which does act there is mass, with all its mechanical consequences, such as weight, mechanical inertia, etc., giving rise to pressures, strains, etc., and that the receptors of this field are adapted for these as stimuli. The other character of the stimulations in this field we held to be that the stimuli are given in much greater measure than in the surface field of reception, by actions of the organism itself, especially by mass movements of its parts. . . . In many forms of animals, e.g., in vertebrates, there lies in one of the leading segments a receptor-organ (the labyrinth) derived from the extero-ceptive field of the remaining segments. This receptive organ, like those of the proprio-ceptive field, is adapted to mechanical stimuli. It consists of two selective parts, both endowed with low receptive threshold and with refined selective differentiation. One part, the otolith organ, is adapted to react to changes in the incidence and degree of pressure exerted on its nerve-endings by a little weight of higher specific gravity than the fluid

otherwise filling the organ. The other part, the semicircular canals, reacts to minute mass movements of fluid contained within it. These two parts constitute the labyrinth. . . . This system as a whole may be embraced within the one term "proprio-ceptive." (Charles Sherrington, *The Integrative Action of the Nervous System,* Yale University Press, New Haven, 1952.)

B. Anatomy of skeletomuscular proprioception

1. Learn Fig. 10-6, the skeletomuscular proprioceptive pathway. It is shared by other modalities. All modalities mediated by this pathway are called *dorsal column modalities.* Study this important pathway until you can reproduce it. First complete the labels along the left side.

* Compare your labels with Fig. 10-2

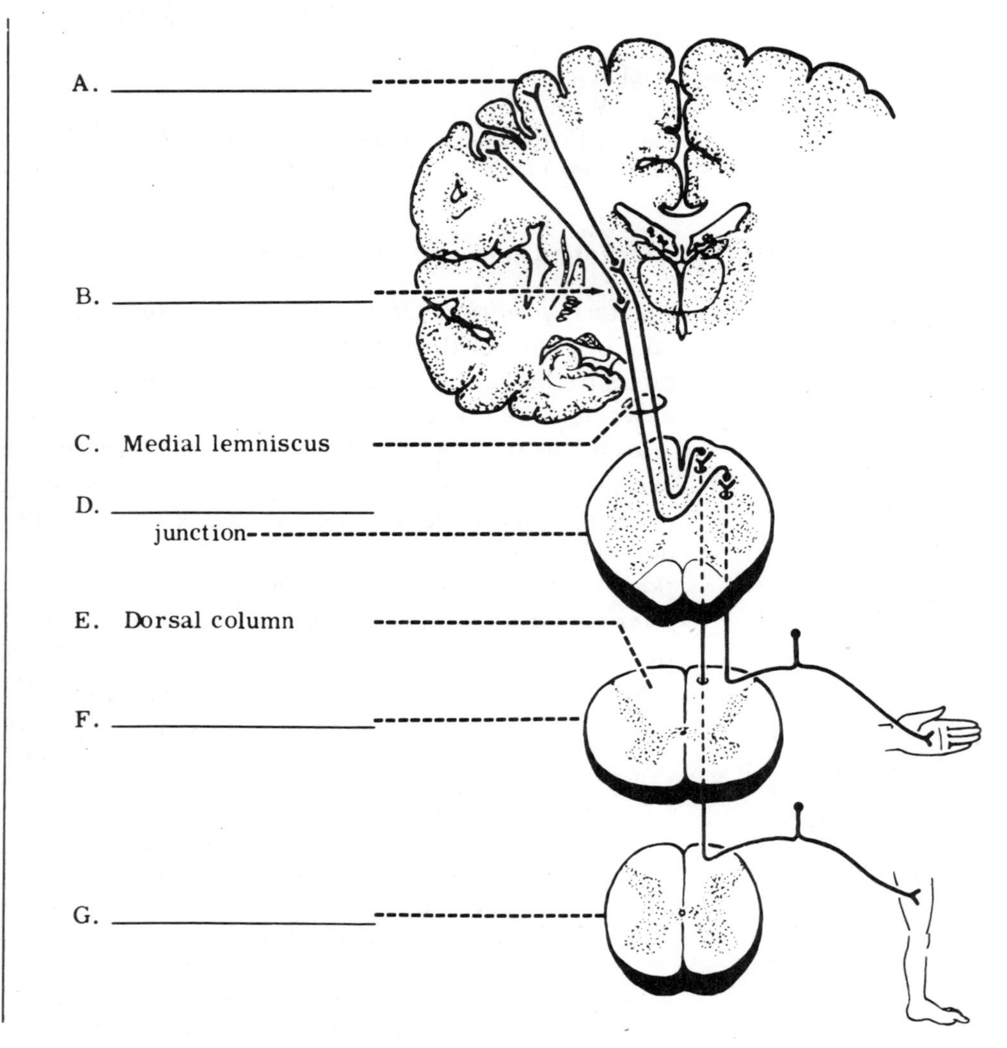

FIG. 10-6. Pathway for dorsal column modalities from periphery to cerebral cortex. Complete labels A through G.

2. Sensory physiologists disagree about the exact receptors for joint position and movement. The muscle spindles would, *a priori,* seem ideal to mediate movement, but no pathway from them to the somesthetic cortex has been found. Some or all of the numerous receptors

dorsal root ganglia

cochlear
vestibular
primary

in the connective tissue of joints and tendons are responsible. The primary proprioceptive neurons, like all primary somatic sensory neurons, are located in the ______________________.

3. Cranial verve VIII has two ganglia which are homologous to dorsal root ganglia, the ______________ ganglion and the ______________ ganglion.
4. The axons ascending in the dorsal columns are from ☐ primary/ ☐ secondary/☐ tertiary neurons.
5. From Fig. 10-6 you can see that the processes of dorsal root ganglion cells extend from the toe to the dorsal column nuclei, the remarkable distance of 170 cm in man, the astonishing distance of 450 cm in a giraffe, and the incredible distance of 2,000 cm in the blue whale.

medial

6. The axons from the foot ascend ☐ lateral to/ ☐ intermingled with/ ☐ medial to those from the arm.
   a. Label the *leg dorsal column* (fasciculus gracilis, column of Goll) and the *arm dorsal column* (fasciculus cuneatus, column of Burdach) in Fig. 10-3.
   ***b.* I prefer the terms *arm dorsal column* and *leg dorsal column,* but use the other terms, if you wish. The trouble is that 2 weeks after you lay aside the text you won't remember which is which if you use the terms *fasciculus gracilis* and *cuneatus.* The sensory homunculus in the dorsal columns is a headless man standing with his feet on the dorsal median septum, as in Fig. 10-7.

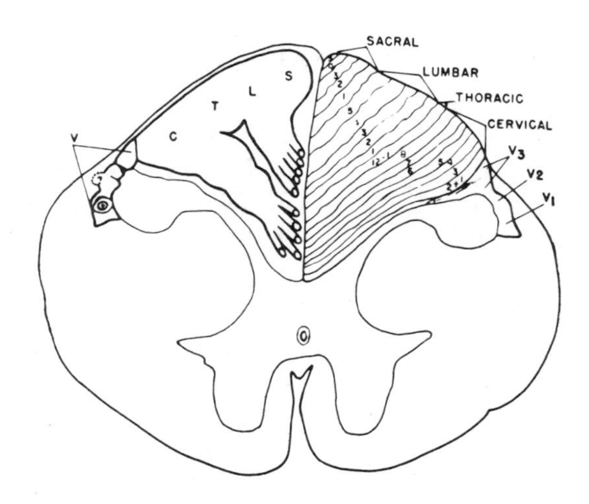

FIG. 10-7. Sensory homunculus in the dorsal column. (*From T. Humphrey: Arch. Neurol. Psychiat.,* 73:36, 1955.)

At the medullo-cervical junction

decussate

lemniscus

7. At what level of the neuraxis is the secondary neuron of the dorsal column pathway? ______________________.
8. The secondary neurons at the medullocervical junction are massed into the *dorsal column nuclei.* What happens to their axons immediately after leaving the nucleus? ______________________.
9. The decussating axons are secondary axons conveying impulses to the thalamus, impulses destined to affect consciousness. The tract they form is called a ______________ (general term).

medial

ventralis posterior

postcentral
parietal

10. The particular name of this lemniscus is the ______ lemniscus.
11. The medial lemniscus terminates in a thalamic nucleus called the nucleus ______.
12. From the nucleus ventralis posterior the pathway for the dorsal column modalities goes to the somesthetic cortex in the ______ gyrus of the ______ lobe.
13. Try the whole thing at once. Wiggle your toe and think through the pathway to the cortex by which you know your toe has wiggled. Can you draw it?

C. The general concept of dorsal column modalities

1. The dorsal columns mediate many sensations besides position and movement. In general, these sensations all depend on receptors deeply placed in the dermis and the connective tissue of the joints, tendons, and muscles. These deep receptors are attuned, as Sherrington said, to mass, inertia, pressure, and movement. Since distance is inherent in the concept of movement, we have the ingredients of classical, Newtonian mechanics. The proprioceptive sensations mediated by the dorsal columns are:
   a. Sense of position
   b. Sense of movement of joints and of body
   c. Sense of vibration
   d. Sense of pressure
2. The discriminative sensations closely allied to the mechanoreceptors and the dorsal column pathway include:
   a. Texture
   b. Localization of touch
   c. Two-point discrimination
   d. Sense of weight
   e. Sense of numbers or letters written on the skin
3. The association of these sensations as basically mechanical stimuli may seem more rational after these considerations:
   a. Vibration is easy to associate with proprioception as mediated by mechanical receptors. Recall that the cochlea, a most sensitive organ for detecting vibration, developed as the phylogenetic brother of the vestibular apparatus, a most sensitive organ for detecting position and motion. Vibration sense is merely the detection of fast changes in the pressure on and position of a minute portion of tissue, the eardrum being the most specialized example.
   b. The sense of weight is the amount of pull on the joint and connective tissue proprioceptors.
   c. To a large extent discriminative touch, such as texture, is based on minute variations in the pressure upon any area of skin. Texture is most prominent when skin is moved over the object, almost a slow vibration sense. Discrimination of characters written on the skin demands first of all the perception of the path traced by an object pressing on the skin, followed by comparison of the

pattern with memory traces. Touch, itself, involves some mechanical displacement, some pressure. Two-point discrimination is the distance between two pressure points. Localization of a touch stimulus depends on comparing the location of a pressure stimulus with the mental image of the body parts. It is essentially the problem of distance. In contrast with all the mechanical sensations of the dorsal column type, you can be burned by an object that does not even touch you, such as the sun, 93,000,000 miles away, and this sensation is mediated by lateral column pathways.

D. *Clinical testing of dorsal column modalities: Position sense*

1. *Procedure:* Position sense is tested by moving the digits of hands and feet up or down from the neutral position.
   a. With one hand, support the part to be tested. With the other hand, grasp the digit by its side and wiggle it up and down, stopping in one direction or the other randomly.
   b. While the patient's eyes are open, instruct him to report whether his finger is "Up" or "Down." This step establishes communication with the patient and reassures him that the test is benign. Then, for the actual testing, have him close his eyes and reply "Up" or "Down" as you test the digits of all four extremities.
   c. Take care not to apply different pressures or use a different tone of voice on the up or down movement. The patient may attend to the wrong stimulus.
   d. When testing position sense, the novice examiner instinctively grasps the thumb, index finger, or large toe. But the greatest challenge to the sense of position comes from using digits three and four. Fig. 10-8 shows why.

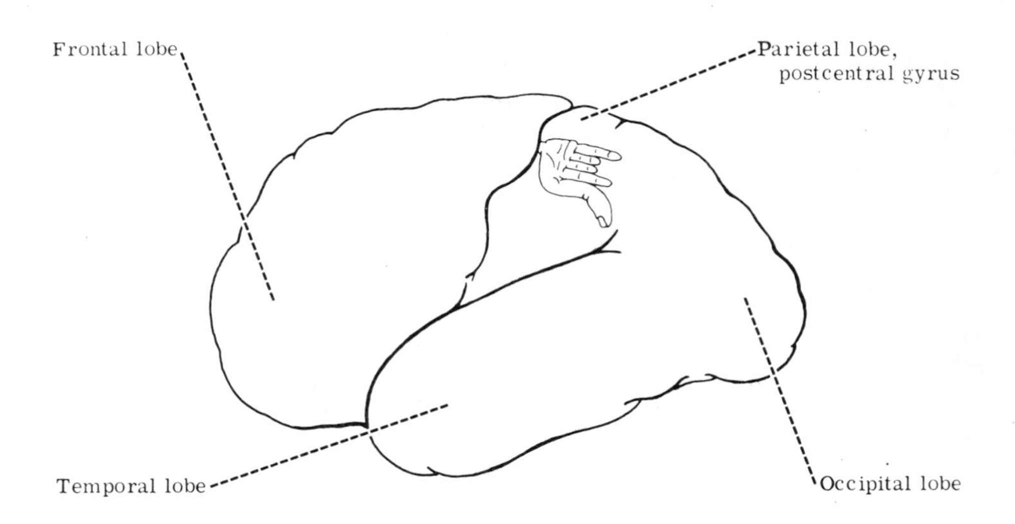

FIG. 10-8. Lateral view of left cerebral hemisphere. The right hand is projected onto the left postcentral gyrus to show the relative area devoted to each of the digits. The face projects to the area immediately inferior to the hand, the trunk and leg superior, just as the representation is in the precentral motor cortex. In reality, the motor and sensory representations somewhat overlap the central sulcus.

e. The first, second, and fifth digits of the hands and feet have the richest innervation and the largest cortical representation. Therefore, the lesion has to be relatively large to interrupt position sense of these digits. You will find it clumsy to use digits three and four, but practice according to Fig. 10-9.

f. When loss of position sense is suggested, always test several digits. Once the patient understands the test, he should make no, *no* errors. Occasionally he will become bored or carelessly reply one direction when he means the other. Immediate repetition and inquiry will disclose whether the error implies carelessness or disease.

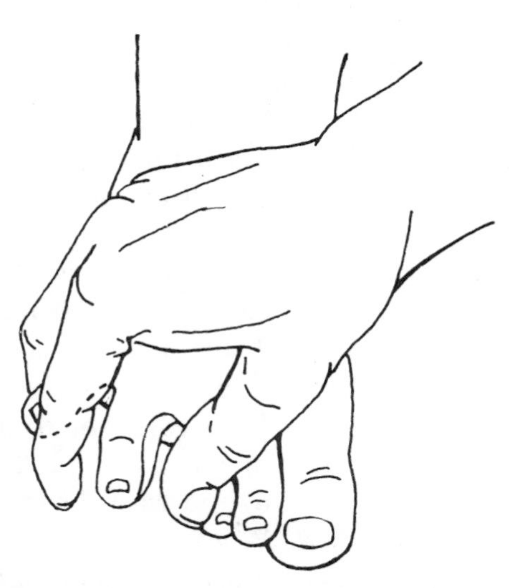

FIG. 10-9. Method of separating the digits to test position sense in the fourth toe. The toe is grasped on the sides and moved by the examiner's other hand.

2. It is convenient to have a single word to speak of loss of position sense. For the moment. we will use the term *statanesthesia* (literally *station, not feeling*).
3. *Interpretation.* The examiner who knows nothing about probability theory misinterprets the responses of the patient with mild or even complete position sense loss. Patients with statanesthesia often give an answer, because they know a reply is expected, and they try to please the examiner.

50 percent

a. If a patient has *no* position sense at all, how many times will he guess the correct direction when his digit is randomly placed up or down? ☐ 0 percent correct / ☐ 25 percent / ☐ 50 percent / ☐ 75 percent.

50

b. The situation is exactly like trying to call heads or tails in flipping a coin. Random calling of heads or tails will win 50 percent of the time, on the average. When given only two choices, up or down, the patient with no position sense at all replies correctly ________________ percent of the time.

c. Next consider impaired but not absent position sense. The patient responds correctly some times because of chance and some times because he correctly identifies the position. The novice

0

examiner may erroneously conclude that these patients are unreliable, because they miss one time and then give several correct responses. If you are satisfied that the patient has not simply made a careless error, you have to remember the rule that the normal person makes ______________ percent errors. If the patient makes even a few noncareless errors, your best interpretation is that ______________________________.

Ans: The patient's position sense is impaired; a few errors are not acceptable as normal. You still have to decide whether the patient is malingering, hysterical, or has a neurologic disease, but you can be certain that something is amiss.

d. The next question is how to reduce the probability of getting the correct answer by chance. How could you accomplish this? ______________________________.

Ans: One method is to give him three alternatives, up, down, **and** straight. **Start by wiggling the finger up and down and then stop** up, down, **or in the** neutral **position, or you can move the digit medially or laterally.**

three

e. By giving three alternatives instead of two, you reduce the chance of guessing the correct answer from one in two, to one in ________.

f. Ordinarily *two*-alternatives testing is easier and faster than *three* alternatives and is reliable. Probability theory sets the minimum numbers of trials to make in *two*-alternatives testing of position sense. You can easily flip a coin, call heads and be right, as you will expect to be one-half of the time. [In mathematical notation, ½ may be written as $(½)^1$.] Now when you try to call the coin twice in a row, the probability of being right is $(½)^2$, or one in four. The probability of calling three in a row would be (½) — or ______.

$(½)^3$
1 in 8.
doubles

g. Each time you try to stretch your luck one more time, the denominator ☐ halves / ☐ doubles / ☐ triples / ☐ quadruples. Soon the odds against chance success are astronomic. Chance success becomes not impossible, but more and more improbable. In testing position sense, the question is where to cut off the trials in order to have confidence that the patient has not succeeded by chance alone, when in fact he has no position sense.

5 trials
$(½)^5 = 1/32$,
which is less than the needed 1/20

h. Statisticians agree that when the probability of an event is one in twenty or less, chance is an unlikely explanation. Thus, in testing position sense, when chance has a 50% success rate, compute the fewest trials the patient must get right to make chance success unlikely: ______________________________.

50%

i. Some mental patients reply exactly opposite to each up or down position, *ipso facto* proving intact position sense. Even with no position sense, a patient just guessing gets ______% right by chance.

j. If position sense is normal distally, it will be normal proximally. If abnormal at the digits, work proximally to test it at the wrist or ankle to establish the severity of the loss.

k. Practice testing position sense on a normal subject, using the *two*- and *three*-alternatives methods and the third and fourth digits.

4. *A final admonition:* In some previous sensory tests, we have implicitly relied on statistical concepts. If we offer coffee as a smell stimu-

lus to an anosmic patient, some will reply because they expect to smell something. Then the question is, how many patients with anosmia will report coffee when in fact they smell nothing? Since the probability of reporting coffee is less than one in twenty, chance is an unlikely explanation for a correct answer. The same consideration holds for taste. In testing pain, we have to consider probability, as well as the fact that some pinpricks do not stimulate pain endings. Hence the patient may report no pain on a particular prick, although you stuck him. Moreover, pain thresholds vary considerably from patient to patient and age to age. Unless the novice practices sensory testing on himself and many other subjects, he fails to appreciate these variables and erroneously concludes that the patient is unreliable.

E. *Clinical testing of position sense by the swaying (Romberg) test*

1. *Procedure*

   Instruct the patient to stand with his heels together. Note whether the patient sways. Then ask the patient to close his eyes, and note whether the swaying increases. Stand up and try this test yourself. Stand on both feet and then on one foot.

2. *Results*

   a. Normal subjects will sway slightly more with the eyes closed than with them open, but they never fall.

   b. Hysterical patients may fall against a convenient support, such as a wall or the examiner, or they may bobble precariously without falling, *ipso facto* proving competent position sense.

   c. Patients with vestibulocerebellar disease may sway some with the eyes open. They will sway slightly more with the eyes closed, but usually do not fall.

   d. Patients with dorsal column lesions sway much worse with eyes closed and may fall unless supported.

3. *Interpretation*

   a. In interpreting the neurologic examination, students have more trouble with this test than with any other one, because they mistake it for a test of cerebellar function. The problem stems, as usual, from failure to analyze the test operationally. Let us see, in terms of the operations of the test, why the patient with dorsal column lesions performs poorly.

   b. After the patient has stood up and placed his feet together, the examiner has one critical comparison to make. The examiner must judge whether the patient sways more ______________________ ______________________.

   when his eyes are closed than when open

   c. Hence a definition of the swaying (Romberg) test is that we compare the degree of swaying when the patient is standing heels together, eyes open, with the degree of swaying after the eyes are closed. This is an ☐ operational / ☐ interpretational definition.

   operational

   d. The critical point in interpretation is that we test the ability of a patient to stand erect when he is deprived of visual cues, for then he must rely solely on proprioception for spatial orientation. The standing posture is maintained by the proprioceptive system (including the vestibular apparatus and cerebellum), basal ganglia, visual system, and pyramidal tracts; in short, an integrated sensorimotor complex. The critical system is the dorsal column proprioceptive system. We know this because dorsal column modality loss, as in tabes dorsalis, causes the most severe swaying with eyes closed.

e. If the patient's eyes are closed, the information required to maintain the standing posture depends on proprioceptive impulses coming through the ________________ columns of the spinal cord.

dorsal

f. Why do you ask the patient to place his heels together for the swaying test? ____

____

____

____.

Ans: Any person with difficulty in balance does worse with a narrow base. In cerebellar disease, the patient automatically compensates with a broad-based stance and gait; hence the tandem walking test. When the patient has to stand with eyes closed, the proprioceptive system is the only source of information to guide the muscular contractions which hold the body upright. The narrow base compounds his difficulty, making the test more sensitive to minimal dorsal column impairment.

g. Why do you ask the patient to close his eyes for the swaying test?

____

____

____.

Ans: To deprive him of visual information for balance and to place the sole responsibility on the proprioceptive system in the dorsal columns of the spinal cord.

h. The patients causing the most difficulty in interpreting the swaying test are hysterically rather than neurologically ill.

(1) The hysterical patient can often be diverted into performing well on the swaying test. Wait until later in the exam, after your first trials of the swaying test. Then have him put his hands straight out in front and put his feet together. Have him touch his finger to his nose, as in ordinary cerebellar testing. Then have him close his eyes. Usually he is so engrossed in the finger-to-nose task that he will maintain his posture without swaying.

(2) A positive swaying test is never the sole manifestation of hysteria. It is only one element in a pattern of psychiatric illness.

i. Just as the swaying test is never the sole manifestation of hysteria, neither is it the sole sign of dorsal column lesions. It is really only a second-best test for pathways tested more directly and specifically by digital position sense, vibration, and other modalities.

F. Clinical testing of vibratory sensation

1. *Procedure*

   a. A tuning fork (256 cps) is struck to set it vibrating. It is applied to bony eminences, such as the malleoli and the distal ends of the radii. Inquire, "Do you feel the buzz?"

   b. As usual, start with the patient's eyes open until communication is established, and then carry out the test with the patient's eyes closed. How would you monitor the patient's suggestibility and reliability in this test? ____.

Ans: Sometimes apply the tuning fork when it is not vibrating. Since the patient will hear you strike the fork to set it into motion, you should stop its vibration after striking the fork. This is accomplished by squeezing the vibrating ends.

2. Strike your tuning fork and apply it to your bony eminences, noting the approximate level of vibration when you no longer feel the buzz.

G. Cerebellar vs sensory dystaxia

sensory

The patient with sensory dystaxia substitutes visual guidance for proprioceptive guidance. When deprived of visual guidance, his performance depends solely on proprioceptors. If proprioceptive information is lacking, his movement is more dystaxic with his eyes closed.

1. Earlier, we stated that the cerebellum could equilibrate only if it had the proper proprioceptive information. If the proprioceptive system is interrupted at dorsal or vestibular roots or spinal cord, the patient has dysequilibrium. The resulting dystaxia of sensory origin must be distinguished from dystaxia of cerebellar origin.
2. In theory, lesions of the corticopontine pathways might be expected to cause dystaxia. In practice, ataxia from corticopontine pathway lesions is rare or nonexistent. Thus, we are left with two types of dystaxia: *cerebellar dystaxia* and *sensory dystaxia.*
3. Sensory dystaxia is partially compensated by visual guidance of movement. Hence, one aid in distinguishing the two types of dystaxia is to have the patient perform with eyes open and closed. Which type of dystaxia, sensory or cerebellar, would be much worse when the patient's eyes were closed? ☐ sensory / ☐ cerebellar.
   Explain: ____.
4. The most reliable differentiation comes from the pattern of cerebellar signs on the one hand, and the pattern of sensory and reflex findings on the other. Complete Table 10-1 by placing plus signs in columns 1 and 2 if the clinical finding in column 3 characterizes or is associated with the type of dystaxia.

Bibliography

Calne, D., and Pallis, C.: Vibratory sense: a critical review, *Brain,* 89:723-746, 1966.

Kornhuber, H. H. (ed.): *The Somatosensory System,* Berlin, Springer-Verlag, 1975.

Schwartzman, R., and Bogdonoff, M.: Proprioception and vibration sensibility discrimination in the absence of the posterior columns, *Arch. Neurol.,* 20: 349-353, 1969.

Sensory	Cerebellar
+	
+	
	+
+	+
+	
	+
	+
	+

TABLE 10-1. Differentiation of Sensory and Cerebellar Dystaxia.

1	2	3
Sensory dystaxia	Cerebellar dystaxia	Clinical finding
		Loss of vibration and position sense
		Areflexia
		Nystagmus
		Hypotonia
		Dystaxia much worse with eyes closed
		Decomposition of movement
		Rebound
		Dysarthria

ventral
dorsal

pain and temperature

H. Touch sensation

1. *Anatomy*

a. Touch has two pathways to the thalamus. One pathway is through the dorsal column route, shown in Fig. 10-6. The second pathway is thought to be in the ventral columns, as shown in Fig. 10-10. In Fig. 10-10, fill in the blanks on the left side before tracing the pathway.

b. Impulses mediating touch sensation may reach the thalamus by traversing either the ______________ or the ______________ columns of the spinal cord.

c. Review the location of the neuron body of the secondary neuron in Figs. 10-3, 6, and 10 before answering this frame. The pathway for touch in the ventral columns most closely resembles the pathway for ☐ pain and temperature / ☐ vibration and position sense.

d. What is the difference in the location of cell bodies of the secondary neurons for the pain and temperature and the ventral column touch pathway as contrasted with secondary neuron bodies for the dorsal column modalities? ______________ ______________.

Ans: The secondary neurons for the dorsal column modalities are gathered together at the cervicomedullary junction. For other modalities the secondary neurons are strung out along the length of the dorsal horn.

lemniscus

spinal

lateral

e. Since the secondary axons for touch ascend to the thalamus, the pathway they form may be called a ______________.

f. Since the secondary axons ascend from the spinal cord to the thalamus, they are part of the ______________ lemniscus.

g. Another name for the touch pathway through the ventral column is the *ventral spinothalamic tract.* Another name for the pain and temperature pathway through the lateral column is the ______________ *spinothalamic tract.*

A. ____________

B. ____________

C. Spinal lemniscus (joins medial lemniscus)

D. ____________ junction

E. ____________

F. ____________

*Compare your labels with Fig. 10-2.

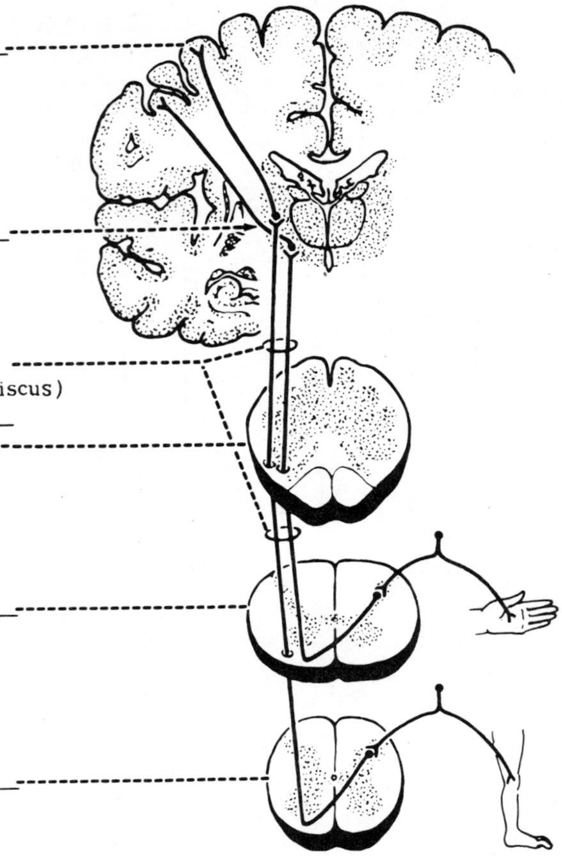

FIG. 10-10. Ventral column pathway for touch sensation. Fill in blanks A through F.

spinothalamic
spinal

h. These two tracts, the ventral and lateral ____________ tracts, taken together form the ____________ lemniscus.

i. All lemnisci unite in the brainstem to travel to the thalamus as one with the medial lemniscus. Complete Table 10-2.

Trigeminal
Lateral
Medial
Spinal

TABLE 10-2. Origin and Name of the Lemnisci

Site of origin of axons	Name of lemniscus
Trigeminal sensory nuclei	
VIIIth nerve nuclei	
Dorsal column nuclei	
Dorsal horn nuclei	

dorsal column
dorsal

j. After the spinal, trigeminal, and medial lemnisci unite, at pontine and mesencephalic levels, the single name *medial* lemniscus is used.

(1) The medial lemniscus proper, at medullary levels, carries only axons from neurons in the ____________ ____________ nuclei.

(2) These axons carry ☐ ventral / ☐ dorsal / ☐ lateral column modalities.

(3) At rostral brainstem levels three lemnisci merge under the single

medial

name of ______________ lemniscus. Thus the medial lemniscus has different components, depending on the level of the brainstem.

secondary
thalamic

k. All the lemnisci carry ☐ primary / ☐ secondary / ☐ tertiary axons to a ______________ nucleus.

l. From the thalamus, the tertiary neurons in the thalamic nucleus relay to various areas of the cerebral cortex.

postcentral
parietal

m. Touch, pain and temperature, and dorsal column modalities relay to the somesthetic cortex in the ______________ gyrus of the ______________ lobe.

occipital
temporal

n. Visual impulses relay to the ______________ lobe, and auditory impulses relay to the ______________ lobe.

lateral
lateral spinothalamic

o. If you wanted to destroy only pain and temperature sensation, you would make a cut in the ☐ ventral / ☐ lateral / ☐ dorsal column to interrupt the ______________ ______________ tract.

No

p. Neurosurgeons make just such a cut in the lateral column of the spinal cord to relieve patients of intractable pain, an operation known as cordotomy. Would a similar cut in the ventral column eliminate touch sensation? ☐ Yes / ☐ No. Explain: ______________

____

____

______________.

Ans: Touch impulses reach the thalamus by two pathways, ventral and dorsal columns. Section of only one pathway does not eliminate touch sensation.

2. *Procedure for testing touch:* The same techniques are used as in testing cranial nerve V.

a. Touch the skin lightly with a wisp of cotton. The patient responds by saying "Touch." He keeps his eyes closed, and sometimes you should not touch him when he expects you to. Do not touch the areas in a definite rhythm, or the patient may respond when he catches the beat.

b. The various skin areas have different thresholds to touch. Hairy areas and thin skin will be more sensitive than horny skin. In manual laborers, the cotton wisp may be subminimal over the palms and fingertips.

c. Practice testing yourself and a companion with a cotton wisp, with a pin, and with a tuning fork. As you test each modality, "think through" the pathway to the cerebral cortex. You must, in particular, review the location of the secondary neuron. The proof that you can "think through" these pathways is to be able to draw them.

Bibliography

DeMyer, W.: Anatomy and Clinical Neurology of the Spinal Cord, in *Clinical Neurology, vol. 3,* Baker, A. B., and Baker, L. H. (eds.), New York, Harper & Row, 1978.

Dyck, P. J., Zimmerman, I. R., O'Brien, P. C., Ness, A., Caskey, P. E., Karner, J., and Bushek, W.: Introduction of automated systems to evaluate touch-pressure, vibration, and thermal cutaneous sensation in man, *Ann. Neurol.,* 4:502-510, 1978.

Gordon, G. (ed.): Somatic and visceral sensory mechanisms, *Br. Med. J.,* 33: 89-182, 1977.

Iggo, A. (ed.): Somatosensory System, in *Handbook of Sensory Physiology, vol. II,* New York, Springer-Verlag, 1973.

Wall, P. D., and Dubner, R.: Somatosensory pathways, in *Annual Review of Physiology,* Palo Alto, Annual Reviews, Inc., 34:315-336, 1972.

Weddell, G., and Verrillo, R.: Common Sensibility, from *Scientific Foundations of Neurology,* Critchley, M. (ed), Philadelphia, F. A. Davis Co., 1972.

IV. The multimodal sensations, the gnosias or knowing sensations

A. *Introduction*

1. We can regard the discriminative sensations as requiring two stages of cortical activity.
   a. The first stage occurs in the primary cortical receptive areas which register the sensory impulses relayed through the thalamus.
   b. The second stage of events is the elaboration of the meaning or significance of the sensory impulses shuttling into the cortex. These impulses must be recognized, compared with stored memories, and finally integrated into the value system of the individual. For example, to know a dime placed in your hand in the dark, you have to recognize its disclike form, its weight, its size and texture, its metallic nature, and finally you have to realize its significance as money.
2. We know little about how the brain associates or integrates primary sensory data into its import, so that we "know" what the sensory data mean. The part of the parietal lobe behind the primary sensory cortex of the postcentral gyrus acts as the association area for somatic sensation. The association areas for sight and sound occupy the zones adjacent to their primary sensory receptive areas in the occipital and temporal lobes. These zones meet and become confluent at the parieto-occipito-temporal junction, a region called the *posterior parasylvian area*. Locate this area in Fig. 10-11.

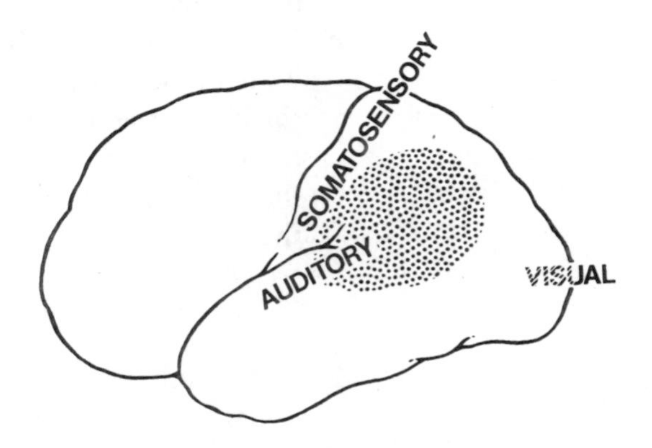

FIG. 10-11. Lateral view of the left cerebral hemisphere. The posterior parasylvian area is shaded.

B. The gnosias, the terminology of knowing

1. A clinical nomenclature of sensation has developed, based on the presumption that the elaboration of sensation into its ultimate meaning depends on association cortex. The sensations that require a high degree of cortical integration, that require a great deal of knowing, we call *gnosias*. Knowledge and gnosia are etymologically related: *diagnosis* is knowing through; *prognosis* is knowing beforehand.

statog*nosia*
station knowing
stereog*nosia*
form knowing
topog*nosia*
graphognosia

2. Sense of position (station) is called *stato-* ______________________.
3. Literally, *statognosia* means ______________________.
4. Sense of form is called *stereo-* ______________________. Literally, it means ______________________.
5. Sense of localization of a skin stimulus is *topo-* ______________________.
6. The *graphic* sense of numbers or letters written on the skin is ______________________.

nosognosia

7. Sense of awareness of a bodily defect is named by using the root *nos* for disease. Hence, nosology is the science of disease classification, and the sense of awareness of disease is ______________________.

position or station
form
place
writing
disease

8. Give the medical meaning of these roots:
   a. *Stato-* means ______________________.
   b. *Stereo-* means ______________________.
   c. *Topo-* means ______________________.
   d. *Grapho-* means ______________________.
   e. *Noso-* means ______________________.

C. The agnosias, the terminology of not knowing

an
a
not knowing

1. The negating prefix to designate lack or absence of, is ______________ before a vowel, or ______________ before a consonant. Hence agnosia literally means ______________________.

astatognosia

astereognosia
atopognosia
agraphognosia
anosognosia

2. If the patient has a gnostic defect because of a lesion in the association cortex or its circuits, we negate the term for the normal sensation:
   a. Loss of position sense, loss of statognosia, becomes *a* ______________________.
   b. Loss of form sense is ______________________.
   c. Loss of cutaneous localization is ______________________.
   d. Loss of the graphic sense is ______________________.
   e. Loss of disease awareness is ______________________.

D. Comparison of the terms to use when the lesion is in association cortex as contrasted to when the lesion is in the sensory pathways

1. Lesions may interfere with the knowing of sensory stimuli in two ways:
   a. If the lesion destroys the receptor, the sensory pathway through nerve or neuraxis, or the primary receptive cortex, the impulses cannot reach the association cortex for interpretation. The patient does not know, because his association cortex receives no impulses.
   b. If the lesion destroys the association cortex, the patient does not know, because he is unable to appreciate the significance of the impulses which reach the cortex.

anesthesia
hypoesthesia, which is contracted to hypesthesia
hyperesthesia
hypalgesia
hyperalgesia

2. How to name a sensory loss to indicate the level of the lesion along the sensory pathway:
   a. If, for example, a peripheral nerve or the spinal cord is cut, the complete loss of sensation is called ________ *esthesia.* If sensation is merely reduced it is *hyp* ________________. Sometimes sensation is excessive, as with an inflamed nerve, and it is called ________ *esthesia* (the opposite of hypo).
   b. Similarly, complete lack of pain sensation is analgesia, reduced pain sensation is ________________, and excessive pain sensation is ________________.
   c. If, for example, position sense is lost because of a lesion in the pathway between receptor and primary sensory cortex, the sensory loss is called *statanesthesia.* If it is lost because of a lesion of the association cortex or its connections with primary sensory cortex, it is called ________________.
   d. If a patient has no hearing because his VIIIth nerve is interrupted he has ☐ deafness / ☐ auditory agnosia.
   e. If a patient has hemianopsia from a lesion in his calcarine cortex, he is said to have ☐ blindness / ☐ visual agnosia in that field of vision.
   f. Explain why we say the patient in *e* is blind, rather than having visual agnosia: ____
   ____
   ____.

astatognosia

deafness

blindness

Ans: Since the lesion is in the calcarine cortex, in the primary receptive area, not in the association cortex, the primary impulses for vision cannot get to association cortex for interpretation. It is improper to diagnose agnosia if impulses fail to reach the association cortex.

   g. It might be supposed that astereognosia would be used to mean complete lack of form perception and hypostereognosia would be used to mean diminished form perception, as in anesthesia and hypesthesia. But not even neurologists like such cumbersome terms as hypostereognosia, and in practice the prefixes *a* or *an* mean either absent or diminished gnostic sensation. Since we do not find a heightened sense of gnosia, as in *hyperesthesia,* the prefix *hyper* is not used with gnosias.

E. Testing for astereognosia

1. Form sense is tested by placing common objects in the patient's hands to be identified without the aid of vision. The patient is given no clue as to what the item is. He is simply instructed to feel it and to identify it.
2. The best items are keys, safety pins, paper clips, and coins. The coins may be a penny, dime, nickle, and quarter. The penny and dime are especially hard to distinguish, and the normal person may miss occasionally.
   a. Stereognosia requires intact touch, position sense, and finally synthesis of the primary modalities into the concept of key, coin, or pin.
   b. Hence, all pathways from the receptor to the parietal cortex must

left

stereoanesthesia

association cortex

statanesthesia

be intact. If you place the object in the patient's right hand you are testing his ☐ left / ☐ right parietal lobe.

3. If the patient has lost his sense of form because of a lesion in the periphery, spinal cord, brainstem, or thalamus, the term *astereognosia* is incorrect. The correct term is *stereo* ______________.
4. The term *agnosia* is correct only if the lesion is in the ☐ nerve / ☐ spinal cord / ☐ brainstem / ☐ thalamus / ☐ association cortex.
5. If a patient has lost position sense because of a spinal cord lesion, the sensory deficit is called ______________.

F. Testing for topognosia and autotopognosia

1. Topognosia is the ability to localize skin stimuli. Autotopognosia is the ability to recognize and orient one's body parts. Autotopognosias such as finger localization (finger gnosia) and right-left orientation become demonstrable in 5 to 6-year-old children. Parietal lobe lesions cause finger agnosia and right-left disorientation.
2. *Method of testing for finger agnosia and right-left disorientation:*
   a. Work out a system of finger identification with the patient. Numbering the fingers 1 to 5 on each hand, beginning with the thumb, is usually the best. The patient closes his eyes. The examiner randomly touches digits on the right or left hand and asks the patient to identify the finger and whether it is the right or left hand. If the patient seems to have right-left disorientation, further commands can be given, such as "Touch your right hand to your left ear," to verify the deficit.
   b. Finger localization is a type of autotopognosia which is easy to test and is sensitive to brain lesions.
3. *Interpretation:*
   a. Agnosias signify lesions of the association areas which extend from the primary sensory receptive areas. For somatic agnosias like atopognosia, the relevant association area extends posterior to the primary somatic sensory receptive area located in the ______________ gyrus of the ______________ lobe.
   b. Finger agnosia and right-left disorientation are commoner with *left* parietal lobe lesions than *right*. The reason for this difference is unclear.
4. *Two-point discrimination:* Discrimination of two points from one when the skin is touched with the tips of calipers is a cortical function closely allied to topognosia. Since two-point discrimination varies with the part of the body tested and the age of the patient, it requires a chart of normal values. It is too time-consuming to be part of the ordinary clinical examination, but it may be used to explore the validity of questionable parietal lobe sensory deficits.

postcentral
parietal

G. Testing for agraphognosia

1. Numbers or letters are traced on the skin of the palm or fingertips. The patient identifies the character with his eyes closed.
   a. The normal person rarely misses the stimulus. The uneducated person, or one unpracticed in numbers, may have some difficulty not due to a brain lesion.

right parietal

graphanesthesia

b. What lobe of the brain do you test in testing for agraphognosia in the left hand? ☐ right/ ☐ left ________________ lobe.

c. In a patient unable to recognize letters written on his skin, whose lesion had destroyed sensory pathways in the brainstem or spinal cord, the correct term would be ________________.

H. Testing for anosognosia

1. Josef Babinski (1857 - 1932) introduced the term *anosognosia* to describe a patient who had left hemiplegia and left-sided sensory loss and who was unaware of his neurologic deficit. The term has been used more generally, but is best restricted to a patient whose brain lesion prevents him from recognizing his deficit. Anosognosia is seen in greatest clarity with right parietal lobe lesions, as originally described by Babinski. It is unusual with left parietal lesions. The reason for this right-left difference is unknown.
2. The most dramatic test is this: Stand on the left side of the patient's bed. Place his hemiplegic arm on the bed, alongside of him. Lay your own arm across his waist. Request him to reach over and pick up his left hand. He will feel across his abdomen, grasp your hand and hold it aloft, triumphantly as it were, never realizing his error. If you ask him whether he can move his arm, he will reply, "Yes," even though it is completely hemiplegic. It is to this unawareness of the deficit that the term ________________ is applied.

anosognosia

I. Testing for tactile inattention

1. In visual field testing, patients sometimes fail to attend to one of two simultaneous stimuli. The same sensory inattention occurs with hearing and with touch or pain.
2. *Method:* Ask the patient to close his eyes and to report where he is touched. Tell him you may touch him in more than one place. Using light pressure, brush the dorsum of both of his hands simultaneously with the tips of your index fingers. The patient reports what he feels. Then alternate, randomly touching only one hand or both, until you determine whether the patient feels both stimuli. Next test cheeks and feet.
3. *Interpretation*
   a. Inattention to simultaneous stimuli is most prominent with right parietal lobe lesions. It is most useful when the lesion spares the postcentral gyrus and its pathways from the thalamus, leaving the sensory thresholds but little altered. If the sensory thresholds are disturbed, the sensory defect is apt to be hypesthesia rather than sensory inattention.
   b. Just why inattention is more common with right parietal lesions is unknown. The patient with such a lesion *inattends* to stimuli from the ☐ right/ ☐ left side when both sides are stimulated. Occasionally, with left parietal lesions, the patient will not attend to the right side on simultaneous stimulation.

left

4. In summary, lesions of *either* parietal lobe may cause contralateral

right

left

astereognosia, astatognosia, agraphognosia, and atopognosia, but inattention and anosognosia are commoner with ☐ right / ☐ left parietal lobe lesions.

5. In contrast, finger agnosia and right-left disorientation are commoner with ☐ right / ☐ left parietal lobe lesions.

J. Practice testing all the parietal lobe gnostic functions on a normal subject

Bibliography

Bender, M.: *Disorders in Perception, with Particular Reference to the Phenomena of Extinction and Displacement,* Springfield, Ill., Charles C Thomas, Publisher, 1952.

Benton, A.: *Right-Left Discrimination and Finger Localization; Development and Pathology,* New York, Hoeber Medical Division, Harper & Row, Publishers, 1959.

Critchley, M.: *The Parietal Lobes,* New York, Hafner Publishing Company, 1966.

Heimburger, R., DeMyer, W., and Reitan, R.: Implications of Gerstmann's syndrome, *J. Neurol. Neurosurg. Psychiat.,* 27:52-57, 1964.

Poeck, K., and Orgass, B.: An experimental investigation of finger agnosia, *Neurology,* 19:801-807, 1969.

Reed, J.: Lateralized finger agnosia and reading achievement at ages 6 and 10, *Child Develop.,* 38:213-220, 1967.

Weinstein, E. A., and Friedland, R. P. (eds.): Hemi-inattention Syndromes and Hemisphere Specialization, in *Advances in Neurology, vol. 18,* New York, Raven Press, 1977.

V. The lobes of the cerebrum

A. We have now reached a point where a closer look at the anatomy of the cerebrum is necessary. Celsus around A.D. 25 stated, ". . . nor can a diseased portion of the body be treated by one who does not know what that part is." This principle remains true today.

B. Learn the names on Fig. 10-12 and the lobes.

C. Subdivisions of the hemispheres into lobes

central

central

frontal
temporal

1. The posterior margin of the frontal lobe is marked by the plane of the ______________ sulcus.
2. The anterior margin of the parietal lobe is marked by the plane of the ______________ sulcus.
3. Notice in Fig. 10-12*B* that the Sylvian fissure extends anterior and posterior to the plane of the central sulcus. In its anterior part, the Sylvian fissure divides the ______________ lobe above from the ______________ lobe below.

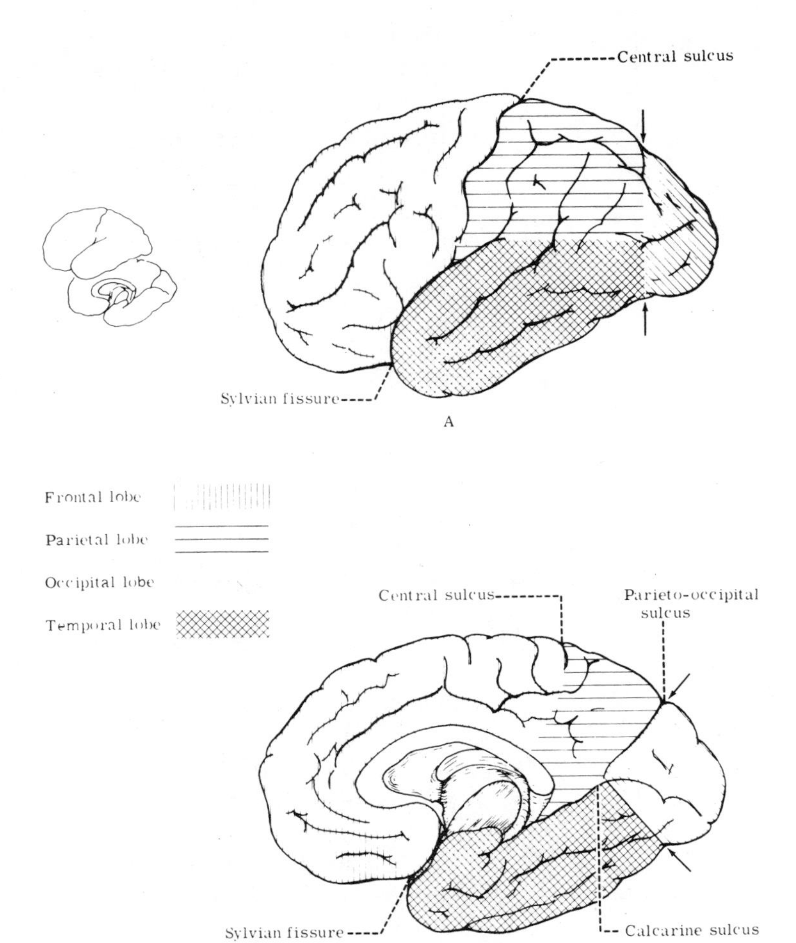

FIG. 10-12. Lobes of the cerebrum. The two cerebral hemispheres have been separated. A. Lateral view of the left cerebral hemisphere. B. Medial view of the right cerebral hemisphere. The arrows in A and B indicate the superior and inferior pre-occipital notches. Label these notches.

parietal temporal	4. In its posterior part, the Sylvian fissure divides the ______ lobe above from the ______ below.
Sylvian	5. On the medial surface, the frontal and temporal lobes are divided by the same fissure as laterally, the ______ fissure.
parietal temporal	6. On the lateral surface, the superior part of the occipital lobe is continuous anteriorly with the ______ lobe, and inferiorly with the ______ lobe.
superior pre-occipital inferior pre-occipital	7. On the lateral surface, the occipital lobe is arbitrarily divided from the parietal and temporal lobes by a line drawn from the ______ notch to the ______ notch.
	8. Taking the midpoint of the line connecting the pre-occipital notches, how do you divide the parietal from the temporal lobe? ______ ______.

Ans: Draw a perpendicular line until it meets the Sylvian fissure.

parieto-occipital

Connect the inf. pre-occipital notch with the junction of the calcarine and parieto-occipital fissures.

parietal

9. On the medial surface of the hemisphere, the occipital lobe is divided from the parietal lobe by a natural boundary, the ____________ ____________ sulcus.
10. Describe how to divide the occipital and temporal lobes on the medial aspect of the hemisphere: ____.
11. If necessary, review Fig. 10-12 before trying to answer this question: If you know one lobe completely, you can fairly well define the boundaries of all lobes. The key lobe is the ____________ lobe.
12. Complete Fig. 10-13*A* and *B* by drawing in the lines which define the parietal, frontal, occipital, and temporal lobes.

* Compare with Fig. 10-12.

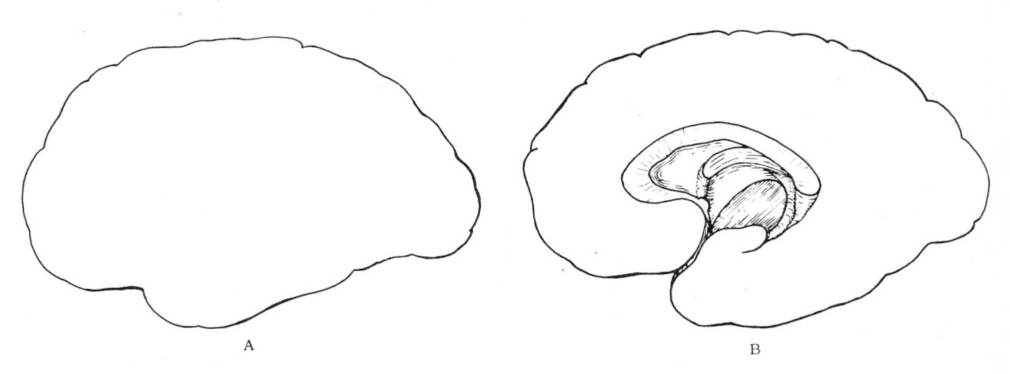

FIG. 10-13. Blank for drawing the boundaries of the frontal, parietal, occipital, and temporal lobes. Shade the lobes with different colors after establishing boundaries. A. Lateral view of the left cerebral hemisphere. B. Medial view of right cerebral hemisphere.

D. The fifth lobe

1. To the traditional lobes, Paul Broca (1824 - 1880) added another lobe of the brain, the limbic lobe. It is shown in Fig. 10-14.

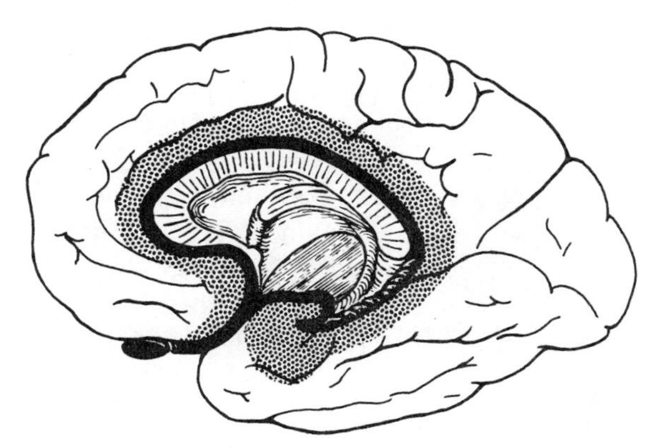

FIG. 10-14. Medial view of left cerebral hemisphere to show the olfactory lobe (black shading) and limbic lobe (light stipple).

limbus

2. Notice that this lobe encircles the junction of the hemispheric wall with the midline structures. Such a junction, as of cornea with sclera at the periphery of the iris, is called a ____________.

limbic

Hence, the junction zone marked in Fig. 10-14 is called the ________ lobe.

3. A sixth lobe can be recognized, the olfactory lobe, as shown in black shading in Fig. 10-14. It and the limbic lobe are sometimes included in the rhinencephalon, but to each his own: every author has a different definition of these structures.
4. The limbic lobe is regarded as being phylogenetically old and originally derived from the olfactory system. It is closely linked anatomically with the hippocampal formation and hypothalamus. You will hear much about this portion of the brain and its pathways as the anatomic substrate of emotion. The hippocampus and its circuits are thought to have special significance for recent memory. At the present time, some clinical use can be made of these speculations, because some disease processes, such as herpes simplex encephalitis, have a predilection for the inferior medial aspect of the temporal lobe. These patients often have disturbances in emotional expression and recent memory, but so do patients with diffuse cerebral disease. In rabies the virus strongly attacks the hippocampus, and emotionality, such as hydrophobia, is prominent in association with the throat spasms of the disease. Deep midline neoplasms, such as gliomas of the septum pellucidum, hippocampus-fornix, and corpus callosum also frequently cause hyperemotionality and loss of recent memory—but so do diffuse cortical diseases. The controversial nature of the limbic lobe and the uncertain clinical correlations go beyond our scope. It is a fascinating chapter, and you are invited into the literature by these authors:

Bibliography

Adey, W.: Recent studies of the rhinencephalon in relation to temporal lobe epilepsy and behavior disorders, *Int. Rev. Neurobiol.,* 1:1-46, 1959.

Alajouanine, Th.: *Les Grandes Activités du Rhinencéphale,* 2 vols., Paris, Masson, 1961.

DiCara, L. V. (ed.): *Limbic and Autonomic Nervous Systems Research,* New York, Plenum, 1974.

Drachman, D., and Arbit, J.: Memory and the hippocampal complex. II. Is memory a multiple process? *Arch. Neurol.,* 15:52-61, 1966.

Hockman, C.: *Limbic System Mechanisms and Autonomic Function,* Springfield, Ill., Charles C Thomas, 1972.

Livingston, K. E., and Hornykiewicz, O. (eds.): *Limbic Mechanisms: The Continuing Evolution of the Limbic System Concept,* New York, Plenum, 1978.

Malamud, N.: Psychiatric disorder with intracranial tumors of limbic system, *Arch. Neurol.,* 17:113-123, 1967.

Reitan, R.: Problems and prospects in studying the psychological correlates of brain lesions, *Cortex,* 2:127-154, 1966.

Victor, M., et al: Memory loss with lesions of hippocampal formation, *Arch. Neurol.,* 5:244-263, 1961.

White, L.: A morphologic concept of the limbic lobe, *Int. Rev. Neurobiol.*, 8:1-34, 1965.

Yakovlev, P. I.: A Proposed Definition of the Limbic System, in Hockman, C. H. (ed.): *Limbic System Mechanisms and Autonomic Function,* Springfield, Illinois, Charles C Thomas, 1972.

Zeman, W., and King, F.: Tumors of the septum pellucidum and adjacent structures with abnormal affective behavior: an anterior midline structure syndrome, *J. Nerv. Ment. Dis.*, 127:490-502, 1958.

VI. Steps in the clinical analysis of a sensory complaint

If the patient has a sensory complaint, consider these points:

A. *Inquire whether the complaint is intermittent or constant*

B. *Inquire about any factors or maneuvers which exacerbate or relieve the complaint.* Ask the patient his opinion as to the cause for his complaint. Frequently you will learn that the patient suffers from fears of cancer or some other dread malady, and you can handle his anxieties better. Even if you learn nothing of immediate clinical value, the patient will appreciate your interest in his observations and opinions. Have the patient demonstrate for you any postures or maneuvers which he thinks exacerbate his complaint.

C. *Ask the patient himself to delineate the area of pain or sensory loss.* If intelligent, observant, and non-psychiatric, he will map it out as well or better than you can with pin and cotton, and much more quickly.

D. *Before each test, establish communication.* Don't equivocate, yet don't suggest response. Ask for "Yes" or "No" responses, or "Is [stimulus] 1 different from [stimulus] 2?"

E. *Isolate modality to be tested from other sensory modalities*

F. *Monitor suggestibility and attentiveness of the patient*

G. *Draw the area of deficit on the patient or on a diagram.* Delineate the borders only as sharply as the results warrant. Repeat the examination on another day to test the reproducibility of the deficit.

H. *Think through the anatomic pathway for the modality.* Know the location of the secondary sensory neuron.

I. *Make a decision on the probable distribution of the sensory complaint as shown in Fig. 10-15.*

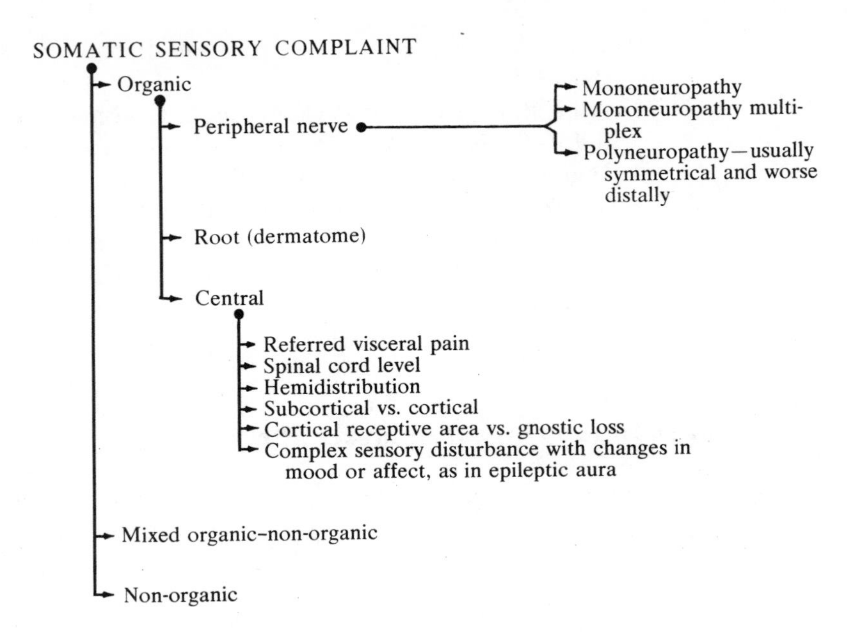

FIG. 10-15. Consider these possibilities to classify the probable nature of the patient's sensory complaint.

VII. Summary of somatic sensory testing

Rehearse section VII, steps A to D, and section VIII, step A, of the Summarized Neurological Examination.

11

The Patient's Mental Status and Higher Cerebral Functions

As not only the disease interested the physician, but he was strongly moved to look into the character and qualities of the patient. . . . He deemed it essential, it would seem, to know the man, before attempting to do him good.

– Nathaniel Hawthorne

I. The mental status examination: a nonprogrammed interlude

A. *Introduction*

1. Most of the information for judging the patient's mental status comes as a natural fallout from the medical history, which is not our primary concern in this text. Moreover, while a rigid routine is advisable for the basic physical examination, the patient's mental status is probed unobtrusively and flexibly. If you blurt out specific questions obviously designed to test the mental status, such as "Do you hear voices," you may frighten and silence a patient who already has fears of insanity. Yet just such a question introduced at the proper time encourages a free discussion of distressing mental experiences, and the patient discloses the voice that repeats, "You have the duty to kill your family." *This is the first point: Technique is everything.*
2. Access to the patient's thoughts cannot be gained by an objective observer, secretly watching the patient's behavior through a one-way glass. An examiner acts as a sounding board, a catalyst, to elicit the patient's mental experiences. To the extent that the examiner's attitudes and techniques determine what the patient says, this part of the examination is subjective and delicate. A mentally disturbed patient may permit you to do a complete physical examination, while at the same time he will strongly resist premature inquiries designed to disclose his stream of thought. This is the second point: Do not try to learn too much too fast.

3. The patient's responses determine the interview technique to use and how far to try to go. As long as the patient talks productively, continue along the line of inquiry. Stop if the patient changes the subject or becomes hostile, evasive, flustered, or silent. You have pressed too hard. The patient does not feel ready to talk about that subject. Patients will talk about whatever problems and anxieties they think about, if they can tolerate the thought and its communication. This is the third point: patients will discuss whatever they need to discuss and can discuss, if you provide a free opportunity.

B. Goals of the mental status examination

1. Consideration for the patient's feelings prevents you from following a strict routine in the mental status examination. However, you must keep the goals of the mental status examination in mind. Without the structure provided by an outline of goals, you will omit or fail to explore areas of inquiry that may provide critical diagnostic information. Thus, learn the goals of the mental status examination listed in Table 11-1.

TABLE 11-1. *Outline of Mental Status Examination*

I. *General behavior and appearance.*	Is the patient normal, hyperactive, agitated, quiet, immobile? Is the patient neat or slovenly? Does the patient dress in accordance with age, peers, sex, and background?
II. *Stream of talk.*	Does the patient converse normally? Is the speech rapid, incessant, under great pressure, or is it slow and lacking in spontaneity? Is the patient discursive and unable to reach the conversational goal?
III. *Mood and affective responses.*	Is the patient euphoric, agitated, inappropriately gay, giggling, or silent, weeping, and angry? Does the mood swing in a direction appropriate to the subject matter of the conversation? Is the patient emotionally labile?
IV. *Content of thought.*	Does the patient have illusions, hallucinations or delusions, and misinterpretations? Is the patient preoccupied with bodily complaints, fears of cancer or heart disease, or other phobias? Does the patient suffer delusions of persecution and surveillance by malicious persons or forces?
V. *Intellectual capacity.*	Is the patient bright, average, dull, or obviously demented or mentally retarded?
VI. *Sensorium.*	A. Consciousness B. Attention span C. Orientation for time, place, and person D. Memory, recent and remote E. Fund of information F. Insight, judgment, and planning G. Calculation.

2. Since many of the items in the mental status examination properly belong to psychiatric history, we will here concern ourselves only with those parts of special significance for organic disease, mainly those portions of the examination encompassed by the term *sensorium.*

C. The sensorium

1. *Introduction to the concept of a sensorium:* For as long as we have had a written history, undoubtedly for as long as we have contemplated ourselves, we have realized that somehow, somewhere within the body a mechanism integrates all the senses, all the memories, all the hopes and desires into a stream of consciousness. The locus of this mechanism, the sensorium, which receives and integrates all the impressions of the indi-

vidual senses, has long been a mystery. To Aristotle (384-322 B.C.) it was the heart. In his *De Partibus Animalium,* he stated, "For the heart is the first of all the parts to be formed; and no sooner is it formed than it contains blood. Moreover the motions of pleasure and pain, and generally of all sensations plainly have their source in the heart and find in it their ultimate termination." Even today we speak of a person in love as having an affair of the heart, or we speak of a person who lacks tender sensibilities as one who has no heart, no organ for a sensorium. Aristotle's confusion on this point is understandable if we realize that in the Athens of his time, human dissection was forbidden. He probably never dissected a human body or saw the human brain in situ, nor was he clear about the difference between nerves and tendons. But even his successor, Theophrastus (371-287 B.C.), cast doubt on the master's locating the sensorium in the heart. The Egyptians, across the Mediterranean, with thousands of years of experience in human dissection, if only for embalming, were free from the Athenian taboos. In Egyptian Alexandria, Herophilus (about 300 B.C.), who was probably only a boy when Aristotle died, located the sensorium in the calamus scriptorius of the fourth ventricle. Another Alexandrian, Erasitratus (310-250 B.C.), opposing on principle the views of his dogmatic senior, Herophilus, shifted the site to the cerebellum, but suggested that the superior intelligence of man was due to the richness of his cerebral cortical convolutions. Nevertheless, Aristotle's views prevailed for 400 years, until the time of Galen (A.D. 130-200?). Galen, apparently during his period of study in Alexandria, resurrected the doctrines of Herophilus and Erasitratus, and from them and his own researches, established forever the brain as the site of the sensorium. *(K. Keele: Anatomies of Pain, Springfield, Ill., Charles C Thomas, Publisher, 1957.)*

In retrospect, it would almost seem as if these early seekers, who suggested that all the individual sensory impressions had to be knit into a single sensorium, anticipated modern studies in sensory deprivation. If a person is kept in a stimulus-free environment, in absolute darkness, with no sound, at constant temperature, with no environmental fluctuation whatsoever, he finds that his sensorium weakens. His thoughts become loosened, detached; he hallucinates; he alternately is bored, then frightened. We can predict that if he were isolated long enough, his sensorium would disintegrate completely. The sensorium requires incessant change, the interplay of light and dark, sound and silence, pain and pleasure, if it is to function. The philosophic ideal of pure thought, free from the fetters of the flesh and its environment, is exposed as a fraud. The sensorium does not function free-floating as a cloud. It functions in respect to particular environments. Thus, in a classroom you behave differently than in a swimming pool, and you survive in both.

We can now offer an interpretational definition of the sensorium commune. *The sensorium commune is the mechanism for consciously perceiving ongoing events, relating them to past experiences, current circumstances, and future goals, and responding with behavior appro-*

priate to one's role in life. Indeed, historically, the term *common sense* derives from the intuition that all normal human beings share this common sense of who, when, where, and what they are, what is happening in daily affairs, and how to respond appropriately.

We can summarize the goal of testing the patient's common sense in one simple question: Does the patient know what's going on? Does the patient know the score? The next section outlines how to find out.

D. *Examination of the sensorium*

1. *Consciousness.* To start with the most elemental consideration, let us ask whether you can make an intelligent response to environmental stimuli when you are asleep. Obviously not. Therefore, the sensorium is a property of the waking, conscious state. For the moment, we will define consciousness interpretatively as awareness of self and environment. (Chapter 13 discusses operational tests of consciousness.) Is the patient aware of self and environment?
2. *Attention span.* If the first aspect of a sensorium is consciousness, the second is attentiveness, the attention span of the individual. Can the patient attend to stimuli sufficiently to comprehend them?
3. *Orientation.* If conscious and attentive, does the patient comprehend *who* he or she is, *where* he or she is, and *when* it is. This orientation as to person, place, and time depends on the ongoing sensory impressions. Have you ever awakened from a deep sleep to find that momentarily you did not know the day, the hour, or where you were? Weren't your mental functions impaired until you became oriented, until all the pieces of the puzzle suddenly fell into place? To judge this function of the sensorium, we find out whether the patient is oriented:
   a. As to *person:* Does the patient recognize him or herself and role as a patient and recognize other people, their roles, and yours as a doctor?
   b. As to *place:* Does the patient understand the nature and geography of the place? Does the patient recognize that he or she is in a hospital, its name, and the name of the city and state?
   c. As to *time:* Does the patient know the time of day, day of week, month, and year?
4. *Memory.* Memory is closely intertwined with orientation and attention. For crude screening purposes appraise it this way:
   a. By noticing how well the patient recalls and relates the events of the medical history.
   b. By inquiring, "Have you been concerned about your memory," or more bluntly, "How has your memory been?" If this appraisal suggests a memory disturbance, say to the patient, "Suppose we try out your memory?" and give him a name, an address, and a color to remember, items that bear no special resemblance to each other. Have the patient repeat the items, to be sure that they have registered with him. Then, at a later time in the interview, ask him to recall them.
   c. By determining whether the patient differs in his ability to recall recent or remote events. Can he give the date of his birth, but

not the present month and year? Recent memory suffers most in aging or brain diseases in general. This difference is easy to remember, because you all know that grandfather cannot remember where he laid his glasses, but he can wax eloquently about the time when he was a small boy and heard Teddy Roosevelt speak at a GAR celebration.

5. *Fund of information.* The patient who is oriented, attentive, and has a good memory, knows what is going on in the world. He should be able to name the President, mention a few of the outstanding news events, and give some coherent viewpoint on current problems. If he cannot, he either has an organic disease of the brain, is culturally deprived, or is so introverted as to need psychiatric care.
6. *Insight, judgement, and planning.* The paraplegic patient who plans to be a carpenter and the individual with a borderline IQ who expects to become a chemist can be said to lack insight, judgement, and planning. Does the patient recognize his illness and its implications? Do his goals and plans match his physical and mental capabilities?
7. *Calculation.* Test calculation by asking whether the patient can balance a checkbook, make change, and subtract sevens serially from 100.
8. *Summary of the questions used to test the sensorium.* Test the patient's sensorium by exploiting the natural questions used when meeting anyone for the first time. The first questions explore the patient's orientation to time, person, place, and role in life. Then several general questions disclose the patient's insight, judgment, and planning, and a few specific questions test memory and calculation. See Table 11-2.

   While Table 11-2 lists the kinds of questions that you should ask during the interview, you do not ask them in any specific order. Do not machinegun the patient with a series of disconnected questions with simplistic answers: "Do you know your name? What city are you in? What is the day, date, and week? Who is the President? Can you subtract serial sevens? What did you do yesterday? Can you remember a name, color, and address?" Yes, if you ask your questions that crudely, the patient quickly realizes that you are testing mental status and often replies (not a little piqued), "What's the matter Doc, are you trying to find out if I'm crazy?" Thus, weave these questions in as they arise naturally during the course of the interview. To the patient it should all seem like an ordinary conversation, not an inquisition. From the clues provided by these screening questions of the patient's mental status, history, and physical findings, you decide whether you should order more extensive, formal neuropsychological testing.
9. *Localizing implications of sensorial defects.* Although sensorial defects usually imply organic disease of the brain, they do not specify the precise location of a lesion. Common sense does not reside snugly in some specifiable series of nuclei and tracts. While memory loss may suggest a lesion of the hippocampal-fornix-mamillary body circuit, and dyscalculia suggests a left posterior hemisphere lesion, in general, sensorial defects represent the effects of diffuse cerebral disease. As a rule, neither defects of the sensorium generally, nor of its arbitrary subdivisions, in particular, predict the site of the lesion, as do sensory and

TABLE 11-2.
Outline of Sample Questions to Screen the Patient's Sensorium

Questions	Area of Sensorium Tested
What is your name? How old are you? When is your birthday? What is your address? Are you staying there now? What kind of work do you do? Do you have a family/wife/husband or children? What are their names/occupations/ages/addresses? Where are they now?	Orientation to person, time and place. Recent and remote memory. Consciousness of self and environment.
Do you happen to know the time of day? Have you been waiting long to see me? What is the day/date/month/year? What is the season/weather? What did you do yesterday?	Orientation to time, recent memory.
What have you come to see me about?, or, How does it come about that you are seeing me? Do you feel that you need any medical help?	Doctor/patient role recognition, insight as to presence of an illness or need for medical attention, and judgment.
What are your plans for the future?, or, How long do you expect you will be off work?	Judgment and planning.
What do you think of . . . (mention some item in the news). How has your memory been? Are you worried about it? Suppose we test it. See whether you can remember . . . (give a name, color, and address) Can you name the last several Presidents?	Recent memory, fund of information, attention span.
Subtract 7 from 100, then take off seven more and continue subtracting 7's. Spell "world" (or other word) backward.	Calculation, attention span.

motor defects. The reason for this disparity is that we know enough about the sensory and motor pathways to use tests that parallel their anatomic and physiologic organization, but we do not know enough about the mind to devise tests that parallel its anatomic and physiologic organization. The operational tests of the sensorium show how well the patient's whole cerebrum functions in processing ongoing events. In general, we test the whole cerebrum with sensorial tests, not just its specific parts.

E. *Affective responses*

Besides being conscious, attentive, and oriented, and having a good memory, a fund of information, and insight judgement and planning, the standard man reacts emotionally to ongoing events. Picture your reaction to a hand grenade thrown onto your table or merely to a cockroach. Neither elicits enthusiasm, but your alarm, your *aversion* differs in the two cases. Affective response should have the appropriate quality and quantity.

1. Assay affective responses not by direct inquiry, but by comparing the observed with the expected reactions. What affect would you expect as a patient discusses her paralyzed arm? What affect would you expect

if the patient complains that the "apparatus" plots to kill him? A blunted, bland, or indifferent affect occurs most commonly in hysteria, schizophrenia, and with bifrontal lobe lesions.

2. If you have cause to cry or laugh, how much provocation does it take you to start and how much time does it take you to get over it? If your patient cries for 15 sec and then starts to laugh when you ask him to tell you a funny story, he has the opposite of affective blunting; he has affective lability. It is common with bilateral cerebral disease, as we have seen in pseudobulbar palsy.

F. Perceptual distortions, illusions, hallucinations, and delusions

1. *Illusions.* You have seen water shimmering on a hot highway on a summer day. The water is an illusion, but suppose you behaved as if water is really there? *An illusion is a false sensory perception, based on natural stimulation of a sensory receptor.* The important thing is that the healthy person realizes it when experiencing an illusion, the sick person may not.
2. *Hallucinations.* Observe that sweating, tremulous man cowering on the bed, screaming about dogs and snakes in the corner of his room. And here is a calm patient with an expressionless face who tells you in a flat voice that God is speaking to her, ordering her to drown her baby. Both patients are having characteristic hallucinations, the man of delirium tremens, the woman of schizophrenia. Before an epileptic seizure, many patients experience visual, auditory, or somatic hallucinations. *An hallucination is a false sensory perception not based on natural stimulation of a sensory receptor.* The mentally ill patient usually does not recognize that the hallucination is a false representation of reality, while the epileptic does.
3. *Delusions.* This patient is eyeing a nurse carrying a tray into the room. He says to you *sotto voce,* "There is one of them now. She's trying to poison me." You make a mistake in responding to this remark if you try to reason with him that she has merely come to take his temperature. Somehow, his psychic economy needs to believe that the nurse is a conspirator, and all the reason in the world will not dispel his belief. *A delusion is a false belief that cannot be dispelled by reason.*
4. The existence of illusions, hallucinations, and delusions seems to have been clear, at least intuitively, to literary geniuses, without medical training. See whether you can identify these perceptual distortions (and get back into training for the programming in the next section):

   a. Here is Macbeth, musing alone after murdering Duncan:

   > Is this a dagger which I see before me,
   > The handle toward my hand? Come, let me clutch thee:
   > I have thee not, and yet I see thee still.
   > Art thou not, fatal vision, sensible
   > To feeling as to sight? or art thou but
   > A dagger of the mind, a false creation,
   > Proceeding from the heat-oppressed brain? . . .

Mine eyes are made the fools o'th'other senses,
Or else worth all the rest: I see thee still. . . .

hallucination

This is an example of ☐ an illusion / ☐ an hallucination / ☐ a delusion, which is defined as ______________________________
______________________________.

Ans: A false sensory perception not based on natural stimulation of a sensory receptor.

b. Here is a passage from Gérard De Nerval's poem, *The Dark Blot:*

He who has gazed against the sun sees everywhere
he looks thereafter, palpitating on the air
before his eyes, a smudge that will not go away.

illusion

This is an example of ☐ an illusion / ☐ an hallucination / ☐ a delusion, which is defined as ______________________________
______________________________.

Ans: A false sensory perception based on natural stimulation of a sensory receptor.

c. Here is Porfiry Petrovitch, a lawyer in Dostoevsky's *Crime and Punishment,* discussing a client:

"Yes, in our legal practice there was a case almost exactly similar, a case of morbid psychology," Porfiry went on quickly. "A man confessed to murder and how he kept it up! It was a regular hallucination; he brought forward facts, he imposed upon every one and why? He had been partly, but only partly, unintentionally the cause of a murder and when he knew that he had given the murderers the opportunity, he sank into dejection, it got on his mind and turned his brain, he began imagining things and he persuaded himself that he was the murderer. But at last the High Court of Appeals went into it and the poor fellow was acquitted and put under proper care."

No

delusion

(1) Was lawyer Petrovitch correct in stating that his client was suffering from "a regular hallucination"? ☐ Yes / ☐ No.
(2) If your answer is *No,* would you call the client's mental aberration ☐ an illusion / ☐ a delusion?
(3) Define a delusion: ______________________________
____
______________________________.

Ans: A delusion is a false belief that cannot be dispelled by reason.

Editorial Note: Lawyer Petrovitch was wrong in diagnosing his delusional client as having hallucinations, but his legal instinct was right. Even in Czarist Russia, a harsh and oppressive society, it was recognized that a confession is insufficient evidence of guilt, because people will confess to crimes they did not commit. Moreover, if the police concentrate too much on obtaining confessions (often by physical and mental duress) they do not concentrate enough on obtaining conclusive, objective evidence of who the criminal is. These facts are reflected by the magnificent insight of the Fifth Amendment against self-incrimination: It protects the person against his own mental quirks as well as against the zeal of his accusors. *(C. Jeffery: Criminal Responsibility and Mental Disease, Springfield, Ill., Charles C Thomas, Publisher, 1967.)*

5. *Localizing significance of hallucinations.* In contrast to most of the abnormalities disclosed by the mental status questions, the presence of

hallucinations may have localizing value. They may appear in a variety of mental illnesses or diffuse metabolic diseases, such as delirium tremens, but a repetitively experienced hallucination may indicate a lesion of the appropriate sensory area of the cortex. A lesion of the occipital cortex might cause hallucinations of vision, in the uncus of smell, and in the postcentral gyrus of somatic sensation. Such hallucinations often constitute part of the aura, or forewarning, of an epileptic seizure produced by a lesion in one of these areas.

II. Agnosia, apraxia, aphasia

I translate into ordinary words the Latin of their corrupt preachers, whereby it is revealed as humbug.

— Bertolt Brecht

A. *Introduction*

Every neurology text is foredoomed to have a section headed by these three mystifying terms of Greek origin. The defects they describe are among the most intriguing consequences of brain lesions, but it has been said that if you want to discourage anyone from studying neurology, turn him loose in the literature on this subject. The difficulty is that too much effort has gone into psychic theory and not enough has gone into rigorous study of the behavioral deficits. Salvation is at hand if we call upon the methods of science, if we ask: what are the operations by which the deficits are disclosed and what are the criteria by which they are recognized?

B. *Agnosia*

1. The root *gnosia* means knowing. Dia*gnosis* means literally *through knowing* or knowing through something. Pro*gnosis* means literally *before knowing* or foreknowledge of what will happen. The term *agnosia* means literally *not knowing.* We may then specify what the patient does not know. Astereo*gnosia* (or stereoa*gnosia,* either is correct) means literally *not form knowing,* or failure of the patient to recognize the form of something held in the hand. If the patient does not recognize letters or numbers written on the palm, it would be called ____________.
2. As a review, list several common types of agnosia tested in the clinical examination:

   a. ________________ *gnosia* *d.* ________________ *gnosia*
   b. ________________ *gnosia* *e.* ________________ *gnosia*
   c. ________________ *gnosia* *f.* ________________ *gnosia*
3. *General definition of agnosia.* Since we know the operations to perform to disclose agnosia (e.g., give the patient certain stimuli to identify), we may attempt a general definition. *Agnosia is the inability to understand the import or significance of sensory stimuli even though the sensory pathways and sensorium are relatively intact.*
4. The necessary conditions to diagnose agnosia are:
   a. The patient's previous skills were sufficient to know the symbolic significance of the stimulus. (Don't expect an Australian aborigine to identify a paper clip.)

agraphognosia or graphagnosia.

astereognosia
agraphognosia
finger agnosia
astatognosia
atopognosia
anosognosia

b. The patient's sensorium is sufficiently intact to understand the stimulus.
c. The patient's sensory pathways are sufficiently intact to feel the stimulus.
d. The patient has an organic cerebral lesion as the basis for the deficit.

5. These conditions eliminate patients with interrupted sensory pathways, profound dementia, mental retardation, and functional mental illness such as hysteria and negativism, for whom agnosia is not meant to apply.

C. *Apraxia will be illustrated as one of the several deficits shown by this patient:*

1. *Medical history.* A 67-year-old right-handed salesman with a college education had noticed dizziness, fatigue, and blurring of vision for three months. Three weeks before hospitalization, he began to have right frontal headaches. For one week he had noticed weakness and numbness of his left extremities. Although he appeared dull and apathetic and did arithmetic poorly, his sensorium was otherwise intact.
2. *Physical examination*

a. Motor examination. The patient could walk, but movements on the left side were moderately weak, except for normal frontalis and orbicularis oculi strength. He had no atrophy, tremor, dystaxia, or involuntary movements. When his left extremities were passively manipulated, they showed an initial catch followed by yielding of the part. His reflex pattern is shown in Fig. 11-1.

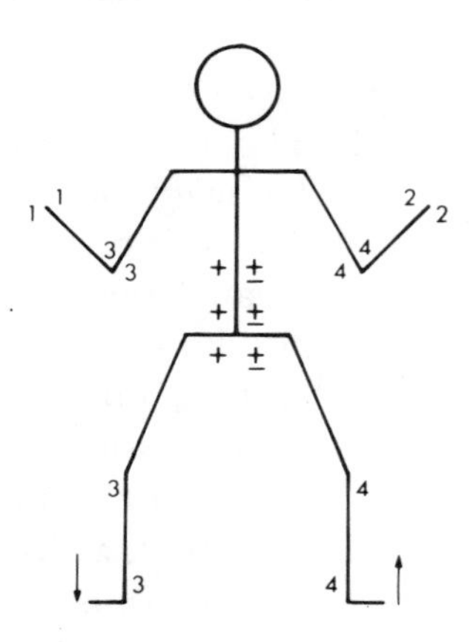

FIG. 11-1. Reflex figurine of the patient.

UMN

(1) His facial weakness was ☐ UMN / ☐ LMN.

Spastic hyperreflexic left hemiparesis with extensor toe sign.

(2) Describe the motor and reflex abnormalities on the left side: ______________________________ ______________________________.

clasp-knife spasticity

(3) The type of hypertonus this patient had is called ______________ ______________.

b. Sensory examination

(1) Although the patient could discriminate the sharp and dull ends of a pin, he reported that the pin felt slightly duller on

hemi*hypalgesia*

the left side. This sensory deficit is called *hemi*___________________________.

(2) He could feel light touch on either side, perhaps less well on the left, but he consistently failed to report a left-sided stimulus when both hands were simultaneously touched. He failed to report left-sided stimuli when simultaneous sound stimuli were presented. This type of sensory deficit is called sensory ____.

inattention or suppression

(3) He recognized coins or a safety pin by vision or when placed in the right hand, but not in the left. This deficit is called ______________________________.

astereognosia

(4) He had difficulty recognizing numbers traced on the left palm, a defect called ______________________________.

agraphognosia

(5) His visual fields are shown in Fig. 11-2. This defect is called ____

complete left homonymous hemianopsia

Left eye Right eye

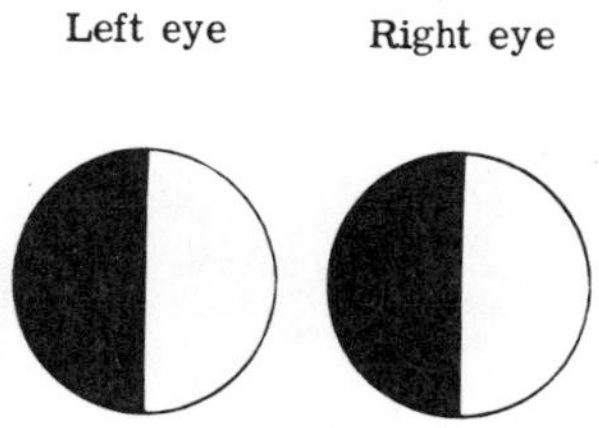

FIG. 11-2. Visual fields of the patient.

(6) Would the patient perceive simultaneous stimuli in the right and left halves of the visual field? ☐ Yes/ ☐ No.

No

(7) Would it be correct to say that the patient had visual agnosia for the left half of space? ☐ Yes/ ☐ No.
Explain ____.

No

Ans: The patient had a left homonymous hemianopsia, which means that he was blind in the left visual field. His lesion had to be in the pathway from the optic tract to, or including, the visual cortex. Since the modality pathway was interrupted, the defect does not qualify as agnosia.

3. *Testing for execution of voluntary acts*

a. The patient was next asked to name a set of figures, which he did correctly, and then to draw them. His drawings are shown in the right-hand column of Fig. 11-3.

b. In Fig. 11-3, study the closure of the patient's figures. In each instance he was unable to complete the ☐ right/ ☐ left side of the figure.

left

c. Here then was a college graduate who could not complete a simple voluntary act such as copying simple geometric figures. Yet he understood what he was to do, and the motility of his right hand was unimpaired. At first thought, you might suspect that his left hemianopsia was responsible for his difficulty, but experience shows that patients with only hemianopsia are able to complete such figures.

(1) The ability to execute a voluntary act is called *praxia*, as in *practice*. If praxia is the ability to do, the inability to do is called ______________.

apraxia

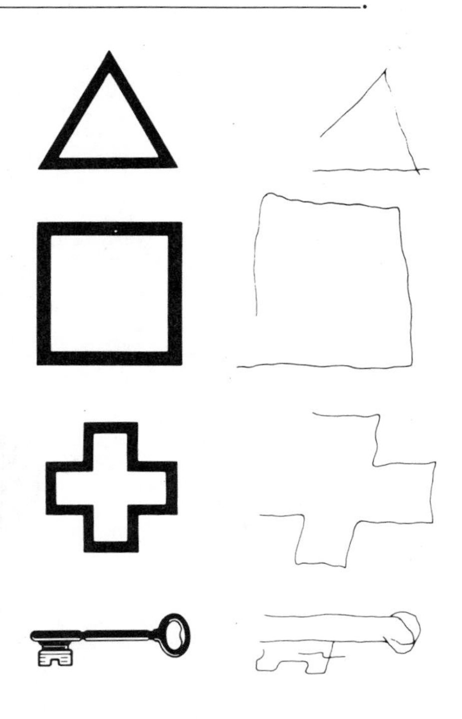

FIG. 11-3. Stimulus figures for patient to name and copy. In the right-hand column are the attempts of the patient to copy the figures after he had named them correctly.

(2) *Apraxia describes the inability of a patient to perform a volitional act even though the motor system and sensorium are relatively intact.*

d. The necessary conditions to diagnose apraxia are:

(1) The patient's previous skills were sufficient for him to do the act.

(2) His sensorium is sufficiently intact for him to understand the act.

(3) His motor system is sufficiently intact to execute the act.

(4) He has an organic cerebral lesion as the cause of the deficit.

e. These requisites are necessary to exclude patients with paralysis, functional mental illness such as hysteria or negativism, profound dementia, or mental retardation for whom the term *apraxia* is not meant to apply. If reading the definition and conditions for diagnosing apraxia gives you the strange illusion of repeating a previous experience (the déjà vu of anterior temporal lobe lesions) we are on the right track. Look back at frames *B*4 and *B*5, which defined agnosia.

f. Since the present patient met all the criteria for apraxia, his deficit in the construction of geometric figures is called *constructional apraxia.*

g. At the end of the examination, the examiner handed the patient his pajama top. Ordinarily, if the patient is disabled, it is courteous to help him dress. In this instance, watching the patient dress was an important part of the examination. He fumbled the garment, repeatedly tried to orient it to put it on and failed. This failure is another example of inability to carry out a volitional act, which in this instance is called dressing ☐ apraxia / ☐ agnosia. Just as there are many varieties of agnosia, so are there many varieties of apraxia.

apraxia

h. Dressing apraxia and constructional apraxia, in which the patient fails to complete the left side of figures, are most frequent with a posterior parietal lesion on the right side of the brain.

(1) Being commoner with right-sided posterior parietal lesions, dressing and constructional apraxia would tend to be associated with ☐ sensory inattention and anosognosia / ☐ finger agnosia and right-left disorientation.

sensory inattention and anosognosia

(2) We call this posterior parietal area, in its confluence with the occipital and temporal lobes, the ______________________________.

posterior parasylvian area

4. *To summarize the patient's clinical deficits:*

a. Motor: Mild spastic, hyperreflexic left hemiparesis with an extensor toe sign. Severe constructional and dressing apraxia.

b. Sensory: Mild left hemipypalgesia and hemiphypesthesia, left-sided astereognosis, left-sided tactile and auditory inattention, and severe complete left homonymous hemianopia.

5. *Localizing significance of the neurologic signs*

a. This patient's motor signs implicate a ______________________ tract lesion.

pyramidal

b. To cause hemiparesis, the pyramidal lesion would have to involve the cervical cord or more rostral levels. If rostral to the cord the lesion might involve brainstem, deep cerebral white matter, or motor cortex. What motor finding locates the lesion at or rostral to the pons? ____ ______________.

UMN facial palsy from interruption of corticobulbar fibers to VII

c. The agnosia and apraxia implicate a lesion at the level of the ☐ sensory pathways / ☐ brainstem / ☐ association areas in the dorsolateral wall of the cerebrum.

association areas

d. The particular types of agnosia and apraxia implicate a lesion of the ☐ right / ☐ left / ☐ both cerebral hemisphere(s), mainly in the ☐ frontal / ☐ parietal / ☐ occipital / ☐ temporal region.

right
parietal

e. While we might account for the patient's left hemiparesis and hemihypesthesia by a brainstem lesion, we now know that his apraxia-agnosia require a lesion of the dorsolateral cerebral wall in the parietal region. Thus, while we might postulate lesions at two levels, brainstem and cerebral wall, we should now invoke one of the most important principles in diagnosis, the principle of parsimony. This principle, otherwise known as Occam's razor (William of Occam, 1280-1349), requires us to try to pare everything down to a single lesion and a single diagnosis. In other words, we seek the simplest, the most *parsimonious,* explanation. Thus, if a single lesion caused the hemiparesis, hemihypesthesia, and agnosia-apraxia, it involves the ☐ brainstem / ☐ thalamus / ☐ dorsolateral cerebral wall.

dorsolateral cerebral wall

f. The complete hemianopia indicates a lesion at some level along the optic pathway. Review the optic pathway in Fig. 4-8 and the course of the optic radiation through the cerebral wall in Fig. 4-9. Hemianopia usually results from a lesion:
(1) ☐ in the retina or optic nerve.
(2) ☐ between the optic chiasm and visual cortex of the calcarine fissure.
(3) ☐ in the anterior part of the temporal lobe.

(2) ☑

g. Applying the principle of parsimony, could the previously postulated lesion of the dorsolateral cerebral wall also interrupt the optic pathway? If so, where (See Fig. 4-9)? ______________________________ ______________________________.

posterior parasylvian area (confluence of the t-p-o lobes)

h. In addition to the agnostic-apraxic deficits, implicating the posterior parietal and parasylvian area, the mild hemihypalgesia and hemihypesthesia implicate the primary somesthetic receptive region of the ______________ gyrus of the ☐ right / ☐ left ______________ lobe.

postcentral
right parietal

i. The mild left hemiparesis implicates the ______________ area along the ______________ sulcus.

motor
central

j. The left-sided auditory inattention implicates the auditory association area in the ☐ anterior / ☐ posterior part of the ☐ right / ☐ left ______________ lobe.

posterior
right temporal

k. Shade Fig. 11-4 to show the presumed extent of the lesion. Use dark shading for the regions which have produced the severest or most complete deficits and lighter shading for the region responsible for the lesser deficits. See frame 4 above for a summary of the deficits.

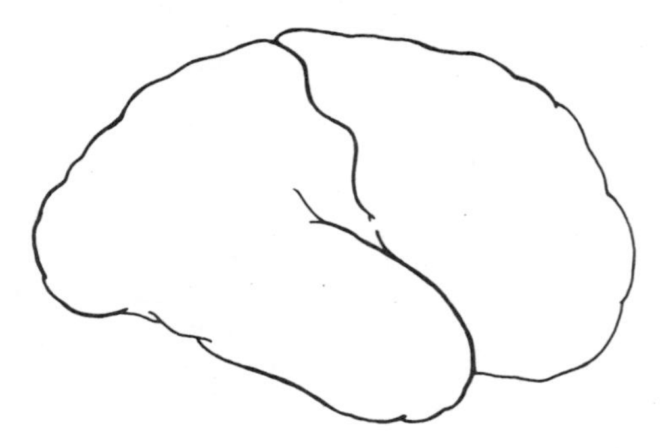

FIG. 11-4. Blank of right cerebral hemisphere to be shaded to show the presumed location of the patient's lesion.

* See next frames and Fig. 11-5.

6. *Neuropathologic considerations*

a. Because of edematous swelling and vascular impingement, lesions may impair the function of surrounding brain tissue. The severest signs usually reflect the site of maximum tissue damage and, therefore, best predict the lesion site. The patient's severest defects, the hemianopia and apraxia, suggested maximum damage to the posterior parasylvian area, with less involvement of the paracentral region.

b. The patient had a craniotomy of the right parieto-occipital region, disclosing a large, expanding neoplasm, with the surrounding brain under pressure. After a biopsy showed a glioblastoma multiforme, the surgeon removed the right occipital lobe, providing internal decompression. Post-operatively, the left hemiparesis disappeared, suggesting that pressure and edema from the neoplasm had caused it rather than direct destruction of the paracentral area by the neoplasm. See Fig. 11-5.

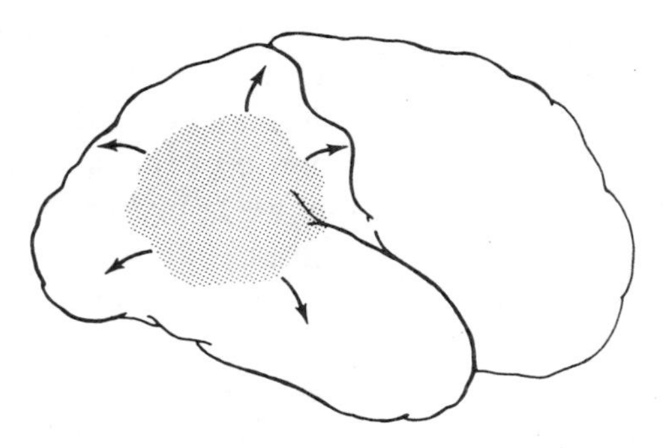

FIG. 11-5. Lateral view of right cerebral hemisphere to show the actual location of the patient's lesion, as determined at autopsy examination. The arrows indicate the surrounding edema of the hemisphere, which led to the clinical signs such as hemiparesis, implicating damage to tissue beyond the immediate confines of the neoplasm.

c. Ordinarily with a lesion in the right posterior parasylvian area, the patient might also have anosognosia. He failed to show this feature before operation, but afterwards he failed to recognize that he had a left hemianopia. Brain-behavior correlations are imperfect, as this patient shows. Anosognosia is more common when the lesion is large and very acute, such as an infarct, than when it evolves relatively slowly, as with a neoplasm.

D. *Additional apraxias*

1. Although all were not shown by the patient just described, some common types of apraxia are:
   a. Constructional apraxia
   b. Dressing apraxia
   c. Gait apraxia
   d. Tongue apraxia
2. Often the apraxic patient can do an act automatically even though he fails on volition. For example, he may be unable to stick out his tongue on command, *tongue apraxia*, but a few seconds later he may lick his lips automatically.
   a. With cerebellar lesions the ability to perform an act is not lost, only the ability to perform it smoothly.
   b. With motor cortex or corticospinal tract lesions, the patient cannot

perform the act because of the paralysis, violating a necessary condition to justify the diagnosis of apraxia. A person may have apraxia and paralysis, but the paralysis precludes recognition of the apraxia.

III. Agnosia and apraxia of language: Aphasia

A. The avenues of language

1. A moment of introspection will disclose that we have four major avenues of language. Normally a person expresses language by *speaking* or *writing,* and receives language by *reading* or *listening.* Thus, we *speak/listen* and *write/read.*
2. Some patients, with cerebral lesions, although neither deaf nor blind, fail to understand the meaning, the symbolic significance, of the words. Thus, instructed by print or voice to hold up a hand, the patient fails to do so, appearing puzzled as if addressed in a foreign language. The general term for failure of a patient with intact sensory pathways to understand the symbolic significance of a stimulus is ______________. Because of the special significance of language for human communication, we apply a special term, *receptive* or *sensory* aphasia, to language agnosia.

agnosia

3. The ordinary avenues of expressing language are ________*ing* and ________*ing.*

speaking
writing

   a. Some patients with cerebral lesions lose their ability to produce the proper words when speaking or writing. If they speak, they utter the wrong syllables or words. If they write, they form the wrong letters or words.

   b. The general term for inability of a nonparalyzed patient to do a voluntary act is ______________.

apraxia

   c. We can recognize then a special form of apraxia, language apraxia, which we call *expressive* or *motor aphasia.*

B. Clinical testing for aphasia

1. Aphasia testing begins when you begin the history. You will appreciate gross defects in language reception or expression from the beginning. The special tests that follow will disclose defects not apparent in ordinary conversation. To test all four avenues of language, require the patient to read, write, name things, repeat words and sentences, and follow written and verbal commands. As part of the screening test for cerebral dysfunction, you also need to test for dyscalculia, constructional dyspraxia, and right-left disorientation. The protocol in Table 11-3, along with Fig. 11-6, provides a standardized way to test all of these things. Don't memorize the table and figure. The Summarized Neurological Examination which you take with you to the bedside includes them. Place the patient's worksheet in the medical chart.
2. Proceed with the Screening Test for Cerebral Dysfunction as follows:

   a. First instruct the patient, "I have a number of things that I want to ask you to do. Some of them are very simple, but even if they are easy for you, I want you to do them carefully and be sure to do your best."

   b. Repeat or amplify instructions as necessary to elicit the patient's best performance, but avoid actual help with any item.

c. Now sit down with a colleague and work through Fig. 11-6 and Table 11-3.

A
B
C
D
E
F
7 SIX 2
G
M G W
H
SEE THE
BLACK DOG.
I
HE IS A FRIENDLY
ANIMAL, A FAMOUS
WINNER OF DOG SHOWS.
J
SQUARE
K
SEVEN
L
85 - 27 =
M
N
PLACE
LEFT HAND
TO RIGHT EAR.
O

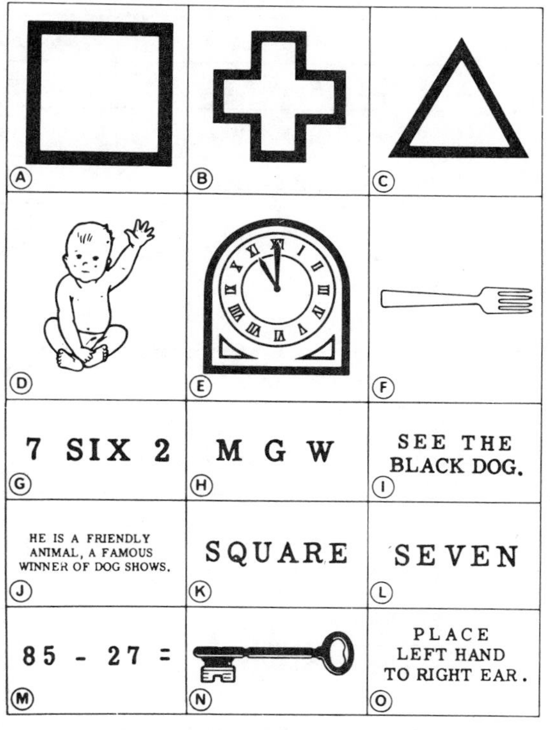

FIG. 11-6. Stimulus figures for testing cerebral functions. This test is the Halstead-Wepman screening test as modified by Dr. Ralph Reitan and currently used in the Neuropsychology Laboratory at Indiana University and many other testing centers.

TABLE 11-3. Instructions for Use with the Stimuli of Fig. 11-6 to Test for Cerebral Dysfunction

Patient's task	Examiner's instructions to the patient
1. Copy SQUARE (A).	FIRST, DRAW THIS ON YOUR PAPER (Point to square, item A). I WANT YOU TO DO IT WITHOUT LIFTING YOUR PENCIL FROM THE PAPER. MAKE IT ABOUT THIS SAME SIZE (Point to square.) Elaborate on the requirement for a continuous line if necessary. If the patient is concerned about making a heavy or double line, point out that only a reproduction of the shape is required. If the patient has obvious difficulty in drawing any of the figures, encourage him to proceed until it is clear that he can make no further progress. If he does not accomplish the task reasonably well on his first try, ask him to try again, and instruct him to be particularly careful to do it as well as he can.
2. Name SQUARE	WHAT IS THAT SHAPE CALLED?
3. Spell SQUARE	WOULD YOU SPELL THAT WORD FOR ME?
4. Copy CROSS (B)	DRAW THIS ON YOUR PAPER. (Point to cross). GO AROUND THE OUTSIDE LIKE THIS UNTIL YOU GET BACK TO WHERE YOU STARTED. (Examiner draws a finger-line around the edge of the stimulus figure.) MAKE IT ABOUT THIS SAME SIZE. (Point to cross.) Additional instructions, if necessary, should be similar to those used with the square.
5. Name CROSS	WHAT IS THAT SHAPE CALLED?

Patient's task	Examiner's instructions to the patient
6. Spell CROSS	WOULD YOU SPELL THAT WORD FOR ME?
7. Copy TRIANGLE (C)	Similar to 1 and 4 above.
8. Name TRIANGLE	WHAT IS THAT SHAPE CALLED?
9. Spell TRIANGLE	WOULD YOU SPELL THAT WORD FOR ME?
10. Name BABY (D)	WHAT IS THIS? (Show baby, item D).
11. Write CLOCK (E)	NOW I AM GOING TO SHOW YOU ANOTHER PICTURE BUT DO *NOT* TELL ME THE NAME OF IT. I DON'T WANT YOU TO SAY ANYTHING OUT LOUD. JUST WRITE THE NAME OF THE PICTURE ON YOUR PAPER. (Show clock, item E).
12. Name FORK (F)	WHAT IS THIS? (Show fork, item F).
13. Read 7 SIX 2 (G)	I WANT YOU TO READ THIS (Show item G). If the subject has difficulty, attempt to determine whether he can read any part of the stimulus figure.
14. Read M G W (H)	READ THIS. (Show item H).
15. Reading I (I)	NOW I WANT YOU TO READ THIS (Show item I).
16. Reading II (J)	CAN YOU READ THIS? (Show item J).
17. Repeat TRIANGLE	NOW I AM GOING TO SAY SOME WORDS. I WANT YOU TO LISTEN CAREFULLY AND SAY THEM AFTER ME AS CAREFULLY AS YOU CAN. SAY THIS WORD: TRIANGLE.
18. Repeat MASSACHUSETTS	THE NEXT ONE IS A LITTLE HARDER BUT DO YOUR BEST. SAY THIS WORD: MASSACHUSETTS.
19. Repeat METHODIST EPISCOPAL	NOW REPEAT THIS ONE: METHODIST EPISCOPAL.
20. Write SQUARE (K)	DON'T SAY THIS WORD OUT LOUD. (Point to stimulus word "square," item K). JUST WRITE IT ON YOUR PAPER. If the patient prints the word, ask him to write it.
21. Read SEVEN (L)	CAN YOU READ THIS WORD OUT LOUD. (Show item L).
22. Repeat SEVEN	NOW, I WANT YOU TO SAY THIS AFTER ME: SEVEN.
23. Repeat-explain, HE SHOUTED THE WARNING	I AM GOING TO SAY SOMETHING THAT I WANT YOU TO SAY AFTER ME, SO LISTEN CAREFULLY: HE SHOUTED THE WARNING. NOW YOU SAY IT. WOULD YOU EXPLAIN WHAT THAT MEANS? Sometimes it is necessary to amplify by asking the kind of situation to which the sentence would refer. The patient's understanding is adequately demonstrated when he brings the concept of impending danger into his explanation.
24. Write: HE SHOUTED THE WARNING	NOW I WANT YOU TO WRITE THAT SENTENCE ON THE PAPER. Sometimes it is necessary to repeat the sentence so that the patient understands clearly what he is to write.
25. Compute 85 − 27 = (M)	HERE IS AN ARITHMETIC PROBLEM. COPY IT DOWN ON YOUR PAPER ANY WAY YOU LIKE AND TRY TO WORK IT OUT. (Show item M).
26. Compute 17 × 3 =	NOW DO THIS ONE IN YOUR HEAD: 17 × 3
27. Name KEY (N)	WHAT IS THIS: (Show item N).

Patient's task	Examiner's instructions to the patient
28. Demonstrate use of KEY (N)	IF YOU HAD ONE OF THESE IN YOUR HAND, SHOW ME HOW YOU WOULD USE IT. (Show item N).
29. Draw KEY (N)	NOW I WANT YOU TO DRAW A PICTURE THAT LOOKS JUST LIKE THIS. TRY TO MAKE YOUR KEY LOOK ENOUGH LIKE THIS ONE SO THAT I WOULD KNOW IT WAS THE SAME KEY FROM YOUR DRAWING. (Point to key, item N.)
30. Read (O)	WOULD YOU READ THIS? (Show item O).
31. Place LEFT HAND TO RIGHT EAR	NOW, WOULD YOU DO WHAT IT SAID?
32. Place LEFT HAND TO LEFT ELBOW	NOW I WANT YOU TO PUT YOUR LEFT HAND TO YOUR LEFT ELBOW. The patient should quickly realize that it is impossible.

3. *Interpretation of test results:*
   a. The normal person with a high school education makes no errors on this test. Illiterate patients will make some spelling errors.
   b. If a patient of previously normal intelligence and a high school education makes errors on this test, he most likely has a cerebral lesion. Expect 100 percent correct answers from a 100 percent intact brain.
4. As an example of how a patient with aphasia performs on the cerebral function test, read Table 11-4, which records the results obtained. Refer to Figs. 11-6 and 11-7 as needed. This patient was a 44-year-old man who formerly had been able to read and write adequately. He had an epileptic seizure and afterwards remained lethargic and his speech was slow and difficult to understand. He had no clinically evident hemiparesis, but on testing with a dynamometer his strength in the right hand was equal to the left whereas it should have been greater, and he was slower on finger tapping with the right hand.

*TABLE 11-4. Test Results on Patient with Severe Aphasia (*An asterisk means to look at Fig. 11-7 to see what the patient did in response to the test item.)*

Patient's task	Patient's response
1. *Copy SQUARE	The patient started to draw on the test booklet. See Fig. 11-7, 1.
2. Name SQUARE	OK.
3. Spell SQUARE	OK.
4. *Copy CROSS	See Fig. 11-7, 4-1 to 3.
5. Name CROSS	"Square" — did not respond to examiner's further questioning.
6. Spell CROSS	"un hu"; "c-r-o-w-s-s-"
7. *Copy TRIANGLE	See Fig. 11-7, 7-1 to 5.
8. Name TRIANGLE	Patient made no response after repeated questioning.
9. Spell TRIANGLE	Patient was asked three times to spell triangle; then asked how the word started: "TR," patient could go no further.

Patient's task	Patient's response
10. Name BABY	OK.
11. *Write CLOCK	Patient took test booklet from examiner and put it sideways. He finally drew Fig. 11-7, 11.
12. Name FORK	OK.
13. Read 7 SIX 2	"Six." (Examiner pointed to the letter.) "7, six and 7 -a four."
14. Read M G W	"Meg-m-i-g"
15. Reading I	Patient had a long pause and then read quickly, "See that dog."
16. Reading II	"He is a" (long pause) "friend of family - oh - woman of a dog." (Read very quickly after pause.)
17. Repeat TRIANGLE	Mushy articulation.
18. Repeat MASSACHUSETTS	Massachuses
19. Repeat METHODIST EPISCOPAL	"Methodiss epis fi tul."
20. *Write SQUARE	See Fig. 11-7, 21.
21. *Read SEVEN	"S s s - sev - s-e-v-e-n." Patient said the word and wrote it although not requested to write. See Fig. 11-7, 22.
22. Repeat SEVEN	"Sevun"
23. Repeat-explain HE SHOUTED THE WARNING.	Repeated the phrase but could not explain its meaning.
24. *Write HE SHOUTED THE WARNING	See Fig. 11-7, 24.
25. *Compute 85 − 27 =	Patient confused — did not know what (—) meant. See Fig. 11-7, 25, 1 to 4. The examiner wrote the problem in 25-5 and the patient answered *9*.
26. *Compute 17 × 3 =	Patient could not compute; See Fig. 11-7, 26-1. Examiner gave 2 × 3; See Fig. 11-7, 26-2. Patient just scribbled.
27. Name KEY	OK with much prompting.
28. Demonstrate use of KEY	Patient could not; "You could show a fellow how."
29. *Draw KEY	Patient turned book upside down to draw. See Fig. 11-7, 29.
30. Read PLACE LEFT HAND TO RIGHT EAR	"Please the left-left hand behind me."
31. PLACE LEFT HAND TO RIGHT EAR	Patient placed right hand to right ear.
32. PLACE LEFT HAND TO LEFT ELBOW	Patient placed right hand to left elbow.

a. This patient showed a type of constructional apraxia different from that shown in Fig. 11-3. In Fig. 11-3, the patient could not complete the left side of objects. In Fig. 11-7, the patient showed a general inability to effect the shape of the objects, but did not show the inattention or neglect of one side of the figure.

b. The performance on the arithmetic part of the test shows severe acalculia. The patient was even unable to multiply 2 × 3.

c. Further diagnostic studies on this patient lead to a left frontopari-

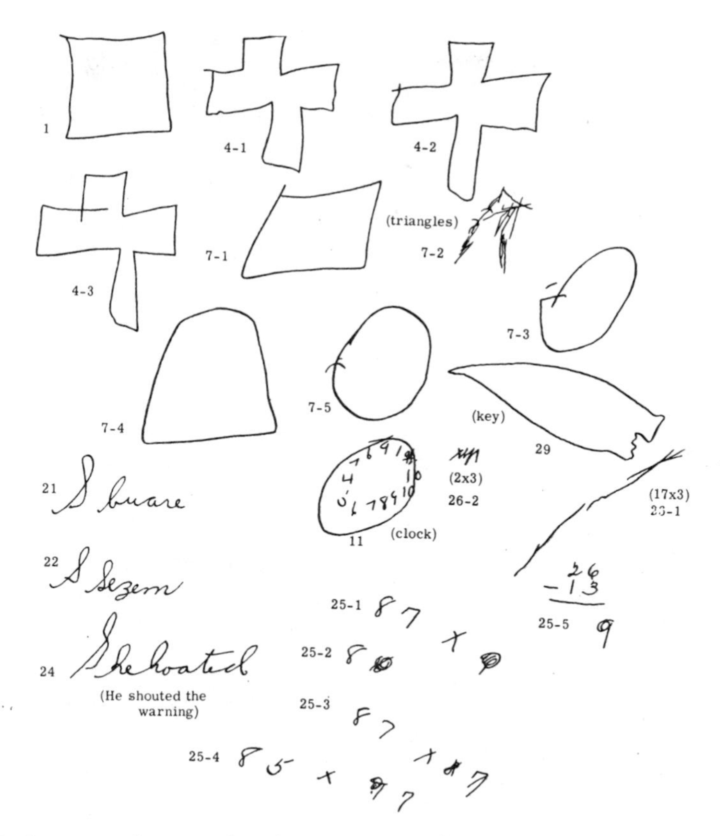

FIG. 11-7. Performance of a severely aphasic patient on the Halstead-Wepman-Reitan screening test for cerebral function. The number beside each figure refers to the number of the test item in Table 11-1. If the number is in two parts, such as 4-2, it refers to the fourth test item, the second attempt of the patient to do the task.

etal craniotomy. Biopsy disclosed a malignant neoplasm. The patient died 28 days after the operation, about a month after the test results given in Table 11-2 and Fig. 11-7 were obtained. He had a large multicentric glioblastoma in the left hemisphere, with one mass of neoplastic tissue in the posterior inferior frontal region and the other in the posterior parasylvian region.

8. Fig. 11-8 gives further examples of aphasic errors in other patients when asked to write, "He shouted the warning."

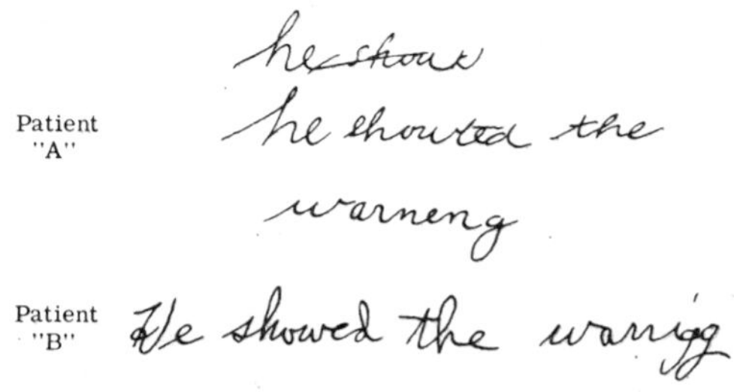

FIG. 11-8. Some typical performances of patients with left hemisphere lesions when attempting to write, "He shouted the warning." The disturbance in letter formation is called *dysgraphia*.

C. A general definition of aphasia and a review of the definition of agnosia and apraxia

1. Now that you know the operational methods to test for aphasia we can

offer a general definition: *Aphasia is the inability to understand or express words as symbols for communication even though the sensory systems, mechanisms of phonation and articulation, and sensorium are relatively intact.*

2. It is now time to take stock and review. Give a general (interpretational) definition of:

   a. Agnosia ____
   ____.

   See frame B3, page 337.

   b. Apraxia ____
   ____.

   See frame (2), page 340.

   c. Aphasia ____
   ____.

   See top of this page.

3. The requisites necessary to distinguish any type of agnosia from other disturbances of sensation, comprehension, or perception are: ____
____.

See frame 4, page 337.

4. The requisites necessary to distinguish any type of apraxia from other disorders of execution are: ____
____.

See frame d, page 340.

D. Nomenclature for and varieties of aphasia

1. *Aphasia versus dysphasia.* To a purist, the term *aphasia* (literally *a* = lack of, and *phasis* = speech) would mean total loss of language. To distinguish partial from total loss, we should use the term *dysphasia* (or dysgnosia and dyspraxia), but you will find that clinicians use the prefixes *a-* and *dys-* interchangeably.
2. *Classification of aphasia.* Traditionally, neurologists have classified aphasia as *receptive, expressive,* or *mixed expressive-receptive* aphasia. Most patients have a mixture of expressive and receptive language deficits, and therefore have a mixed type of aphasia. Mixed aphasia, when it involves all four avenues of language, constitutes *global* aphasia. Such a patient may have little or no remaining language function.

   Some authors prefer to classify aphasia as *fluent* or *nonfluent,* rather than according to the traditional expressive-receptive scheme (Geschwind, 1971).

   a. The patient with nonfluent aphasia speaks telegraphically and sparsely. The patient may use nouns and verbs, but omits small connecting words, conjunctions such as *but, or,* and *and,* or articles such as *a, an,* or *the.* In fact, an excellent sentence to ask the aphasic patient to repeat is "No *if's, and's, but's,* or *or's.*" A patient with nonfluent aphasia loses the normal rhythms and inflections of speech, and thus has *dysprosody* as well as dysphasia.

   b. The fluent aphasic patient produces a plentiful or even an excessive number of words, many of them wrong. The patient crams in numerous word substitutions, circumlocutions, and neologisms, perhaps best described as a word salad or word potpourri, which robs the speech of meaning. Yet the jargon may retain normal prosody, normal rhythm, and inflection.

3. *Relative language deficits in aphasia:*
   a. Although most patients have a mixed type of aphasia, some have a relatively pure deficit in speaking, writing, or comprehending spoken or written words. A patient with relatively pure visual agnosia for words is said to have *alexia* or *dyslexia*. The numerous other terms for the varieties of aphasia become so confusing that they will not be offered in this introductory text.
   b. In judging relative loss of receptive and expressive language functions, you should understand that language expression is a more active process than receiving it. It is harder to give than to receive. Therefore, the average aphasic patient (as contrasted for example to the dyslexic), will retain more comprehension of language than expression. Not only do aphasic patients differ in their ease of expressing or receiving language, but they also differ in the degree to which they can express the content of speech.

   Some speech serves mainly to communicate the emotional state of the moment. Other speech serves to communicate ideas. Emotional speech tends to come forth spontaneously, unwilled, and automatically, with little deliberation, forethought, or planning: "Ouch." We communicate ideas in the form of propositions. A proposition states something that was, is, or could be. "Here is my proposition. . . ." It is preeminently deliberate, measured, planned, and wilful. The aphasic patient loses this propositional speech out of proportion to the loss of emotional—particularly expletive—speech. Thus after struggling to produce a propositional statement and failing miserably, the patient heaves a sigh and announces spontaneously with perfect clarity, "Oh damn, I can't do it." Yet when asked to repeat the automatically uttered sentence, now become propositional or wilful speech, the patient fails again. This fact demonstrates that the brain uses different circuitry for propositional as contrasted to emotional speech.

E. Localizing implications of aphasia

1. *Localization to the dominant hemisphere.* Almost all right-handed and most left-handed patients with aphasia have a lesion of the left cerebral hemisphere. Therefore we say that the left hemisphere is usually dominant for language function. Operationally what we mean by a dominant hemisphere for language is that it is the hemisphere which, if damaged, will result in aphasia.
2. *Localization within the dominant hemisphere.* The lesion which causes aphasia is most frequently located in the parasylvian region of the left hemisphere. Rarely the lesion occupies the parasylvian region of the right hemisphere. See Fig. 11-9.

   The type of aphasia fairly well predicts the location of the lesion

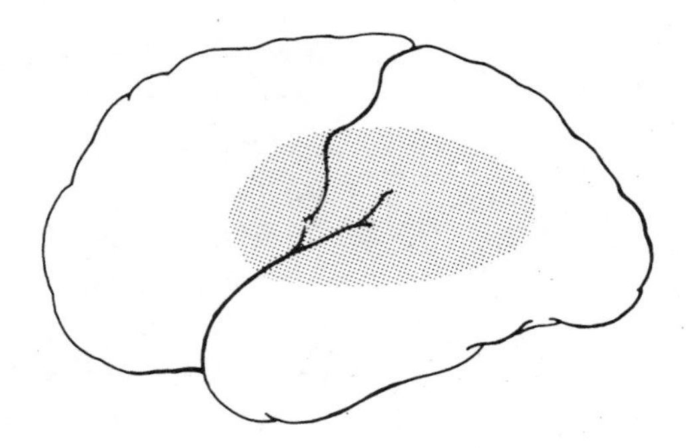

FIG. 11-9. Lateral view of the left cerebral hemisphere to show the expected lesion site when the patient is aphasic.

within the aphasic zone. It has, however, become evident that everyone who studies aphasia must, compulsively it seems, disagree with the classification and localization of their predecessors. (Compare, for example, Mohr, et al., 1978; Benson and Geschwind, 1971; and Brown, 1972.) Thus, take the simplified scheme given here for what it is: a useful approximation for the clinician, not immutable dogma. In order to prove that you know the location of the aphasic zone, shade it in Fig. 11-10.

a. A relatively pure expressive aphasia or nonfluent aphasia suggests a lesion of the anterior part of the aphasic zone in the posterior inferior part of the frontal lobe (Broca's area). This region abuts on the classical motor area and correlates with the predominantly motor function of this region of the cerebrum. Because of the inverted representation of the body in the motor strip, the face area abuts on the aphasic zone. Thus the aphasic patient with an anterior lesion will usually also have at least an upper motor neuron palsy of the right side of the face, if not a frank hemiplegia.

b. When the patient has relatively pure alexia, the lesion usually occupies the posterior end of the aphasic zone, toward the occipital lobe, which contains the primary visual receptive area. This statement applies to the dyslexic patient with an acquired brain lesion. Developmental dyslexia, as seen in children, constitutes a different problem (Critchley, 1964).

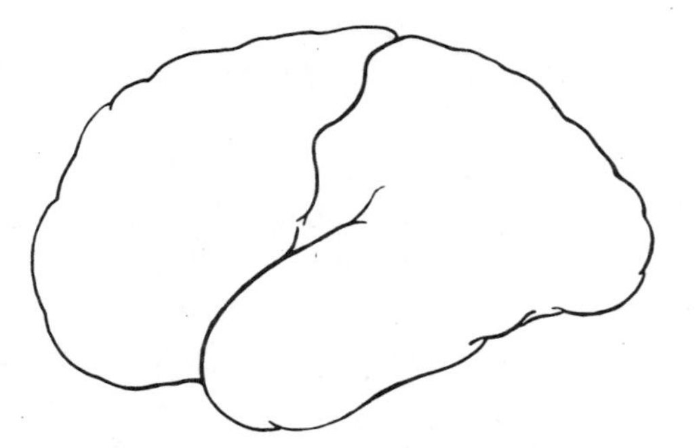

FIG. 11-10. Blank of the left cerebral hemisphere to be shaded to show the expected lesion site when the patient is aphasic.

*See Fig. 11-9.

c. When the patient has relatively pure auditory aphasia, the lesion tends to occupy the posterior part of the superior temporal gyrus next to the primary auditory receptive area in the transverse gyri of that gyrus.

d. When the patient has fluent aphasia accompanied by prominent auditory word agnosia, dyslexia, dysgraphia, and dyscalculia, the lesion usually occupies the region around the posterior end of the Sylvian fissure at the confluence of the parietal, occipital, and temporal lobes (Wernicke's aphasia).

Thus, the lesion in the fluent aphasic patient tends to affect the aphasic zone more posteriorly and temporally than nonfluent aphasia. It disconnects the auditory cortex in the superior temporal gyrus from the rest of the posterior parasylvian area, the word association area. In addition to losing the ability to audit the words of others, these patients lose the ability to audit their own words. They cannot use their auditory feedback to correct their own errors in word production, resulting in their barrage of word errors.

e. Large lesions of the entire parasylvian zone, or its total destruction, cause a severe type of global expressive and receptive dysphasia which may rob the patient of virtually all communication by words.

f. The neurologic deficits associated with aphasia will vary depending on the location of the lesion within the aphasic zone. A lesion in the anterior part of the zone will be adjacent to the motor area, while a more posterior lesion may affect the optic radiation (geniculocalcarine tract). (Review Fig. 4-9 if necessary.)

g. The patient with nonfluent aphasia would more likely have ☐ hemiparesis/ ☐ hemianopsia/ ☐ right-left confusion, because the lesion is located ____
____
____.

hemiparesis
anteriorly in the aphasic zone, next to the motor area

h. The patient with fluent aphasia would more likely have ☐ hemiparesis/ ☐ hemianopsia/ ☐ anosognosia because the lesion is located ____
____
____.

hemianopsia
posteriorly in the aphasic zone, overlying the geniculocalcarine tract

i. The patient with ☐ fluent/ ☐ nonfluent aphasia would most likely have a severe receptive aphasia because the lesion is located ________
____
____.

fluent
posteriorly in the aphasic zone, in the auditory and visual word association region

F. *Four levels of speech disturbance*

We have now distinguished four levels of disturbance in speech production: dys*phonia,* dys*arthria,* dys*prosody,* and dys*phasia.* At the lowest level, dysphonia consists of a disturbance in the production of sounds in the larynx. At the highest level, dysphasia consists of a disturbance in the understanding or expression of words as symbols for communication. Review (if you wish, write out) the definitions of these terms and check your definitions against the ones given in Sec. III of the Summarized Neurological Examination.

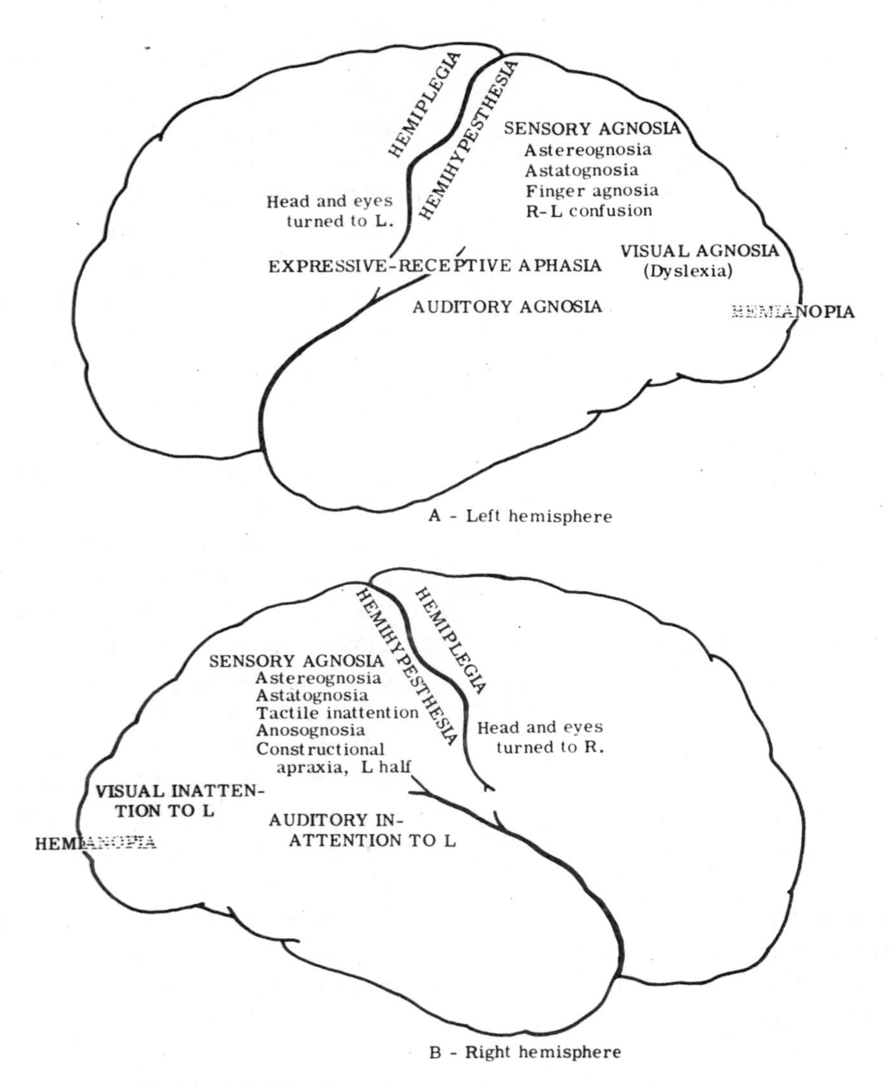

FIG. 11-11. Summary of the signs and symptoms that occur with focal destructive lesions in the right or left cerebral hemispheres. *A*. Lateral view of left cerebral hemisphere. *B*. Lateral view of the right cerebral hemisphere. Notice that some signs and symptoms, such as hemiplegia, are common to both hemispheres, but that others are different. Thus, the syndrome of the right cerebral hemisphere can be distinguished from the syndrome for the left.

G. A resumé of cerebral localization

1. The philosopher seeks to localize functions in the brain, to find the seat of mind and emotion. The practicing physician seeks to localize lesions in the brain. Sometimes the philosopher-physician gets things turned around. He thinks that because he can localize a lesion from the deficit of function he has localized the function. He has merely indulged in circular reasoning:

   Sequence 1:

   Child: "Daddy, why do things fall to the ground?"

   Daddy: "Why that's simple, because there is gravity."

   Sequence 2:

   Child: "Daddy, why do you say there is gravity?"

   Daddy: "Why that's simple, because things fall to the ground."

2. Fig. 11-11 does not imply that functions localize in the regions labeled. It means that given a clinical deficit, determined according to a specific test procedure, we can expect a lesion in a particular cerebral area. We do not concern ourselves with localizing functions if we recall the operational steps: Give a test, executing it and judging the results according to standard procedure. Match the results against the site of brain lesions and note with what consistency particular deficits correlate with particular lesion sites. That is how Fig. 11-11 was constructed.

   We cannot now answer and cannot ever answer the questions of the Book of Job: But where shall wisdom be found? And where is the place of understanding?

H. Significance of deficits of the sensorium, agnosia, aphasia, and apraxia

1. After you have finished interviewing and examining any patient you have to make a critical judgement: you have to set up some tentative diagnosis to guide you in selecting ancillary diagnostic tests. You then confirm or reject your tentative diagnosis, depending on subsequent findings.
2. Diagnosis can be regarded as a process of making a series of dichotomies as though proceeding through a labyrinth in which each turr you take depends on the evidence you accumulate. See Fig. 11 - 12.

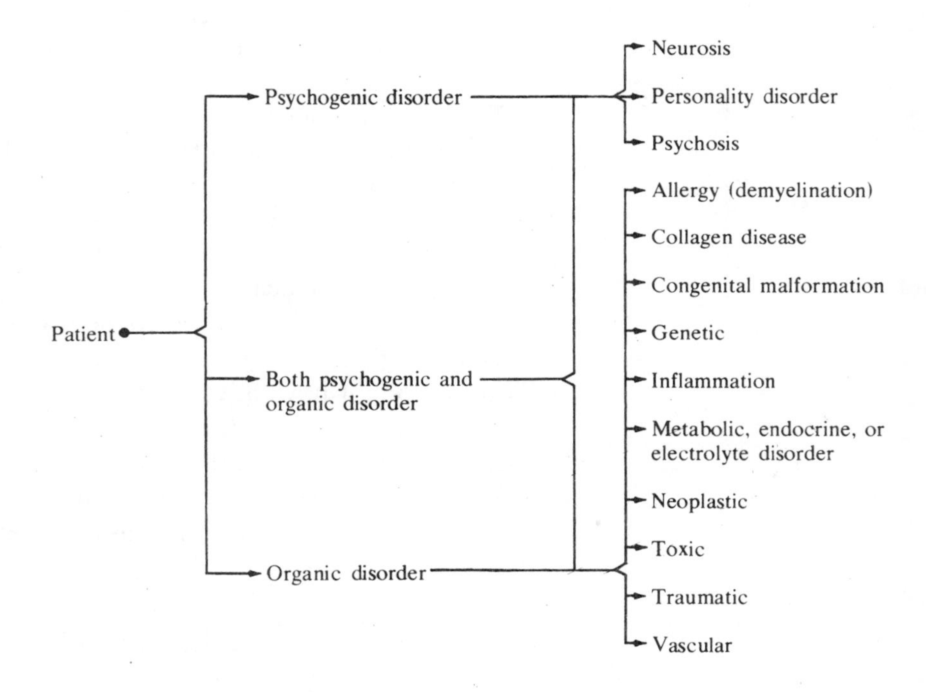

FIG. 11 - 12. The initial diagnostic impression to guide in selecting further studies. Each of the end stations in this dendrogram can be subdivided to generate the gamut of diagnostic possibilities. (Reference only.)

3. To pass through each filter or diagnostic category of the dendrogram, you must have firm evidence from the history, physical examination,

and laboratory tests. The first diagnostic dichotomy involves a decision as to whether the patient most likely has an organic or a so-called functional (emotional) disorder. If you realize that a large percentage of patients seeking medical help have emotional disorders — perhaps as many as 50 percent of the adults who will come to your office — you will see how important it is to make the first dichotomy in diagnosis correctly.

4. In essence you must answer these questions:
   a. Does the patient have a lesion?
   b. Where is the lesion?
   c. What is the lesion?
   d. What are the critical diagnostic procedures to be done?

organic

5. If the patient has frank neurologic signs, such as hemiplegia or hemianopsia, the first diagnostic dichotomy is easy; he has ☐ organic/ ☐ functional disease.

organic

6. He may, however, have defects of the sensorium and no frank signs. Brain lesions impair memory, orientation, consciousness — sensorial functions. Therefore, sensorial defects indicate ☐ organic/ ☐ functional disease.
7. Most functional diseases spare most of the sensorium. Therefore, the average neurotic or mildly psychotic patient has little or no sensorial defect.
8. You will find that disturbances of consciousness, orientation, and memory are the sensorial changes which are easiest to ascertain and most reliable.

organic

   a. When consciousness, orientation, or memory are disturbed in a mentally disturbed patient, he most likely has ☐ organic/ ☐ functional disease.

functional

   b. When consciousness, orientation, or memory are not disturbed in a mentally disturbed patient, he most likely has ☐ organic/ ☐ functional disease.
9. And listen to this: The absence of sensorial defects and frank neurologic signs never guarantees that the patient has no organic brain lesion. The disease may not have advanced far enough to exceed the safety factor of the tissue. The function has not yet deteriorated to the range for disclosure by testing, although it does produce symptoms which the patient or his associates recognize. We often walk the fine edge between triumph and disaster in trying to assay cerebral function for "organicity."

Bibliography

Aphasia and Alexia

Adams, R. D., and Victor, M.: *Principles of Neurology,* New York, McGraw-Hill Book Company, 1977.

Benson, D.: The third alexia, *Arch. Neurol.,* 34:327-331, 1977.

Benson, D., Brown, J., and Tomlinson, E.: Varieties of alexia, *Neurology,* 21: 951-957, 1971.

Benson, D., and Geschwind, N.: The aphasias and related disturbances, in *Clinical Neurology,* Baker, A. B. (ed.), New York, Harper, 1971.
Brown, J.: *Aphasia, Apraxia, and Agnosia: Clinical and Theoretical Aspects,* Springfield, Ill., Charles C Thomas, 1972.
Critchley, M.: *Developmental Dyslexia,* London, William Heinemann Medical Books, Ltd., 1964.
Drew, A.: A neurological appraisal of familial congenital word-blindness, *Brain,* 79:440-460, 1956.
Friedlander, W. J. (ed.): Current reviews of higher nervous system dysfunction, in *Advances in Neurology, vol. 7,* New York, Raven Press, 1975.
Geschwind, N.: Aphasia, *N. Engl. J. Med.,* 284:654-656, 1971.
Gloning, I.: Eine Klassifizierung der Aphasie aufgrund einer quantitativ-experimentellen Untersuchung, *Fortschr. Neurol. Psychiatr.,* 38:246-264, 1970.
Goodglass, A., and Kaplan, E.: *Assessment of Aphasia and Related Disorders,* Philadelphia, Lea & Febiger, 1972.
Head, H.: *Aphasia and Kindred Disorders of Speech,* New York, Stechert-Hafner, Inc., 1963.
Hecaen, H., and Ajuriaguerra, J.: *Left-Handedness, Manual Superiority and Cerebral Dominance,* New York, Grune & Stratton, Inc., 1964.
Kertesz, A., Lesk, D., McCabe, P.: Isotope localization of infarcts in aphasia, *Arch. Neurol.,* 34:590-601, 1977.
Mehegan, H., and Freifuss, F.: Hyperlexia, *Neurology,* 22:1105-1111, 1972.
Mohr, J. P., Pessin, M. S., Finkelstein, S., Funkenstein, H. H., Duncan, G. W., and Davis, K. R.: Broca aphasia: Pathologic and clinical, *Neurology,* 28:311-324, 1978.
Nielsen, J. M.: *Agnosia, Apraxia, Aphasia: Their Value in Cerebral Localization,* New York, Stechert-Hafner, Inc., 1962.
Penfield, W., and Roberts, L.: *Speech and Brain Mechanisms,* Princeton, Princeton University Press, 1959.
Reitan, R. M., and Davison, L. A.: *Clinical Neuropsychology: Current Status and Applications,* New York, John Wiley & Sons, 1974.
Russell, W., and Espir, M.: *Traumatic Aphasia,* London, Oxford University Press, 1961.
Weisenburg, T., and McBride, K. E.: *Aphasia: A Clinical and Psychological Study,* New York, Stechert-Hafner, Inc., 1964.
Wheeler, L., and Reitan, R.: Presence and laterality of brain damage predicted from responses to a short aphasia screening test, *Percept. Motor Skills,* 15:783-799, 1962.

Other Cerebral Dysfunctions

Allison, R.: *The Senile Brain: A Clinical Study,* London, Edward Arnold (Publishers) Ltd., 1962.
Bender, M., and Feldman, M.: The so-called visual agnosias, *Brain,* 95:173-186, 1972.
Benson, D., and Blumer, D.: *Psychiatric Aspects of Neurological Disease,* New York, Grune & Stratton, 1975.
DePaulo, J. R., and Folstein, M. F.: Psychiatric disturbances in neurological patients: Detection, recognition, and hospital course, *Ann. Neurol.,* 4:225-228, 1978.
Galaburda, A. M., LeMay, M., Kemper, T. L., and Geschwind, N.: Right-left asymmetries in the brain, *Science,* 199:852-856, 1978.

Jenkyn, L. R., Walsh, D. B., Culver, C. M., and Reeves, A. G.: Clinical signs in diffuse cerebral dysfunction, *J. Neurol. Neurosurg. Psychiatry,* 40:956-966. 1977.

LeDoux, J. E., Wilson, D. H., and Gazzaniga, M. D.: A divided mind: Observations on the conscious properties of the separated hemispheres, *Ann. Neurol.,* 2:417-421, 1977.

Luria, A. R.: *Higher Cortical Functions in Man,* New York, Basic Books, 1966.

Strub, R. L., and Black, F. W.: *The Mental Status Examination in Neurology,* Philadelphia, F. A. Davis Company, 1977.

Weinstein, E. A., and Friedland, R. P. (eds.): Hemi-inattention syndromes and hemisphere specialization, in *Advances in Neurology, vol. 18,* New York, Raven Press, 1977.

Wells, C. E. (ed.): *Dementia,* in *Contemporary Neurology Series, vol. 15,* 2nd ed., Philadelphia, F. A. Davis Company, 1977.

IV. Summary of tests for cerebral functions

A. *Rehearsal time again:* Give a definition of the sensorium, state the seven areas of the sensorium and give an example of a question designed to test each of the areas.

B. *Distinguish between an illusion, a hallucination, and a delusion*

C. *Define agnosia, aphasia, and apraxia, and describe tests for each*

D. *Work through the cerebral function screening test with a partner, using sections VIII, steps A and B, of the Summarized Neurological Examination.* Be familiar with the procedures but do not try to memorize the test. Use the instruction sheet each time you give the test.

12

Examination of the Patient Who Has a Disorder of Consciousness

I may speak alike to you and my own conscious heart.
— Percy Bysshe Shelley

I. Consciousness

A. *Introduction*

1. Among the endless philosophic definitions of consciousness, let us choose one: *consciousness is the awareness of self and environment.* To determine the patient's awareness of self and environment, physicians use operational criteria, based on inspection, conversation, or, if necessary, painful stimuli.
   a. *Inspection:* Does the patient respond to the ongoing visual and auditory stimuli of the environment?
   b. *Conversation:* Does the patient respond to conversational voice or loud commands and questions?
   c. *Stimulation:* Does the patient respond to pain?
2. Besides making a qualitative judgment as to the presence or absence of consciousness, the physician needs a simple quantitative scale to grade the level of consciousness during the course of an illness. The trend lines derived from standardized grading of the responses to standardized stimuli graphically disclose any deterioration or improvement. In the Glascow Coma Scale (Teasdale and Jennett, 1974) shown in Fig. 12-1, the trend lines show a declining level of consciousness in a patient with cerebral edema. After intravenous administration of mannitol, a hyperosmolar agent that reduces edema, the trend lines document the abrupt improvement.

   Several other scales have similar merit (Albert et al., 1976; Subczynski, 1975). The greatest value of a grading scale is that it forces you to observe systematically and accurately. I guarantee that the challenge of grading a response, as in eliciting muscle stretch reflexes,

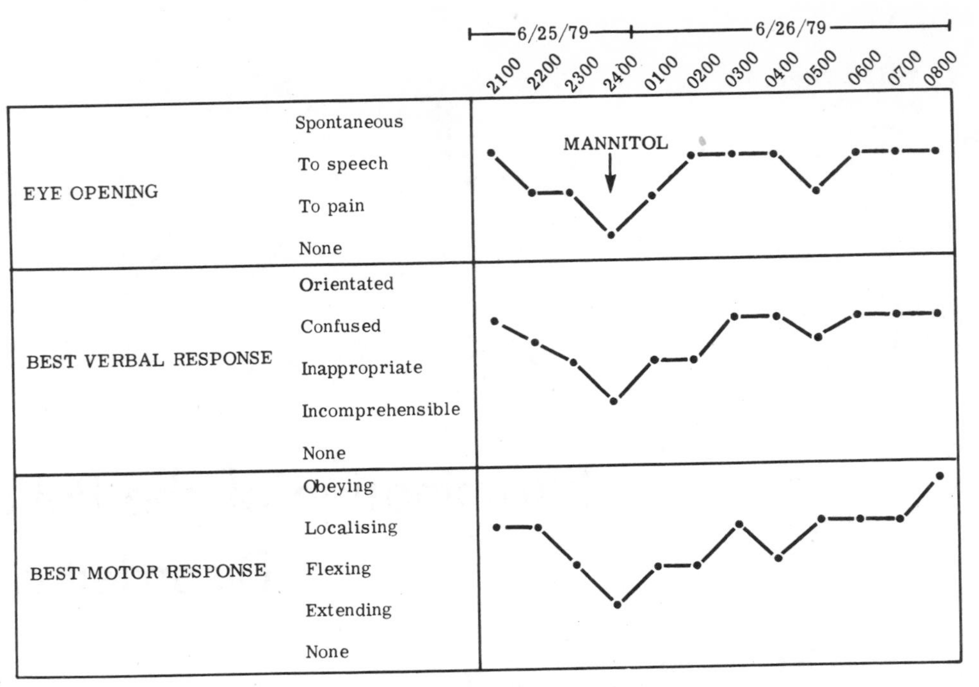

FIG. 12-1. The Glascow coma scale. Notice the declining level of consciousness until after treatment with mannitol, which reduces brain edema.

makes you observe more carefully than if you do not face such a reckoning.

Depend on it sir, when a man knows he is to be hanged in a fortnight, it concentrates his mind wonderfully.

Samuel Johnson

B. *The anatomy of consciousness*

1. *Parts of the neuraxis unnecessary for consciousness.*

To emphasize the parts of the neuraxis necessary for consciousness, we will start by asking what parts we can cut away and discard as unnecessary for consciousness. The text will describe a series of gross surgical cuts through or into the neuraxis. To follow the text, you must know the gross subdivisions of the neuraxis. Make a large, lateral-view drawing of these subdivisions as shown in Fig. 3-1, page 73. Then use scissors to make the cuts in your drawing as the text describes them.

In our search for the neural parts unnecessary to consciousness, we could start either at the extreme caudal or rostral tips of the neuraxis. Let us select the caudal tip of the sacral cord. Surgical transection of the neuraxis at any level from the sacral region to the midpons spares consciousness (if we artificially maintain breathing and blood pressure). Complete removal of the cerebellum spares consciousness. Scissor these parts off of your drawing. (Go ahead and do it. This is not busywork. It will teach you something.) Thus we can discard the spinal cord, medulla, caudal half of the pons, and cerebellum as unnecessary for consciousness. But now, any complete transection at *any* level between the midpons and the rostral end of the midbrain will completely and irreversibly abolish consciousness. Next, instead of completely transecting the pons and midbrain, let us confine the operations to partial transections to determine whether we can dispense with additional parts of these structures. To appreciate the additional knife cuts, draw the generalized cross section of the brainstem, Fig. 3-13, page 91. Again, actually scissor the parts off of your drawing as called for.

We find that we can completely transect, or even remove, the entire basis of the midbrain or pons bilaterally without abolishing consciousness. If we start with an intact nervous system, bilateral destruction of the basis of pons or midbrain produces an individual with complete paralysis of all volitional movements of the trunk, extremities, and all cranial nerve muscles except for vertical eye movements. Such a person retains full sensation and full consciousness and can communicate that consciousness if the examiner works out a code for the vertical eye movements: *up* for *yes* and *down* for *no*. This patient, locked in by the nearly total paralysis, has the locked-in syndrome. Common causes include basilar artery occlusion, tumor, or demyelinating diseases. Thus, snip off the basis bilaterally, and place on the discard heap.

After transecting the basis, we can insert the knife blade a little deeper to transect the medial and lateral lemnisci. The person loses the sensation mediated by these pathways, but consciousness remains. We can then start in dorsally on the brainstem and transect or remove the tectum. Consciousness remains. Next, core out the cranial nerve motor nuclei. Consciousness remains. Thus, cut away from your brainstem drawing the tectum, lemnisci, and cranial nerve motor nuclei, and add them to the discard heap. Now, if we transect the tegmentum bilaterally at any level between midpons and rostral midbrain, the individual becomes abruptly and irreversibly unconscious. For consciousness the pontomesencephalic tegmentum must remain intact and in continuity with the cerebrum at the diencephalon. Yet we have discarded all other parts of the neuraxis caudal to the cerebrum.

From your original drawing you now have remaining in your hand a cerebrum with its midbrain in continuity with the rostral half of the pons. We will next examine the role of the cerebrum in consciousness by progressing rostrally to transect or ablate it bit by bit. We will begin by transecting the diencephalon and basal ganglia, the masses of gray matter that extend the brainstem into the deep white matter of the cerebral hemispheres. We will have to insert the knife through the bottom of the cerebrum to transect these gray masses without disturbing the surrounding white matter or cortex. Bilateral transection of the diencephalon at any level permanently and irreversibly abolishes consciousness. As we extend more rostrally into the basal ganglia, the evidence becomes a little less secure because of the lack of pure lesions in human disease. Tentatively, we can state that bilateral destruction of the globus pallidus and caudate nuclei also abolishes consciousness, at least if the lesion extends a little into the neighboring diencephalon or septal region, as it usually does, or into the neighboring medial hemispheric wall (Freemon, 1971). Thus, we find that bilateral brainstem lesions at any level, from the pontomesencephalic tegmentum up through diencephalon and basal ganglia to the medial hemispheric wall, abolish consciousness.

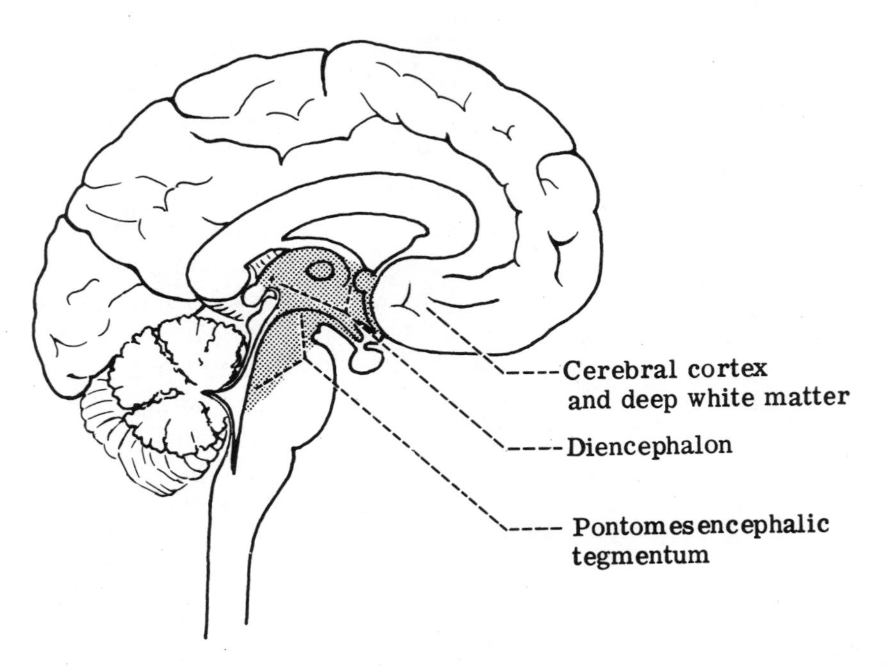

FIG. 12-1.1. Sagittal section of the brain. The stippled area includes the part of the pontomesencephalic tegmentum and diencephalon in which bilateral lesions abolish consciousness.

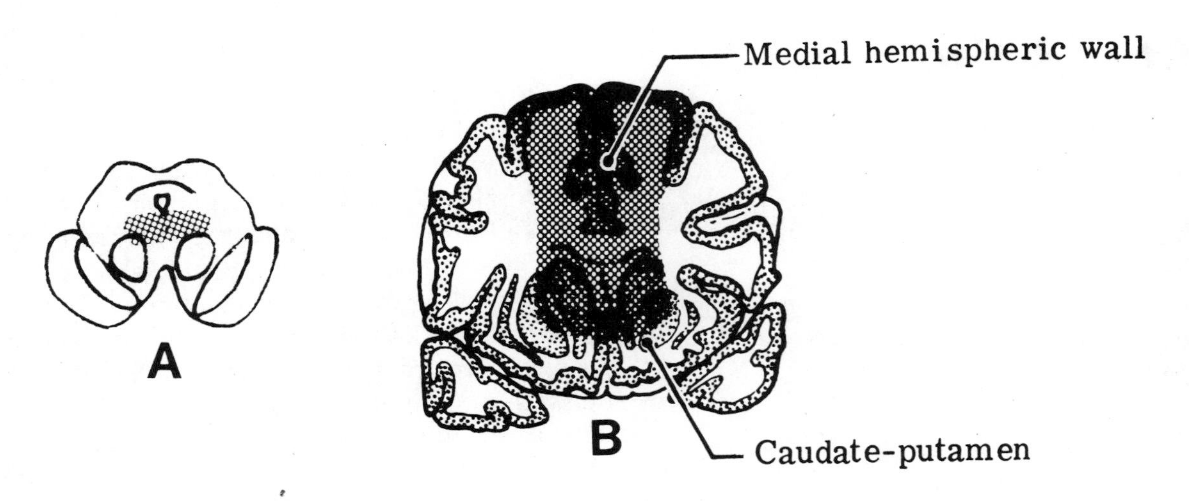

FIG. 12-1.2. Coronal section of the midbrain (A) and of the cerebrum (B) at the level of the caudate nuclei. The shaded area shows the sites and comparative sizes of lesions that abolish consciousness.

Notice in Figs. 12-1.1 and 12-1.2 that as the lesions involve the more rostral structures, particularly basal ganglia and medial hemispheric wall, they must become increasingly larger than those required in the pontomesencephalic tegmentum and diencephalon.

The next anatomical region surrounding the diencephalon-basal ganglia consists of the deep white matter, which conveys axonal circuits between those neuronal masses and the cortical neurons. If we destroy the deep white matter of a hemisphere, or scrape off all of its cerebral cortex, or remove both white matter and cortex by a hemispherectomy,

the patient can retain consciousness (see, however, Albert et al., 1976). Thus, add either one of the two cerebral hemispheres to the discard heap. Actually trace a hemisphere from Fig. 12-1.1 and cut it out for the discard heap. The discard heap of the gross parts unnecessary for consciousness thus includes: ______________________________
____
____.

Ans: The entire spinal cord, medulla, caudal half of the pons, the cerebellum, entire basis and tectum of pons and midbrain, the lemnisci and cranial nerve motor nuclei, and either one of the two cerebral hemispheres.

Although we can dispense with either one of the two cerebral hemispheres, we cannot dispense with both. If we scrape the cerebral cortex off of both hemispheres, or destroy it by hypoxia or hypoglycemia, the patient becomes permanently unconscious. If we suck out the deep white matter from both hemispheres, leaving the cortical shell and brainstem intact, the patient becomes permanently unconscious. Such severe, bilaterally destructive decorticating or demyelinating lesions stand in direct contrast to the tiny, confined bilateral tegmental-diencephalic lesions that exquisitely and selectively abolish consciousness with little effect on functions mediated through other pathways.

2. *Summary of the parts of the neuraxis necessary and unnecessary for consciousness.*

We conclude from these observations that full consciousness requires the pontomesencephalic tegmentum and diencephalon of at least one half of the brainstem, and one (or at least most of one) cerebral hemisphere. This may, just may, constitute the minimum amount of brain required to function as a person. Although a necessary condition for consciousness, integrity of the pontomesencephalic tegmentum is not a sufficient condition, or at least not sufficient to provide operational evidence of consciousness. That requires, in addition, a cerebral hemisphere.

To justify your having learned the structures unnecessary for consciousness, note this supreme fact: If a patient has a lesion of one of these structures and is or becomes unconscious, you must find another explanation for the unconsciousness. The usual explanation is that the lesion has herniated or shifted the brain to compress one of the structures indispensable for consciousness. The patient will die unless you can intervene. A subsequent section discusses these internal brain herniations and their clinical recognition.

3. Now, to summarize this section, do these things:

   a. Enumerate the parts of the neuraxis that we can discard without abolishing consciousness: ______________________________
   ____
   ____.

Ans: Spinal cord, medulla, and caudal half of pons (but we must artificially support breathing and blood pressure); cerebellum; tectum; basis; lemnisci; cranial nerve nuclei of the brainstem; and one cerebral hemisphere (and maybe a little of the other hemisphere).

b. Enumerate the various locations of lesions within the neuraxis that will abolish consciousness. Assume artificial support of breathing and blood pressure so that the loss of consciousness is from the neural lesion, not secondary to hypoxia or ischemia: ______________
____
____
____.

Ans: Make the lesions bilaterally at any level from the rostral pontine midbrain-tegmentum, diencephalon, basal ganglia, or medial hemispheric wall, including the septal region. Or destroy bilaterally the cerebral cortex or the deep white matter.

c. State where to put the most restricted lesions that will most selectively abolish consciousness: ______________________________
____
____.

Ans: Place the lesion bilaterally in the rostral pontine-midbrain tegmentum or diencephalon. See Fig. 12-1.2A.

d. Describe the motor function and level of consciousness of a patient with bilateral destruction of the midbrain-pontine basis (the locked-in syndrome): ______________________________________
____
____.

Ans: The patient remains fully conscious but has paralysis of all volitional movements except for vertical eye movements and convergence.

e. Explain why the patient with the locked-in syndrome retains volitional vertical eye movements: ______________________________
____
____.

Ans: The cortical efferent axons for volitional vertical eye movements run directly to the IIIrd and IVth nerve nuclei from the internal capsule without descending into the basis. The horizontal movement pathways descend through the internal capsule into the basis (along with all other cortical efferent pathways for volitional movements), before entering the lateral conjugate gaze center in the pontine tegmentum. Review the MLF, page 134, if you missed this.

4. Microscopically, the critical region for consciousness in the pontomesencephalic tegmentum consists of the reticular formation. The reticular formation is an intermixture of nerve fibers and neurons which are more or less randomly arranged or loosely nucleated. It fills in, so to speak, the interstices of the tegmentum not occupied by long tracts, cranial nerve, and supplementary motor nuclei. See Figs. 3-13 to 3-17. The reticular formation, as anatomically defined, extends through the tegmental core of the brainstem from the rostral part of the cervical cord into the diencephalon. Reticular formation neurons are connected by numerous short axonal pathways. They receive collaterals from many ascending and descending pathways of the brainstem.
5. The reticular formation, as anatomically defined, subserves many functions in addition to consciousness, such as respiration, pulse rate and blood pressure, posture and muscle tone, and temperature

rostral part (Review Figs. 12-1.1 and 12-1.2 if you missed.)

regulation. The critical part of the reticular formation for consciousness is the ☐ caudal part in the medulla and caudal pons/ ☐ rostral part in rostral pons and mesencephalon.

C. *Operational demonstration of the pathways for consciousness*

1. Insert a *stimulating* electrode into the rostral part of the reticular formation of an animal.
2. Apply *recording* electrodes over the scalp. The record obtained from the scalp electrodes is called an electroencephalogram (EEG).
3. When the animal is asleep, stimulate the reticular formation and observe:
   a. That the animal opens his eyes and looks around. This is the fundamental observation.
   b. That the EEG shows a distinct change in the electrical activity of the brain. This is the correlative observation. See Fig. 12-2.

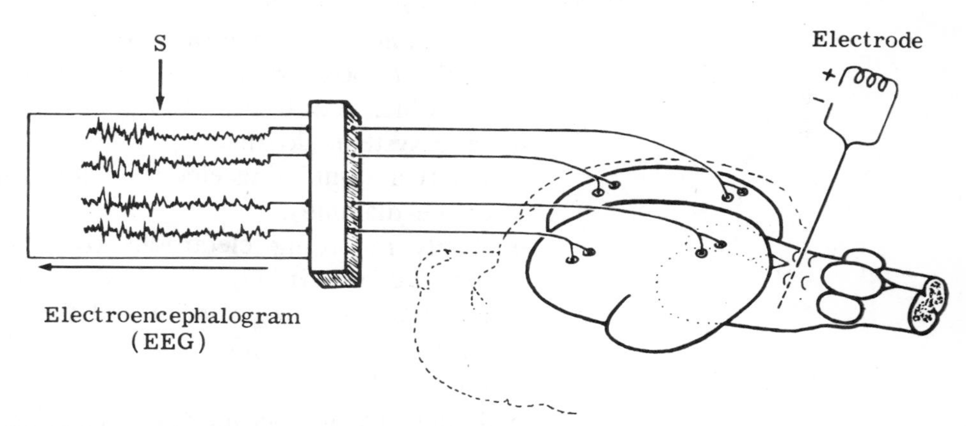

FIG. 12-2. Experimental arrangement to show an alerting response from stimulation of an electrode which has been inserted into the rostral reticular formation. The animal initially is asleep. *S* is the point of stimulation during the EEG recording. Notice the abrupt change from the high amplitude slow waves of sleep to the low amplitude, fast activity of the waking state.

4. Once having awakened the animal with a stimulus to the reticular formation, you can greatly increase the current to make an electrolytic lesion around the tip of the electrode. The animal will lapse into unconsciousness.
5. If the stimulating needle is inserted into the thalamus, into the midline and intralaminar nuclei, a similar alerting response is obtained.
6. *Interpretation of the experiment*
   a. When the electrode is first stimulated, the result is like throwing on a master switch: the whole brain lights up.
   b. Since the whole cortex is affected, we say that a diffuse or nonspecific ascending pathway has been stimulated. Since some or most of these impulses run through the thalamus, we conclude that the experiment demonstrates an ascending reticulothalamocortical pathway. For convenience, we will call this pathway the *ascending reticular activating system* (ARAS). Although the physiologic evidence for the thalamocortical component of the ARAS is strong, the anatomic basis has as yet eluded demonstration.
   c. As operationally defined, the ARAS consists of those neuronal

increases
decrease

assemblies in the rostral part of the brainstem in which stimulation ☐ increases / ☐ decreases consciousness and in which destructive lesions ☐ increase / ☐ decrease consciousness.

d. Notice that the operational definition of the ARAS is based on two lines of evidence: Consciousness is heightened if the ARAS is ______________, and consciousness is abolished if the ARAS is ________.

stimulated
destroyed

7. Give an operational definition of the ARAS based on the effects of stimulation or destruction: ____
____
____.

Ans: The ARAS consists of the neuronal groups in the pons-midbrain tegmentum and diencephalon which increase consciousness when stimulated and decrease it when destroyed.

D. Demonstration of specific thalamocortical pathways

1. The thalamocortical pathways of the sensory nuclei have a very specific, point-to-point relation to the cerebral cortex, in contrast to the ARAS which is diffuse or nonspecific. To demonstrate this contrasting, specific system, do this:
   a. Insert a stimulating electrode into one of the sensory relay nuclei of the thalamus.
   b. Apply recording electrodes over the cortical receptive area of the nucleus. In Fig. 12-3, the stimulating electrode is placed in nucleus ventralis posterior and the recording electrodes are placed over the somesthetic receptive area in the postcentral gyrus. Study Fig. 12-3.
2. Although the diffuse, nonspecific pathway of the ARAS to the cortex has not been anatomically defined, the specific system can be traced anatomically. The specific system is so specific that a discrete locus

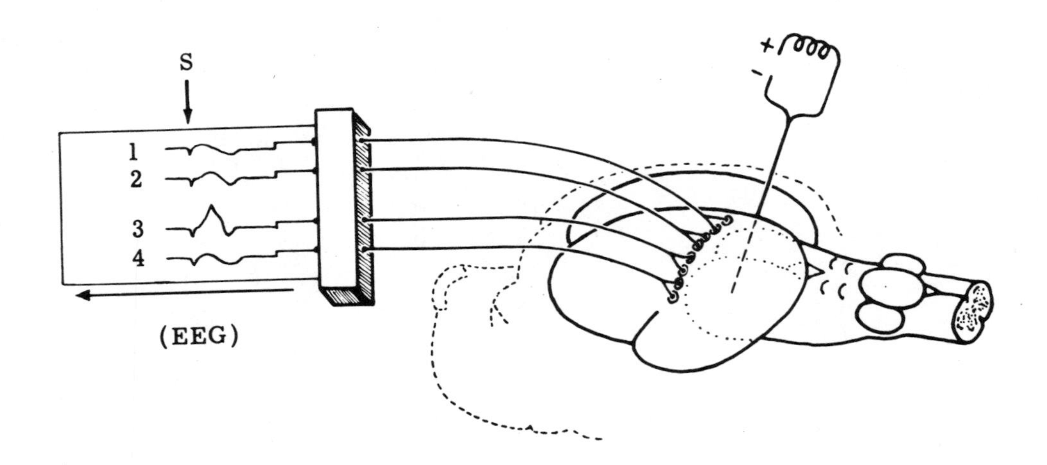

FIG. 12-3. Experimental arrangement to show the specific point of cortical excitation after stimulating a thalamic sensory relay nucleus. Notice in the EEG that a large potential was recorded only from the cortex under the third electrode. Computer averaging is necessary with scalp recording to separate the signal from the noise.

of electrical activity in the cortex can be recorded following stimulation of minute retinal areas, from discrete sound frequencies, or from stimulating the skin of individual digits. Complete Table 12-1 to review the specific thalamic sensory relay nuclei and their cortical projection areas.

1. Lateral geniculate body, occipital

2. Medial geniculate body, temporal

3. N. ventralis posterior, parietal

TABLE 12-1. Specific Sensory Relay Nuclei of the Thalamus

Modality	Thalamic nucleus	Cortical receptive area
Vision		Calcarine cortex in ______ lobe
Hearing		Superior temporal gyrus in ______ lobe
Somatic sensation		Postcentral gyrus in ______ lobe

nonspecific

specific

3. The nonspecific thalamocortical pathway of the ARAS can be contrasted with the specific thalamocortical pathways of the sensory nuclei. The general state of consciousness is mediated through the □ specific / □ nonspecific thalamocortical pathways, whereas the consciousness of particular sensory events is mediated through the □ specific / □ nonspecific thalamocortical pathways.

E. Pathologic alterations in the level of consciousness

1. Consciousness may be altered in one of two directions. It may be elevated or depressed.
2. *Elevation of consciousness*
   a. Insomnia
   b. Agitation
   c. Mania
   d. Delirium (delirium tremens is the classical clinical example of excessive consciousness: insomnia, tremulousness, agitation, anxiety, hallucinations, and the final outcome of any excessive cerebral excitation, convulsions.)
3. *Depression of consciousness*
   a. Normal depression. Drowsiness and sleep at appropriate times.
   b. Pathologic depression
      (1) Somnolence, or pathologic sleep, is sleep that comes on at inappropriate times, but the patient can be aroused to a normal level of awareness. Narcolepsy (literally, *narco* = stupor, as in *nar*cotic, and *lepsy* = to seize, as in epi*lepsy*) is a form of pathologic sleep often associated with other vegetative disturbances, such as a ravenous appetite (polyphagia).
      (2) *Semicoma* (lethargy, stupor). The patient may be aroused to some degree, but cannot reach or sustain a normal level of consciousness.

(3) *Coma.* The patient cannot be aroused. Coma can be graded into *partial* coma, in which the patient is unarousable but retains reflexes, and into *deep* coma, in which even the reflexes are lost.

c. Put S (somnolence), SC (semicoma) or C (coma) before the appropriate statements in Table 12-2.

C

S

SC

S

S

C

TABLE 12-2. *Characteristics of Depressed Consciousness*
________ Patient is areflexic.
________ Patient can be aroused to normal consciousness.
________ Patient can be partially aroused but lapses quickly.
________ Inappropriate as to time of occurrence only.
________ Frequently occurs with polyphagia (megaphagia).
________ Pupils unresponsive to light.

Bibliography

Albert, M. L., Silverberg, R., Reches, A., and Berman, M.: Cerebral dominance for consciousness, *Arch. Neurol.,* 33:453, 1976.

Cairns, H.: Disturbances of consciousness with lesions of the brain-stem and diencephalon, *Brain*, 75:8-146, 1952.

Evans, B. M.: Patterns of arousal in comatose patients, *J. Neurol. Neurosurg. Psychiatry,* 39:392-402, 1976.

Freemon, F. R.: Akinetic mutism and bilateral anterior cerebral artery occlusion, *J. Neurol. Neurosurg. Psychiatry,* 34:693-698, 1971.

Jefferson, G.: *Selected Papers,* Springfield, Ill., Charles C Thomas, Publisher, 1960.

Karp, J., and Hurtig, H.: "Locked-in" state with bilateral midbrain infarcts, *Arch. Neurol.,* 30:176-178, 1974.

Plum, F.: Organic Disturbances of Consciousness, from *Scientific Foundations of Neurology,* Critchley, M. (ed), Philadelphia, F. A. Davis Co., 1972.

Skinner, J., and Lindsley, D.: Electrophysiological and behavioral effects of blockade of the nonspecific thalamo-cortical system, *Brain Research,* 6:95-118, 1967.

Subczynski, J. A.: State of consciousness scoring system, *J. Neurosurg.,* 43:251, 1975.

Teasdale, G., and Jennett, B.: Assessment of coma and impaired consciousness. A practical scale, *Lancet,* 2:81-84, 1974.

Teasdale, G., Knill-Jones, R., and van der Sande, J.: Observer variability in assessing impaired consciousness and coma, *J. Neurol. Neurosurg. Psychiatry,* 41:603-610, 1978.

Valdman, A. (ed.); Pharmacology and Physiology of the Reticular Formation, *Progress in Brain Research,* vol. 20, Amsterdam, Elsevier Publishing Co., 1967.

II. The neurologic signs of rostral brainstem lesions

A. *Impaired consciousness from brain herniations*

1. Many lesions, cerebral contusions, hematomas, abscesses and neoplasms, either by their nature or by inciting edema, increase the volume of the intracranial contents. With characteristic jargon, clinicians call these *space occupying lesions.* When lesions increase intracranial pressure or shift the brain, the brainstem may become compressed, interfering with life sustaining functions of respiration, blood pressure control, and temperature regulation. In preparation for learning how space occupying lesions kill patients, study Figs. 12-4 and 12-5. Note these facts:
   - *a.* How the falx cerebri and tentorium cerebelli partition the intracranial space.
   - *b.* How the transected brainstem remains *in situ* after removal of the cerebral hemispheres.
   - *c.* How the posterior cerebral artery passes over the free edge of the tentorium to reach the temporo-occipital portions of the cerebrum.

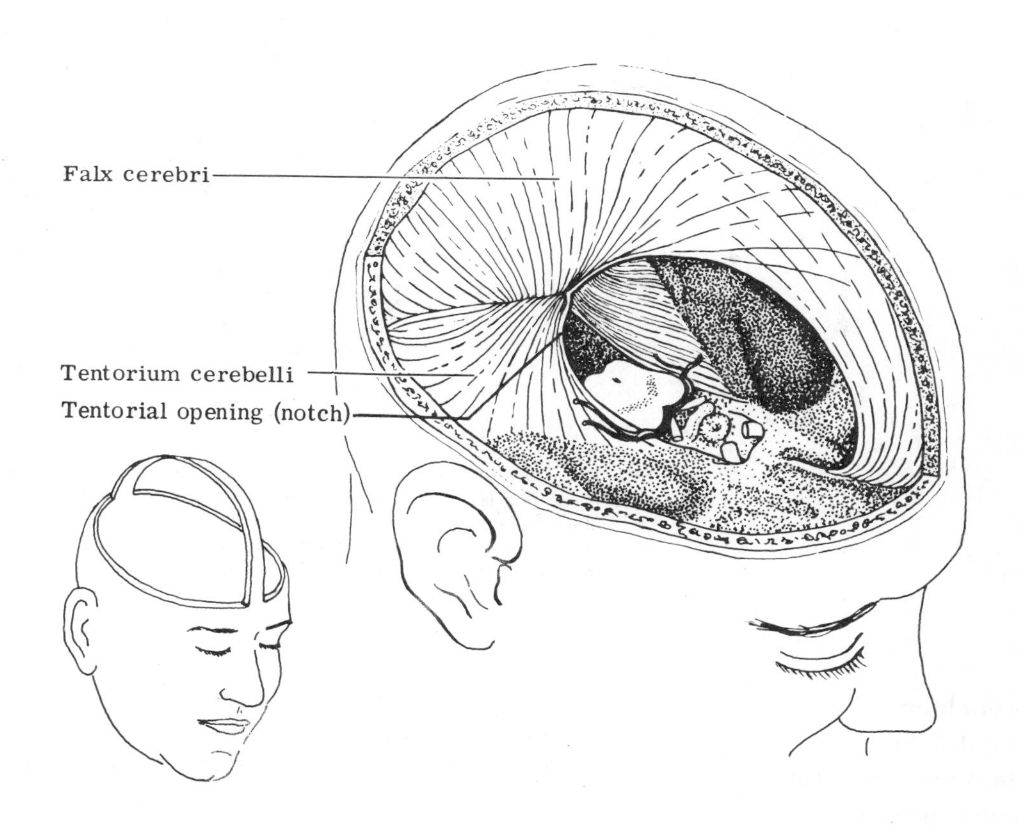

FIG. 12-4. Basket handle dissection of the head, with removal of the cerebral hemispheres. Notice the partitioning of the intracranial space by the falx cerebri and tentorium cerebelli, folds of the dura mater. Notice how the brainstem has been sectioned at the mesencephalon and left *in situ.* Locate the IIIrd nerve issuing from the mesencephalon, going under the posterior cerebral artery, and piercing the dura. Notice the posterior cerebral artery then passing over the free edge of the tentorium to reach the overlying temporo-occipital portions of the cerebrum.

d. How the IIIrd nerve issues from the mesencephalon and passes under the posterior cerebral artery.

falx
tentorium
sagittal

2. The cranial cavity is divided by tough, thick dural partitions called the ______________ cerebri and the ______________ cerebelli.
3. The falx is the dural partition in the ______________ plane of the skull.

cerebellum

4. The tentorium cerebelli forms a tent over the hemispheres of the ______________.

vermis

5. The part of the cerebellum which protrudes through the tentorial notch is the ______________.

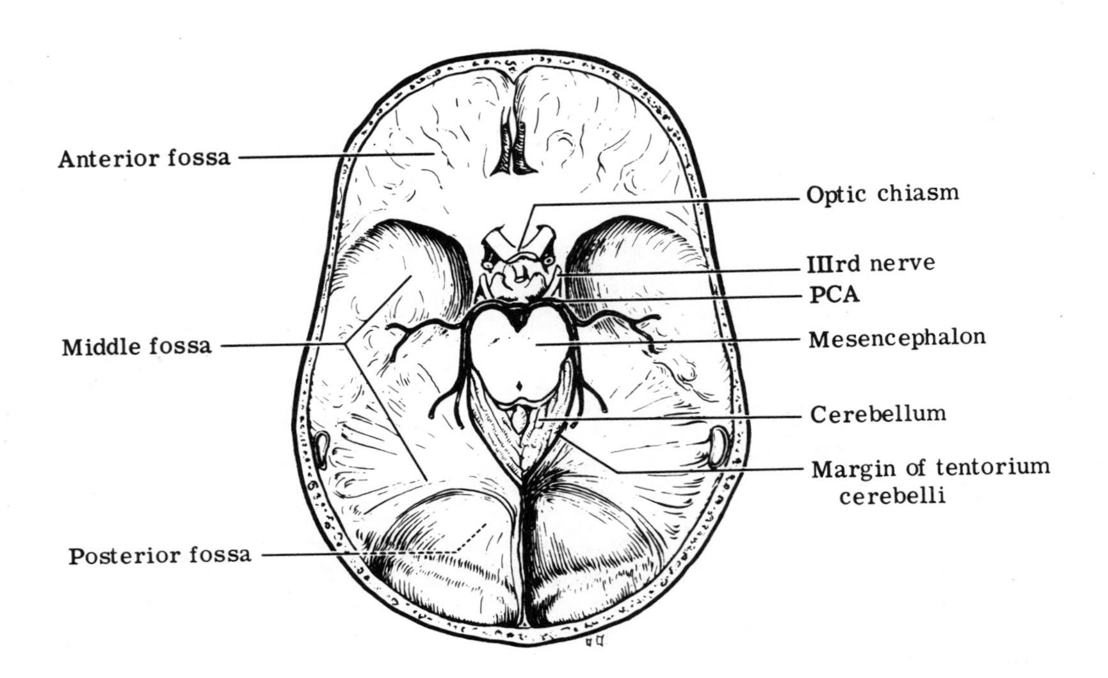

FIG. 12-5. Base of the skull after removal of the basket handle and its attached falx cerebri. The mesencephalon is still *in situ*, as in Fig. 12-4. Notice that the cerebellar vermis occupies the apex of the tentorial opening. Notice that the posterior fossa is under the tentorium. Notice the IIIrd nerve traveling under the posterior cerebral artery (PCA). (*Redrawn from F. Plum and J. Posner: The Diagnosis of Stupor and Coma, Philadelphia, F. A. Davis Company, 1966.*)

cerebellum
occipital or temporo-occipital
notch (opening)
mesencephalon

6. The tentorium cerebelli is inserted between the ______________ below and the ______________ lobes above.
7. The free, medial edges of the tentorial halves form the tentorial ______________, surrounding the mesencephalon.
8. The edges of the tentorial notch surround the ☐ pons / ☐ mesencephalon / ☐ diencephalon.
9. Fig. 12-6 shows a coronal section through the head at the level of the tentorial notch.
10. With a space-occupying lesion in one hemicranium, as shown in Fig. 12-6, the bony wall of the skull prevents herniation or decompres-

falx cerebri

tentorium cerebelli

sion outward. The only place the hemisphere can go is medially or downward.

a. Opposing *medial* shift of the brain is one of the dural membranes, the ____________ ____________.

b. Opposing *downward* shift of the brain is another dural membrane, the ____________ ____________.

11. Brain tissue is about 90 percent water. Brain water is physically incompressible and biologically relatively immobile, since it is confined within the tissue. This relatively immobile brain water can be

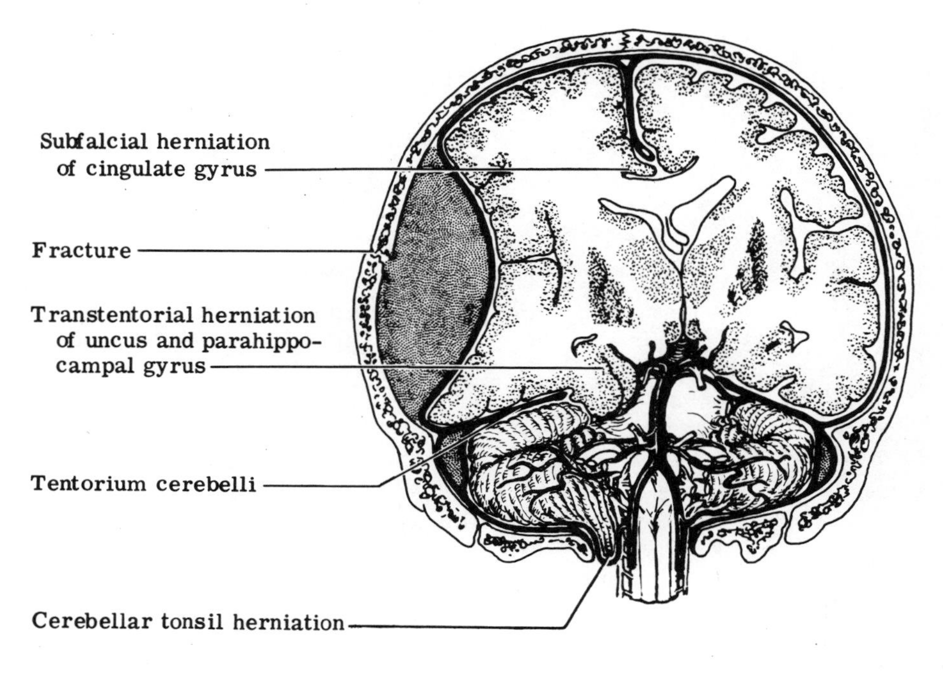

FIG. 12-6. Coronal section of the head; ventral view of the brainstem and cerebrum. A large epidural hematoma has shifted the brain from right to left. Notice that the uncus has herniated over the tentorial edge on the right. Follow along the vertebral and basilar arteries to their terminal branches, the posterior cerebral arteries. Notice how the posterior cerebral artery on the right impinges on the IIIrd nerve. (*Redrawn from F. Netter: Ciba Symposia, vol.* 18, *plate* XI, 1966.)

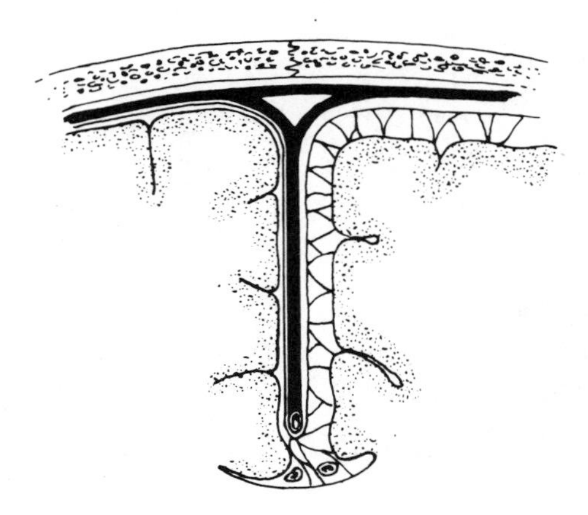

FIG. 12-7. Coronal section through falx and adjacent portions of the cerebrum along the interhemispheric fissure. Notice that the swollen hemisphere (reader's left) has collapsed the subarachnoid space and that the cingulate gyrus is beginning to herniate under the falx.

	contrasted to two rapidly mobile fluid pools of the intracranial space, the *intravascular blood* and the *cerebrospinal fluid* (CSF). When brain tissue swells what would happen to the lumen of the veins and capillaries? ________________.
collapse	12. Study Figs. 12-6 and 7 to describe what pressure does to the ventricle, sulci, and subarachnoid space of a swollen hemisphere: ________________.
collapses them	13. Thus, the first compensation for increased pressure depends on the two rapidly mobile intracranial fluid pools, the ________________.
CSF and intravascular blood	14. The infant has an additional method of compensating for increased intracranial pressure, manifested by the following physical signs: ________________
bulging fontanels, split sutures, and increased OFC	15. As the skull matures, it no longer yields to increased intracranial pressure. If you find split sutures on a skull radiograph of a mature patient you can assume that the increased pressure must have been present before the age of ________________.
puberty (10 to 12 yrs)	16. If the hemispheric swelling exceeds the compensatory mechanisms in infant or adult, the only escape for the displaced hemisphere is to herniate out of the hemicranium. Study Fig. 12-6 and state the only *two* places the shifting hemisphere can go: *a.* ________________. *b.* ________________.
medially under the falx, or downward over the edge of the tentorial notch	17. The combining term *trans* means *over* or *across*; hence, *trans*continental. Since part of the swollen hemisphere has shifted *across* the free edge of the tentorium cerebelli, this event is called ________*tentorial* herniation. Since part of the swollen hemisphere has shifted *under* the falx cerebri, this event is called *sub*________ herniation.
*trans*tentorial sub*falcial* (The x becomes c.)	18. Hence, the two internal herniations of a swollen hemisphere are called ________ herniation and ________ herniation.
transtentorial subfalcial	19. The part of the brain that undergoes subfalcial herniation is the ________ gyrus, while the parts of the brain that undergo transtentorial herniation are the medial parts of the temporal lobe, namely the ________ and ________ gyrus.
cingulate uncus, parahippocampal (See Fig. 12-6 if you missed.)	20. Fig. 12-8 is the brain of a patient, as freshly removed at autopsy. Fill in the labels, and in the blanks below, describe what is wrong. ________________
The left uncus and parahippocampal gyrus have herniated across the tentorial notch, compressing the IIIrd nerve and midbrain.	21. After subfalcial or transtentorial herniation, the diencephalon and mesencephalon become compressed and torqued. Because of interference with the ARAS, the patient suffers a change in his level of consciousness. He may have a transient phase of elevated consciousness, with excitement or delirium, but more typically he descends gradually through the three levels of decreased consciousness, ________
somnolence, semicoma,	

coma

posterior cerebral, IIIrd

constrict

increases
The pupillodilator muscle (sympathetic) enlarges it.

* A. IIIrd nerve
B. Uncus
C. Parahippocampal gyrus
D. Mesencephalon
E. Tentorial notch

__________, ____________________, and ______________.

22. As transtentorial herniation increases, the uncus displaces the ______________ artery and ______________ cranial nerve.
23. The IIIrd nerve contains parasympathetic fibers which when stimulated cause the pupil to ______________.
24. After interruption of the IIIrd nerve, what happens to the pupillary size? ______________. Explain: ______________

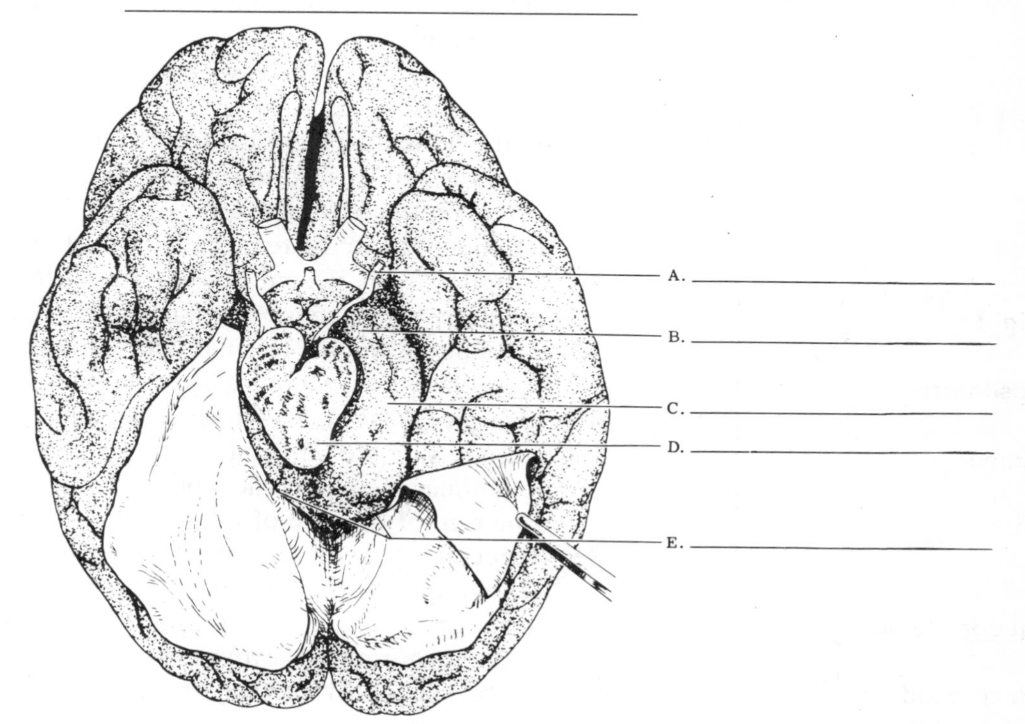

FIG. 12-8. Ventral view of the cerebrum with the tentorium cerebelli reflected on the left side. Complete the labels on the right side. (*Redrawn from T. Peele: The Neuroanatomic Basis for Clinical Neurology, 2nd ed., New York, McGraw-Hill Book Company, 1961.*)

25. Since the pupilloconstrictor fibers occupy the superomedial part of the IIIrd nerve, they suffer compression by the caudally displaced PCA when the temporal lobe herniates. See Fig. 12-9.

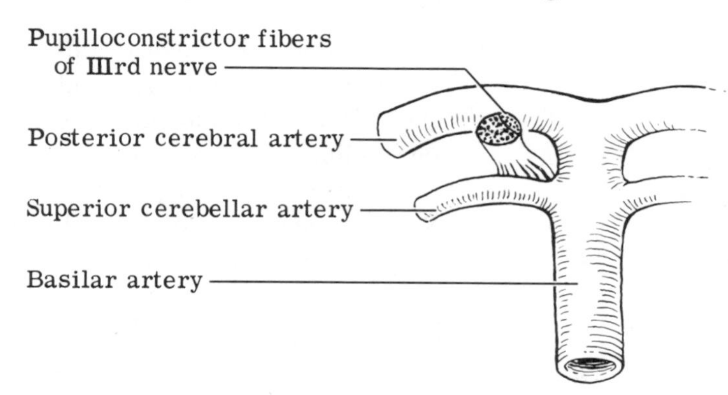

FIG. 12-9. Relation of pupilloconstrictor fibers of cranial nerve III to the posterior cerebral artery. To orient this illustration, see Figs. 12-6 and 3-21.

Transtentorial herniation, brainstem compression, death!

26. In a patient suspected of a space-occupying lesion, what does an increasing pupillary size and a decreasing level of consciousness imply? ______________________________

____

27. As transtentorial herniation advances, both of the IIIrd nerves may cease to function. Both pupils become *dilated* and *fixed*, no longer responding to light. Whereas a unilateral dilated and fixed pupil announces danger requiring prompt or even heroic intervention, bilateral dilated and fixed pupils from brainstem compression are almost synonymous with death.

left

28. Consider now a patient with a large acute right hemisphere lesion. It would cause a ______________-sided hemiplegia.
29. As the herniating right hemisphere compresses the mesencephalon, the left basis gets pushed across against the opposite free edge of the tentorium on the left side. Notice in Fig. 12-5 the close relation of the basis mesencephali to the tentorial edges, affording virtually no safety factor.

right

ipsilateral

30. If the left basis is compressed, the UMN fibers are unable to transmit impulses. The patient now shows a ______________-sided hemiplegia, in addition to his original left hemiplegia. The new hemiplegia is ☐ ipsilateral / ☐ contralateral to the right hemisphere lesion.

same

31. Such an ipsilateral hemiplegia is called a *paradoxical* hemiplegia because it is on the ☐ same / ☐ opposite side as the hemispheric lesion. Sometimes the paradoxical hemiplegia appears first and is a false localizing sign of the side of brain herniation.

quadriplegia

32. Hence, if a patient started out with a large right hemispheric lesion and left hemiplegia, and he then had right hemiplegia, he has double hemiplegia or ______________plegia.

decreased or absent

33. If the quadriplegia evolves very rapidly, the patient might display cerebral shock. What would happen to the MSRs and tone? ______________

______________________________.

34. Thus, depending on the rapidity of evolution of the lesion, the MSR's and tone vary, and they may vary from moment to moment and from side to side.

B. A summation, part-way through the neurologic consequences of rostral brainstem lesions

1. To this point we have discussed the effect of rostral stem lesions on the IIIrd nerve, the pyramidal tracts in the basis mesencephali, and the ARAS. Remaining for consideration are the sensory tracts, the cerebellum, and the regulatory mechanisms for respiration, pulse, blood pressure, and posture.
2. Sensory systems are tested by inflicting pain and watching for movement of the extremities or grimacing.

No

3. Could you test for cerebellar function in a comatose patient? ☐ Yes / ☐ No. Explain: ______________________________

____

______________________________.

Ans: The cerebellum has no known role in consciousness or mentation. It func-

tions when the voluntary motor system functions. Since the comatose patient makes no voluntary movements, cerebellar function cannot be tested.

4. Next we will consider the effects of rostral brainstem lesions on posture and on respiration, blood pressure, and pulse.

C. *Decerebrate rigidity, a postural syndrome of rostral brainstem lesions*

1. Either transtentorial herniation or intrinsic lesions of the rostral part of the brainstem may cause a diagnostic postural syndrome called *decerebrate rigidity*. Surgical transection of the midbrain produces the posture in experimental animals.

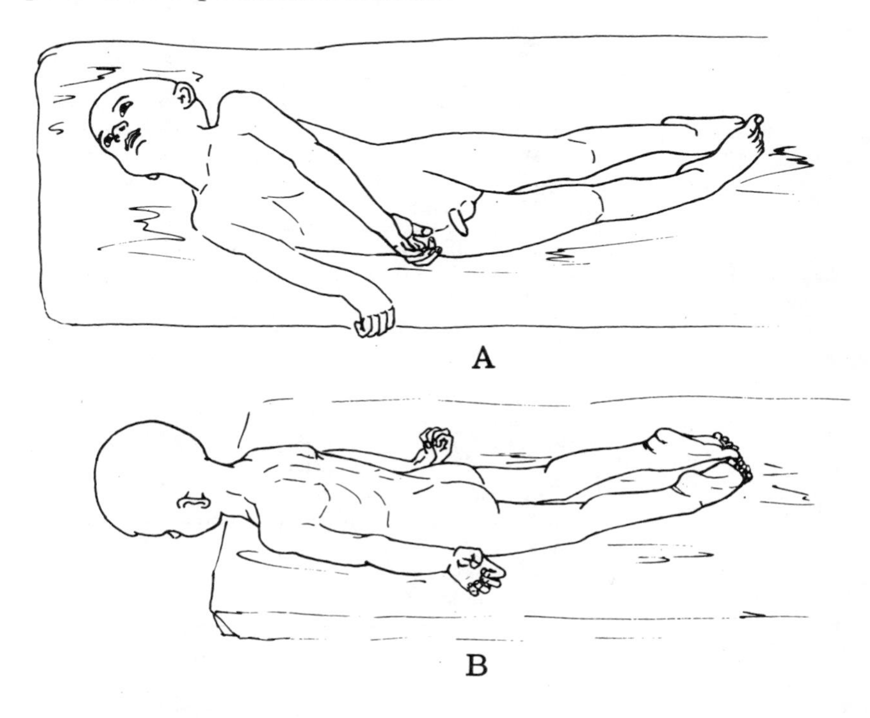

FIG. 12-10. Decerebrate posture. A. The patient is on his side. B. The patient has been placed with his head over the edge of the table to show the rigid extension of his neck. (*Redrawn from W. Penfield and H. Jasper: Epilepsy and the Functional Anatomy of the Human Brain, Boston, Little, Brown and Company, 1954.*)

closed

extended

extended

extended, internally rotated

flexed

flexed

extended, internally rotated

plantar flexed, inverted (equinovarus)

plantar flexed

TABLE 12-3. Posture in Decerebrate Rigidity
The mouth is ☐ open / ☐ closed.
The head is ☐ extended / ☐ flexed.
The trunk is ☐ extended/ ☐ flexed.
The arms are ______________________.
The wrists are ______________________.
The fingers are ______________________.
The legs are ______________________.
The feet are ______________________.
The toes are ☐ plantar flexed/ ☐ dorsiflexed

2. Study Fig. 12-10. Assume the decerebrate posture yourself. Is it a natural, easy posture to maintain?
3. After you have carefully inspected the patient in Fig. 12-10, test your powers of observation by completing Table 12-3.
4. As a prelude to interpreting the posture in decerebrate rigidity, review the strength of the muscle actions listed below. It is best to actually test them again on a normal subject to complete Table 12-4.

TABLE 12-4. Comparative Strength of Postural Deviations in Decerebrate Rigidity

Action	Stronger than/	Weaker than/	Action
1. Jaw closure is	☐	☐	jaw opening
2. Head extension is	☐	☐	head flexion
3. Trunk extension is	☐	☐	trunk flexion
4. Arm extension is	☐	☐	arm flexion
5. Forearm pronation when the arm is extended is	☐	☐	supination
6. Wrist flexion is	☐	☐	wrist extension
7. Finger flexion is	☐	☐	finger extension
8. Leg extension is	☐	☐	leg flexion
9. Inversion of the foot is	☐	☐	eversion
10. Ankle flexion is	☐	☐	ankle extension
11. Toe flexion is	☐	☐	toe extension

Test a normal subject. If you did and you tested carefully, you should have checked the *stronger than* column every time.

strongest (antigravity)

5. To generalize we can say that the posture assumed by the decerebrate patient is determined by the direction of pull of the ________ muscles.
6. If you test muscle tone, you would find that the extremities are rigidly extended, but if you once bend the part, it will yield like a clasp knife. Hence the tonic disturbance is a mixture of spasticity and rigidity.

extension
flexion
internally

7. A descriptive definition of decerebrate rigidity is that it is an involuntary posture of rigid ☐ extension/ ☐ flexion of the proximal joints, with rigid ☐ extension/ ☐ flexion of distal joints, and with the forearms and legs ☐ internally/ ☐ externally rotated.
8. If you examine a quadruped animal with decerebrate rigidity, you would observe the posture of Fig. 12-11.

transect the mesencephalon

9. What operation would you do to the animal to produce the posture of Fig. 12-11? ________
10. If a quadruped with decerebrate rigidity is set on its feet, it will stand. The extended head, tail, and extremities, and the closed jaw, indicate that all muscles maintaining the posture are acting against gravity. Hence, decerebrate rigidity is interpreted as that posture maintained by rigidity of the antigravity muscles of the quadruped. Removal

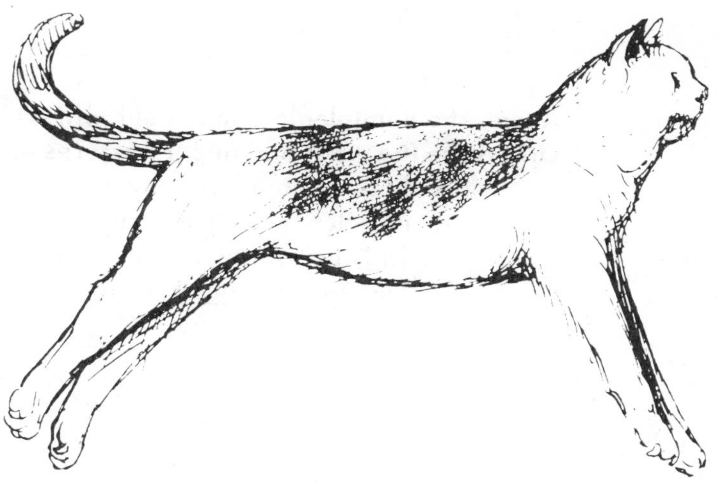

FIG. 12-11. Decerebrate posture in cat. (*From L. Pollock and L. Davis: The reflex activities of a decerebrate animal, J. Comp. Neurol., 50:377-411, 1930.*)

of the rostral cerebral and diencephalic influences on the caudal brainstem releases the primitive, supporting, antigravity postures, whether the animal is a quadruped, or a biped such as man.

It is a new behavior released after interruption of descending motor pathways.

11. Interruption of the pathways descending through the midbrain results in the decerebrate posture. Explain whether to classify the decerebrate posture as a deficit or release phenomenon: ____.

12. Like any release phenomenon, decerebrate rigidity not only requires a lesion to release it, but an intact neural mechanism to produce and perpetuate it. Sherrington showed that the central lesions which abolished decerebrate rigidity transected the vestibulospinal tracts, meaning that activity via these tracts drives the decerebrate posture. Dorsal or ventral root transection also abolish it.

mesencephalon
vestibulospinal tract and dorsal and ventral roots

13. In order for decerebrate rigidity to appear, the critical neural structure transected or compressed is the ______________; the critical neural structures which must remain intact are the ____.

clasp-knife

14. In decerebrate rigidity the term *rigidity* indicates that the limbs are rigidly extended, but it differs from Parkinsonian rigidity since you would perceive a ☐ clasp-knife / ☐ lead-pipe sensation when you attempt to flex the limbs.

clasp-knife
lead-pipe

15. Hypertonus occurs in decerebrate rigidity, Parkinsonism, and chronic hemiplegia. Although the term *rigidity* has the sanction of custom, in the decerebrate patient the hypertonus most closely resembles the ______________ spasticity of chronic hemiplegia rather than the ______________ rigidity of Parkinsonism.

16. It is instructive to compare the posture of decerebrate rigidity with chronic hemiplegia after the stage of cerebral shock or diaschisis in acute hemiplegia has passed. See Fig. 12-12.

17. What is the major difference in the posture of the arm in decerebrate rigidity vs hemiplegic spasticity? ______________

____

____

______________________________.

Ans: The hemiplegic arm is held in flexion at the elbow, rather than extension. Otherwise the wrist and finger postures are similar (as is the leg posture).

quadruped

quadruped (Review Table 12-4 if you missed.)

18. In decerebrate rigidity, the rigidity expresses itself in the true antigravity muscles of a ☐ quadruped/ ☐ biped.
19. In general, the strongest muscles of man are the true antigravity muscles of a ☐ quadruped / ☐ biped.

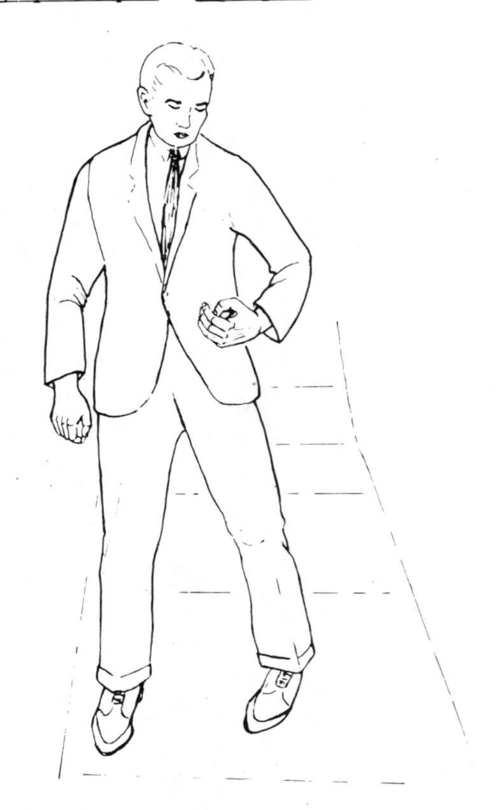

FIG. 12-12. Posture in chronic adult hemiplegia. Compare the arm position with Fig. 12-10.

20. Give a succinct description of the decerebrate posture. Be sure to separate observation from interpretation: ______________________________

____

____

Ans: The decerebrate posture consists of rigid extension of the neck, trunk, arms, and legs, with wrist pronation and wrist and finger flexion, and ankle and toe flexion with internal rotation of the feet.

21. What is the pathophysiologic interpretation of decerebrate rigidity?

____

____

____

Ans: It is a release of the antigravity posture of the quadruped, maintained by the vestibulospinal system and dorsal root afferents, after mesencephalic transection.

22. Some unconscious patients show decerebrate posturing only in response to pain. To elicit the posture, press the ball of your thumb or a knuckle hard for several seconds against the patient's sternum.

D. Respiratory effects of the brainstem lesions and transtentorial herniation

1. Different respiratory dysrhythmias correlate with lesions at various levels along the brainstem. Transtentorial herniation, by external compression, caudal displacement, and kinking of the brainstem, causes respiratory dysrhythmias similar to brainstem lesions. The one type of dysrhythmia seen with intrinsic brainstem lesions but not with transtentorial herniation is apneustic breathing, *C* of Fig. 12-13 (Plum and Posner, 1972). Learn Fig. 12-13.

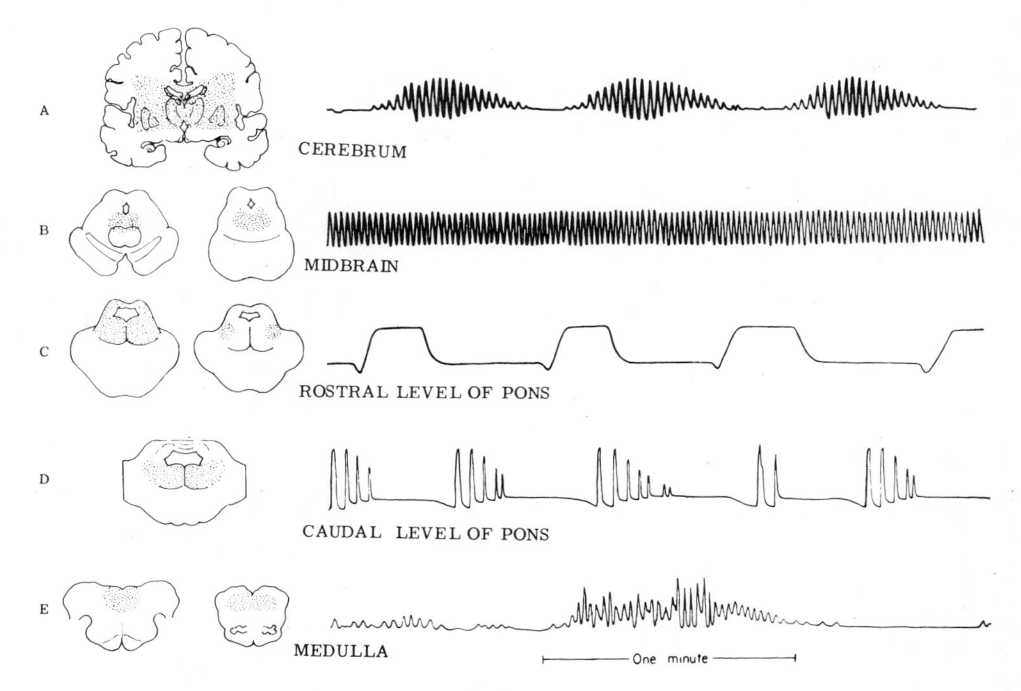

FIG. 12-13. Correlation of intraaxial brainstem lesions at successive levels, with the type of respiratory dysrhythmia. A. Cheyne-Stokes respiration. B. Central neurogenic hyperventilation. C. Apneustic breathing. D. Cluster breathing. E. Ataxic breathing. (*Redrawn from P. Plum and J. Posner: The Diagnosis of Stupor and Coma, Philadelphia, F. A. Davis Company, 1966.*)

2. The effect of transtentorial herniation or other brainstem lesions on blood pressure and pulse is variable, like that on respiration. While either hypertension or hypotension and tachycardia or bradycardia may occur, the typical picture is one of a slowing pulse rate and an increasing blood pressure. Many factors, such as the ventilatory efficiency, may alter this formula. Thus, the important feature is to look for variability of these vital signs and to detect such trends as may occur.

E. Bilateral transtentorial herniation

1. So far, we have considered the transtentorial herniation syndrome as caused by a unilateral expanding lesion in a hemicranium. Many pathologic conditions cause *bilateral* expansion of the brain, usu-

ally by cerebral edema. Trauma, encephalitis, and metabolic disorders such as uremia, hepatic coma, and lead poisoning are common offenders. Of the structural lesions, head injury, hydrocephalus, multiple metastatic neoplasms or abscesses, and intracranial hemorrhage lead the list. If both hemispheres swell, the unci and parahippocampal gyri of both sides try to squeeze through the tentorial notch. The ring of swollen tissue acts exactly as if you had placed a ligature around the mesencephalon, tied a slip knot, and pulled both ends.

2. The *coup de grâce* to the patient with transtentorial herniation, either bilateral or unilateral, from any cause, is mesencephalic and pontine hemorrhage. As the brainstem vessels become stretched and compressed, the blood flow to the stem and to the vessel walls themselves is interrupted. The walls become necrotic and rupture. This brainstem hemorrhage is usually the terminal event which causes the patient to die. See Fig. 12-14.

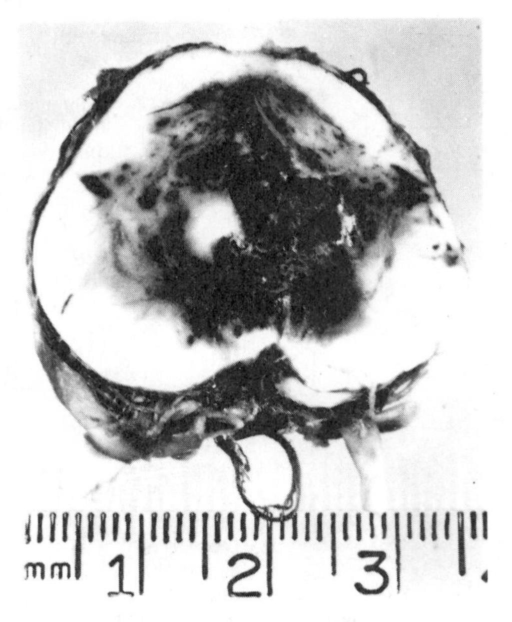

FIG. 12-14. Transverse section of the mesencephalon showing hemorrhages secondary to transtentorial herniation. The third nerves are seen, exiting ventrally. The caudal displacement of the brainstem by the expanding cerebrum stretches and compresses the brainstem vessels until they rupture, killing the patient.

F. Transforaminal herniation

1. The diffusely swollen brain or the hydrocephalic brain may impose the death penalty by another mechanism. As increased pressure pushes the intracranial contents caudally, the cerebellum and medulla are displaced into the foramen magnum. This aperture is designed to accommodate only the medulla at its transition to the ______________________________.

spinal cord

2. The caudalmost part of the cerebellum is called the *tonsil,* in clinical jargon. It is the part of the cerebellum to herniate. This type of brain herniation is called *tonsilar herniation,* or *transforaminal herniation* as we shall term it, because the herniated brain is jammed

foramen

through the ______________ magnum. See the herniated right cerebellar tonsil in Fig. 12-6.

3. Transforaminal herniation may be caused by expanding *supra*tentorial lesions, as of the cerebrum, or by expanding *infra*tentorial lesions, as of the cerebellum.
4. The clinical syndrome of transforaminal herniation mimics transection of the neuraxis at the level of the medullocervical junction. The patient becomes quadriplegic and anesthetic. He has complete respiratory arrest, because the cervical LMNs which innervate the diaphragm and the thoracic LMNs which innervate the intercostal muscles receive no UMN impulses from the brain.

Subfalcial, transtentorial, and transforaminal

5. Name the common internal herniations of the brain: ______________ ______________ ______________.

Cingulate gyrus; parahippocampal gyrus and uncus; cerebellar tonsil

6. Name the parts of the brain which herniate in each case: ______________ ______________ ______________.

By impairing vital functions like breathing, P rate, and BP, and causing brainstem compression and hemorrhage

7. State, in principle, how brain herniations kill the patient: ______________ ______________ ______________.

G. Brain herniations: a summation

1. When any modern gladiator, a boxer, a football player, or a race driver dies after a head injury, in sacrifice to our appetite for brutality, you can surmise that the mechanism of death was brain herniation. If we do not as a people value above all else the preciousness and fragility of life, one might suppose that we would at least value the organ of advantage. (For the brain is not, as you might have misbelieved, an organ of intelligence; it is as Szent-Györgyi said, an advantage-seeking organ.) The "private eye" or TV hero who gets hit on the head and bounces right back to great heights (or depths) of performance is not only a cultural travesty, but also an egregious error in medical management. The patient with any head injury or who is even suspected of a space-occupying intracranial lesion must be recognized as the most imperative type of medical emergency, as imperative as cardiac arrest, respiratory arrest, or hemorrhage, which are often also present. Anyone can recognize when the patient is in coma. The physician must read the clinical warnings to anticipate when coma threatens. That is to say, we must deal with prediction, the most difficult of all the arts. To predict the predictable and prevent the preventable, you must know how brain lesions kill and read the evolving signs that can lead to death.
2. When a patient with a potential brain herniation is identified, he must be carefully watched and *all* physical signs must be recorded: vital signs, such as blood pressure and pulse, and physical signs such as the pupillary diameters in millimeters. Given a patient with a head injury and left hemiparesis who is initially conscious, outline the sequence of events, in order, that will predict transtentorial herniation, and list the sequence of events to death:

Answer given in next frame.

a. Consciousness: ______________________________

____

b. Condition of extremities: ______________________________

____

c. Pupillary changes: ______________________________

____

d. Respiration: ______________________________

____

e. Pulse and blood pressure: ______________________________

____

f. Final pathologic change in brainstem:

____

3. Answers to frame 2:
   a. May have some excitement, then pathologic sleep, semicoma, and coma.
   b. Left hemiparesis may worsen, right hemiparesis appears, then quadriplegia, often followed by decerebrate rigidity and then complete flaccidity just preceding death.
   c. The right pupil becomes dilated and fixed, then the left.
   d. Cheyne-Stokes, central neurogenic hyperventilation, apneusis, cluster breathing, and ataxic respiration, finally respiratory paralysis.
   e. Pulse and blood pressure may fluctuate, but tendency to increasing blood pressure with decreasing pulse rate.
   f. Hemorrhage into the brainstem, secondary to stretching of the brainstem vessels.
4. The time to help such a patient has already been lost when he has reached the stage of bilateral pupillary dilation, decerebrate rigidity, and coma. At that point he is irretrievable. The patient's increased pressure and potential for herniation must have been recognized early by the attending physician who must call for neurological help. If the physicians can relieve the pressure early, the patient recovers, If not he dies: that is why you have to understand the physical signs and mechanisms we have just studied.

Bibliography

Brain herniations

Azambuja, N., Lindgren, E., and Sjögren, S.: Tentorial Herniations. I. *Anatomy Acta. Radiol.,* 46:215-223, 1956.

Emery J.: Kinking of the medulla in children with acute cerebral oedema and hydrocephalus and its relationship to the dentate ligaments, *J. Neurol. Neurosurg. Psychiat.,* 30:267-275, 1967.

Feindel, W., Penfield, W., and McNaughton, F.: The tentorial nerves and localization of intracranial pain in man, *Neurology,* 10:555-563, 1960.

Finney, L., and Walker, A.: *Transtentorial Herniation,* Springfield, Ill., Charles C Thomas, Publishers, 1962.

Friede, R., and Roessmann, U.: The pathogenesis of secondary midbrain hemorrhages, *Neurology.* 16:1210 - 1216, 1966.

Hassler, O.: Arterial pattern of human brainstem: Normal appearance and deformation in expanding supratentorial conditions, *Neurology,* 17:368-375, 1967.

Howell, D.: Upper brain stem compression and foraminal impaction with intracranial space-occupying lesions and brain swelling, *Brain,* 82:525, 1959.

Norris, F., and Fawcett, J.: A sign of intracranial mass with impending uncal herniation, *Arch. Neurol,* 12:381-386, 1965.

Plum, F., and Posner, J.: *The Diagnosis of Stupor and Coma,* Philadelphia, F. A. Davis Co., 2nd ed., 1972.

Walker, A.: The syndromes of the tentorial notch, *J. Nerv. Ment. Dis.,* 136:118-129, 1963.

Decerebrate rigidity and other brainstem signs of coma

Brendler, S. J., and Selverstone, B.: Recovery from decerebration, *Brain,* 93:381-392, 1970.

Cravioto, H., Silberman, J., and Feigin, I.: A clinical and pathologic study of akinetic mutism, *Neurology,* 10:10-21, 1960.

Feldman, M.: Physiological observations in a chronic case of "locked-in" syndrome, *Neurology,* 21:459-478, 1971.

Freemon, F.: Akinetic mutism and bilateral anterior cerebral artery occlusion, *J. Neurol. Neurosurg. Psychiat.,* 34:693-698, 1971.

Halsey, J., and Downie, A.: Decerebrate rigidity with preservation of consciousness, *J. Neurol. Neurosurg, Psychiat.,* 29:350-355, 1966.

Kemper, T., and Romanul, F.: State resembling akinetic mutism in basilar artery occlusion, *Neurology,* 17:74-80, 1967.

Pollock, L., and Davis, L: The reflex activities of a decerebrate animal, *J. Comp. Neurol.,* 50:377-411, 1930.

Roberston, R., and Pollard, C., Jr.: Decerebrate state in children and adolescents, *J. Neurosurg.,* 12:13-17, 1955.

Sherrington, C.: *The Integrative Action of the Nervous System,* New Haven, Yale University Press, 1947.

Westmoreland, B. F., Klass, D. W., Sharbrough, F. W., and Reagan, T. J.: Alpha-coma, *Arch. Neurol.,* 32:713-718, 1975.

Zeman, W., and Youngue, E.: Decortication as a result of widespread circulatory and anoxic damage, *J. Neuropath. Exp. Neurol.,* 16:492-506, 1957.

III. Neurologic examination of the comatose patient

A. For the most difficult diagnostic challenge of all, I would give you a patient brought in comatose off the street, with no history available. In the differential diagnosis, you will immediately want to see whether the patient has an ascertainable neurologic lesion. I must assume that you will do a complete *general* physical examination. Here are the *special* features of the neurologic examination.

B. Inspection of the comatose patient

1. Check for respiration and record the type. An open airway is the first rule in coma.
2. Inspect and palpate the head for bruises, swellings, or depressions.
3. Record the size of the pupils in millimeters and the position of the eyes.

ipsilateral
contralateral (If you missed, review pages 134 - 136.)

☑ to

VI and VII

away from

a. If the eyes persistently deviate to one side, in the absence of convulsions, you would expect a destructive lesion in the conjugate gaze center in the ☐ ipsilateral / ☐ contralateral posterior frontal region or in the ☐ ipsilateral / ☐ contralateral half of the pons.

b. If the lesion were in the hemisphere, the eyes would deviate ☐ to / ☐ away from the side of the lesion.

c. State which cranial nerve(s) would most likely be paralyzed with a pontine lesion that affected the conjugate lateral gaze center ______________.

d. If the lesion were in a pontine center, the eyes would deviate ☐ to / ☐ away from the side of the lesion.

4. Look for asymmetry of spontaneous facial movements.
5. Look for asymmetry of spontaneous extremity movements.
6. Strip off all the clothes, search the clothing for suicide notes or medication, then look for injuries, injection scars in the arm veins, and hypodermic scars from drug or insulin injection.
7. Roll the patient over and look at back and buttocks. (Maybe he is in shock from rectal bleeding.)

C. Smelling the comatose patient's breath

1. The alcoholic breath of the alcoholic patient.
2. The fruity breath of the diabetic in coma.
3. The "bitter" breath of the dehydrated patient.
4. The death smell from the gangrenous lung of the patient in pulmonary coma.

D. Signs of hemiplegia in the comatose patient

1. Detection of hemiplegia in the unconscious patient depends, in principle, on detecting asymmetry of movement and muscle tone.
2. Detect asymmetry of movement by inspection. Unless deeply comatose, the patient moves all extremities spontaneously or in response to pain stimuli. Absence of spontaneous or pain-induced movements on one side indicates hemiplegia, provided you exclude local disorders such as a dislocated shoulder or broken hip.
3. Detect asymmetry of muscle tone by inspection and by passive manipulations. The acute, severe lesions that cause unconsciousness usually cause flaccid hemiplegia (cerebral shock). The face and extremities on the intact side continue to show some muscle tone.
4. When the comatose hemiplegic exhales, one cheek puffs out more than the other. It will be on the ☐ hemiplegic / ☐ nonhemiplegic side. Explain: ____
____
____.

hemiplegic

Ans: The buccinator and other facial muscles on the hemiplegic side have a flaccid paralysis from cerebral shock. Facial muscles on the other side have tone. Therefore, the cheek on the hemiplegic side puffs out.

5. *The eyelid release test*

a. Make a drawing to show the UMN and LMN innervation of the right side of the face in Fig. 12-15.

b. Recall that the LMNs for the orbicularis oculi muscle may be innervated by many crossed UMNs. Hence, in acute hemiplegia, when UMN axons are suddenly interrupted, the eyelid shows ☐ flaccid/ ☐ spastic weakness. The eyelid release test demonstrates it.

flaccid

Compare with Fig. 6-3.

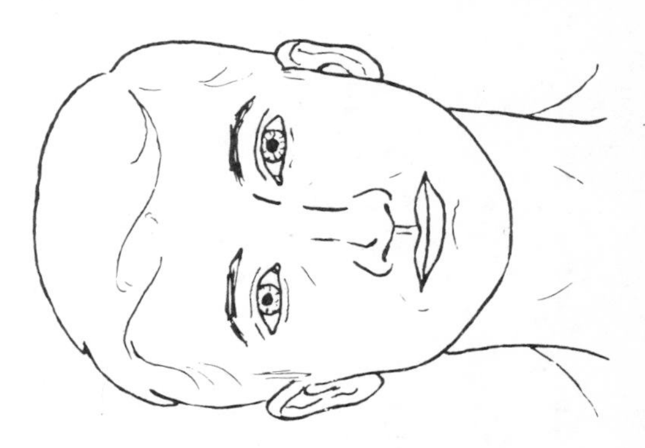

FIG. 12-15. Blank to draw in the UMN innervation of the VIIth nerve nucleus and the LMN innervation of the facial muscles.

c. Procedure for eyelid release test. Gently pull both eyelids up with your two thumbs and then release them simultaneously, as in Fig. 12-16.

d. Results. The eyelid of the hemiplegic side glides down slowly while the opposite lid usually closes rapidly, unless the patient is deeply comatose. Why does the eyelid on the nonhemiplegic side close faster? ____

____.

Ans: The orbicularis oculi muscle of the normal side is not paralyzed and retains muscle tone.

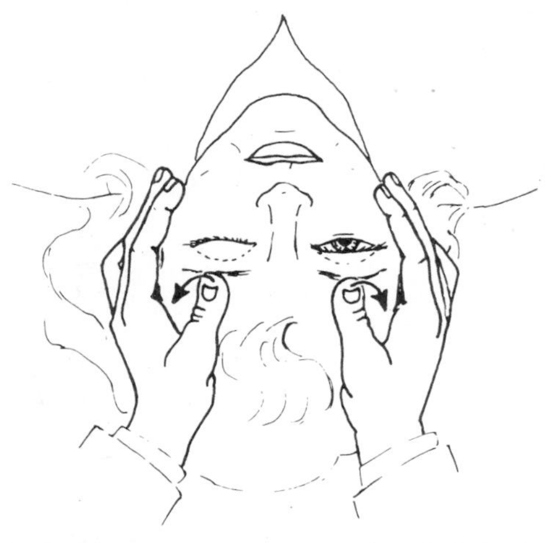

FIG. 12-16. Eyelid release test in a comatose patient with right hemiplegia. The examiner stands at the head of the patient. The patient's eyelids are elevated by the examiner's thumbs and released simultaneously. The lid of the hemiplegic side closes slowly, and the lid of the normal side closes briskly.

6. *The limb-dropping tests.* Flaccid paralysis of the extremities is verified by the *limb-dropping tests.*
   a. *The wrist-dropping test.* Grasp both of the patient's forearms just proximal to the wrist. Hold the forearms vertical, as in Fig. 12-17. The hemiplegic wrist drops at right angles, while the nonhemiplegic wrist remains to some degree vertical.

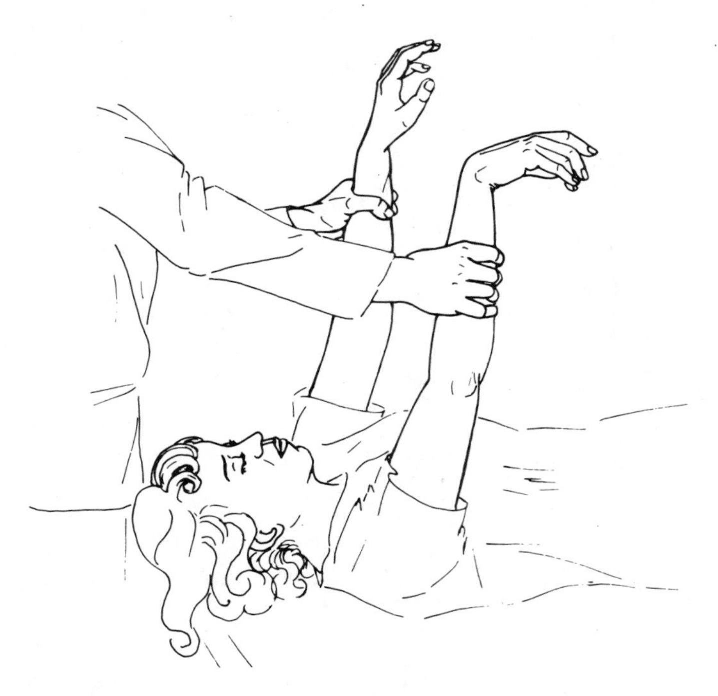

FIG. 12-17. The wrist-dropping test for flaccid hemiplegia in a comatose patient with right hemiplegia.

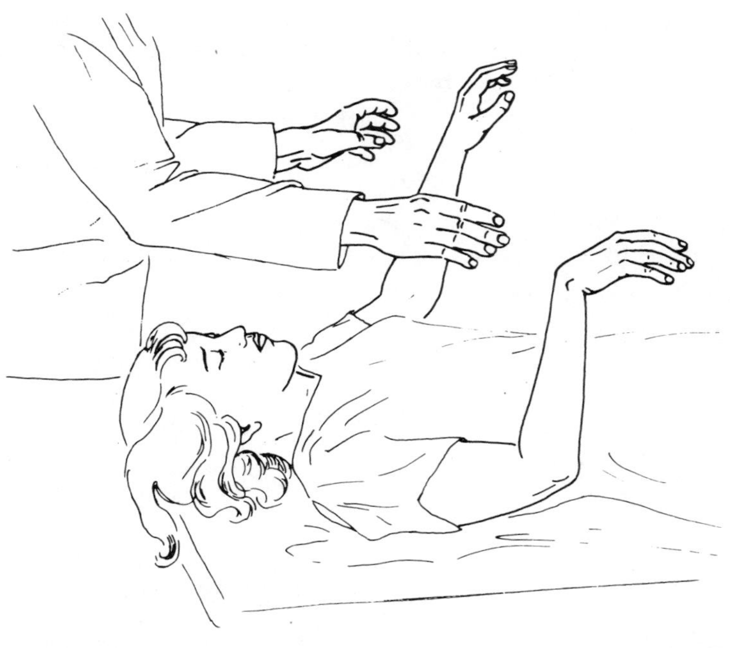

FIG. 12-18. The arm-dropping test for flaccid hemiplegia in a comatose patient with right hemiplegia.

b. *The arm-dropping test.* Grasp both forearms, as in the wrist-dropping test, and release them simultaneously. The hemiplegic arm drops limply, while the normal arm glides or floats down. See Fig. 12-18. Lift the arm only a few inches—beware of ulnar nerve injury.

c. *The leg-dropping test.* Crook the patient's knees on your arm, as in Fig. 12-19. Extend first one leg, then the other and drop them.

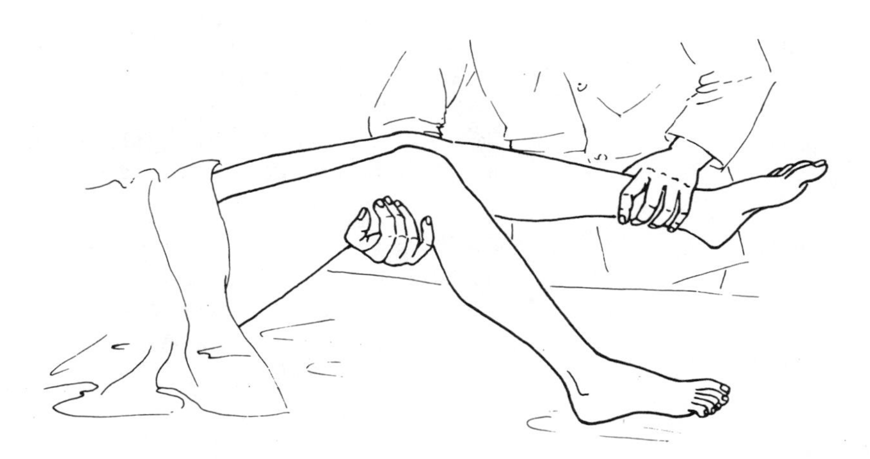

FIG. 12-19. The leg-dropping test for flaccid hemiplegia in a comatose patient with right hemiplegia.

You can both see and hear the difference as the hemiplegic leg drops more rapidly to strike the bed.

tone

d. The dropping tests depend on the principle of asymmetry of muscle ________________.

coma

e. For correct interpretation, the nonhemiplegic side must have some muscle tone. Hence, the tests are invalidated if the patient is completely *atonic.* They are useless in deep ________________, when reflexes and tone are lost on both sides.

7. Summarize the methods of detecting acute hemiplegia in a semicomatose or comatose patient: ____.

Ans: Inspect for asymmetry of movement and puffing out of one cheek. Test for asymmetry of muscle tone by manipulation of the extremities and by the eyelid and extremity-dropping tests.

E. Resistance to movement: paratonia

1. *Paratonia* is a resistance to movement of any part of the body in all directions. It is common in semicoma or light coma. It is as if the patient divines every movement you impose and automatically counteracts it.

coma

2. Paratonia, like any resistance dependent on muscular contraction, would not appear on the side of acute flaccid hemiplegia or if the patient were in deep ________________, when all tone is lost.

decreased

3. The novice often misidentifies the nonhemiplegic side as hemiplegic because he mistakes paratonia for the increased tone of an UMN lesion. In the unconscious patient with acute hemiplegia, the tone on the hemiplegic side is usually ☐ increased / ☐ decreased.
4. Paratonia or other rigidities are common complications of tranquilizer drugs, such as prochlorperazine (Compazine), and may be seen in lesions of the extrapyramidal system, hysteria, senility, and mental confusion.

F. Resistance to movement: nuchal rigidity and meningeal irritation signs

1. *Nuchal rigidity*

   Definition: The term *nucha* refers to the back of the neck. If you cannot flex the patient's head because of reflex spasm of the nuchal (extensor) muscles, we say that the patient has nuchal rigidity. Nuchal rigidity indicates an irritative lesion of the subarachnoid space, most commonly meningitis or hemorrhage.
2. *The mechanism of spasm of the extensor muscles of the neck*
   a. Once you appreciate the mechanics involved, the signs of meningeal irritation are easy to understand, and you get a bonus: you learn how to position a patient who has suffered a vertebral fracture. Study Figs. 12-20 and 21.
   b. The bar in Fig. 12-20 impales the neuraxis. It acts as a lever with the fulcrum at the top of the vertebral column. Thus, when the head is flexed, the spinal cord is ☐ relaxed / ☐ extended.

extended

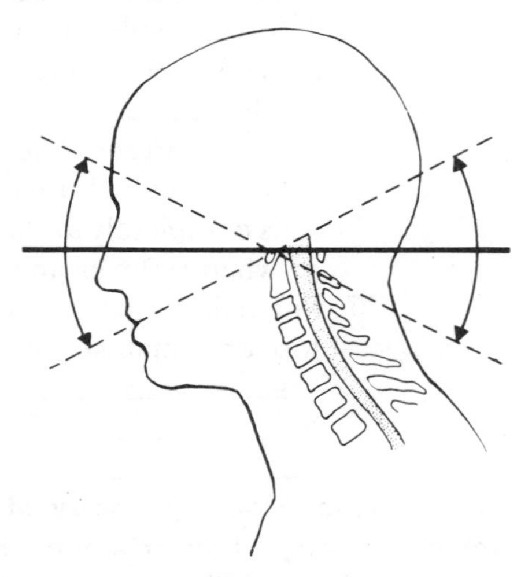

FIG. 12-20. Sagittal section of the head to show the effect of head extension and flexion in tightening and relaxing the spinal cord. Imagine a steel rod driven through the head, as indicated by the solid black line. It acts as a lever with the fulcrum over the vertebral bodies.

   c. Neck flexion and extension is more complicated than Fig. 12-20 shows. Movement occurs not only between the skull and first cervical vertebra, but also between all other cervical vertebra. The neck does not flex as though hinged at one point: it bends like a sapling. Fig. 12-21*A* and *B* shows the actual changes in vertebral angulation with flexion-extension and the accompanying changes in tension on the nerve roots and spinal cord.

d. The cord is held in position by its attachment to the brain and by suspensory ligaments, the dentate ligaments. The cord is tethered to some extent by the nerve roots and also it is buoyed by the surrounding CSF. See the dentate ligaments in Fig. 12-22.

e. During ordinary movement, little or no traction is placed on cord or roots, according to Breig's studies. Between extension and flexion, the cord changes from a relaxed accordion-like wrinkling to simple straightening. When, however, roots, meninges, and cord are in-

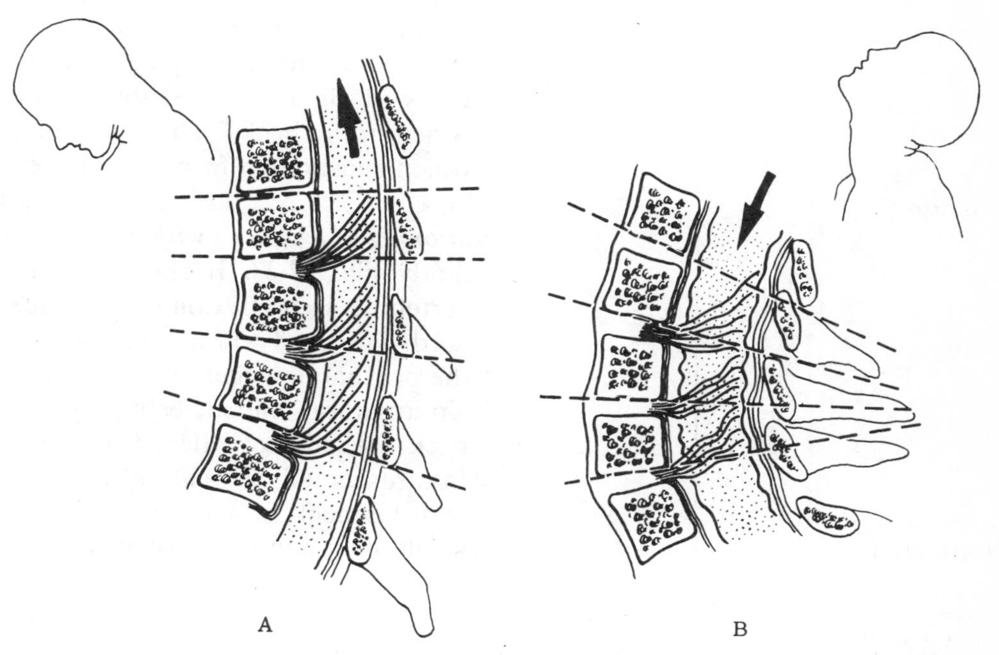

FIG. 12-21. Sagittal sections through the cervical spinal cord and vertebrae. *A.* Head flexion. *B.* Head extension. Notice that the spinal cord and nerve roots are stretched and lengthened in *A* and relaxed and pleated in *B*.

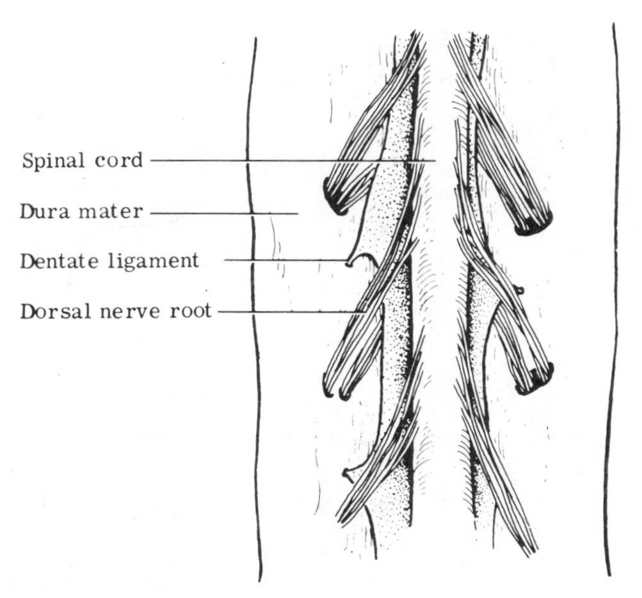

FIG. 12-22. Dentate ligaments. The dura has been slit open to expose the dorsal surface of the cord.

flamed and swollen, the ordinarily innocuous act of flexing the head puts tension on the inflamed structures. It is perhaps much like pressing on a boil. As long as the part with the boil is still, it doesn't hurt much. Movement of the part, placing tension on the swollen tissues, causes intense pain. Any pain of this type elicits immediate muscle spasm, which acts to prohibit the painful movement. If you have ever tried to take a deep breath when you had a "stitch" in your side from a pleuritic rub, you will know how effectively pain inhibits the muscular contraction which causes it. Other examples of pain-avoiding muscle spasm are the abdominal wall rigidity of peritonitis, and back rigidity from sprains, a "crick in the back." Thus, with inflammed meninges, the movement which causes pain from tension on the cord and nerve roots would be ______________________ of the neck.

flexion

3. *Positioning of a patient with known or suspected cervical cord injury*
   a. Study Fig. 12-23. It shows a fracture dislocation of the cervical vertebrae. Head flexion would place tension on the swollen, softened cord. The cord will impinge on the protruding bone, compounding the original damage.
   b. Your natural tendencies urge you to place an injured person on his back with his head flexed on a pillow, exactly the wrong position. In a suspected cervical cord injury, splint and transport the patient with his neck in a position to reduce tension on the cord, which would be a neutral or slightly ______________________ position.

extended

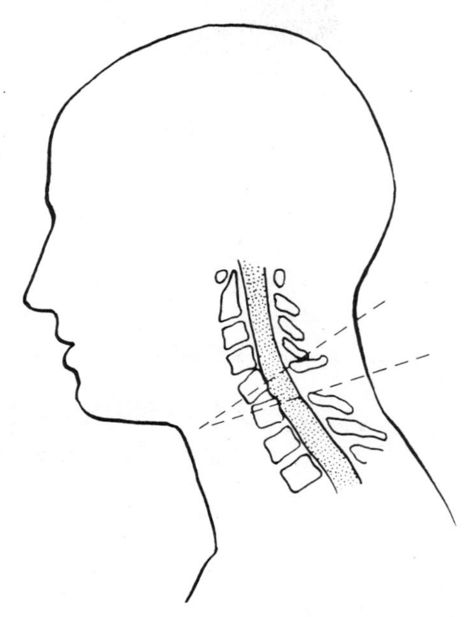

FIG. 12-23. Fracture-dislocation of C_5 on C_6. The cord has been contused and is swollen.

4. *Differential diagnosis of nuchal rigidity from cervical rigidity*
   a. Cervical rigidity means any resistance to neck movement, in contrast to nuchal rigidity. Fig. 12-24 summarizes some of the numerous causes.

b. Because true nuchal rigidity indicates meningeal irritation, most commonly from meningitis or subarachnoid hemorrhage, you must distinguish it from other forms of cervical rigidity. Nuchal rigidity means that only the muscles of the nucha, the nape of the neck, the extensor muscles, resist movement. The other neck movements, rotation, and extension are free.

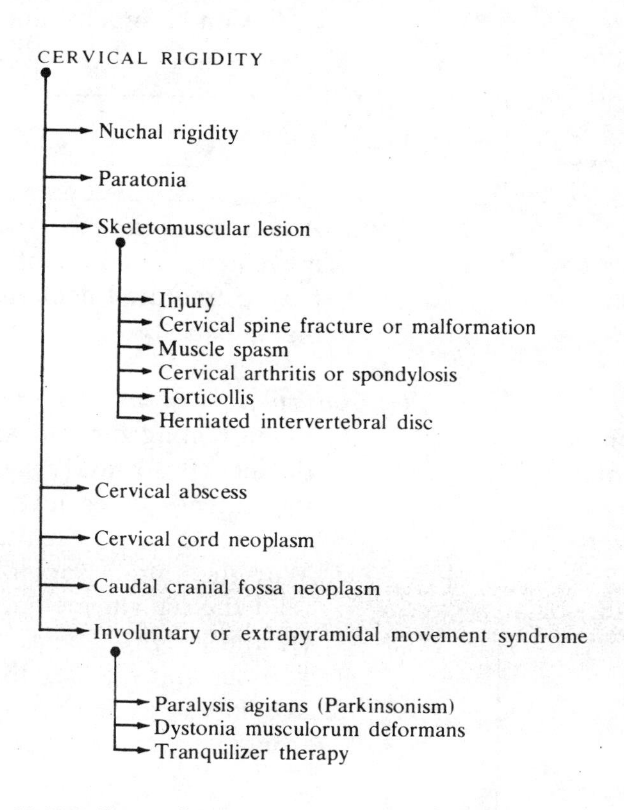

FIG. 12-24. Differential diagnosis of cervical rigidity. (Reference only.)

c. Technique of testing for nuchal rigidity. Have the patient supine and relaxed. Place your hand under his occiput and gently attempt to flex his neck. Normally, it bends freely. If severe, nuchal rigidity enables you to pick up the patient's head and trunk as though he were a block or statue. Next, to demonstrate that rigidity affects only the nuchal muscles, place the patient's head on the pillow and, with your hand on his forehead, passively roll the patient's head side to side to demonstrate free head rotation. Then, lift the patient's shoulders to let his head fall backwards, testing for freedom of extension.

d. When, and only when, the neck resists flexion but moves freely in the other directions do we call it ____________ rigidity.

e. Then, and only then, do we accept it as a reliable sign of an irritative process in the ____________ space, the commonest causes of which are ____________ and ____________ ____________.

nuchal

subarachnoid
meningitis
and subarachnoid hemorrhage

flexion

paratonia

With patient on back, roll the head from side to side and lift the shoulders to show free movement in other directions.

f. In nuchal rigidity, the neck moves freely in all directions except for ______________.

g. If the head of the patient with decreased consciousness resists movement in all directions and the extremities do likewise, then he has the generalized hypertonia called ______________.

h. State the maneuvers to show that a patient with resistance to neck flexion has nuchal and only nuchal rigidity. ______________

____

____

____

____

______________.

5. *A note of caution in testing neck movements:* Be gentle! Do not force movement. The patient may resist movement for good cause: he may have a fractured neck and you may shear off his spinal cord by your manipulations.

G. Confirmatory signs of meningeal irritation

relaxes tension on cord and roots (Review nerve root stretching tests, page 298, if you missed.)

No

1. When testing for nuchal rigidity, watch for adduction and flexion of the legs (Brudzinski's sign) as you attempt to flex the head. Why would the patient's knees flex? ______________

______________.

2. With the patient supine, flex the thigh on the abdomen and try to extend the leg. In meningeal irritation, the patient resists leg extension (Kernig's sign). The same resistance is obtained when the straight leg is raised so as to flex the hip.

3. Would you expect a deeply comatose patient with meningeal irritation from infection or subarachnoid blood to show nuchal rigidity? ☐ Yes / ☐ No. Explain. ______________

____

______________.

Ans: In deep coma, all reflexes and all muscle tone are absent; therefore, the meningeal signs, which depend on reflex muscle spasm, are absent.

4. The usual meningeal irritation signs may fail to occur in three circumstances: infancy, senility, and coma. In these patients, you have to tap the subarachnoid space with a needle to diagnose inflammation or hemorrhage.

H. Opisthotonos, another postural syndrome (ŏp′is-*thŏt*′ō-nŭs)

1. The extensor hypertonus of the neck seen in decerebrate rigidity or meningeal irritation may advance to involve all of the muscles of the back. The patient assumes a bowed position of hyperextension called *opisthotonos,* as shown in Fig. 12-25.

2. Opisthotonos has many causes and many mechanisms. At least three different mechanisms cause opisthotonos as seen in meningeal irritation, decerebrate rigidity, and tetanus and strychnine intoxication. Opisthotonos also occurs in hysteria and catatonic schizophrenia, conditions without a demonstrable lesion. See Fig. 12-26.

a. In meningeal irritation, opisthotonos results from spasm of the powerful extensor muscles, splinting the neck and back against flexion, which causes pain. We can regard it as a pain-protective reflex posture in these cases.

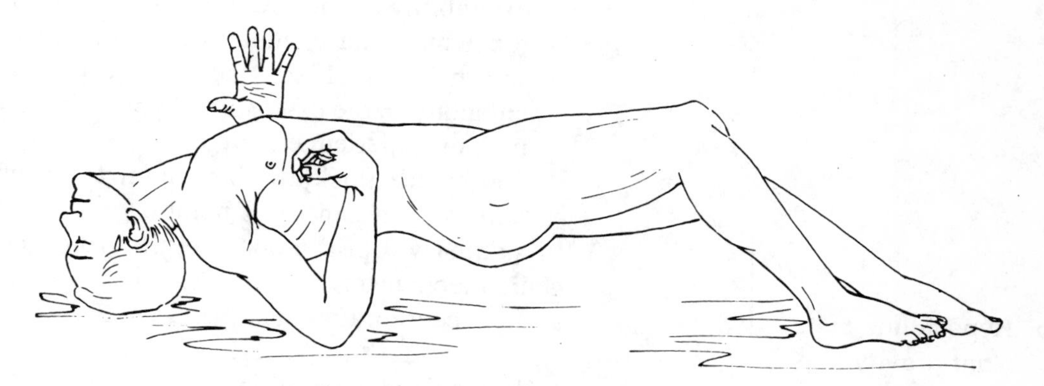

FIG. 12-25. Severe opisthotonus. (Redrawn from *Dorland's Illustrated Medical Dictionary*, Philadelphia, W. B. Saunders Co., 1965.)

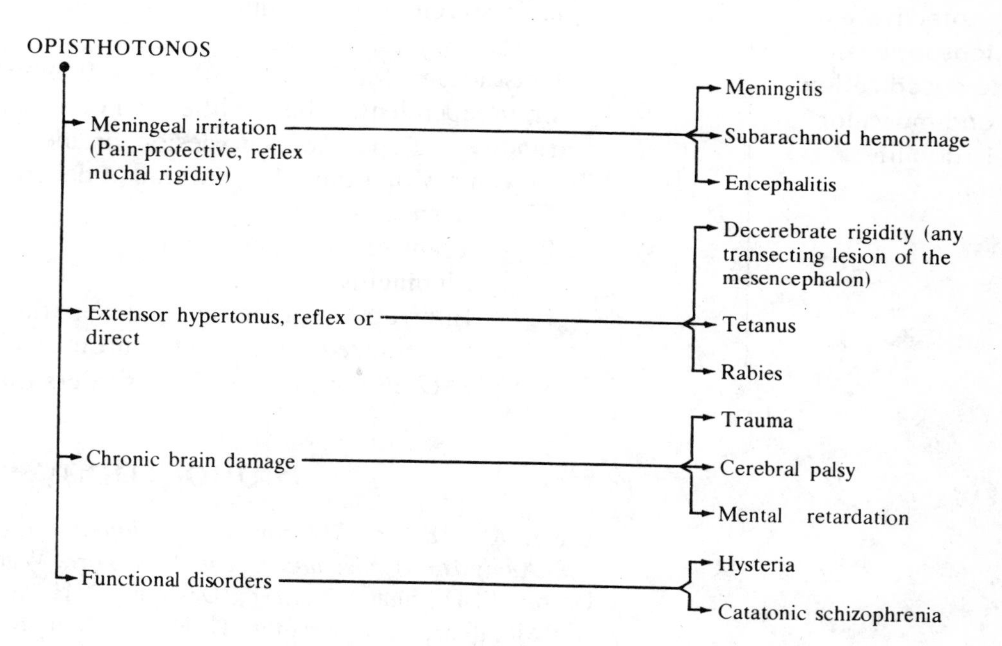

FIG. 12-26. Some causes of opisthotonus. (Reference only.)

antigravity

b. In decerebrate rigidity, the opisthotonic posture results from the hypertonus of the quadrupedal ______________ muscles. We can regard it as a release of the quadrupedal antigravity supporting mechanism, driven by the vestibular system, appearing when a transecting mesencephalic lesion removes the inhibitory influences coming from the cerebrum.

c. In tetanus and strychnine intoxication, muscle stretch reflexes and LMN excitability increase tremendously. All skeletal muscles become extremely hypertonic. Tetanus toxin, in addition to its central excitatory effects, also has a direct contractile action on muscles, causing them to remain cramped even after transection of their nerves. When all muscles contract maximally, the strongest muscles dictate the posture by overpowering their weaker antagonists. However, in tetanus in particular, local factors based on variability in the excitability of the LMN pools and the direct cramping action of the toxin may cause violations of the strongest muscle law. Thus, as shown in Fig. 12-25, the arm flexors may overcome their stronger antagonists, the extensors. If you want to know what the opisthotonic patient experiences, lay down, extend your neck and legs, clench your teeth (lockjaw), and contract every muscle in your body as hard as you can for 1 minute.

3. In summary, opisthotonos results from at least three different pathogenic mechanisms.
   a. In decerebrate rigidity: ______________________
   b. In meningeal irritation: ______________________
   c. In strychnine or tetanus intoxication: ______________________

a. Hypertonus of antigravity muscles.
b. Reflex pain protective extensor spasm.
c. Increased reflex and muscular irritability.

4. Opisthotonos, thus, appears as a fragment of decerebrate rigidity, or independently, but neither it nor other fragments of decerebrate rigidity are specific as to lesion or mechanism. On the other hand, we can say that the full syndrome of decerebrate rigidity indicates:
   ☐ *a.* A specific lesion type
   ☐ *b.* Transtentorial herniation
   ☐ *c.* Meningitis
   ☐ *d.* Interruption of mesencephalic pathways
   ☐ *e.* Generalized increase in neuromuscular irritability due to a toxin

☑ d.

5. See Fig. 12-26 for some of the disorders that cause opisthotonos.

Bibliography

Breig, A.: *Adverse Mechanical Tension in the Central Nervous System: An Analysis of Cause and Effect,* New York, Wiley and Sons, 1978.

Dastur, F. D., Shahani, M. T., Dastoor, D. H., Kohiyar, F. N., Bharucha, E. P., Mondkar, V. P., Kashtap, G. H., and Nair, K. G.: Cephalic tetanus: Demonstration of a dual lesion, *J. Neurol. Neurosurg. Psychiatry,* 40:782-786, 1977.

O'Connell, J.: The clinical signs of meningeal irritation, *Brain,* 69:9-21, 1946.

Thorner, M.: Modification of meningeal signs by concomitant hemiparesis, *Arch. Neurol. Psychiat.,* 59:485-495, 1948.

Toomey, J.: Stiff neck and meningeal irritation, *J.A.M.A.,* 127:436-439, 1945.

Wartenberg, R.: The signs of Brudzinski and Kernig, *J. Pediat.,* 37:679-684, 1950.

I. Sensory examination of the unconscious patient

1. Just as in testing an alert patient, you test the sensory system of the comatose patient systematically, starting with the rostralmost cranial nerves and proceeding caudally over the body. Cranial nerve I cannot be tested.

IIIrd

mesencephalon

2. *Cranial nerve II* is tested indirectly by the pupillary light reflexes. Since the pupilloconstrictor fibers run in the ______________ nerve, both it and II are tested simultaneously.
   a. The IIIrd cranial nerve nucleus is located in the tegmentum of the □ diencephalon / □ mesencephalon / □ pons.
   b. In Fig. 12-27, draw the pupilloconstrictor reflex pathway. Start, as usual, at the receptor and trace through the pathway.

* Compare with Fig. 4-2

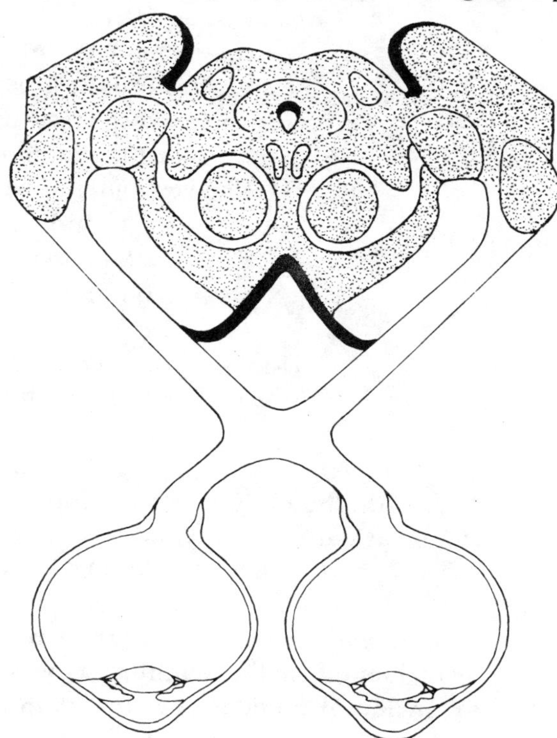

FIG. 12-27. Blank for drawing the pathway of the pupilloconstrictor reflex. Start with a retinal neuron.

3. *Cranial nerve V* is tested by reflexes, just as II and III.
   a. Testing somatic sensation in the unconscious patient requires observing some motor response to a stimulus, usually pain. To test the afferent arc of the Vth nerve requires VIIth nerve function to express a trigemino-facial reflex. The two reflexes involved are the corneal reflex and grimacing to supra-orbital pressure. Either anatomic interruption of the VIIth nerve or an upper motor neuron palsy with cerebral shock may block a response. Then you do not know which limb of the reflex arc, the afferent or efferent, has failed.
   b. Hence, in the stage of flaccid hemiplegia after an acute cerebral lesion, the corneal reflex is □ increased/ □ decreased or absent.
   c. Test the corneal reflex as usual. Test the other V-VII reflex by pressing your fingernail into the eyebrow over the superciliary notch. The expected response in a stuporous or semicomatose patient is a facial grimace *ipsilateral* to the side of stimulation. Hence, each half of the face can be tested separately. In the comatose patient with acute hemiplegia, the grimace would

decreased or absent

hemiplegic

be weaker on the ☐ hemiplegic / ☐ nonhemiplegic side. Explain: ____

Ans: With acute UMN lesions, the excitability of reflexes is temporarily reduced during the phase known as cerebral shock. The pain stimulus which ordinarily would elicit facial movement is insufficient to activate the LMNs.

4. *Cranial nerve VIII*
   a. Hearing cannot be tested unless the patient is sufficiently conscious to show a startle response to loud sound. Clang a pan or clap.
   b. Vestibular responses can be tested and provide a very valuable means to test the integrity of the tegmental core of the brainstem.
      (1) The vestibular nuclei connect with cranial nerve nuclei ________, ________, and ________, which innervate the eye muscles.
      (2) The tract coursing through the tegmental core of the brainstem and conveying vestibular impulses to these nuclei is called the ________.
   c. How do you stimulate the vestibular system? Give details of position and materials to be used. ____.

III, IV, VI

MLF

Ans: With the patient supine, flex his head 30°. Irrigate the auditory canals with 100 ml of water at 30 or 44°C over a period of 40 sec or with 5 ml of ice water.

   d. What precaution do you take before irrigating? ________________________.

Ans: If you have already done a complete general physical examination you have looked in the auditory canals. The patient's coma might have come from extension of a middle ear infection into the brain.

   e. If no response is obtained from either ear after caloric irrigation, how do you interpret the result? ____.

See next frame

   f. Think through the reflex arc: either the stimulus is inadequate, in which case use colder water and irrigate longer, or the patient's labyrinths are inexcitable, or the VIIIth nerve is interrupted, or the MLF is interrupted, or the oculomotor nerves are interrupted, etc. Obviously if you get a response bilaterally, you have more useful information than no response. All systems, afferent and efferent, have to be *GO* to get a caloric response. Thus, in the comatose patient, a lesion at any level of the reflex pathway from the labyrinth to ocular muscles may prevent a response.
   g. Depending on the degree of unconsciousness, caloric irrigation may produce only conjugate deviation of the eyes, without the nystagmus seen in the alert patient.
   h. *The doll's eye test.* If you have an old-fashioned doll around the house, hold it up in front of you. If you turn the doll's head down, the eyes will turn up to remain looking you in the eye. If you turn

the doll's head up, the eyes will rotate down and will close when the doll is laid down. The eyes are counterweighted to cause this *contraversive* movement.

(1) The patient in coma can be tested in the same way for proprioceptive contraversive eye movements by moving his head up and down and side-to-side. The patient's head is held in your hands in a neutral position and briskly rotated up, down, or to the sides. The eyes move *contraversively*, opposite to the direction of head turning, if proprioceptive impulses get through from the neck and labyrinth to the nuclei of III, IV, and VI via the MLF. After the movement, the eyes return quickly to their resting position.

(2) *A note of caution.* If the patient has a head injury, he may also have a fractured neck. If you fail to recognize it you may shear off his spinal cord if you move the head too forcefully in doing the doll's eye test. Should the patient resist head movement, *cease* and *desist*. His cervical rigidity may be splinting a neck fracture.

i. Name the two methods of testing the comatose patient for the integrity of the MLF in its course through the tegmental core of the brainstem.

(1) ______________________

(2) ______________________

1. Caloric irrigation
2. The doll's eye test

5. *Cranial nerves IX and X* are tested by the gag reflex. Only a persistent asymmetry of response is significant. You must be careful not to stimulate too strongly since gagging and reflex vomiting may lead to aspiration of stomach contents into the lungs.

6. *Somatic sensation*

a. Pain tests the somatic pathways in unconscious patients. Test for a generalized pain response by pressing a knuckle or the ball of your thumb against the sternum. Observe for an arousal response with eye opening or decerebrate posturing.

b. Test for a localized pain response by stimulating each extremity by pinching the patient's fingernails or toenails hard, or by pressing them with the rubber tip of a pencil. Grade the response as localizing (by which is meant appropriate avoidance as by brushing away), flexing, extending, or no response (Teasdale and Jennett, 1974).

c. As alternative pain stimuli, try pinching the skin. Avoid too much pinpricking or use of your fingernails which may leave wounds. Try the various ways of testing facial and body pain on yourself to gain an appreciation of the proper strength of stimulus to use.

J. MSRs and toe signs in the comatose patient

You may wonder why I have waited until the last to discuss the MSRs and toe signs, which are so valuable in the alert patient. Because of the problem of cerebral shock, the MSRs may be decreased, equal, or increased. If the MSRs are unequal you don't know whether one side is pathologically depressed or the other pathologically hyperactive. Extensor toe signs may be present bilaterally when consciousness is depressed from any cause, or they may be absent in deep coma. This is not to say that the MSRs and toe signs are valueless and need not be tested. They may well fall into a diagnostic pattern which supports conclusions from inspection and testing for muscle tone. It is to say that in coma, neither the presence nor the absence of the typical UMN signs have the significance that they do in the alert patient.

Bibliography

Carmichael, E., Dix, M., and Hallpike, C.: Observations upon the neurological mechanism of directional preponderance of caloric nystagmus resulting from vascular lesions of the brain-stem, *Brain,* 88:51 - 74, 1965.

Plum, F., and Posner, J.: *The Diagnosis of Stupor and Coma*, Philadelphia, F. A. Davis Co., 2nd ed., 1972.

Rodríguez Barrios, R.: The study of ocular motility in the comatose patient, *J. Neurol. Sci.,* 3:183 - 206, 1966.

IV. Intermittent disturbances of consciousness: syncope or fainting

A. Introduction

1. *Definition.* Syncope is a sudden temporary loss and return of consciousness, not caused by epilepsy. The mechanism is usually cerebral ischemia, induced most commonly by:
   a. Vagal inhibition of the heart, causing bradycardia-asystole
   b. Inhibition of vasoconstrictor tone
   c. Mechanical disturbances in blood flow or cardiac output
   d. Cardiac dysrhythmias
2. Syncope is the final common denominator, the end result, of numerous factors, some psychogenic, others organic in origin.
   a. Psychogenic syncope is the end result of emotional illness. It is never the sole manifestation. It is only one shadow in a pattern of emotional maladjustment. Look at the emotional background of the patient.
   b. Neurogenic syncope is the end result of an identifiable sensory stimulus. Look for the inciting stimulus.
   c. Mechanical syncope is the end result of an impedance or short-circuiting of blood flow. Look for the mechanical insufficiency in the heart and vessels.
   d. Cardiac dysrhythmia syncope is the end result of a disturbance in impulse conduction or transmission in the heart. Look for the heart disease underlying it.

B. Historical factors

1. Since syncope has so many causes, the history must be relied upon to help delimit the proper steps to take in the physical examination.
2. The most important point in the history or observation of any blackout spell is to learn the mode of onset. The critical question is: what

are the patient's symptoms, posture, activities, and social circumstances when the attacks come on? Are they the same for all attacks? Is the patient standing, sitting, moving, changing position, coughing, urinating, hyperventilating? Is he alone or with people?

3. Usually the most difficult decision is whether the syncope is psychogenic or organic.
   a. If the attacks are psychogenic, the patient usually does not hurt himself when he falls. Often, as in doing the swaying test, the patient conveniently falls into the observer's arms. In organic attacks, the patient often injures himself when he falls. This distinction is by no means absolute.
   b. Hysterical attacks are most apt to occur when the patient is with people emotionally entangled with him. At the end of the examination, call in the family to see how the family and patient interact. He may faint on the spot, thus clinching the diagnosis. Organic syncope is not "socially dependent."
4. The point made in the preceding frame is critical: After you have completed the history and routine examinations, try to reproduce, as closely as possible, the circumstances of the attack. If the patient reports that a posture, such as head turning, elicits an attack, have him turn his head.
   a. If hyperventilation precedes the attack, have him ______________________.
   b. If he faints after coughing have him ____________________.
   c. If he faints in the presence of his mother, observe him when he is with his ____________________.

hyperventilate

cough

mother

C. *Observation of the patient during an attack*

1. If you are fortunate enough to observe the beginning of an attack, have the patient describe his symptoms — dizziness, weakness, nausea, and so on. Prepare to protect the patient during the unconscious phase.
   a. Place him on a soft surface.
   b. Be sure he is breathing and has an open airway.
   c. If he vomits, turn his head to prevent aspiration into his lungs.
   d. Check vital signs, blood pressure, pulse, respiratory rate, pupillary size, muscle tone, and reflexes.
   e. If the history suggests one of the rarer, metabolic causes of syncope or loss of consciousness, such as hypoglycemia or hypocalcemia, draw a blood sample. In fact it is usually wise, until the diagnosis is established, to draw a blood sample if you observe any attack.
2. Usually the patient is pallid and sometimes sweaty. His pupils may dilate in unconsciousness from any cause, and once the patient is unconscious, he usually shows no pathognomonic signs that identify the cause. In hysterical or feigned unconsciousness, he may show paratonia, eyelid fluttering or forceful resistance to eyelid opening, or he may assume bizarre postures. Unfortunately for differential diagnosis, the organic patient in the "twilight zone" of unconscious-

ness may also show any or all of these signs. The clue to the cause is more often learned from what initiates the attack rather than what ends it.

D. As a prelude to the special features of the physical examination in patients with intermittent unconscious spells, consider this dendrogram (Fig. 12-28):

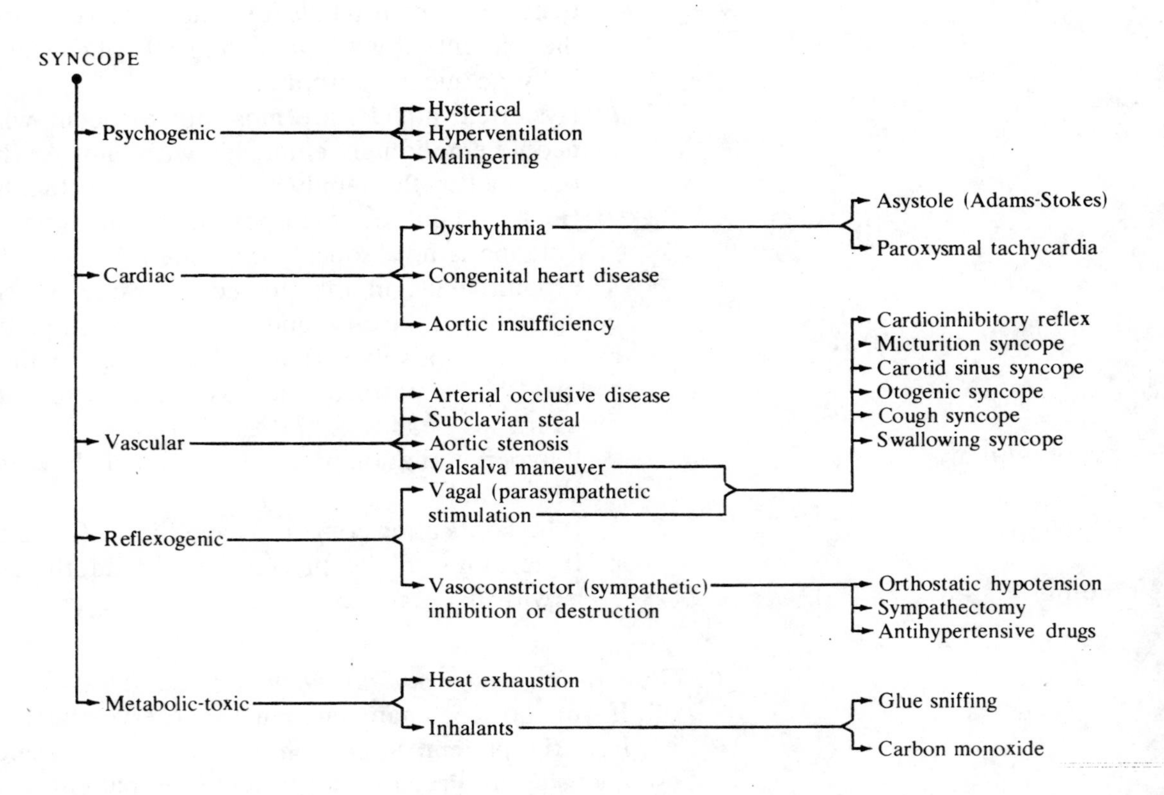

FIG. 12-28. Common types of syncope. (Reference only.)

E. Reflexogenic syncope from coughing, swallowing, ear disease, or micturition

1. *Swallowing or glossopharyngeal syncope*
   a. The patient complains of syncope associated with spontaneous pain in the ear and throat (glossopharyngeal neuralgia analagous to trigeminal neuralgia) or with swallowing.
   b. The mechanism of syncope apparently is a vagal reflex cardiac inhibition. Thus, this type of syncope involves cranial nerves numbers ______________.

IX and X

2. *Cough syncope*
   a. The patient, usually one with lung disease, has syncope after prolonged coughing.
   b. The mechanism of syncope may be from vagal afferent stimulation with cardiac inhibition or from the Valsalva effect.
3. *Otogenic syncope*
   a. While the Vth cranial nerve innervates the skin over the tragus

VII, IX, X

and crus helix, and the C_2 dermatome the rest of the external ear, the origin of the ear from the branchial arches causes it to have sensory twigs from the other branchial arch nerves. Considering V as the first branchial arch nerve, the other three branchial arch nerves with a superficial sensory component also supply twigs. These nerves are ________, ________, ________.

b. The patient may faint when his external auditory canal is stimulated, or as a result of ear disease. The mechanism is probably cardiac inhibition through the Xth nerve.

4. *Micturition syncope*
   a. The patient complains that when he has a full bladder and urinates, he faints.
   b. The mechanism is probably mechanical, in analogy with the Valsalva effect. With a full bladder, the abdominal wall is splinted by reflex abdominal muscle spasm. When the bladder is emptied, a large volume of fluid is suddenly released from the abdominal cavity, and the abdominal wall muscles relax. The sudden decrease in intraabdominal pressure causes pooling of blood in the tributaries of the inferior vena cava, curtailing venous return to the heart. The same mechanism causes syncope when ascitic fluid is removed too rapidly from the abdomen.

cerebral ischemia from hypotension (inadequate cardiac output)

5. Whether reflex vasodilation from inhibition of sympathetic vasoconstrictor tone contributes to these types of syncope is unknown. At any rate, the final reason the patient faints, whether from cardioinhibitory reflexes, inhibition of vasoconstrictor tone, or Valsalva effect is ________________
6. Since cerebral ischemia disrupts brain metabolism, the patient not only may faint, but he may also have a convulsion, an epileptic seizure, as part of his attack of syncope.

F. Reflexogenic syncope from carotid sinus hypersensitivity

1. An increase in blood pressure stimulates receptors in the carotid sinus. As a consequence, homeostatic reflexes cause vasodilation or cardiac inhibition, opposing the hypertension. If the carotid sinus is hypersensitive, cardiac output is decreased too much, causing syncope.

IXth

Xth

   a. The carotid sinus is innervated by the ________ cranial nerve.
   b. Cardiac inhibition is a parasympathetic effect mediated through the ________ cranial nerve.
   c. If carotid sinus hypersensitivity causes syncope by bradycardia-asystole, it is called *cardioinhibitory syncope.*
   d. If carotid sinus hypersensitivity causes syncope from inhibition of sympathetic vasoconstrictor tone, the syncope is called *vasodepressor carotid sinus syncope.*
   e. A third, controversial type of carotid sinus syncope is the *cerebral type* in which neither the pulse nor the blood pressure changes radically. The mechanism (and even the existence) of this type of syncope is disputed.
2. Complete Table 12-5.

Decreased sympathetic vasoconstrictor tone

Reflex asystole or bradycardia

Unknown

TABLE 12-5. Mechanisms of Carotid Sinus Syncope

Type of carotid sinus syncope	Mechanism of syncope
Vasodepressor	
Cardioinhibitory	
Cerebral	

3. *Role of head turning in syncope*
   a. A patient with a hypersensitive carotid sinus or with swollen lymph nodes may faint when he turns his head, mechanically stimulating the carotid sinus.
   b. Another cause of fainting from head turning is temporary mechanical occlusion of a carotid or vertebral artery. In a normal young person, occlusion of a major cerebral artery may cause no symptoms or signs. In the elderly, hypertensive, or arteriosclerotic patient with occlusive arterial disease, the other arteries are incompetent to supply the brain when one is occluded. Furthermore, one artery may have occluded "silently" and then, as the occlusive disease advances, blood flow through the remaining patent arteries is reduced by head turning (see Fig. 12-29).

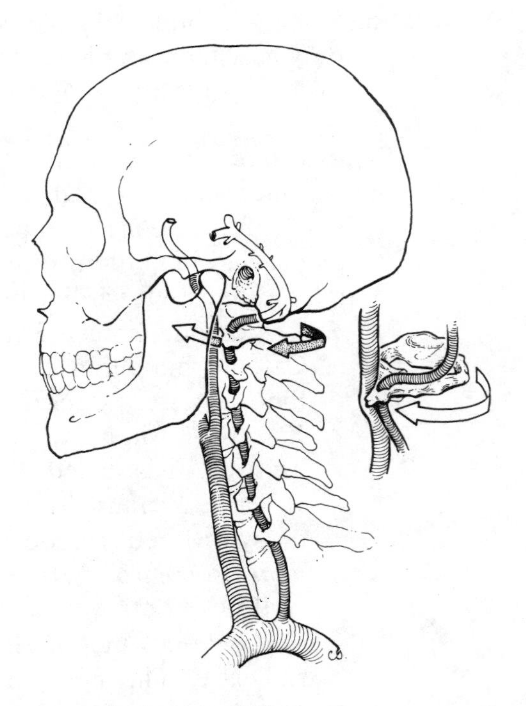

FIG. 12-29. Diagram to show how turning of the head may kink or compress the carotid or vertebral arteries, interfering with blood flow to the brain.

G. *Carotid sinus massage test for carotid sinus sensitivity*

1. A special test such as carotid sinus massage is only done after the routine examination is completed. You must first learn whether the patient has contraindications for the test.
2. *Contraindications are:*
   a. The test is not done if the patient is hypertensive, elderly, or arteriosclerotic, unless he can be monitored by EKG and EEG. Cardiac asystole or hypotension may cause death or a brain infarct. Ideally every patient tested should have EEG-EKG monitoring, but practically it is impossible.
   b. The test is not done in a patient with known or suspected heart disease.
   c. The test is not done if one carotid artery fails to pulsate.
3. *Indications*
   a. A patient with lapses of consciousness for which the history and physical examination disclose no cause.
   b. A patient whose syncope is precipitated by head turning or who has enlarged cervical lymph nodes.
   c. A patient who has none of the contraindications.
4. *Procedure for carotid sinus massage test*
   a. If the patient gives a history of some posture or maneuver that causes his syncope, have him repeat the maneuver. Always listen to what the patient thinks causes his attacks and reproduce, if possible, the conditions under which the attacks occur.
   b. Position the patient upright in a chair. If he is standing he may fall. If he reclines, he may not have sufficient hypotension to faint even though a hypersensitive carotid sinus is causing his attacks.
   c. Since you already have completed a general physical and neurologic examination, you have palpated the neck for nodes and listened over the head and neck for bruits.
   d. Tell the patient you are going to rub his neck, but do not instruct him as to the possible outcome.
   e. Select any point on the neck, except over the carotid sinuses, and massage gently for 15 sec. If the patient faints, it is psychogenic syncope. Since psychogenic syncope is the commonest type, a control test for suggestibility must be included.
   f. Locate the carotid sinus by palpating the bulb at the carotid bifurcation. It is found by pressing your fingers gently backward, just below the angle of the mandible and anterior to the sternocleidomastoid muscle. Stop and record the blood pressure and pulse. Massage the carotid bulb for 15 sec and record pulse and blood pressure. A modest drop in pulse and BP is normal.
   g. Wait 5 min and massage the other carotid bulb.
   h. While it is merely reprehensible to miss an untreatable disorder, it is criminal to miss a treatable disorder. Carotid sinus hypersensitivity can be treated by surgical denervation of the sinus or by parasympathetic blocking agents. Therefore, this treatable cause of syncope should never be overlooked.

5. Name two mechanisms by which head turning can cause loss of consciousness: ____
____
____
____.

Ans: Stimulation of a hypersensitive carotid sinus or occlusion of a major cerebral artery.

old person, arteriosclerosis, heart disease, occlusion of one carotid artery

6. Name the contraindications to the carotid sinus massage test: ______________
____
____.

sitting

7. What is the position of the patient for the carotid sinus massage test? ☐ sitting / ☐ standing / ☐ reclining. Explain ______________________
____
____.

Ans: If standing, the patient may fall. If reclining, he may not faint even though his carotid sinus is hypersensitive.

Bibliography

Corbett, J. J., Butler, A. B., and Kaufman, B.: "Sneeze syncope" basilar invagination and Arnold-Chiari type I malformation, *J. Neurol. Neurosurg. Psychiatry,* 39:381-384, 1976.

Duvoisin, R.: Convulsive syncope induced by the Weber maneuver, *Arch. Neurol.,* 7:219-226, 1962.

Engel, G.: *Fainting,* 2d ed., Springfield, Ill., Charles C Thomas, Publisher, 1962.

Gauk, E., Kidd, L., and Prichard, J.: Aglottic breath-holding spells, *New Eng. J. Med.,* 275:1361, 1362, 1966.

Kubala, M., and Millikan, C.: Diagnosis, pathogenesis, and treatment of "Drop Attacks," *Arch. Neurol.,* 11:107-113, 1964.

Lukash, W., Sawyer, G., and Davis, J.: Micturition syncope produced by orthostasis and bladder distention, *New Eng. J. Med.,* 270:341-344, 1964.

Lyle, C., et al.: Micturition syncope. Report of 24 Cases, *New Eng. J. Med.,* 265:982-986, 1961.

North, R., et al.: Brachial-basilar insufficiency syndrome, *Neurology,* 12:810-820, 1962.

Page, I., and McCubbin, J.: One facet of neural regulation, *New Eng. J. Med.,* 276:335-338, 1967.

Reese, C., Green, J., and Elliott, F.: The cerebral form of carotid sinus hypersensitivity, *Neurology,* 12:492-494, 1962.

Sheehan, S., Bauer, R., and Meyer, J.: Vertebral artery compression in cervical spondylosis, *Neurology,* 10:968-986, 1960.

V. The summarized neurologic examination of the unconscious patient

Examination of the unconscious patient requires a different protocol from the one designed for the conscious patient. Work through the Neurologic Examination of the Unconscious Patient, pages XV-XVIII, which follow the Summarized Neurologic Examination.

13

Ancillary Neurodiagnostic Procedures

We have instruments of precision in increasing numbers with which we and our hospital assistants at untold expense make tests and take observations, the vast majority of which are but supplementary to, and as nothing compared with, the careful study of the patient by a keen observer using his eyes and ears and fingers and a few simple aids.

— Harvey Cushing

I. The cerebrospinal fluid (CSF) examination

A. *Introduction.* By some quirk of habit, evaluation of the CSF is usually regarded as a laboratory procedure, but make no mistake on this point: CSF examination is part of the physical examination. The attending physician himself makes the first and most important observations.

B. *Origin and circulation of the CSF*

1. According to traditional theory, CSF is formed by the choroid plexuses of the lateral, third, and fourth ventricles. It escapes from the interior of the brain by flowing out of foramina in the fourth ventricle, the *L*ateral foramina of *L*uschka and the *M*edian formen of *M*agendie. Study Fig. 13-1 to learn the course of CSF circulation.
2. After flowing from the foramina, the fluid is in the subarachnoid space, between the arachnoid and pia mater. It may then percolate down around the spinal cord or up over the cerebral hemispheres to the region of the superior sagittal sinus. Here Pacchionian granulations indent the sinuses and permit absorption of the fluid into the venous system. See Fig. 13-2.
3. Trace a drop of CSF from the temporal horn of the lateral ventricle to its absorption into the blood. ______________________

____

____

____

____

Temporal horn, anterior horn, interventricular foramen, IIIrd ventricle, IVth ventricle, subarachnoid space, Pacchionian granulations.

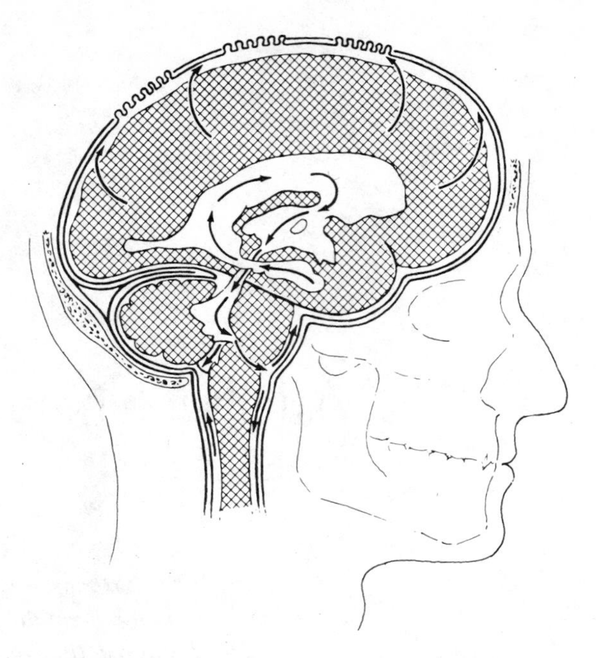
FIG. 13-1. Lateral view of the ventricular system and cerebrospinal fluid (CSF) circulation. Beginning in the temporal horn, trace a drop of CSF through the ventricular system, into the subarachnoid space, and up over the convexity of the hemisphere to the Pacchionian granulations along the superior sagittal sinus.

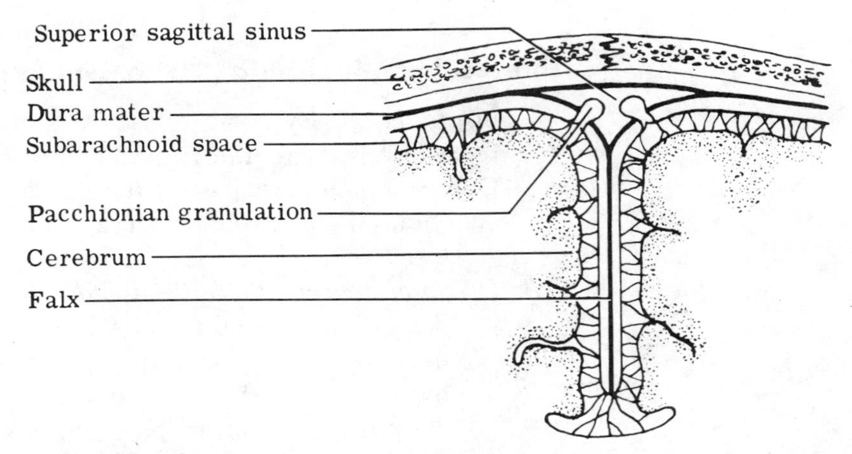

FIG. 13-2. Coronal section through the cerebral falx to show how the Pacchionian granulations project directly into the superior sagittal sinus. CSF passes through the granulations into the venous blood of the sinus.

C. Hydrodynamics and composition of the CSF

1. The most common clinical problem in CSF dynamics is increased CSF pressure, with or without hydrocephalus. Low CSF pressure sometimes occurs. Increased pressure has two common causes:
   a. Expanding lesions within the craniovertebral space, such as neoplasms, abscesses, and brain edema. Rarely, increased production of CSF may cause increased pressure.
   b. Occlusive lesions which impede the flow of CSF from the ventri-

cles to the subarachnoid space and through the Pacchionian granulations. The occlusion commonly occurs at any point where the aperture for CSF flow is critically small, where the fluid passageway can easily be blocked.

(1) Interventricular foramina (usually neoplastic lesion).
(2) Aqueduct (usually congenital atresia or stenosis, inflammatory adhesions, or neoplastic compression).
(3) Fourth ventricle and its outlets (usually posterior fossa neoplasms or inflammatory adhesions).
(4) Subarachnoid space (usually adhesions after meningitis or subarachnoid hemorrhage).
(5) Pacchionian granulations (usually adhesions, high CSF protein, or superior sagittal sinus thrombosis).

2. The CSF is about 100 percent water. The CNS is about 80 percent water. Students who are only familiar with the stiff, unyielding, formalin-fixed brain of the cadaver have difficulty appreciating the supple softness of the living brain. It is compliant, like a balloon (the pia-arachnoid) filled with viscid molasses. Therefore, a physicist, in studying the hydrodynamics of the CSF might, without doing too much violence to reality, regard the CNS and the CSF as a single homogeneous fluid. In Fig.13-3 the CNS and CSF have been replaced by a single fluid, as shown by the stippling. Subsequently we shall use the term *CNS-CSF* for the combined CNS and CSF, regarded as a single fluid. To duplicate biologic conditions with our model, the blood vessels which surround and honeycomb the CNS must be included. These are depicted in Fig. 13-3.
3. The CNS-CSF fluid in the craniovertebral space is incompressible. According to Pascal's law, pressure exerted on a fluid in a closed container is transmitted equally in all directions, The pressure transmission is independent of the size or shape of the container.
4. *Measurement of CNS-CSF pressure by needling the lumbar subarachnoid space*
   a. The patient is placed on his side with his legs drawn up and his head and trunk bowed forwards. This position of universal flexion is called the *fetal position.* In this position, the distance between the dorsal processes and lamina of adjacent vertebrae is ☐ increased/ ☐ decreased, because the spine is flexed. Spine flexion thus increases the target area for the needle.

   increased (Review Fig. 12-21 if you erred.)

   b. Scrub the skin with antiseptic and, under sterile technique, insert a 20 guage needle in the interspace between the dorsal processes of vertebrae $L_{4\text{-}5}$ or L_5-S_1. Angle the needle slightly cephalad. If the history or opthalmoscopic examination indicate the likelihood of a space-occupying lesion or increased pressure, do not do a lumbar puncture unless you have signs of meningeal irritation and suspect meningitis or subarachnoid hemorrhage. If the history or ophthalmoscopic examination indicates merely the remote possibility of a space-occupying lesion or increased intracranial pressure, proceed this way: Insert a needle through the skin but stop it just before it

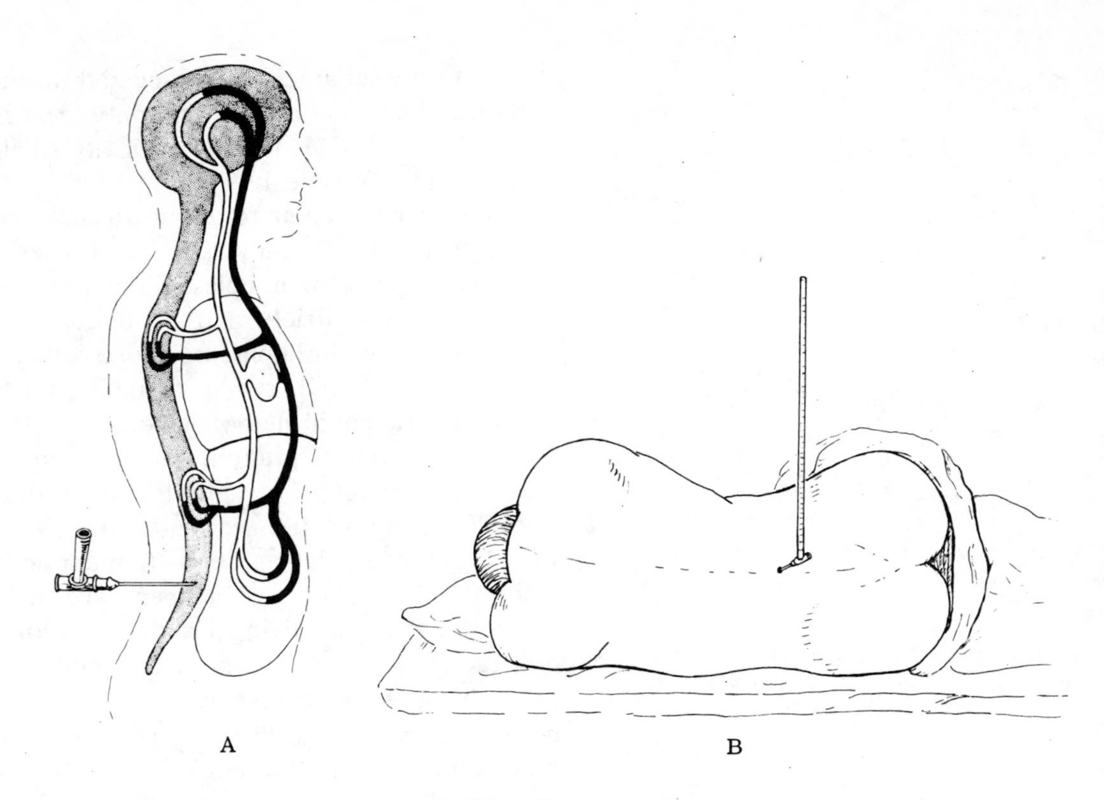

FIG. 13-3. Diagram to show the continuity of vessels inside and outside of the craniovertebral cavity. A needle has been inserted into the lumbar subarachnoid space, and a vertical manometer has been attached. A. For this and subsequent illustrations, the patient is to be regarded as lying on his left side with the manometer vertical (see B). B. Patient in left lateral position with legs and neck flexed.

reaches the subarachnoid space. Attach a manometer. When the manometer is in place, advance the needle into the subarachnoid space. With your examining finger over the open bore at the top of the manometer, allow the fluid to fill the manometer slowly. If no space-occupying lesion or increased pressure is indicated by the history and ophthalmoscopic examination, you may insert the needle with its regular stilet in place and quickly attach the manometer when the stilet is withdrawn.

c. The normal pressure is 80 to 180 mm water. A graph of the fluctuations of the CSF fluid level in the manometer is shown in Fig. 13-4.

d. The pressure maintains a mean value of about 120 mm water, but it fluctuates around this mean. Let us see why the fluctuations occur. From Fig. 13-3, notice that the intracranial-intraspinal veins communicate directly with the extracranial veins. These communicating channels have no valves. If the pressure in the extracranial veins increases or decreases, the pressure within the craniovertebral space also increases or decreases.

e. Notice in Fig. 13-3 that the craniovertebral veins communicate with the intrathoracic veins. When a person inhales air, the CNS-CSF pressure ☐ increases/ ☐ decreases/☐ does not change.

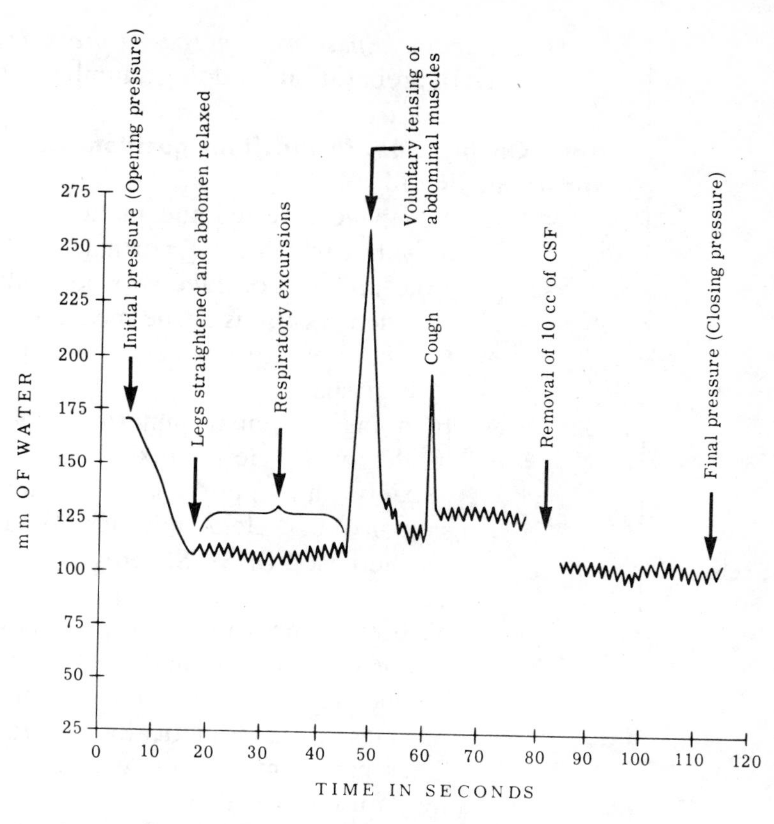

FIG. 13-4. Graph of cerebrospinal fluid pressure, as measured by manometry. Starting at the left, read through the legends just above the arrows.

Ans: Decreases. The intrathoracic pressure decreases with inspiration. Blood is sucked from the CNS veins and the CNS-CSF pressure drops during inspiration.

respiration

(1) The rhythmic excursions at the rate of 16 per min, as shown in Fig. 13-4, are caused by ______________________.

heart beat (pulse)

(2) Smaller excursions at the rate of 72 per min (not shown in Fig. 13-4 because of their small amplitude) are caused by the ______________________.

increases

f. When a patient contracts his abdominal muscles, the CNS-CSF pressure ☐ increases / ☐ decreases / ☐ does not change. Explain: ____
____.

Ans: The increased intraabdominal pressure is reflected backwards through the intervertebral veins. This dams up the outflow of blood from the CNS, but the arterial input continues. Therefore, the CNS-CSF pressure must increase.

120

g. Since much of the arterial pressure is absorbed by the arterial walls, the CNS-CSF pressure is most closely dependent on the capillary and venous pressure. If the CNS-CSF pressure reflected the arterial blood pressure, it would fluctuate between 80 to 120 mm of *mercury* rather than fluctuating around a mean of ______________ mm of *water.* (Mercury is about 13 times heavier than water. The normal CNS-CSF pressure would be about 11 times greater if it reflected arterial pressure.)

D. Clinical evaluation of increased pressure as registered by CSF manometry

1. In preparation for doing a lumbar puncture, position the patient ________________________________.

Ans: On his side, in the fetal position, i.e., with his legs drawn up, and head and trunk flexed.

high

2. You have inserted the manometer and obtain a reading of 240 mm of water, which is ☐ normal / ☐ low / ☐ high.
3. You have to consider two possibilities:
   a. The pressure is a true measure of the intrinsic CNS-CSF pressure.
   b. The pressure is a reflection of factors extrinsic to the craniovertebral space.

abdominal muscle tension

4. In doing a lumbar puncture, you have literally stabbed the patient in the back. He is anxious and apprehensive about the procedure. Anxiety and apprehension usually are manifested by increased tension in the skeletal muscles. What, then, is a simple extrinsic cause for increased CNS-CSF pressure? ________________________________.
5. To determine whether the supposition of abdominal muscle tension is correct, you induce the patient to relax his abdominal muscles by having him straighten out his legs slightly, since the abdominal muscles are automatically contracted when the legs are drawn up. Then have him take a few deep breaths, which causes the tense abdominal muscles to relax.

high

6. In our patient this maneuver caused the pressure to drop to 200 mm of water. This value is ☐ normal / ☐ low / ☐ high.
7. You must then look for another cause for extrinsic pressure. When a person tucks up into the proper position, he flexes his head on his chest, and it may be bent somewhat to the side if his pillow is not the right height. The jugular veins may be compressed if the head is flexed or turned. To test for this supposition, you should have the patient straighten his head and readjust it on the pillow.

intrinsic

8. If the maneuvers to relax the abdominal muscles and to relieve jugular compression fail to cause the pressure to return to normal, you conclude that the increased intracranial pressure is ☐ intrinsic / ☐ extrinsic to the CNS-CSF.
9. If the CNS-CSF pressure is increased because of an intrinsic cause, say an expanding intracranial lesion, let us visualize what happens if you remove fluid from a lumbar tap before measuring pressure. See Fig. 13-5.

transtentorial
transforaminal

10. The patient may have early or impending internal herniation of his brain from increased intracranial pressure. The system may be delicately balanced, with his uncus and parahippocampal gyrus poised, ready to plunge over the edge of the tentorium, or his cerebellar tonsils poised, ready to plunge over the edge of the foramen magnum. These two potentially fatal herniations are called ________________ and ________________ herniation.
11. If fluid is withdrawn from the lumbar region, the brain, being 80 percent water, will flow down toward the point of low pressure, according

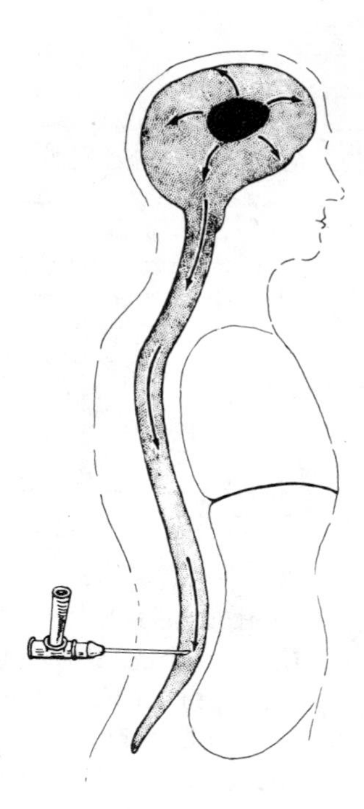

FIG. 13-5. This patient has an expanding intracranial lesion (oval black mass) which has caused increased intracranial pressure. The pressure is exerted equally in all directions. If fluid is allowed to escape through a lumbar needle, the pressure within the craniovertebral space is lowered. The brain flows (herniates) toward the region of lowered pressure.

die

Withdraw the needle immediately!

to Pascal's law. The potential herniation is converted to actual herniation. The patient will ______________

12. If, after careful measurement, you decide that the patient truly has intrinsic increased intracranial pressure, what should you do? ☐ Withdraw fluid rapidly/ ☐ Withdraw fluid cautiously/ ☐ Withdraw the needle immediately.
13. Describe the maneuvers you use to ensure that a high spinal fluid pressure reading is not due to extrinsic factors: ______________
____
____
______________.

Ans: Have the patient straighten his legs and take several deep breaths. Extend the patient's head and reposition it on the pillow.

E. *Cessation of CSF flow*

1. A frequent problem during lumbar puncture is that the initial CSF pressure appears to be normal, yet the flow of fluid stops when the manometer is removed to collect the CSF for laboratory studies. Very rarely, the cause of arrested flow is that transforminal herniation has suddenly occurred and the pressure in the spinal subarachnoid space drops rapidly after a small amount of fluid has drained out. In this case, the patient shows dramatic signs of stupor or coma, and quadriplegia. Most commonly, the cause is far more benign and mundane: something has blocked the flow of fluid through the needle. The most likely causes and their remedies are shown in Table 13-1.

TABLE 13-1. Common Causes for Cessation of CSF Flow and Their Remedies	
Cause	Remedy
Blood clot in the needle lumen.	Replace stilet to ream out the needle.
Nerve root has fallen over the bevel of the needle.	Rotate the shaft of the needle.
Displacement of the tip of the needle from the subarachnoid space or incomplete penetration.	If you think the needle tip is too deep, withdraw it slightly or if too shallow, insert it further.

respiration

2. After trying the maneuvers in Table 13-1, the manometer may be re-attached to measure the pressure. If the needle is patent from the subarachnoid space to the manometer, you should be able to see excursions at the rate of 16 per min, caused by ______________.
3. If respiratory excursions are small, you can test for the patency of the CSF-needle-manometer system by using a safe method of extrinsic pressure to see whether it is reflected in the CNS. What would be a safe method to raise the extrinsic venous pressure to test for a rise and fall in the manometer, indicating patency of the system, but without the peril of promoting brain herniation?

____

____.

Ans: Press on the patient's abdomen. You do not want to raise the intracranial pressure, for fear of brain herniation. Therefore, abdominal pressure is the only safe test. If you answered that you would have the patient perform the Valsalva maneuver (forceful exhalation against a closed glottis), you erred. This maneuver would increase jugular pressure and therefore intracranial pressure.

(1) Replace and withdraw the stilet
(2) Rotate the shaft of the needle
(3) Advance or withdraw the tip slightly
(4) Replace manometer and watch for respiratory excursions or press on abdomen

Watching for a rise of fluid in the manometer after *abdominal* compression

4. Another situation in which fluid will flow poorly or not at all from the needle is when a lesion occludes the vertebral canal, as in Fig. 13-6.
   a. If the vertebral canal is occluded by a lesion, only a small amount of fluid can be obtained. The patency of the system is tested just as before. Thus, you would (list in proper order):
   (1) ______________
   (2) ______________
   (3) ______________
   (4) ______________
   b. If the CSF-needle-manometer system is patent, only one of the tests in the preceding frame will prove it conclusively when the vertebral canal is blocked at the level shown in Fig. 13-6. That test is ______________.

F. The jugular compression (Queckenstedt) test

1. If the abdominal compression test has proven the patency of the system, the jugular compression test may be done if you:

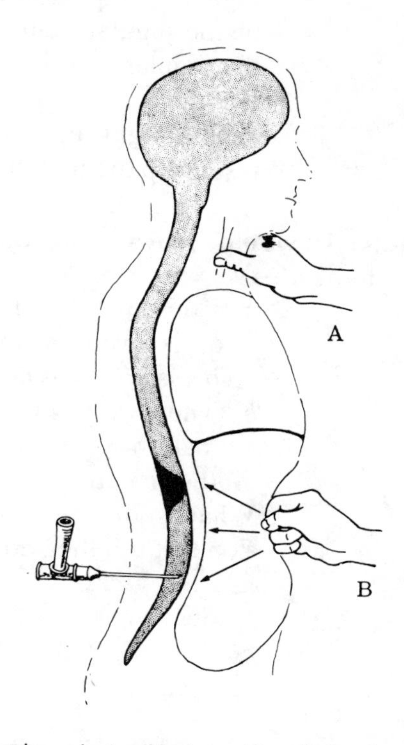

☒ abdominal compression only

FIG. 13-6. This patient has a lesion (black mass) occluding his vertebral canal. A. Compression of jugular vein. B. Compression of abdomen. Which will cause a rise of fluid in the manometer or cause a few drops of CSF to flow from the needle? ☐ jugular compression only / ☐ abdominal compression only.

a. Have a reason to suspect a space-occupying lesion caudal to the foramen magnum.
b. Have no reason to suspect increased intracranial pressure or an intracranial lesion.

2. *Procedure:* One or both jugular veins are occluded by digital compression. Thus, the intracranial pressure increases, and according to Pascal's law, so will the pressure at the lumbar needle, causing the fluid to rise promptly in the manometer. When the jugular pressure is released, the fluid level in the manometer will ______________ promptly.

   drop

   a. Thus, a normal result of the test would be a prompt ______________ in pressure upon jugular compression and a prompt ______________ after release of jugular compression.

   rise
   drop

   b. Operationally what you learned is whether increased intracranial pressure from above is transmitted to your needle below, according to Pascal's law.
3. In Fig. 13-6 a lesion has occluded the vertebral canal. What will be the effect of jugular compression on the fluid level in the manometer? ______________.

   no effect
4. In Fig. 13-6 what would be the effect of the abdominal compression test on the fluid level in the manometer? ______________.

   increase it
5. The validity of the jugular compression test rests on the ability of

Previous thrombosis or congenital abnormality

jugular compression to raise the intracranial pressure. What lesion(s) of the jugular vein might prevent a rise in intracranial pressure when the jugular vein is compressed? ______________________

____

6. What might be the unfortunate effect of the jugular compression test in a patient with early transforaminal herniation? ______________________

____

Ans: It would convert the early herniation to late herniation, too late—the patient dies.

a. Consequently, if the patient has increased intracranial pressure or is even *suspected* of an intracranial lesion, the jugular compression test is *never* done.

kill

b. The test is not done because you cannot gain *any* useful information, and because you might ______________ the patient.

When you suspect a lesion that occludes the vertebral canal

7. What is the *only* type of CNS lesion in which the jugular compression test is indicated? ______________________

____

In increased intracranial pressure or suspected space-occupying intracranial lesion

8. Under what condition is the jugular compression test *absolutely* contraindicated? ______________________

____

G. The syndrome of low CSF pressure

low

1. Suppose that the CSF pressure is 50 mm water, and all tests show a patent system from CSF to manometer. This CSF pressure is ☐ low/ ☐ high/ ☐ normal.
2. Low CSF pressure may be seen after head injuries and in severe dehydration. The temptation when the CSF is low and the physician wants a CSF sample is to put a syringe on the needle and withdraw fluid. This should not be done. You invite catastrophe, either by sucking a nerve root up into the needle or the brain down through the foramen magnum.

H. The appearance of the CSF. Proper inspection of CSF after the sample is collected is often as important as inspection of the patient. It is the attending physician's responsibility, not the laboratory technician's. The fluid is collected by allowing 5 ml to drip into each of three tubes. The normal fluid is sparkling clear. The commonest gross changes are *cloudiness, redness (erythrochromia),* and *yellowness (xanthochromia).*

1. *Cloudiness* usually signifies an increased cell count in the CSF. Rarely it is due to numerous bacteria. The normal cell count is less than 5 white blood cells (WBCs) per mm^3. If the polymorphonuclear white blood cells are more than 300 per mm^3, or if the lymphocyte count is more than 500 per mm^3, the fluid will be visibly cloudy, if properly inspected. If the CSF contains 600-800 WBCs per mm^3 or more, the cloudiness is easy to see. In order to detect minimal cloudiness, when the cell count is in the range of several hundred WBCs per mm^3, here is what to do:

a. Obtain a tube of the same manufacture as the tubes used to collect the CSF. Add the same amount of water to this control tube as is in the CSF tube. A control tube of the same make as the CSF tube is necessary because tubes of different manufacture are slightly different in color, translucency, and refractive index.

b. Hold the control and CSF tubes side-by-side against a white sheet of paper, then against a dark background, and then against a light source. Use daylight if at all possible. Compare the CSF with the water by looking through the sides of the tubes and by looking down through the bore of the tubes, as in using a colorimeter. Normally the CSF collected in each of the three tubes should look equally clear. The direct, side-by-side comparison will disclose cloudiness or color changes which cannot be read unless a matched control tube is used, as described.

(1) Students often grumble that this is all unnecessary because you are going to send the specimen to the lab for the "official" examination and cell count anyway, so why bother? Well, if you are a good physician, you will do the cell count yourself, on the spot, before the cells have undergone autolysis, and to gain the information quickly and reliably. In the second place, your visual inspection gives you a rough check against the accuracy of the laboratory, and believe me that check is necessary. (See the article by Kaufman and Vanderlinde.)

(2) If the lab technician returns a count of 20 WBCs per mm^3 and you saw a cloudy fluid, you know the laboratory is in error. If the patient has meningitis, you simply cannot tolerate an error on this critical point.

2. *Erythrochromia* means a red or pink CSF. It is detected by the technique of controlled inspection, just described in frame b. Erythrochromia is caused by red blood cells (RBCs) in the CSF. It can be detected when the RBC count is more than 100-300 RBCs per mm^3. The normal RBC count is zero.

a. RBCs get into the CSF at one of two times in relation to the tap:

(1) From *preexisting* bleeding caused by a ruptured blood vessel, injury, or other CNS lesion.

(2) From *inadvertent* bleeding caused by the needle puncture, a "traumatic tap."

b. Preexisting bleeding is of the most serious import, while the traumatic tap is inconsequential. The problem is to distinguish the two sources of blood. It is done this way:

(1) Compare the amount of discoloration in the three tubes of CSF. If the first is pink and the last is clear, the blood cannot have been freely admixed with CSF and must be due to a traumatic tap.

(2) If the three tubes are uniformly bloody, centrifuge one, decant the supernatant fluid, and compare it with the control tube of water. If the supernatant CSF is sparkling clear, the blood is of recent origin, either coming from preexisting bleeding

that occurred less than 4 to 6 hr before the tap or from the tap itself. Discoloration of the supernatant fluid of a bloody CSF specimen means that the RBCs have been in the CSF more than 4 to 6 hr and have undergone disintegration. The color of the supernatant fluid is from free hemoglobin, or, if the bleeding occurred several days before the tap, the color is partially from bilirubin, a degradation product of hemoglobin.

(3) Crenation of RBCs as demonstrated by microscopy once was thought to prove preexisting bleeding, but the greater osmolarity of CSF always tends to crenate cells, making this criterion false. The only microscopic proof of preexisting blood comes from the demonstration by sedimentation cytology of RBCs within macrophages.

3. *Xanthochromia* is a yellowish discoloration of the CSF, detected by controlled comparison of the CSF sample with water. It is caused most commonly by free hemoglobin-bilirubin or by high protein. The two possibilities are distinguished this way:
   a. The fluid that is xanthochromic because of high protein will usually clot quickly on standing (Froin's syndrome).
   b. Wet a piece of Hemastix and a piece of Ictotest tape (Ames Laboratories) with the CSF sample. If hemoglobin is present, the Hemastix tape is positive; if bilirubin is present the Ictotest tape is positive, and if only protein is increased, neither tape will be positive.

I. Laboratory examination of the CSF. After the physician himself has inspected the CSF and done the cell count and differential, the fluid is sent to the laboratory. The laboratory tests to be done routinely are sugar, total protein, and serologic test for syphilis. If the cell count is over 5 WBCs per mm^3 the fluid should be smeared on a slide, stained and examined for organisms, and cultured. Many physicians are in the habit of ordering chloride determination, but it is of no value on the routine specimen. Depending on the diseases suspected clinically, the fluid is stained with India ink for fungi, and the cellular content is studied by the sedimentation method which will disclose neoplastic as well as inflammatory cells. Protein and globulin content of the CSF is studied by the colloidal gold test, agar or polyacrylic gel electrophoresis, immuno-electrophoresis, and serologic tests for viruses. The array of commonly used tests is shown in Fig. 13-7.

J. Summary of indications and contraindications for diagnostic lumbar puncture. The major indications for a diagnostic LP consist of identifying or excluding meningitis, encephalitis, subarachnoid hemorrhage, and demyelinating diseases.

The major contraindications to an LP consist of the presence of or suspicion of increased intracranial pressure or a mass lesion that threatens to herniate the brain. Posterior fossa lesions which may cause transforaminal herniation pose the greatest threat. The commonest mass lesions which threaten to cause herniation consist of neoplasms, hematomas, abscesses,

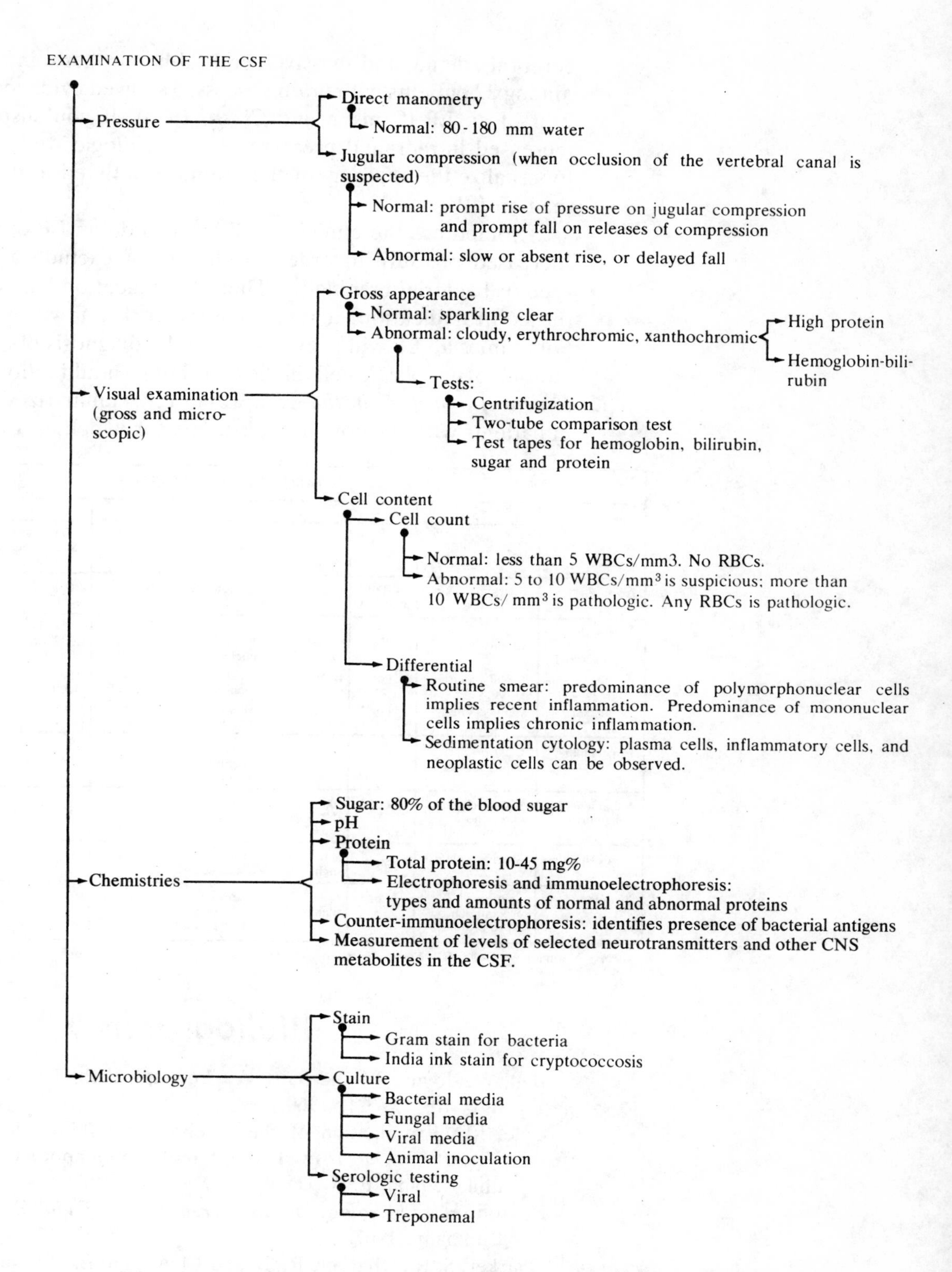

FIG. 13-7. Commonly used methods of examination of cerebrospinal fluid. (Reference only.)

cerebral edema, and massive cerebral hemispheric infarction. For example, among 22 patients with brain abscess, 5 showed evidence of herniation within 2 hr of an LP (Samson and Clark, 1973). If you suspect a mass lesion or increased intracranial pressure, do a radiologic study, usually a CAT scan to visualize the anatomy of the brain, as outlined in the next section, rather than an LP.

Sometimes the clinician will elect to do an LP even in the presence of increased pressure in order to identify or exclude a specifically treatable type of bacterial meningitis. Then the indication has to be weighed against the contraindication, a type of guesswork known as "clinical judgment." Sometimes an LP will prove useful in the diagnosis of a neoplasm by demonstration of neoplastic cells in the CSF, but it should follow other investigations.

K. *Diagnostic profiles in the CSF.* Table 13-2 summarizes the usual LP findings in patients with the common disorders for which an LP is indicated.

TABLE 13-2. Typical CSF Profiles

	Color	Pressure	Cytology			Chemistry		Immuno-electro-phoresis
			Cell count/mm³	Cell type	Stained smear or culture	Glucose: % of blood sugar	Total protein	
Normal	Sparkling clear	80-180 mm H_2O	<5	Mononuclear	No bacteria	≈66% of blood	10-40 mg%	Normal
Meningitis Acute bacterial	Cloudy	↑	500 to 1000's	Polymorphonuclear	Bacteria present	<50% of blood	↑	†CIE shows bacterial antigens
Tuberculous	Cloudy, xanthochromic	*N or ↑	10-500	Mostly mononuclear	Bacteria present	<50% of blood	↑	Not diagnostic
Fungal	Cloudy, xanthochromic	N or ↑	<500	Mostly mononuclear	Fungi present	<50% of blood	↑	Not diagnostic
Encephalitis	Clear to faintly cloudy	N or ↑	<500	Mononuclear after first hours	Stain negative	N	N to moderate ↑	Use serologic testing
Subarachnoid hemorrhage	Erythrochromic or xanthochromic	N or ↑	100's to 1000's to 10,000's	RBCs	Negative	N	Varies with amount of bleeding	Not helpful
Demyelinating diseases	Sparkling clear	N	N or slight ↑	Mononuclear, plasma cells	Negative	N	N to slight ↑	Increased γ-globulin
Neoplasm	Sparkling clear or xanthochromic if protein↑	N or ↑	N or slight ↑	Neoplastic cells sometimes present	Negative	N	N to slight ↑	Normal or nondiagnostic

*N = Normal †CIE = Counter-immunoelectrophoresis

Bibliography

Bell, W., Joynt, R., and Sahs, A.: Low spinal fluid pressure syndromes, *Neurology,* 10:512-521, 1960.

Cole, M.: Examination of the cerebrospinal fluid, in *Special Techniques for Neurologic Diagnosis,* Toole, J. (ed), Contemporary Neurology Series, vol. 3, Philadelphia, F. A. Davis, 1969.

Davson, H.: *Physiology of the Cerebrospinal Fluid,* Boston, Little, Brown and Company, 1967.

Dharker, S. R., Dharker, R. S., and Chaurasia, B. D.: Lactate dehydrogenase and aspartate transaminase of the cerebrospinal fluid in patients with brain tumors, congenital hydrocephalus, and brain abscess, *J. Neurol. Neurosurg. Psychiat.,* 39:1081-1091, 1976.

Gomez, D. G., Chambers, A. A., DiBenedetto, A. T., and Potts, D. G.: The spinal cerebrospinal fluid absorptive pathways, *Neuroradiology,* 8:61-66, 1974.

Greensher, J., Mofenson, H. C., Borofsky, L. G., and Sharma, R.: Lumbar puncture in neonate, *J. Pediatr.,* 78:1034-1035, 1971.
Johnson, R.: Cerebrospinal Fluid, in *Scientific Foundations of Neurology,* Critchley, M. (ed), Philadelphia, F. A. Davis Co., 1972.
Kaufmann, W., and Vanderlinde, R.: Medical-laboratory evaluation, *New. Eng. J. Med.,* 277:1024-1025, 1967.
Kolar, O. J., and Burkhart, J. E.: Neurosyphilis, *J. Ven. Dis.,* 53:221-225, 1977.
Kutter, D.: Bedside test for the chemical examination of spinal fluid, *Helv. Pediat. Acta.,* 19:490-495, 1964.
Lakke, J.: *Queckenstedt's Test.,* Amsterdam, Excepta Medica Foundation, 1970.
Lups, S., and Haan, A.: *The Cerebrospinal Fluid,* Amsterdam, Elsevier Publishing Company, 1954.
Oehmichen, M. L.: *Cerebrospinal Fluid Cytology: An Introduction and Atlas,* Philadelphia, W. B. Saunders Company, 1976.
O'Reilly, S., and Kwa, G.: Examination of the cerebrospinal fluid, *Resident Physician,* 13:51-62, 1967.
Plum, F., and Price, R. W.: Acid-base balance of cisternal and lumbar cerebrospinal fluid in hospital patients, *N. Engl. J. Med.,* 289:1346-1351, 1973.
Samson, D. S., and Clark, K.: A current review of brain abscess. *Am. J. Med.,* 54:201-210, 1973.
Scarff, J.: Treatment of hydrocephalus: an historical and critical review of methods and results, *J. Neurol. Neurosurg. Psychiat.,* 26:1-26, 1963.
Van Der Meulen, J.: Cerebrospinal fluid xanthochromia: An objective index, *Neurology,* 16:170-178, 1966.

II. Neuroradiology

A. *Introduction*

In principle, radiology depends on the fact that biologic tissues absorb or transmit radiation differentially. Thus bone, a radiodense tissue, transmits less radiation than fluid or gas, which are radiolucent. Soft tissues, like brain, have an intermediate radiolucency. After the radiation passes through the tissue, it then strikes film containing a silver salt. The silver reduces to blackened grains, it tarnishes, in proportion to the amount of radiation transmitted through the tissues. Basically, then, an x-ray film records the amount of radiation transmitted to its different areas. When developed, the film shows the radiodense tissues as light areas (few blackened grains of reduced silver), and the radiolucent tissues as dark areas (many blackened grains of reduced silver). Normal brain, CSF, blood vessels, and most lesions do not differ sufficiently in radiation absorption to show up on plain radiographic films. Several artifices can increase the contrast of the soft tissues so as to visualize them. Air, injected into the CSF of the ventricles and subarachnoid spaces, outlines their anatomy by its radiolucency, as contrasted to brain, spinal cord, or bone. A radiopaque fluid injected into the CSF also outlines the ventricles and subarachnoid spaces of the brain or spinal cord. Similarly, a radiopaque fluid can be injected into blood vessels to display them. The newest method combines tomography with computer enhancement of the absorption differences of tissues, a procedure called *computerized axial tomography,* or the CAT scan. This method enhances the minimal existing differences in radioabsorption by the soft tissues. Thus, CAT scan shows the actual brain tissue, its cavities, and subarachnoid spaces, and several of its lesions without injecting any air or radiopaque material into the body. CAT scanning can also be done after injecting radiopaque fluid into the blood vessels. To appreciate the array of neuroradiologic procedures, study Table 13-3 and Fig. 13-8.

TABLE 13-3. Summary of Neuroradiologic Procedures

Neuroradiologic examination	Procedure for performing	Risk	Structures visualized and advantages of procedure
1. *Plain Film Radiography*			
a. Plain skull films. See Fig. 13-8A.	Positioning only	Radiation	Bone shown in great detail but no soft tissues unless calcified
b. Plain spine films	Positioning only	Radiation only, unless neck broken or other cervical lesion present	Bone but no soft tissues unless calcified
2. *Computerized Axial Tomography, the CAT scan*. See Fig. 13-8B.	Positioning for plain CAT scan or injection of radiopaque fluid into vessels to enhance them by positive contrast, the "enhanced CAT scan"	Radiation and rare adverse reaction to the radiopaque fluid. Almost risk-free	Soft tissues of the brain and spinal cord, ventricles and subarachnoid space. Enhanced scans fail to show the detail of regular angiography, but much safer
3. *Negative Contrast Radiography* (injection of air into cavities to outline their anatomy by radiolucency)			
a. Pneumoenceph-alography. See Fig. 13-8C.	Injection of air into lumbar subarachnoid space with positioning of patient to trace the air through subarachnoid space of spinal cord or brain and into brain ventricles	Radiation plus infection, cardiorespiratory arrest, brain herniation. Most patients suffer headache, nausea, and vomiting	Shows ventricles and subarachnoid spaces in much greater detail than CAT
b. Ventriculography	Direct injection of air into ventricles by needle puncture of brain	As above plus hemorrhage	Shows lateral and IIIrd ventricles, but may not show aqueduct or IVth ventricle. Bypasses danger of brain herniation from doing an LP
c. Pneumomyelog-raphy (air myelography)	Lumbar puncture	As for pneumo-encephalography	Generally not as successful as positive contrast myelography. See below
4. *Positive Contrast Radiography* (injection of radiopaque substance into cavities, spaces or vessels to outline them by radiodensity)			
a. Angiography (brain or spinal cord). See Fig. 13-8D.	A radiopaque fluid is in-jected into the blood vessels	Radiation plus vascular occlusion with infarc-tion, hemorrhage, sep-sis, allergic reactions, and cardiorespiratory arrest	Visualizes arterial, capil-lary, and venous circula-tion. Shows occluded, displaced, ballooned, or malformed vessels
b. Myelography	Lumbar puncture with injection of radiopaque fluid into subarachnoid space	Infection, allergic reac-tion, cardiorespiratory arrest, arachnoiditis, quadriplegia, or paraplegia	Best for outlining sub-arachnoid space of spinal cord
c. Cisternography	Lumbar puncture with positioning to run radiopaque fluid up into the subarachnoid space, the cisterns at the base of the brain	As above	Rivals, or better than, pneumoencephalog-raphy to show basal cisterns

TABLE 13-3. *Summary of Neuroradiologic Procedures* (continued)

Neuroradiologic examination	Procedure for performing	Risk	Structures visualized and advantages of procedure
d. Ventriculography	Direct needle puncture of the brain to inject radiopaque fluid into the lateral ventricle	As above, plus hemorrhage	Bypasses danger of causing brain herniation from doing an LP. Shows IIIrd and IVth ventricles and aqueduct better than air ventriculography. Can be used when air does not enter IVth ventricle during pneumoencephalography
5. *Radioisotope Radiography*			
a. Dynamic radioactive brain scan (flow study)	After injection of a radioactive element or gas into the blood, radiation counters over the head register brain blood flow by taking serial counts at 2 sec intervals for 10-50 sec	Radiation, venipuncture with very rare sepsis	Gives crude estimate of cerebral blood flow and shows areas of decreased or increased blood flow
b. Static radioactive brain scan. See Fig. 13-8E.	As above but single rather than serial images are made at 2 or more hr after injection to detect residual radioactivity in brain	As above	Displays areas of increased blood-brain barrier permeability, usually caused by destructive lesions
c. Radioactive cisternography and ventriculography. See Fig. 13-8F.	After injection of a radioactive substance into the CSF at lumbar levels, radiation counts are made over vertebral column and head as fluid percolates through the subarachnoid space and refluxes into ventricles	As above	Records the dynamics of the CSF circulation and outlines subarachnoid spaces, ventricular size, and exchange of CSF with ventricles

B. *Use of neuroradiologic procedures by the non-specialist*

When to order one neuroradiologic test over another, its value in relation to other tests, its limitations, false positive and false negative results, in short, the *epistemology* of neuroradiologic tests (to use an ostentatious word) exceed the ken of the general physician. The generalist simply cannot judge the pros and cons that balance effectiveness, risk, and cost of the various procedures. The generalist might reasonably expect to achieve some understanding of when to order plain films of the skull and spine, and the CAT scan.

Because the nonspecialist does not personally have to do or interpret the radiologic tests and subsequent procedures described in this chapter, I have chosen not to program them.

C. *Plain skull and spine radiographs*

1. *Information provided:* Skull radiographs show the bones of the skull, their contours, thickness, density, integrity, sutures, foramina and canals, air-filled cavities, and vascular markings. Plain skull radiographs do not show normal brain, ventricles, or subarachnoid spaces, nor do they show most lesions unless they calcify. They show normal calcification as in the pineal gland or choroid plexuses, and abnormal calcification in

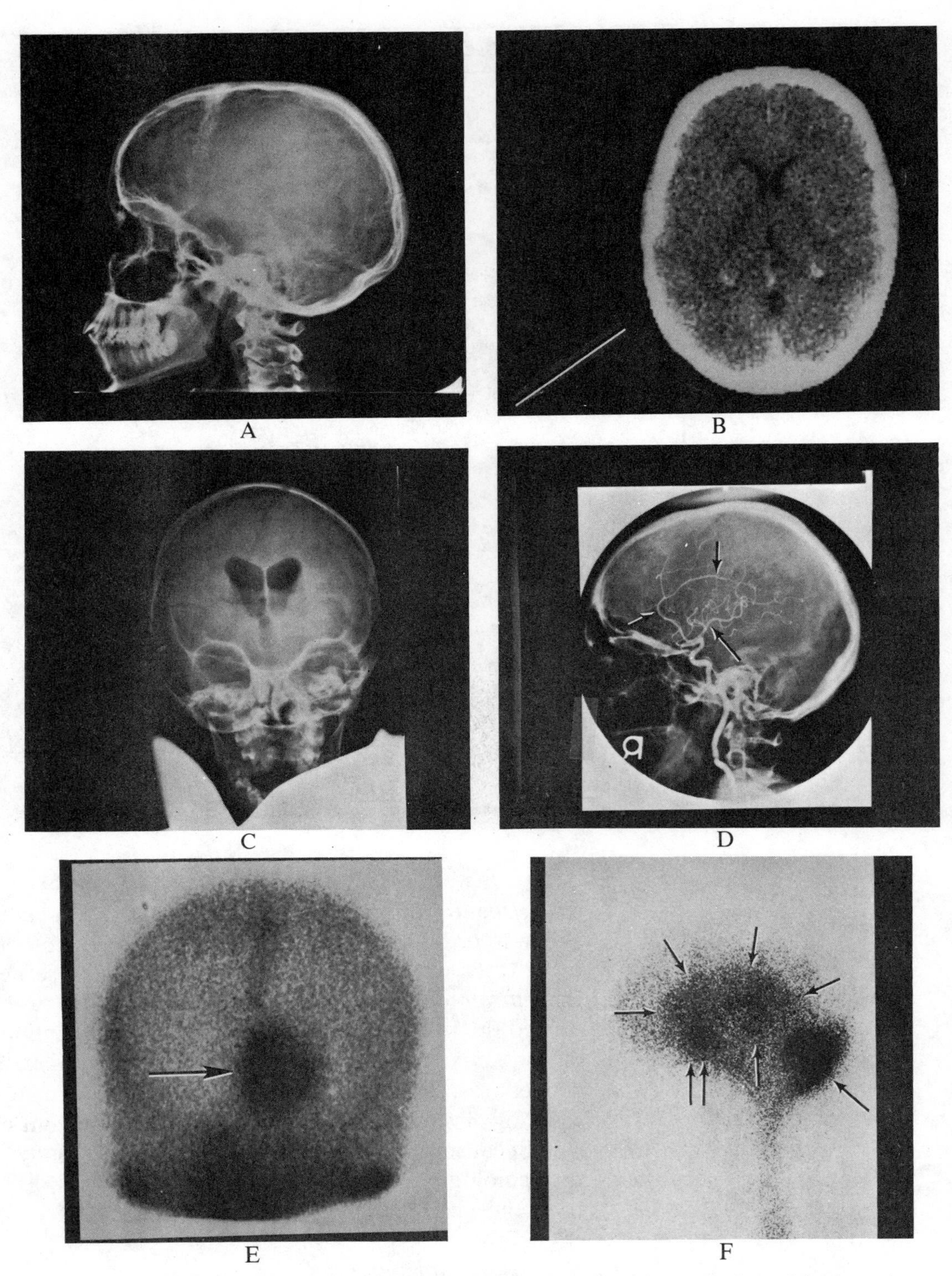

FIG. 13-8. Various neuroradiologic diagnostic procedures. On all lateral views the front of the patient's head is to the reader's left. *A.* Plain skull radiograph, lateral view, normal. *B.* Computerized axial tomogram (CAT scan), horizontal view, normal. *C.* Pneumoencephalogram, posterior-anterior view, showing slightly dilated lateral ventricles. *D.* Angiogram, lateral view, showing normal middle cerebral artery (single long arrow) and anterior cerebral artery (short arrow). *E.* Static radioactive brain scan, frontal view, showing meningioma with dense concentration of radioactive tracer (arrow). *F.* Cisternogram, lateral view, showing concentration of radioactive tracer in cisterna magna cerebelli (single arrow, right lower), third ventricle (double arrows), and lateral ventricle (multiple arrows). The ventricles are enlarged.

the basal ganglia, blood vessels, and some space-occupying lesions. Calcification occurs in longstanding lesions of soft tissue, as reviewed in Table 13-4.

TABLE 13-4. Chronic Brain Lesions Which May Calcify and Show on Plain Skull Radiographs

1. Chronic abscesses or other scars from inflammation. 2. Scars from traumatic injury. 3. Slowly growing neoplasms.	4. Some vascular lesions such as chronic hematomas, and arteriovenous malformations. 5. Some metabolic-degenerative diseases cause basal ganglia calcification.

In addition to calcified lesions, plain radiographs may show soft tissue lesions that contain fat (lipomas) or gas, which appear radiolucent, or penetrating, radiopaque objects such as bullets and wire, and depressed or sequestered bone fragments. Plain skull radiographs also show inflammation in the sinuses and mastoid air cells, if those cavities fill with fluid or show thickening of their mucosal lining.

Soft tissue lesions that impinge on bone affect it in one or two ways, uncommonly by causing bone proliferation (hyperostosis), and more commonly by eroding it (osteolysis). Bone yields to soft tissue pressure, particularly neoplasms, or pulsating soft tissues, like aneurysms. For example, neoplasms of nerves, such as optic nerve gliomas or acoustic nerve neurinomas, erode their bony foramina. In obstructive hydrocephalus, with increased intraventricular pressure, the ballooned base of the brain continually pulsating against the posterior clinoid processes erodes them. Thus osteolysis or hyperostosis on the plain films may provide evidence of long-standing soft tissue lesions or increased intracranial pressure.

2. *Indications:* Order plain skull radiographs when the patient has symptoms or signs that could be of intracranial origin, if the lesion *suspected* or to be *excluded* could affect the skull bones, or calcify. Common indications include seizures, headaches of unexplained origin, changes in mental status, or neurologic signs of brain disease. Table 13-5 reviews the kinds of lesions that plain films help to identify or exclude.

   Some authors have legitimately questioned the overuse of plain radiographs (see Bell and Loop, 1971; and Delaney, 1976 in Section 2 of the Radiology Bibliography). However, such studies fail to give sufficient weight to one simple fact: the kind of information you need *before* you make the diagnosis differs entirely from what you find you could have

TABLE 13-5. Kinds of Lesions That Plain Radiographs Help to Identify or Exclude

1. Changes in the density, integrity, contour, and thickness of skull bones. 2. Erosions of flat bones, skull base, or clinoid processes by tumors, aneurysms, inflammatory lesions, or hydrocephalus. 3. Separated or prematurely closed sutures.	4. Penetrating radiopaque objects such as bullets, or depressed skull fractures. 5. Inflammation of sinuses or mastoid air cells. 6. Long-standing lesions that may calcify. 7. Congenital malformations of bone.

dispensed with *after* the diagnosis. While I am groping to make the diagnosis, I need negative information. I need to know what the patient does *not* have in order to focus on and direct me to the studies that will be positive. The decision to proceed with the final test that establishes the diagnosis often comes from knowing which tests have failed.

D. *Plain spine radiographs*
Obtain plain spine radiographs on the basis of the same principles as govern skull radiographs: whenever the history and physical examination suggest a lesion that may affect the density, contour, integrity, and processes of the vertebra, the size of the vertebral canal and the intervertebral foramina, or the spaces between the vertebral bodies occupied by the intervertebral discs.

E. *Computerized axial tomography (CAT)*
Order a CAT scan when the history and physical examination raise the question of a lesion that may distort the size and shape of the brain or spinal cord, the ventricles or subarachnoid space, the blood vessels, or that may alter the radiopacity of the neural tissue itself. Order a CAT scan before doing an LP in a patient who may have increased intracranial pressure or a potential brain herniation. The major exception to this rule is when the patient may have bacterial meningitis that may require a specific type of antibiotic treatment. The major classes of pathologic processes disclosed by CAT consist of neoplasms, abscesses, hematomas, infarcts, aneurysms or vascular malformations, demyelination, brain edema, brain atrophy or enlargement, congenital malformations, and hydrocephalus. See Fig. 13-9.

With present techniques, CAT scan least effectively shows lesions at the base of the brain and in the posterior fossa. Although CAT scan does show the basal subarachnoid spaces (cisterns), cerebellum, and IVth ventricle fairly well, other neuroradiologic procedures listed in Table 13-3 show them better.

F. *Radioisotope brain scans*
1. *Information provided:* The static brain scan (see Table 13-3) shows a darkened area of radioactivity at sites of increased blood-brain barrier permeability where the radioactive substance has leaked into, and remains in, the tissue (see Fig. 13-7*E*). Most lesions which show unequivocally in CAT scans are destructive: neoplasms, abscesses, and infarcts (after several days), contusions, and subdural hematomas. Radioisotope scans work best with large destructive lesions near the brain surface and least well with small, relatively slowly progressive, less destructive lesions deep in the brain or at the base of the skull. Dynamic radioisotope scans disclose gross disturbances in cerebral blood flow.
2. *Indications:* When available, CAT scan is usually the procedure of choice for visualizing brain lesions. Use static radioisotopic scans to survey the brain for destructive lesions in lieu of CAT scan, or when the CAT scan or other procedures leave some doubt as to the presence of a lesion. Use dynamic brain scans to document gross disturbances in

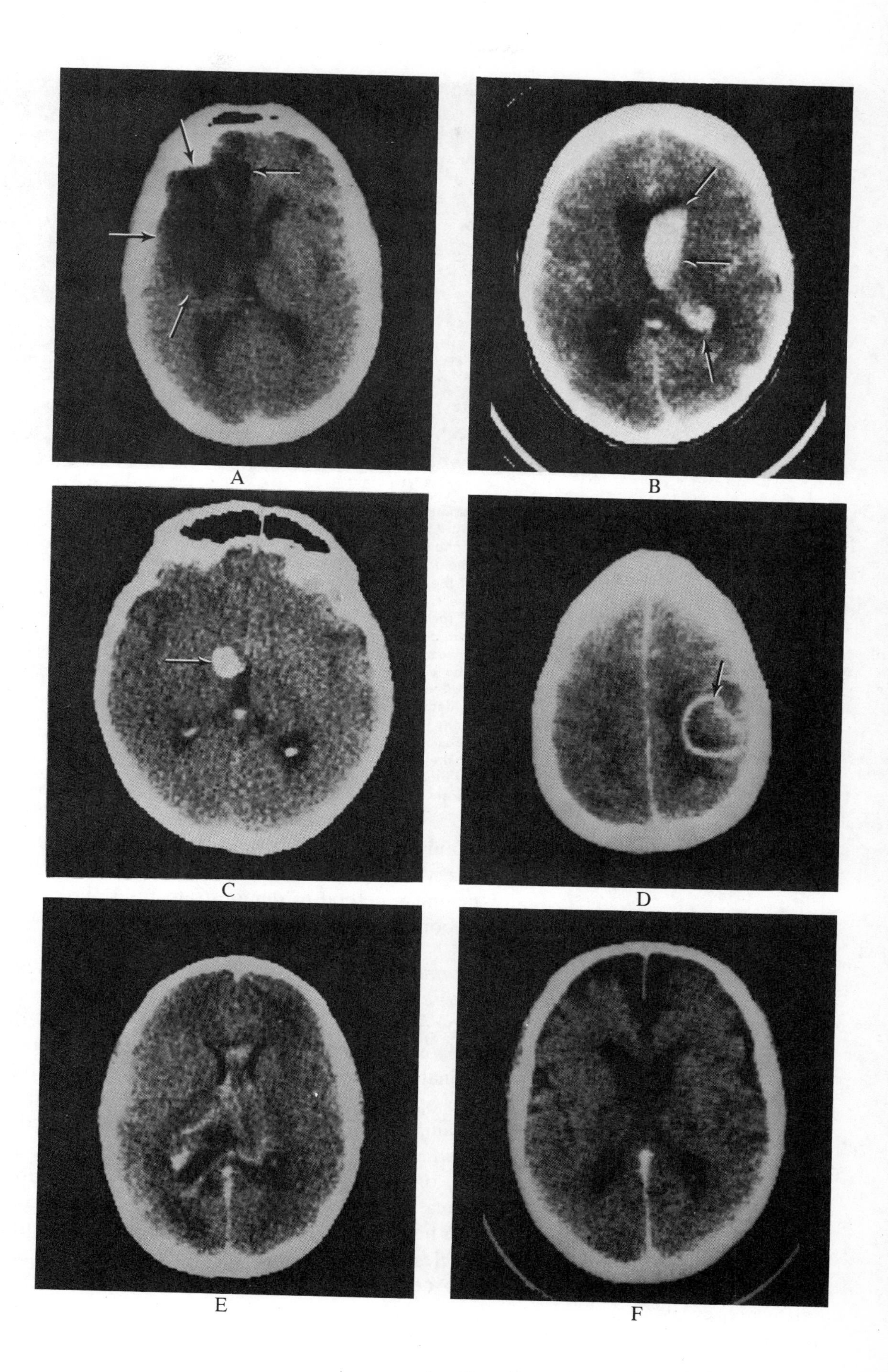
A
B
C
D
E
F

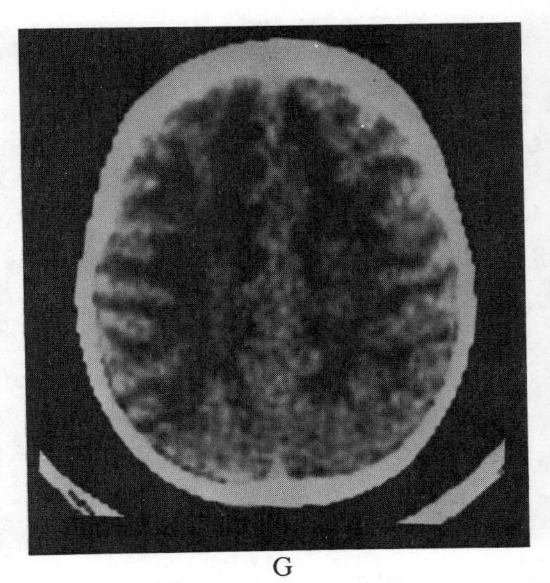

G

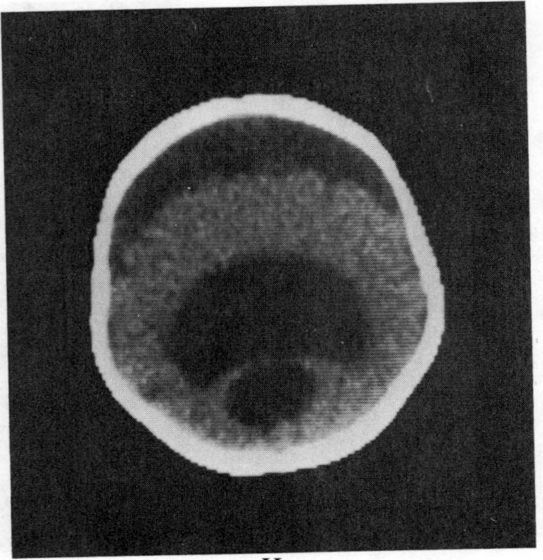

H

FIG. 13-9. Various lesions shown by CAT scans. All illustrations are horizontal scans with the front of the head toward the top of the page. See Fig. 13-8B for a completely normal CAT scan. A. Old infarct, left anterior and middle cerebral artery distributions. The destroyed tissue, replaced by fluid, leaves a large, radiolucent cavity (arrows). B. Intraventricular hemorrhage on the right (arrows), with distension of the ventricular system. C. Aneurysm of left internal carotid artery (arrow), enhanced scan. D. Abscess, right parietal lobe, enhanced scan showing the radiodense ring of vascularity in the abscess wall (arrow). The lucent region around the abscess ring is edema. E. Glioblastoma of the fornix, septum pellucidum, and corpus callosum, enhanced scan, showing mottled areas of radiodensity from vascularity of the neoplasm. Notice the widened, tumor-infiltrated septum pellucidum separating the anterior horns of the lateral ventricles. Compare this scan with the normal one in Fig. 13-8B. F. Cerebral atrophy in presenile dementia with widening of the interhemispheric fissure anteriorly, widening of the sulci, and enlargement of the ventricular system. G. Diffuse demyelinating encephalopathy (leukodystrophy) with destruction of and extreme radiolucency of the white matter. Notice the preservation of the gyral pattern by the rim of intact cerebral cortex. H. Congenital malformation of the brain with monoventricle and incomplete separation of the cerebrum into mirror-image halves (holoprosencephaly). Notice that the space anteriorly, between the anterior curve of the brain and the skull, contains radiolucent cerebrospinal fluid, as does the monoventricle.

blood flow in cerebrovascular disease such as venous sinus or major artery occlusion, or in suspected subdural hematomas, and as a supplementary method to demonstrate total absence of cerebral blood flow to confirm brain death.

G. To summarize this section on neuroradiology, state the neuroradiologic procedure

1. To best visualize bone of the skull or vertebrae, do __________.
2. To visualize the anatomy of the brain, its ventricles and lesions, and the spinal cord, with the least risk and discomfort, do __________.
3. To optimally visualize the anatomy of the subarachnoid spaces of the brain, or the IIIrd and IVth ventricles and aqueduct, do __________ or __________.
4. To optimally visualize the anatomy of the subarachnoid space of the spinal cord, do __________.
5. To best visualize the flow of CSF in the subarachnoid space and ventricles, do __________.
6. To best visualize details of the cerebral or spinal blood vessels, do __________.

plain radiographs
CAT scan

pneumoencephalography or positive-contrast cisternography, or ventriculography
positive contrast myelography
radioisotope cisternography
angiography

dynamic radioisotope scan
static radioisotope scan

7. To visualize gross disturbances in cerebral blood flow without doing angiography, do ______.
8. To visualize regions of increased blood-brain barrier permeability, do ______.

Bibliography

General Texts for Neuroradiology

DeBlanc, H. J., and Sorenson, J. A. (eds.): *Noninvasive Brain Imaging: Computed Tomography and Radionuclides,* Acton, Mass., Publishing Sciences Group, Inc., 1975.

Decker, K., and Backmund, H.: *Pediatric Neuroradiology,* E. H. Burrows, trans., Acton, Mass., Publishing Group, Inc., 1975.

Harwood-Nash, F.: *Neuroradiology in Infants and Children,* 3 vols., St. Louis, The C. V. Mosby Company, 1976.

Kaufmann, H. J. (ed.): Skull, Spine, and Contents: vols. 5 and 6, *Progress in Pediatric Radiology,* Basel, S. Karger, 1975.

McClure, W.: *The Anatomic Foundation of Neuroradiology of the Brain,* 2nd ed., Boston, Little, Brown and Company, 1972.

Newton, T. H., and Potts, D. G. (eds.): *Radiology of the Skull and Brain,* vol. 1, Books 1 and 2, The Skull; vol. 2, Book 1, Technical Aspects; Book 2, Arteries; Book 3, Veins; Book 4, Specific Disease Processes, vol. 3, Anatomy and Pathology, St. Louis, The C. V. Mosby Company, 1974.

Peterson, H., and Kieffer, S.: Neuroradiology, in *Clinical Neurology,* Baker, A., and Baker, L. (eds.), New York, Harper & Row, 1977.

Ruggiero, G., Bories, J., Calabro, A., et al.: *Radiological Exploration of the Ventricles and Subarachnoid Space,* New York, Springer-Verlag, 1974.

Salamon, G., and Huang, Y. P.: *Radiologic Anatomy of the Brain,* New York, Springer-Verlag, 1976.

Taveras, J. M., and Wood, E. H.: *Diagnostic Neuroradiology,* vols. 1 and 2, 2nd ed., Baltimore, The Williams & Wilkins Company, 1976.

Plain Skull Radiographs

Bell, R. S., and Loop, J. W.: The utility and futility of radiographic skull examination for trauma, *N. Engl. J. Med.,* 284:236-239, 1971.

Chaster, C.: *Atlas of Roentgen Anatomy of the Newborn and Infant Skull,* St. Louis, Warren H. Green, Inc., 1972.

Delaney, J. F.: Routine skull films in hospitalized psychiatric patients, *Am. J. Psychiatry,* 133:93-95, 1976.

DeBoulay, G.: *Principles of X-ray Diagnosis of the Skull,* Washington, Butterworths, 1965.

Epstein, B., and Davidoff, L.: *An Atlas of Skull Roentgenograms,* Philadelphia, Lea & Febiger, 1953.

Etter, L. E.: *Atlas of Roentgen Anatomy of the Skull,* Springfield, Ill., Charles C Thomas, Publisher, 1955.

Schmitz, A., Haveson, R., and Hanna, D.: *Illustrative Cranial Neuroradiology,* Springfield, Ill., Charles C Thomas, Publisher, 1967.

Selman, J. (ed.): *Skull Radiography: A Simplified System,* Springfield, Ill., Charles C Thomas, Publisher, 1966.

Computerized Axial Tomography

Abrams, H. L., and McNeil, B. J.: Medical implications of computed tomography ("CAT scanning"), Part I, *N. Engl. J. Med.,* 298:255-261, 1978. Part II, ibid., 310-318.

Clifford, J. R., Connolly, E. S., and Voorhies, R. M.: Comparison of radionuclide scans with computer-assisted tomography in diagnosis in intracranial disease, *Neurology,* 26:1119-1123, 1976.

Gonzales, C. F., Grossman, C. B., and Pulucios, E.: *Computed Brain and Orbital Tomography,* New York, John Wiley and Sons, 1971.

Henderson, S. D.: *Pathology in Computed Tomography of the Brain,* Springfield, Ill., Charles C Thomas, Publisher, 1978.

Jabbour, J. T., Ramey, D. R., and Roach, S.: *Atlas of Computerized Tomography Scan in Pediatric Neurology,* Garden City, Medical Examination Publishing Co., Inc., 1977.

Naidich, T. P., Pudlowski, R. M., and Leeds, N. E., et al.: The normal contrast-enhanced computed axial tomogram of the brain, *Journal of Computer Assisted Tomography,* 1:16-29, 1977.

New, P. J.: Computed tomography: A major diagnostic advance, *Hosp. Prac.,* 10:55-64, 1975.

Oldendorf, W. H.: The quest for an image of the brain: A brief historical and technical review of brain imaging techniques, *Neurology,* 28:517-533, 1978.

Penn, R. D., Belanger, M., and Yasoff, W. A.: Ventricular volume in man computed from CAT scans, *Ann. Neurol.,* 3:216-223, 1978.

Radioactive Brain Scan

Glasauer, F. E., Alker, Jr., G. J., and Leslie, E. V.: Isotope cisternography and ventriculography, *Am. J. Dis. Child.,* 120:109-114, 1970.

Handa, J. (ed.): *Dynamic Aspects of Brain Scanning,* Baltimore, University Park Press, 1972.

Harbett, J.: *Cisternography and Hydrocephalus: A Symposium,* Springfield, Ill., Charles C Thomas, Publisher, 1972.

Lassen, N. A., Ingvar, D. G., and Skinhoj, E.: Brain function and blood flow, *Sci. Am.,* 239:62-71, 1978.

Mealey, P. R., and Campbell, J.: Scintillography of infantile subdural effusions and its clinical application, *Acta Radiol.,* 5:871-883, 1966.

Penning, L., and Front, D.: *Brain Scintigraphy,* Excerpta Medica American Elsevier, New York, 1975.

Rowan, J.: Radioisotopes in diagnosis, in Critchley, M., O'Leary, J., and Jennett, B. (eds.): *Scientific Foundations of Neurology,* Philadelphia, F. A. Davis Company, 1972.

Angiography of the Brain

Krayenbuhl, H., and Yasargil, M.: *Die Zerebrale Angiographie: Lehbuch fur Klinik und Praxis,* Stuttgart, Georg Thieme Verlag, 1968.

Leeds, N. E., and Taveras, J. M.: *Dynamic Factors in Diagnosis of Supratentorial Brain Tumors by Cerebral Angiography,* Philadelphia, W. B. Saunders Company, 1969.

Newton, T. H., and Potts, D. G. (eds.): *Radiology of the Skull and Brain,* vol. 2, Book 1, Technical Aspects; Book 2, Arteries; Book 3, Veins; St. Louis, The C. V. Mosby Company, 1974.

Nomura, T.: *Atlas of Cerebral Angiography,* New York, Springer-Verlag, 1970.

Szikla, G., Bouvier, G., Hori, T., and Petrov, V.: *Angiography of the Human Brain Cortex,* New York, Springer-Verlag, 1977.

Takahashi, M.: *Atlas of Vertebral Angiography,* Baltimore, University Park Press, 1972.

Wolpert, S. M.: *Angiography of Posterior Fossa Tumors,* New York, Grune and Stratton, 1976.

Pneumoencephalography and Ventriculography

Davidoff, L., and Dyke, C.: *The Normal Encephalogram,* 3rd ed., Philadelphia, Lea and Febiger, 1951.

Davidoff, L., and Epstein, B.: *The Abnormal Pneumoencephalogram,* 2nd ed., Philadelphia, Lea and Febiger, 1955.

DiChiro, G.: *An Atlas of Detailed Normal Pneumoencephalographic Anatomy,* Springfield, Ill., Charles C Thomas, Publisher, 1961.

——: *An Atlas of Pathologic Pneumoencephalography,* Springfield, Ill., Charles C Thomas, Publisher, 1967.

Epstein, B.: *Pneumoencephalography and Cerebral Angiography,* Chicago, Year Book Medical Publishers, 1966.

Heimburger, R.: Positive-contrast cerebral ventriculography using water-soluble media, *J. Neurol. Neurosurg. Psychiatry,* 29:281-290, 1966.

Robertson, E.: *Pneumoencephalography,* 2nd ed., Springfield, Ill., Charles C Thomas, Publisher, 1967.

White, Y., Bell, D., and Mellick, R.: Sequelae to pneumoencephalography, *J. Neurol. Neurosurg. Psychiatry,* 36:146-151, 1973.

Plain Spine Radiography

Epstein, B.: *The Spine, A Radiological Text and Atlas,* Philadelphia, Lea and Febiger, 1955.

Hardy, J. H. (ed.): *Spinal Deformity in Neurological and Muscular Disorders,* St. Louis, The C. V. Mosby Company, 1974.

Schmorl, G.: "The Human Spine in Health and Disease: Anatomicopathologic Studies." In H. Junghanns (ed.), *Clinicoradiologic Aspects* (S. P. Wilk, and L. S. Goin, trans.), New York, Grune and Stratton, 1959.

von Torklus, D., and Gehle, W.: *The Upper Cervical Spine: Regional Anatomy, Pathology, and Traumatology: A Systematic Radiological Atlas and Textbook,* New York, Grune and Stratton, 1972.

Wackenheim, A.: *Roentgen Diagnosis of the Craniovertebral Region,* New York, Springer-Verlag, 1974.

Wilkinson, M.: *Cervical Spondylosis: Its Early Diagnosis and Treatment,* Philadelphia, W. B. Saunders Company, 1971.

Myelography

Shapiro, R.: *Myelography,* 3rd ed., Chicago, Year Book Medical Publishers, 1975.

Valentino, V.: *Myelography,* Springfield, Ill., Charles C Thomas, Publisher, 1965.

Angiography of the Spinal Cord

Djindjian, R.: *Angiography of the Spinal Cord,* Baltimore, University Park Press, 1970.

Doppman, J., DiChiro, G., and Ommaya, A.: *Selective Arteriography of the Spinal Cord,* St. Louis, Warren H. Green, Inc., 1969.

III. Echoencephalography

A. *Principle.* Ultrasound beamed through the head reflects off of interfaces in the brain and meninges. The pattern of reflection of the ultrasound discloses the midline structure of the cerebrum. As techniques improve, we can expect to detect other normal structures and some lesions with ultrasound.

B. *Risk.* None known.

C. *Clinical use.* Echoencephalography provides a quick method of locating the midline of the cerebrum. Use it whenever you suspect that a unilateral cerebral lesion may have shifted the cerebrum across the midline, threatening transtentorial herniation. Obtain an echoencephalogram in head injuries, coma of unknown origin, or whenever knowledge of the location of the cerebral midline may prove useful to management of the patient. Safe and noninvasive, echoencephalography can be used repeatedly on the same patient to follow the course of any lesion which shifts the cerebrum.

Bibliography

McKinney, W.: Echoencephalography, in *Special Techniques for Neurologic Diagnosis,* Toole, J. (ed), Contemporary Neurology Series, vol. 3, Philadelphia, F. A. Davis, 1969.

IV. Electroneurodiagnosis

A. *Electroencephalography (EEG)*

1. *Principle.* Fluctuations in the electrical activity of the brain can be recorded by electrodes attached to the scalp. The potentials are amplified and the voltage fluctuations are recorded as lines on a paper. The voltage fluctuations have a rhythmic character which varies with the region of the cerebrum and the age and the level of alertness of the patient. The electroencephalographer notes the frequency of the electrical fluctuations in cycles per second, the contour or configuration of the waves, and searches for pathologic alterations characterized by waves that are too high or too low, or too fast or too slow. He describes the location, whether focal, unilateral, or diffuse, of the abnormal wave forms and compares the amplitude of the waves from the two sides of the head. See Fig. 13-10.
2. *Risk.* None.
3. *Clinical use.* The EEG is most helpful in diagnosing epilepsy, space-occupying lesions, and, on occasion, coma.

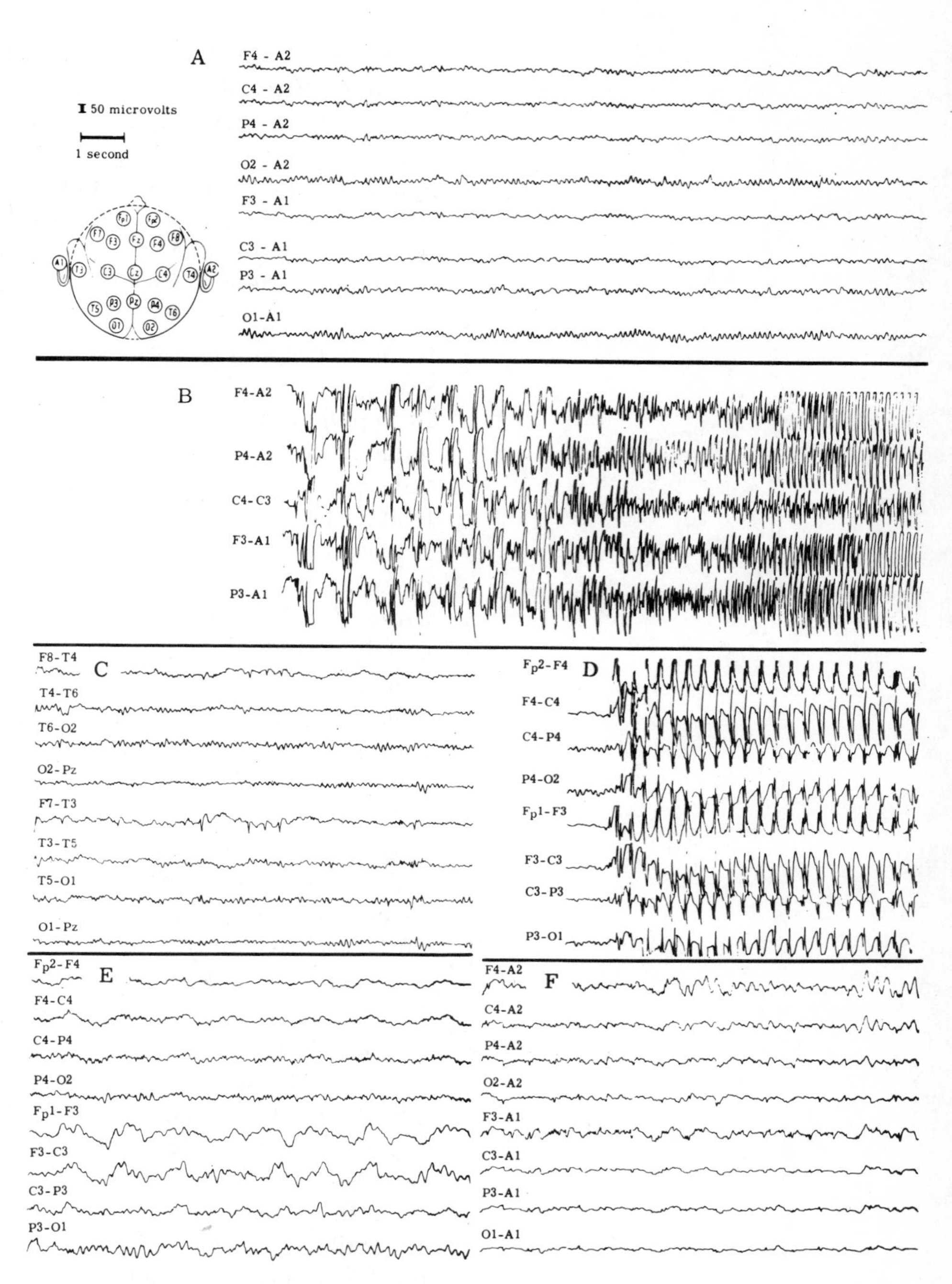

FIG. 13-10. Electroencephalograms. The inset at the upper left shows the calibration signals and the position of the electrodes on the head. A large number of combinations of electrodes are possible, but only a few are used in routine work. The electroencephalograph is simply an X-Y recorder (kymograph). Each line on the EEG represents the difference in electrical potential between a pair of electrodes. Excepting record B, the first four lines in each record (even numbers) are from the right side of the head, the second four (odd numbers) are homologous leads from the left side. The way to read the records is to mentally "pick up" the top four lines and superimpose them on the bottom four lines. A. Normal record with symmetrical 10 cps (alpha) rhythm in the occipital leads. B. High amplitude, symmetrical hypersynchronous discharge during a generalized motor seizure. The first portion of the record shows a few myoclonic jerks, the mid-portion shows the tonic phase, and the last portion of the record shows the clonic phase. The patient had received succinylcholine to block the skeletal muscular action, permitting a record to be obtained which is free from movement and muscle action potentials. C. Spike focus in the left frontotemporal region. This type of focal abnormality usually indicates a chronic, epileptogenic lesion. D. Three cps generalized hypersynchronous (Continued)

a. Most epileptic patients have abnormal EEGs in the interval between seizures. Virtually all epileptics have abnormal EEGs during a seizure, when high amplitude, hypersynchronous waves appear. See Fig. 13-10.

b. *Space-occupying lesions* such as infarcts, neoplasms, abscesses, and contusions cause focal slow waves over the lesion site. Like the brain scan, the EEG gives localizing information, but it does not identify the histologic type of lesion.

c. *Coma* of metabolic origin, such as uremic or diabetic, or of infectious origin, such as encephalitic, or of most diffuse brain lesions, causes diffuse slowing. The EEG is of little differential help. In hepatic coma, the EEG may show triphasic waves and in drug-induced coma, as with barbiturates, the EEG may show low-amplitude fast rhythms superimposed on the slow background waves. Unilateral flattening in a comatose patient suggests a subdural hematoma, a massive necrotizing process such as a large infarct, or exhaustion of the neurons after a focal seizure.

d. *Brain death* results in complete absence of recordable electrical activity. Most institutions have established brain death protocols consisting of clinical and EEG criteria. Recognition of brain death makes further therapeutic efforts, such as artificial support of ventilation and blood pressure, futile. The physician then discontinues these efforts in acknowledgment of brain death. Any salvageable organs may then be transplanted to a living recipient. Laboratory aids to confirm brain death, in addition to EEG, consist of a dynamic radioisotope scan or regular angiography, neither of which show any cerebral blood flow. CSF examination shows extremely high levels of degradative enzymes.

e. *To summarize:* Sharp waves or spikes imply an epileptogenic lesion, usually of static type, as a brain scar, or a slowly advancing lesion. Slow waves, if focal, imply a focal destructive lesion; if generalized, slow waves imply reduction of consciousness or a generalized brain disease. Flattening of the waves, if not postseizure, suggests a substance, such as fluid, between the brain and skull, or absence or complete destruction of the cerebral wall.

f. *Activating procedures during EEG.* Several procedures may activate epileptiform discharges, consisting of spikes or spikes and waves, in the EEG. These procedures increase the likelihood that any given interictal EEG will show an epileptiform abnormality that will aid in establishing the diagnosis of epilepsy, and in fact may precipitate an actual seizure. Without activation, the interictal EEG sometimes appears normal, and thus gives no support to the clinical diagnosis of a seizure disorder.

---

burst usually associated with transient loss of consciousness without a generalized convulsion. E. Random slow (delta) waves of 1 to 3 cps in the left anterior and central regions. This wave form usually indicates an acute destructive lesion such as an infarct, neoplasm, abscess, or contusion. F. Amplitude asymmetry with flattening of the waves over the left hemisphere and some generalized slow activity. The patient had a subdural hematoma with a large amount of blood over the left hemisphere.

The routine procedures consist of hyperventilation for 3 to 5 min., photic stimulation, and sleep. Hyperventilation drives off CO_2, producing an alkaline change in the blood. This change increases the likelihood of a spike or spike-wave discharge, particularly in patients with petit mal seizures. Photic stimulation of the eye with different flash frequencies activates the occipital cortex and may bring out an epileptiform discharge or clinical seizure. Sleep may also activate a spike focus.

4. *Clinical indications for EEG.* Obtain an EEG when the patient's signs raise the question of a brain disorder that could alter the electrical activity of the brain. Table 13-6 summarizes the major indications.

TABLE 13-6. Summary of Clinical Indications for an Electroencephalogram
1. Intermittent disorders of brain function, especially episodic disturbances of consciousness or the mental state.
2. Unconsciousness of unexplained origin.
3. Clinical suspicion of a focal brain lesion or diffuse encephalopathy of unknown origin.
4. Disturbances of the sleep-wake cycle.
5. Suspected brain death.

5. *Editorial note:* The field of electroencephalography seems to have attracted at least its fair share of speculative physicians and psychologists (a few of whom are simply entrepreneurs). You cannot read a person's thoughts from the EEG or match him with the proper marriage partner. Some interesting correlation has been achieved between learning and the EEG. In general the correlation of the EEG with mental activity and behavior has been poor, in fact downright disappointing. Undoubtedly, correlations will improve in the future, but for the present, EEG reading is a visual art, not an objective science. The difficulty of the art does not prevent incompetent readers from entering the field with great aplomb. As a general rule, with some exceptions, the EEG is worse than useless unless it is read by a physician:
   a. Who is trained in neurology.
   b. Who personally diagnoses, treats, and is responsible for the care of a wide variety of neurologic patients.
   c. Who continually matches his diagnoses and interpretations against the clinical course and ultimate diagnosis of the patient.
   d. Who regularly subjects his opinions and conclusions to the corrective influence of knowledgeable colleagues.
   e. Who is familiar with the structure of the brain, understands its pathologic reactions, and regularly attends autopsy sessions to make rueful note of his errors.

   In fact, you see that these criteria, with slight change, characterize not only the good electroencephalographer, but any good physician.

Bibliography

Bennett, D. R., Hughes, J. R., Korein, J., et al.: *Atlas of Electroencephalography in Coma and Cerebral Death: EEG at the Bedside or in the Intensive Care Unit,* New York, Raven Press, 1976.

DeMyer, W., and White, P.: EEG in holoprosencephaly (arhinencephaly). *Arch. Neurol.,* 11:507-520, 1964.

Goldensohn, E. S., and Koehle, R.: *EEG Interpretation: Problems of Overreading and Underreading,* Minneapolis, American Academy of Neurology, 1975.

Hill, D., and Parr, G. (eds.): *Electroencephalography,* New York, The Macmillan Company, 1963.

Kiloh, L., and Osselton, W.: *Clinical Electroencephalography,* 2d ed., Washington, Butterworths, 1966.

Kooi, K.: *Fundamentals of Electroencephalography,* New York, Harper & Row, Publishers, 1971.

Werner, S. S., Stockard, J. C., and Bickford, R. G.: *Atlas of Neonatal Electroencephalography,* New York, Raven Press, 1977.

White, P., DeMyer, W., and DeMyer, M.: EEG abnormalities in early childhood schizophrenia: A double-blind study of psychiatrically disturbed and normal children during Promazine sedation, *Amer. J. Psychiat.,* 120:950-958, 1964.

B. *Evoked potentials*

Stimulation of a peripheral nerve causes electrical impulses in the appropriate pathways of the spinal cord, brainstem, and in the sensory areas of the cerebral cortex. With ordinary surface recording, as in routine EEG, only photic stimulation produces an easily definable response. To see the less obvious sensory impulses, to pick out the signal from the noise of the ongoing background of impulses, requires computer averaging, a CAT scan, but this time the acronym stands for computer of average transients, not computerized axial tomography. The computer of average transients remembers and displays those electrical wave forms that follow the stimulus at any regular interval of time after hundreds or thousands of stimuli are applied. By knowing that the wave does follow the stimulus by a regular time interval, the observer then learns to recognize normal and abnormal wave patterns, and can even work out a computer program to assist in this decision. At present, brainstem auditory evoked responses (BAER) and photic driving are the most useful sensory evoked responses, but surface recording of somatic sensory impulses from the spinal cord and parietal cortex offers promise of clinical application.

Bibliography

Cusick, J. F., Myklebust, J. B., Larson, S. J., and Sances, A.: Spinal cord evaluation by cortical evoked responses, *Arch. Neurol.,* 36:140-143, 1979.

Davis, A. D., and Wada, J. A.: Lateralization of speech dominance by spectral analysis of evoked potentials, *J. Neurol. Neurosurg. Psychiatry,* 40:1-4, 1977.

Hashimoto, I., Ishiyama, Y., and Tozuka, G.: Bilaterally recorded brainstem auditory evoked responses, *Arch. Neurol.,* 36:161-167, 1979.

Jones, S. J.: Investigation of brachial plexus traction lesions by peripheral and spinal somatosensory evoked potentials, *J. Neurol. Neurosurg. Psychiatry,* 42:107-116, 1979.

Naunton, R. F., and Fernandez, C. (eds.): *Evoked Electrical Activity in the Auditory Nervous System,* New York, Academic Press, 1977.

Starr, A., and Acher, L. J.: Auditory brainstem responses in neurological disease, *Arch. Neurol.,* 32:761-768, 1975.

Stockard, J. J., Stockard, J. E., and Sharbrough, F. W.: Detection and localization of occult lesions with brainstem auditory responses, *Mayo Clin. Proc.,* 52: 761-769, 1977.

C. Electronystagmography (ENG)

ENG provides a quantitative method for recording nystagmus, either spontaneous or evoked by caloric stimulation, positional change, rotation, or by an optokinetic drum. The method depends on the fact that the eye is polarized (with the cornea positive in reference to the fundus). Skin electrodes placed on either side of the eye record the electrical changes as the polarized eyeballs move. An X-Y recorder, as with EEG or EKG, then records the movements as waves on a strip of moving paper.

ENG proves helpful in the analysis of patients with the complaint of dizziness or who have symptoms or signs of VIIIth nerve or brainstem disease.

Bibliography

Electronystagmography

Baloh, R. W., Konrad, H. R., Dirks, D., et al.: Cerebellar-pontine angle tumors, *Arch. Neurol.,* 33:507-512, 1976.

Naunton, R. F. (ed.): *The Vestibular System,* New York, Academic Press, 1975.

Rubin, W., and Norris, C. H.: *Electronystagmography: What is ENG?,* Springfield, Ill., Charles C Thomas, Publisher, 1974.

Uemura, T., Suzuki, J-I., Hozawa, J., et al.: *Neuro-otological Examination,* Baltimore, University Park Press, 1976.

D. Electromyography (EMG)

1. *Principle.* Electrical potentials derived from contracting muscle fibers are recorded from a needle electrode and are displayed on an oscilloscope screen. See Fig. 6-14.
2. *Risk.* If, as is customary, needle electrodes are used, the insertion of the needle is painful, but only rarely leads to complications.
3. *Clinical use.* EMG is only of value when a disease of the LMN or muscle is suspected. It is of no value for UMN or cerebral lesions. The two essential questions the EMG can answer are: Is there evidence of denervation, such as of fibrillations, fasciculations and giant polyphasic motor units, or is there evidence of a myopathy, such as decreased amplitude of muscular potentials, or myotonic potentials? Unless the clinical evidence suggests neuromuscular disease, don't order an EMG (see Bibliography after E, next section).

E. *Nerve conduction velocity and nerve trunk stimulation*

1. *Principle.* A stimulating electrode is applied over a large motor nerve trunk and the response is recorded from one of its muscles. From the distance and the time elapsed between stimulus and response, the velocity of impulse conduction in the nerve can be calculated. Ideally, stimuli can be applied at two points along the nerve and the time for the shorter distance subtracted from the longer, to cancel out the delay for neuromuscular transmission.
2. *Risk.* Moderately uncomfortable to the patient.
3. *Clinical use.* Conduction velocity determinations or direct stimulation are of help in diagnosing peripheral neuropathies, nerve compression syndromes, and myasthenia gravis.
   a. In *peripheral neuropathies*, the nerve conduction velocity is less than 75 percent of normal. The test only establishes that the nerve is diseased. It gives little differential information as to whether the disease is toxic, metabolic, or heredofamilial in origin.
   b. In *nerve compression syndromes*, stimulation of nerve trunks can be of decisive value in localizing the lesion site. For example, it is sometimes difficult to decide whether a patient who has tingling in his thumb and index finger has compression of his C_6 nerve root or compression of his median nerve at the wrist, in the carpal tunnel. Delayed conduction across the wrist establishes the carpal tunnel syndrome, rather than a nerve root compression syndrome.
   c. In *myasthenia gravis*, repetitive supramaximal stimulation of a nerve trunk and recording of the muscular response gives objective evidence of decrementing muscular strength.

Bibliography

Aminoff, M. J.: *Electromyography in Clinical Practice,* Menlo Park, Addison-Wesley, 1978.

Cohen, H. L., and Brumlik, J.: *Manual of Electroneuromyography,* 2nd ed., New York, Harper & Row, 1976.

Desmedt, J. E. (ed.): *New Developments in Electromyography and Clinical Neurophysiology,* New York, S. Karger, 1973.

Dorfman, L. J., and Bosley, T. M.: Age-related changes in peripheral and central nerve conduction in man, *Neurology,* 29:38-44, 1979.

Goodgold, J., and Eberstein, A.: *Electrodiagnosis of Neuromuscular Disease,* Baltimore, The Williams & Wilkins Company, 1972.

Hansen, S., and Ballantyne, J. P.: A quantitative electrophysiological study of motor neurons disease. *J. Neurol. Neurosurg. Psychiatry,* 9:773-783, 1978.

Littman, B.: Peripheral nerve maturation in premature infants, *Neuropaediatrie,* 6:284-291, 1975.

Martinez, A. C., Barrio, M., Perez Conde, M. C., et al.: Electrophysiological aspects of sensory conduction velocity in healthy adults. 1. Conduction velocity from digit to palm to wrist, and across the elbow, as a function of age, *J. Neurol. Neurosurg. Psychiatry,* 41:1097-1101, 1978.

Schwartz, M. S., and Stalberg, E.: Single fibre electromyographic studies in myasthenia gravis with repetitive nerve stimulation, *J. Neurol. Neurosurg. Psychiatry,* 38:678-682, 1975.

Thiele, B., and Stalberg, E.: Single fibre EMG findings in polyneuropathies of different aetiology, *J. Neurol. Neurosurg. Psychiatry,* 38:881-887, 1975.

V. Biopsy

A. Introduction

1. *Principle.* Biopsy is the process of surgically removing a tissue sample from the living patient for the purpose of laboratory examination.
2. *Risk.* Possibility of hemorrhage, infection, or anesthetic complication.
3. *Clinical use.* Biopsy may be regarded as *mandatory* or *elective.*
   a. If the biopsy is done with the expectation of making a diagnosis to guide therapy for the individual patient, the biopsy is considered mandatory.
   b. If the biopsy is done with the expectation to diagnose an untreatable disease to gain information for optimum general management, prognosis and family counseling, or to advance scientific understanding of the disease process, the biopsy is considered elective. In these instances, the biopsy is not expected to be of immediate benefit to the individual patient.

B. Brain biopsy

The most common indications for brain biopsy are in diagnosing mass lesions of unknown histologic type, mainly neoplasms, and in diagnosing or recovering viruses in patients suspected of encephalitis. Both slow-virus encephalitides—such as subacute sclerosing panencephalitis—and acute viral encephalitides, such as herpes simplex, may require biopsy for confirmation. Virus can be demonstrated by serologic testing, fluorescent antibodies, culture, and electron microscopy.

Knowing the specific type of virus raises the possibility of using specific antiviral treatment. Specific antiviral treatment of herpes simplex currently shows some promise.

In the past, elective brain biopsies were done frequently to diagnose metabolic-degenerative diseases of the brain. Recent advances in biochemical tests and tissue culture of non-neural cells have greatly reduced the frequency of elective brain biopsy. For further discussion of elective biopsy, see the first or second editions of this text.

Bibliography

Adams, H.: Brain biopsy, in *Scientific Foundations of Neurology,* Critchley, M. (ed), Philadelphia, F. A. Davis Co., 1972.

Moossy, J.: Diagnostic cerebral biopsy, in *Special Techniques for Neurologic Diagnosis,* Toole, J. (ed), Contemporary Neurology Series, vol. 3, Philadelphia, F. A. Davis, 1969.

Whitley, R. J., Soont, S-j., Dolin, R., et al.: Adenine arabinoside therapy of biopsy-proved herpes simplex encephalitis, *N. Engl. J. Med.,* 297:289-294, 1977.

C. *Muscle biopsy*

1. *Principle.* A sample of tissue is taken from a muscle that is neither too diseased nor too healthy, according to clinical and electromyographic criteria. Part of the tissue is fixed in formalin for histologic stains, in glutaralydehyde for electron microscopy, and unfixed tissue is frozen for enzyme histochemistry, biochemistry, and immunoelectrophoresis.
2. *Risk.* Wound infection, bleeding, and anesthetic complication.
3. *Clinical use.* The biopsy is of value in distinguishing muscular weakness of *neuropathic, myopathic,* or *inflammatory* origin.
   a. *Neuropathic* disease of the LMNs or peripheral nerves is indicated by atrophy of the muscle fibers of individual fascicles of the muscle. A fascicle of muscle fibers which has lost its axon undergoes degeneration, while the neighboring fascicles of muscle fibers which have retained their axons are healthy.
   b. *Myopathic* disease is indicated by relatively uniform involvement of all muscle fibers with hypertrophic or retrogressive changes. The process is not limited to individual fascicles.
   c. *Inflammatory* disease is indicated by an inflammatory reaction of the tissue, mainly perivascular lymphocytes, granulomas, or parasitic cysts.

Bibliography

Adams, R., Denny-Brown, D., and Pearson, C.: *Diseases of Muscle: A Study in Pathology* (3rd ed.), New York, Hoeber Medical Division, Harper & Row. 1975.

Bethlem, J.: *Myopathies,* New York, North-Holland Publishing Company, 1977.

Brooke, M. H.: *A Clinician's View of Neuromuscular Diseases,* Baltimore, The Williams and Wilkins Company, 1977.

Dubowitz, V., and Brooke, M. H.: *Muscle Biopsy: A Modern Approach,* Philadelphia, W. B. Saunders, 1973.

Engel, W.: *Current Concepts of Myopathies.* Philadelphia, J. B. Lippincott, 1965.

McComas, A. J.: *Neuromuscular Function and Disorders,* London, Butterworths, 1977.

Walton, J. (ed.): *Disorders of Voluntary Muscle,* 3rd ed., Boston, Little, Brown, and Company, 1974.

D. *Nerve biopsy*

1. *Principle.* A few diseases cause pathognomic or highly suggestive changes in peripheral nerves, changes which can be demonstrated by the appropriate histologic technique. Sensory nerves are biopsied.
2. *Risk.* Wound infection and anesthesia in the nerve distribution.
3. *Clinical use.* Peripheral nerve biopsy may provide useful information in many types of neuropathies, particularly of metabolic or heredofamilial type. It provides valuable information not only for diagnosis but also for understanding the problems of pathogenesis, degeneration, and

regeneration of nerves. The procedure requires the teamwork of surgeon, neurologist, and neuropathologist. It provides the most information in connection with muscle biopsy, EMG, and nerve conduction velocity studies. The pulp nerve of deciduous or carious teeth provides a convenient source of peripheral nerve in some patients.

Bibliography

Dyck, P.: Pathologic alterations of the peripheral nervous system of man. In Dyck, P., Thomas J., and Lambert, E.: *Peripheral Neuropathies,* Philadelphia, W. B. Saunders Co., 1975.

Gardner, D. and Zeman, W.: Biopsy of the dental pulp in the diagnosis of metachromatic leucodystrophy, *Devel. Med. child. Neurol.,* 7:620-627, 1965.

VI. A perspective for the use of laboratory procedures is provided by these perceptive words of Robert Wartenberg:

> Careful history taking and interpreting, minute and repeated clinical examinations are time consuming. It is particularly the busy physician who is inclined to delegate the diagnosis to the laboratory in the vain hope of saving time. Too many irrelevant technical procedures often confuse the issue, cloud the essential point and broaden the margin for error. Time invested in clinical examination might have paid greater dividends.
>
> The main point is this: laboratory procedures often seem necessary because the clinical examination has not been adequate. They are all too often superfluous, and a thorough clinical examination would have provided grounds for correct management of the patient. The more clinical neurology we know, the less need there is for laboratory procedures and the more valuable these procedures become when they are necessary. . . .
>
> Before any technical procedure is used, the following points should be considered carefully. (1) Some methods are time consuming. Valuable and irretrievable time may be lost through their use. (2) Some methods are expensive and to some patients may be an incommensurate economic burden. (3) Some methods are not always harmless, are often painful and sometimes fraught with danger. (4) The objective findings depend on the integrity of delicate mechanical apparatus. (5) The interpretation may be equivocal. (6) Even if by laboratory procedures the presence of a definite pathological process has been established, it does not mean that the finding is clinically significant or that it can account for the patient's present condition. (7) The information obtained, however interesting, may not influence the clinical diagnosis and may be completely irrelevant to the actual management of the patient. (8) The correct evaluation of the most informative and illuminating laboratory findings is possible only when correlated with the findings of a complete clinical examination, for which there is no substitute. The laboratory cannot tell the whole story; it can give only a brief passage. (9) The more thorough and exact the neurological examination, the more informative and helpful are the results of the necessary laboratory procedures. (10) If the laboratory findings contradict the clinical findings, it is, in the last analysis, best to base the diagnostic decision on the clinical findings. — Robert Wartenberg (*Diagnostic Tests in Neurology. A Selection for Office Use,* Chicago, Year Book Medical Publishers, 1953.)

14

A Synopsis of the Neurologic Investigation and a Formulary of Neurodiagnosis

I. The routine screening neurologic examination when the patient has no symptoms likely to be neurologic in origin

A. Whenever seeing the patient for the first time or doing a periodical physical check up, the physician should include a basic minimum screening examination of all body systems. Beyond a certain invariant minimum check of each system, you tailor the examination to each patient, for you need not and should not do every test on every one. If a patient comes to you for a sore throat, having no history suggesting neurologic disease, you squander time if you test smell and taste, do caloric irrigation, a complete aphasia examination, and tug against every muscle. You can learn to do a screening neurologic examination on an intelligent, cooperative patient who has no neurologic symptoms in about 6 minutes. This statement presupposes a thorough history. The longer the history, the more you can shorten the examination.

B. Mandatory minimum screening examination for patients who have no history suggestive of neurologic disease.

1. When taking the history, appraise mental status, speech, and posture. Look for tremors and involuntary movements and inspect facial features, including eyes, palpebral fissures, and ocular movements.
2. Inspect head shape, palpate the head and neck. Record the head circumference in every pediatric patient. Attempt transillumination in all young infants.
3. *Visual system*
   a. Test visual acuity (central fields) and peripheral fields
   b. Pupillary light reflexes
   c. Ophthalmoscopy
   d. Follow finger through full range of ocular movements
4. Test motor cranial nerves V, VII, IX, X, XI and XII.
5. Test hearing by tuning fork (Rinné test), or by finger rustling.

6. *Somatic motor examination*
   a. Undress the patient
   b. Inspect for somatotype, muscle atrophy, fasciculations, and neurocutaneous stigmata, tremors, and involuntary movements.
   c. Test gait by free walking, toe, heel, and tandem walking, and deep-knee bend.
   d. Test strength of abduction of shoulder, wrist dorsiflexion, grip, hip flexion, and foot dorsiflexion.
   e. Test cerebellar function by finger-to-nose and heel-to-knee tests.
   f. Elicit muscle stretch reflexes of biceps, triceps, quadriceps femoris, and triceps surae.
   g. Elicit abdominal and plantar reflexes.
7. *Sensory examination*
   a. Test superficial sensation by light touch and pinprick on face and hands and feet.
   b. Test deep sensation by position sense in fingers and toes, vibration sense at ankles, and use coins to test for stereognosis.

C. *Recording the routine neurologic examination*

Of the many printed forms and checkoff lists offered to record the neurologic examination, I have found nothing better than a series of statements (best dictated and typed). Here is what to write down for the average patient who has no neurologic signs:

1. *General appearance and mental status.* The patient is a well-developed, well-nourished __________ year-old male / female. He / she is oriented, intelligent, cooperative, has appropriate affect, and gives an apparently reliable history.
2. *Head.* Normocephalic—no bruits, exostoses, tenderness, or depressions. The OFC is __________. The pupils are equal, __________ mm in size, and react to light and in accommodation. The ocular movements are full, no nystagmus. Fundi and visual fields are normal. Tongue, jaw, and palate midline. Facial movements symmetrical. Hearing intact per tuning fork tests.

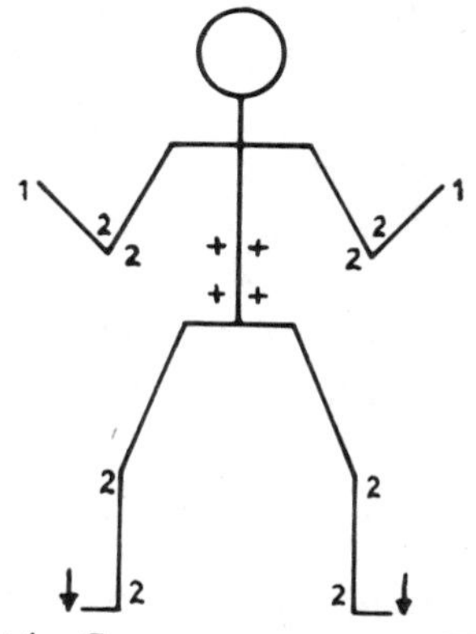

3. *Motor system.* Gait and station normal. No atrophy or fasciculations. No tremor at rest or during movements. No involuntary movements. Strength of neck, shoulder girdle, dorsiflexors of hands and feet, and grip is normal.
4. *Sensory system.* Touch and pinprick normally perceived over face, hands, and feet. Position and vibratory sensation intact. Coin recognition normal.

5. *Skin.* No lesions.
6. *Case summary.*
7. *Clinical impression.*
8. *Recommendations.*

__________________________ M.D.

D. The six-minute neurological examination
Ah me, I can hear it now. You are going to say, "But I don't have time to do all of that." If you practice it over and over, you will find that you can complete the whole examination in about six minutes in the mentally normal, cooperative patient who has no neurologic disease. When you can do it all in six minutes, you will know when you have practiced it enough. Examination of the neurologically ill patient of course takes much, much longer. But remember that when you do the clinical examination you use the most efficient method known for the detection of disease. In taking sufficient time to examine the patient properly, you function at maximum efficiency, at what your professional training prepares you to do best.

II. The neurologic investigation when the patient has signs or symptoms which may be neurologic in origin

A. When the history or physical examination suggest neurologic disease, the examination must include every clinical test for the integrity of neural structures in the vicinity of the suspected lesion. Achieving a provisional diagnosis becomes the immediate goal of the medical investigation. To reach a provisional diagnosis, the physician poses numerous diagnostic hypotheses while he pursues the history, physical examination, and laboratory workup. He accepts or rejects his provisional diagnostic hypotheses until he has secured the most likely one, which he terms the final diagnosis. From the best provisional diagnosis or the final diagnosis, the physician plans the optimum management to meet the needs of the patient, his family, and society.

B. The diagnostic catechism: In formulating the hypotheses which lead to the final diagnosis, the physician works through five fundamental questions, which we will call the *diagnostic catechism.*

1. Does the patient have a lesion?
2. If so, where is the lesion?
3. What is the lesion or the simplest provisional diagnosis?
4. What tests clinical or laboratory will confirm or reject the provisional diagnosis and establish the final diagnosis?
5. What is the optimum management?

III. What the questions of the diagnostic catechism encompass

A. Is there a lesion? A considerable number of patients who come to see you will have no identifiable lesion. Does the patient have an emotional disorder, an organic disorder, or both? You cannot avoid this first and often the most difficult question because you must tailor your clinical examination and laboratory tests to provide a basis for an answer. To answer "Yes" to the question, "Is there a lesion?" you hope to find at least one sign. One firm sign clamors louder than a multitude of symptoms. If the patient's history or signs raise the question of neurologic disease, think through Fig. 14-1 to start generating the possibilities in your mind.

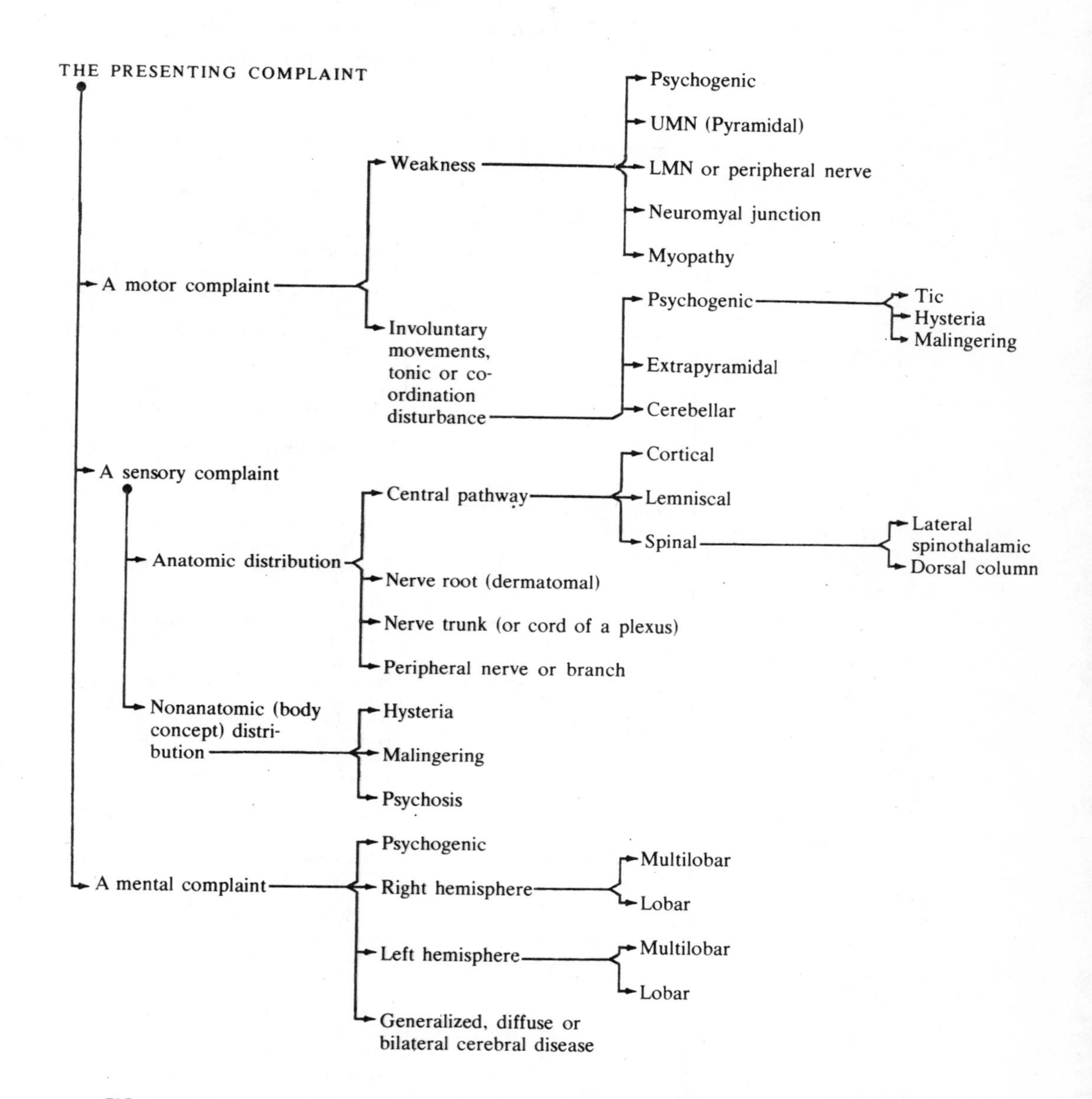

FIG. 14-1. Consider these preliminary possibilities when the patient has a complaint suggesting neurologic disease.

B. *Where is the lesion?* If the clinical evidence suggests a lesion, ask these questions:

1. Is the lesion in the structure or biochemistry of the patient?
2. Is it at the level of gene, chromosome, or cell? Is it at the level of blend-

ing of cells into tissues or of tissues into organs, or of organs into systems, or of systems into the general somatotype of the patient? In other words, do the findings constitute a morphologic or biochemical syndrome?

3. Can a decision be made as to the organ or organs, system or systems involved by the lesion?

   If the lesion appears to involve the nervous system:

   a. Is it intra-axial or extra-axial?

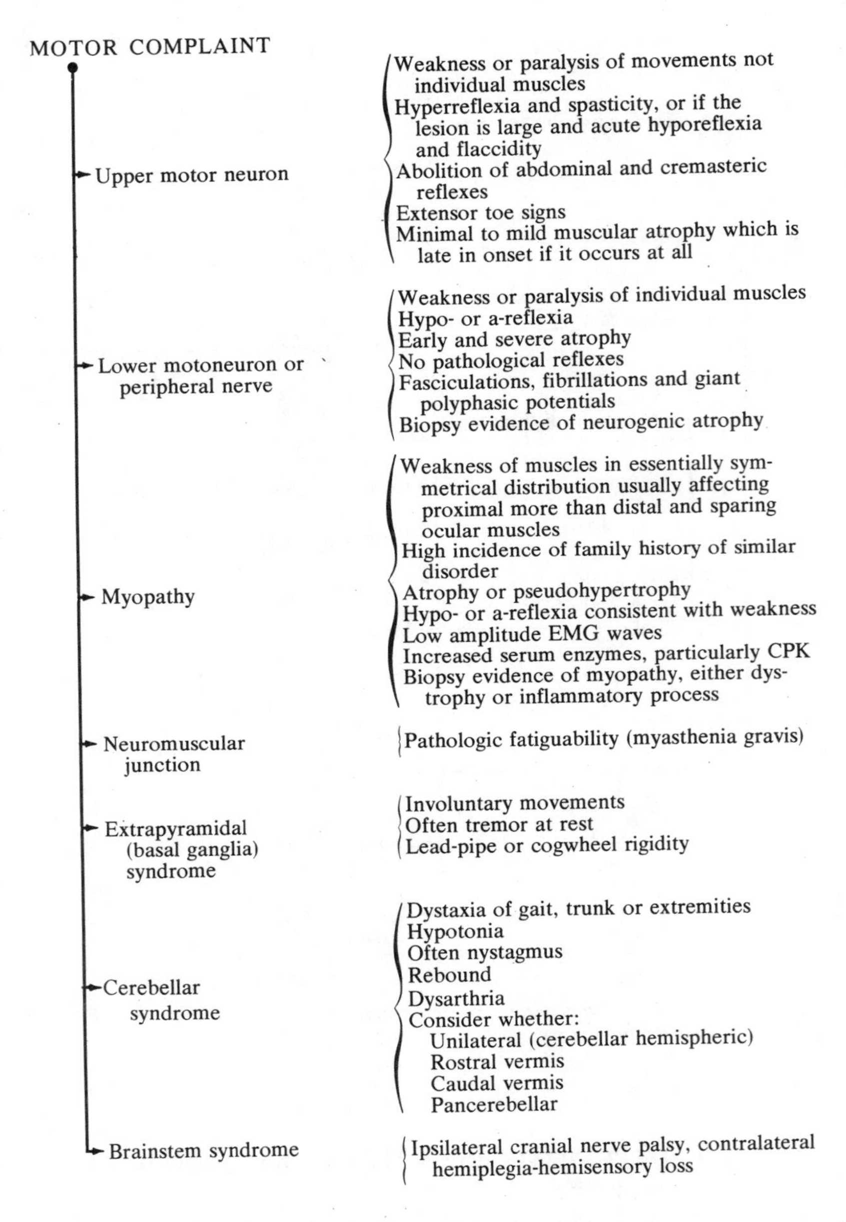

FIG. 14-2. Consider these neuronal systems to localize the lesion in a patient with symptoms and signs suggesting an organic motor system disorder.

b. If intra-axial, is it focal, in cerebrum, ventricular cavities or passageways, basal ganglia, brainstem, cerebellum, or spinal cord. Or is it multifocal, diffuse, or generalized?

c. If it could be extra-axial is it:

(1) In a meningeal or bony covering?

(2) In a meningeal space: epidural, subdural, or subarachnoid?

(3) In a nerve root, plexus, peripheral nerve, neuromyal junction, or muscle?

4. When the patient has a complaint likely to be of neurologic origin, try to classify it as motor, sensory, sensorimotor, headache, or organic mental syndrome. Then:

a. If motor, see Fig. 14-2 to locate the neuronal system affected, or if an involuntary movement syndrome, see Fig. 14-3.

b. If sensory, see Fig. 14-4.

c. If a headache, see Fig. 14-5.

d. If an organic mental syndrome, see Fig. 14-6.

C. *What is the lesion?*

Having hypothesized the neuronal system or systems involved and the lesion site, you next have to hypothesize *what* the lesion is. For this purpose, sys-

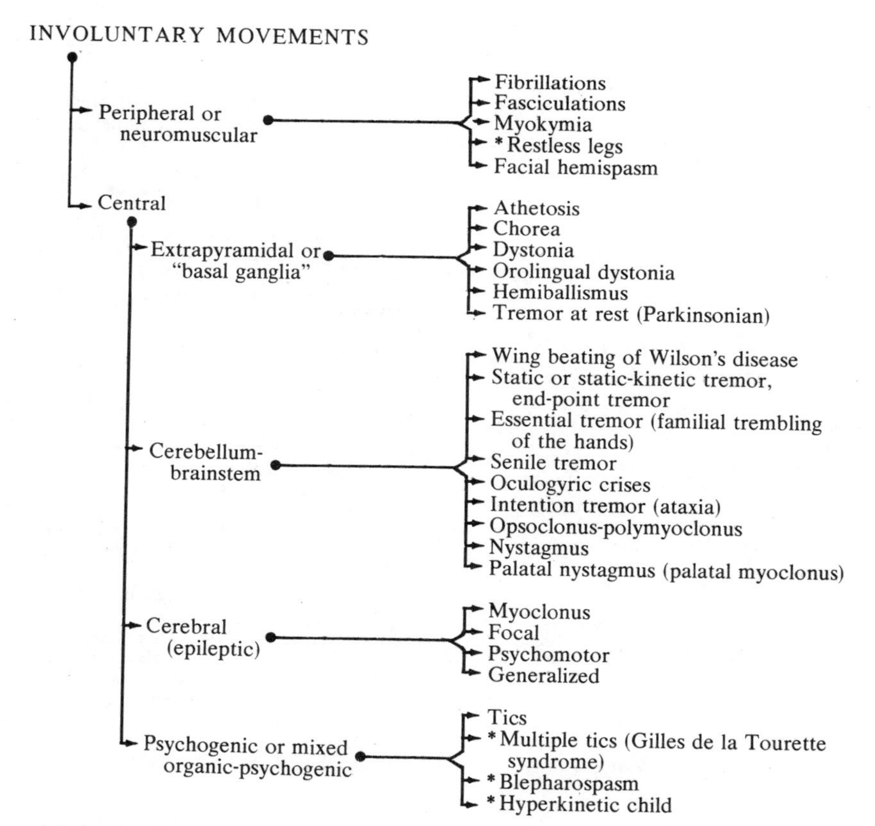

FIG. 14-3. Consider these possibilities when a patient has involuntary movements.

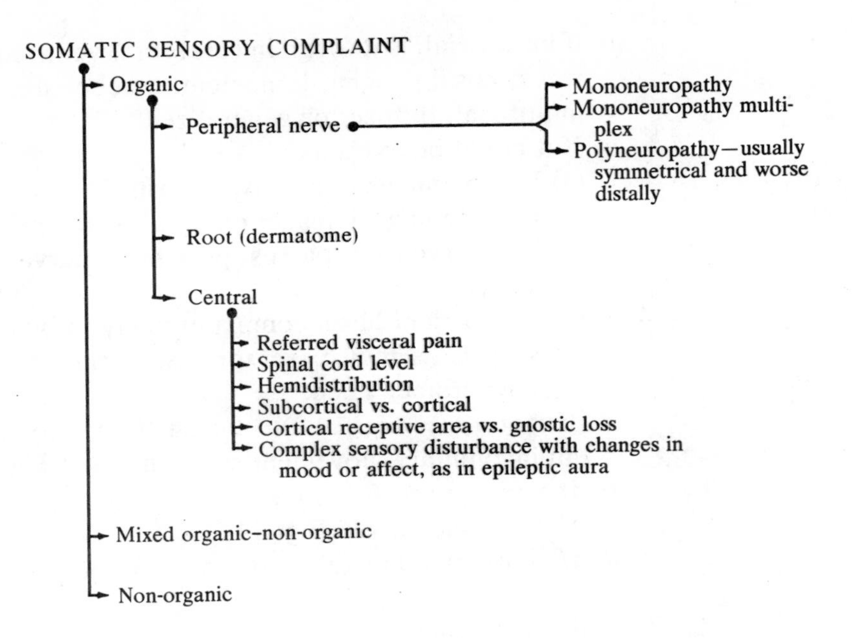

FIG. 14-4. Consider these possibilities to classify the probable nature of the patient's sensory complaint.

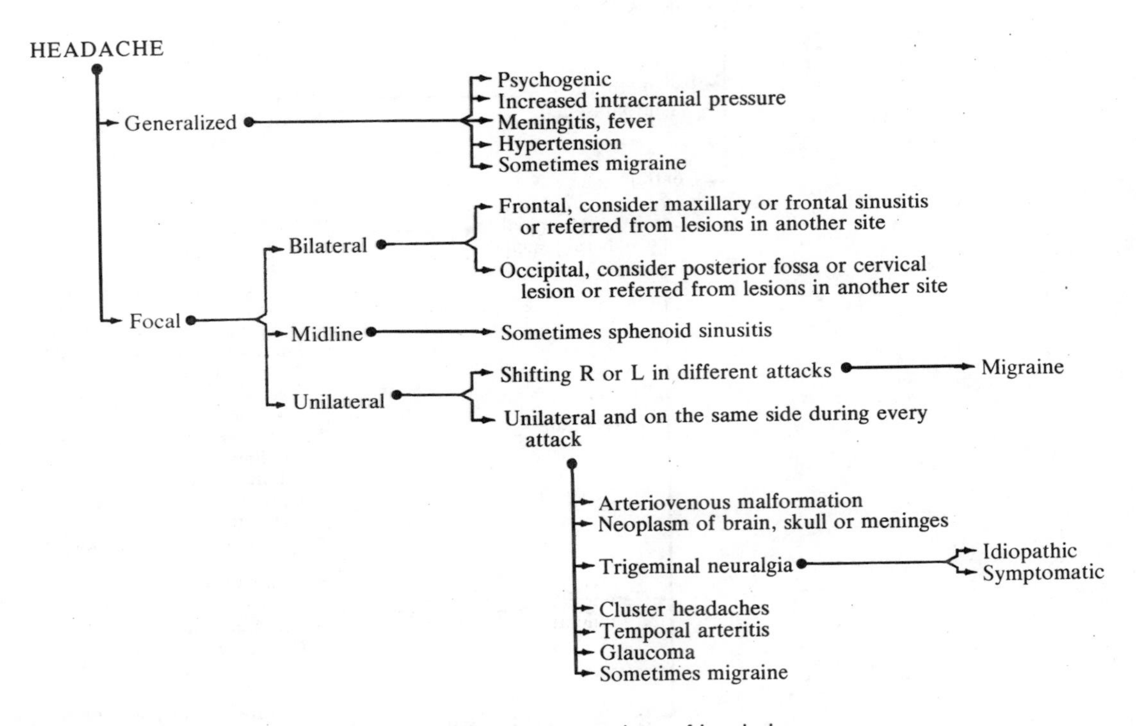

FIG. 14-5. Consider these possibilities when the patient complains of headaches.

tematically think through the entities in Fig. 14-7. Then state a provisional diagnosis. State the provisional diagnosis according to the principle of parsimony: the simplest diagnosis that will explain the signs and symptoms.

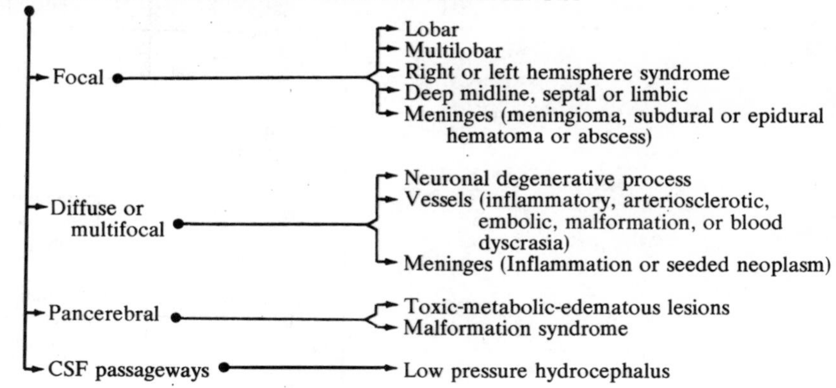

FIG. 14-6. Consider these possibilities when the patient has mental, emotional or intellectual deficits which suggest an organic neurologic disorder.

An explicit diagnosis offers a basis for an argument to establish its validity over the other diagnostic possibilities. Settle the argument from the data disclosed by clinical and laboratory tests which support or deny the provisional diagnosis.

D. *What tests, clinical or laboratory, will confirm or reject the provisional diagnosis and establish the final diagnosis?*

1. If your hypothesis is correct, what corollary findings should you look for? Can you do any other clinical tests? If not, select laboratory procedures, according to these principles:
   a. Can the test provide critical evidence to support or reject the provisional diagnosis?
   b. Is the test the simplest, safest, and cheapest one?
   c. When faced with a hopeless or untreatable disorder, have you taken all reasonable steps to exclude a treatable disorder?
2. *Neurodiagnostic procedures of minimal or no risk which the general physician can order or do:*

a. Radiographs of skull or spine: plain films, tomograms, foramen, magnum, optic foramen, or sinuses and CAT scan.
b. Echoencephalogram.
c. Electroencephalogram.
d. Radioactive brain scan.
e. Electromyogram, nerve conduction velocity, and Jolly test.
f. Lumbar puncture.
g. Subdural puncture (infants only).
h. Neuropsychological testing.
i. Visual fields mapping.
j. Audiometry and BAER.
k. Electronystagmography.
l. Urinary screening for amino acids, mucopolysaccharides, and reducing substances.
m. Biochemical-endocrine tests of blood and urine.
n. Serological testing.
o. Serum electrophoresis.
p. Serum enzyme determinations.
q. Bone marrow examination.
r. Edrophonium (tensilon) test.

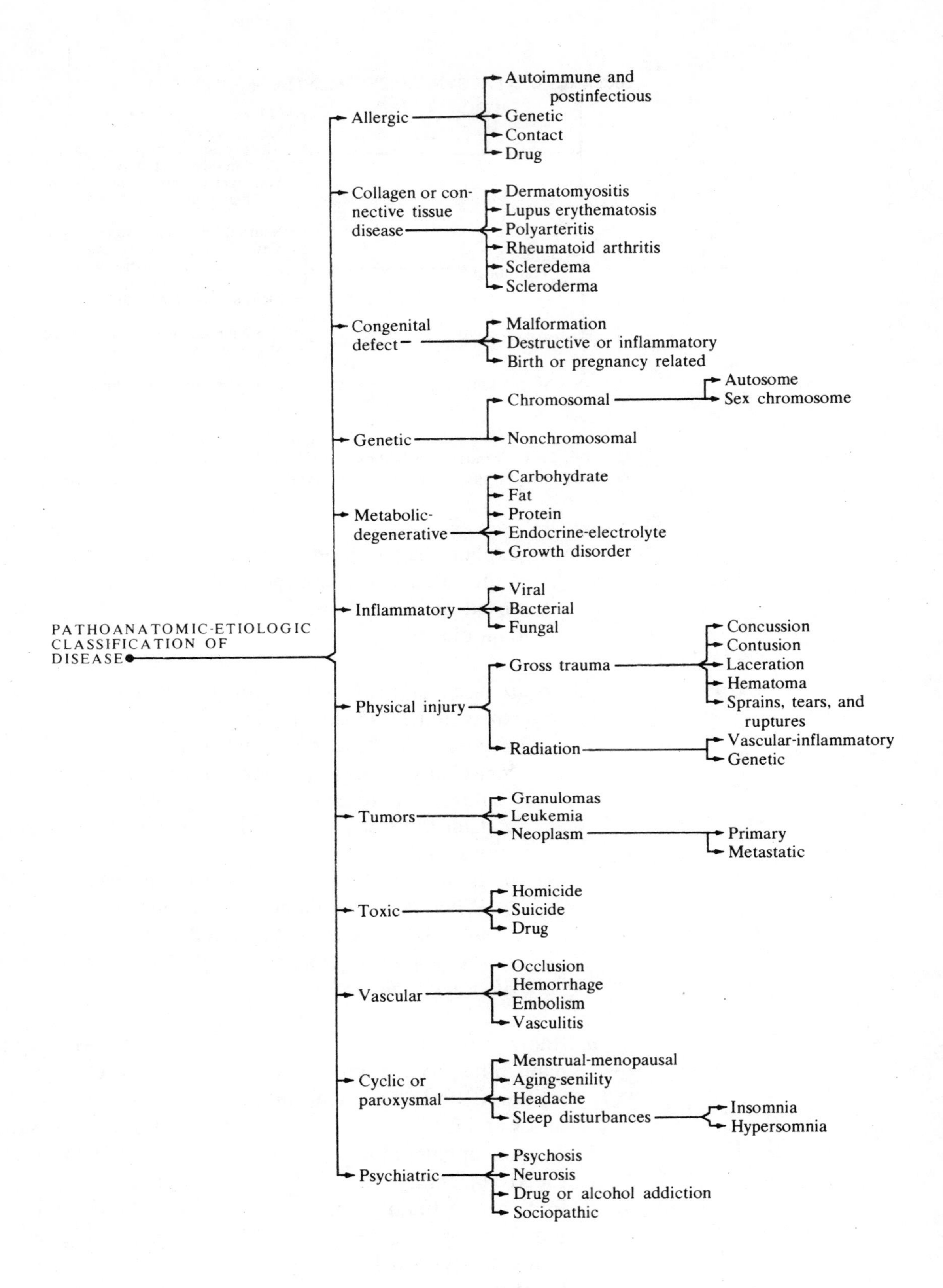

FIG. 14-7. Pathoanatomic-etiologic classification of disease. Review systematically for each patient in order to generate the gamut of diagnostic possibilities that might explain the clinical findings. The branching of the dendrogram to the right can be continued almost endlessly. (Reference only.)

3. *Neurodiagnostic procedures ordered or done by the neurologic specialist:*

a. Pneumoencephalography.
b. Ventriculography.
c. Myelography.
d. Angiography.
e. Biopsy of nerve, muscle, or brain.
f. Cisternal puncture.
g. Tissue culture of fibroblasts for determination of enzyme defects or chromosome analysis.

E. What is the optimum management?

1. State therapeutic goals and how to meet them. (Yes, just what can you hope to do for the patient?)
2. What emotional, educational or socio-economic perils does the patient face because of his illness? What agencies or institutions might help him?
3. What other persons are known to be at risk now that you have identified the patient's illness? How can they be identified and what prophylactic measures can be offered? Consider for patients with environmentally induced, contagious-infectious, or hereditary diseases.
4. Follow the patient to insure that your final diagnosis is indeed final and that the subsequent course of the patient continues to confirm its finality.

IV. Hysteria: Use of the clinical and laboratory techniques of the neurologic examination to distinguish hysteria from neurologic disease

A. Introduction

This section reviews the use of neurologic techniques to distinguish hysteria from neurologic disease. To the neurologist, hysteria means a mental illness which alters sensory or motor function but without a lesion in the parts of the nervous system that anatomically and physiologically should mediate the symptoms.

Hysteria may closely mimic organic disorders of mentation, sensation, and motor function. Because of no definable lesion in the parts of the nervous system manifesting the hysterical symptoms, we say the hysterical patient has a *functional* (psychogenic) rather than *organic* disorder. Every practitioner will, on occasion, mistake functional for organic disease, or organic disease for functional. However, in most instances, certain principles make the diagnosis relatively easy.

B. Distinction between hysteria and malingering

Psychiatrists assume that an hysterical symptom represents an *unconscious* mental mechanism for the relief of anxiety. The symptom provides a *primary* gain and *secondary* gains for the patient. The primary gain consists of the relief of anxiety. The secondary gains consist of relief from duties and responsibilities and the achievement of manipulative control over the emotional responses of other persons. The origins of the symptom and the purposes it serves are presumed to remain at a subconscious level in hysteria.

In contrast, the malingerer is presumed to be purposefully and consciously faking disease to achieve some immediate goal. The goals most frequently consist of monetary compensation in a lawsuit with the patient as plaintiff, or to appear mentally ill in a criminal action with the patient as defendant. Either patient, hysteric or malingerer, has a serious mental problem. I will not belabor the issue of trying to enter the patient's mind to decide just how conscious or unconscious the symptom is. That is not the physician's task. The physician must respond as helpfully as possible, as to any other clinical phenomena rather than to make any metaphysical, punitive, or pejorative judgments. The rest of this chapter refers mainly to hysteria, but the principles apply to malingering or other so-called functional mental disorders.

C. *Criteria for the diagnosis of hysteria*

1. *Explicit criteria*
   a. Presence of symptoms that do not match organic patterns of illness. The symptoms reflect the patient's notions of bodily arrangements and functions.
   b. Absence of signs of organic illness. Symptoms are maximal but signs are absent.
   c. History of psychiatric illness or stresses.
   d. Full remission of the symptom with time.
2. *Historical criteria*
   The overt, pseudoneurological symptoms of hysteria usually manifest in patients between 10 to 30 years of age. The patient usually has a long history of a disordered personality. Some immediate emotional stress precedes and precipitates the hysterical symptom. For example, a young woman may display hysterical paraplegia as an unconscious defense against sexual temptation or sexual activity. The history of longstanding emotional problems and the precipitating event is essential to the diagnosis of hysteria. For goodness sake, don't diagnose hysteria in a previously well adjusted 60-year-old patient with the sudden onset of neurologic symptoms that could be organic.
3. *Mental status criteria for hysteria*
   The hysterical patient often appears blandly indifferent (la belle indifférence) to the hysterical disability and rarely seems concerned or asks about the cause or prognosis. For example, the hysterical paraplegic seems, good naturedly as it were, to accept the paraplegia. Organic paraplegic patients experience it as a very disturbing and threatening illness. Since the symptom serves as a defense against overt anxiety, the patient feels more comfortable with the symptom than the anxiety that it masks. With some hysterical symptoms, particularly sensory ones such as pain, the patient overreacts with much wailing or dramatic prostration. The art of diagnosis, the art is to recognize the *disproportionate* reaction in either case.

   When interviewing or examining the hysterical patient, the physician will find that while focusing on the disability such as a tremor, the disability gets worse. The disability also gets worse in the presence of family members or acquaintances. During such periods, the patient may also hyperventilate. In other words, the symptom varies with the attention directed to it or the presence of emotionally significant people. It is socially dependent. Remember, however, that emotional stress may similarly enhance organic tremors and involuntary movements.

D. Patterns of sensory dysfunction in hysteria

1. *Hysterical disorders of vision*

   Hysterical visual disorders usually consist of diminished vision or blindness, visual field defects, or monocular diplopia.

   a. Hysterical visual fields defects

   The typical hysterical visual field defect consists of concentric constriction, producing tunnel or tubular vision, as if the person were looking through a tunnel. A closely allied phenomenon is the *spiral visual field* in which the size of the field diminishes on successive trials. In tunnel vision the visual field remains the same size at various visual target distances. Normally the field expands with the increasing distance of the target from the eye. See Fig. 14-8.

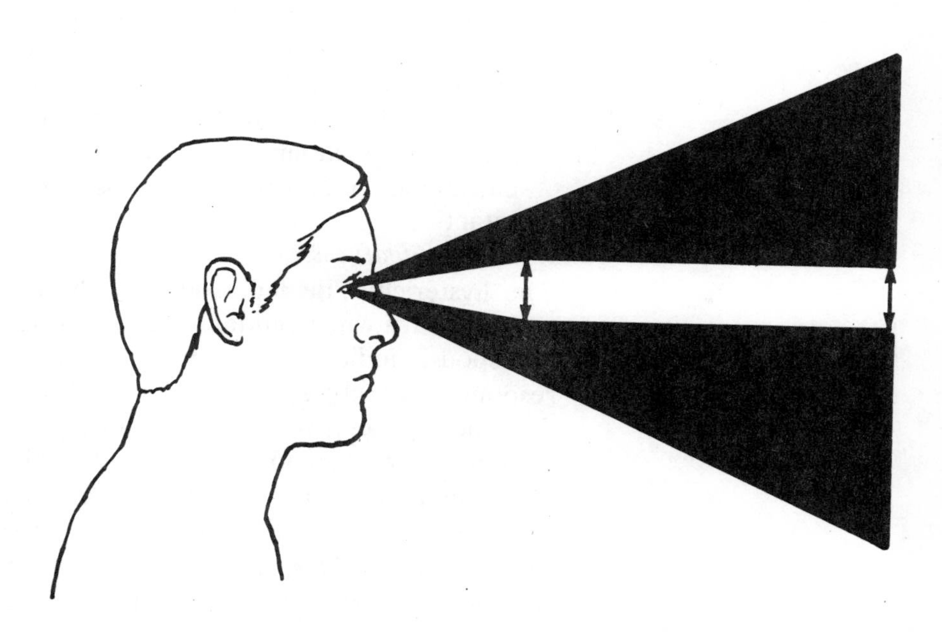

FIG. 14-8. Illustration of tunnel vision in a patient with hysteria. The normal visual field expands. In tunnel vision the field remains the same size for targets at different distances.

   b. Monocular diplopia

   Hysterics may complain of monocular diplopia. The diplopia will not follow any of the laws of diplopia and the patient shows no ocular malalignments.

   Caveat: True, organic monocular diplopia can occur from a dislocated lens, retinal fold, detachment or elevation, or hole in the iris, but the ocular examination and ophthalmoscopy differentiate these conditions easily.

c. *Hysterical blindness*
The eyes of the hysterically blind patient often will show fixation upon and attraction to moving objects. The patient retains pupillary light reactions, and has a fundus that appears normal. Most patients will show optokinetic nystagmus (railroad nystagmus) when exposed to a rotating drum or moving stripes. However, the patient can inhibit optokinetic nystagmus. Its presence thus establishes integrity of the retino-geniculocalcarine pathway and the efferent optomotor pathway to the brainstem from the occipital cortex, but the absence of response does not prove that the patient has a lesion. The electroretinogram in hysterics remains normal, the electroencephalogram shows a photic driving response, or more refined evoked potential studies prove that impulses reach the visual cortex (see Chapter 13). In monocular hysterical blindness the patient may be induced to see double by prisms or canthal compression, proving that the blind eye has vision.

Caveats: Acute retrobulbar neuritis can cause complete blindness in one eye and a normal appearing fundus before optic atrophy sets in. The direct and consensual pupillary light reflexes from that eye will be absent, but the pupil of the afflicted eye will constrict consensually with illumination of the opposite pupil. In Anton's syndrome, a bilateral or at times even unilateral, occipital lobe lesion causes bilateral cortical blindness, yet the pupillary responses remain intact.

2. *Hysterical deafness*
The hysterically deaf person may show a startle response to sudden sound or turn when suddenly addressed from the side. The presence of a response indicates an intact auditory pathway, but absence of a response does not establish organic disease. An electroencephalogram done during sleep will show an alerting response to sound, establishing the integrity of the auditory pathway. Audiologists have several methods of manipulating sound to recognize hysterical loss of hearing. Objective measurement of cochlear potentials, the brainstem auditory evoked response (BAER) test (Chapter 13), and evoked potentials recorded over the auditory cortex, all document the integrity of the auditory pathways.

Caveat: Some patients with acute viral illness suddenly lose hearing even though they may show no other evidence of neurologic disease.

3. *Hysterical disorders of somatic sensation*
Patients with hysterical somatosensory disorders usually complain of anesthesia, paresthesia, hyperesthesia, or pain. The anesthesia usually affects all sensory modalities. If the patient loses only one modality, it is usually touch or pain. Hysterics virtually never complain solely of loss of vibration or position sense.

The nonanatomical distributional pattern of the sensory loss gives the best immediate clue to hysteria. Hysterical sensory losses conform to the patient's mental image of the body, not the actual anatomic pattern of innervation by peripheral nerves, nerve roots, or central pathways. For example, organic facial anesthesia from a Vth-nerve lesion spares the angle of the mandible, which receives its sensory innervation from C2. Review Fig. 9-13, page 292. The hysteric includes the angle of the mandible: it belongs with one's *mental image* or *body scheme* of the face. See Fig. 14-9, A and B.

In hysterical anesthesia of an extremity, the loss usually includes the hand or foot and extends proximally to stop abruptly at a joint line or skin fold. In hysterical anesthesia of the arm, the loss stops at the shoulder joint, in conformity with one's mental image of an arm, but not in conformity with the actual innervation by dermatomes or peripheral nerves. See Fig. 14-9, C and D. In hysterical lower extremity anesthesia, the proximal border often falls at the gluteal fold posteriorly and the inguinal line anteriorly. See Fig. 14-9, E and F. In hysterical

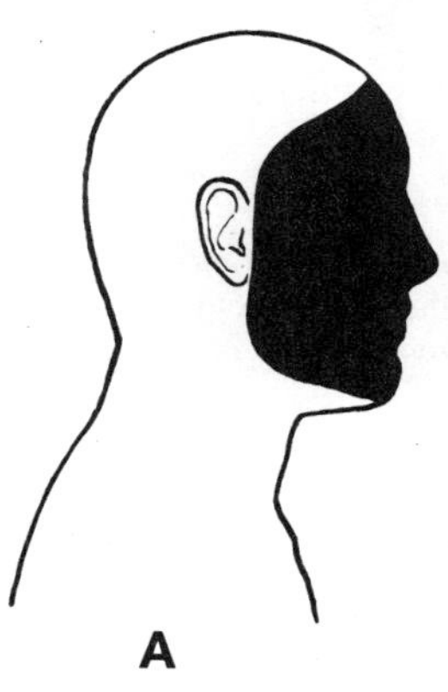

A. Functional facial anesthesia usually includes the angle of the mandible and may stop at the hairline.

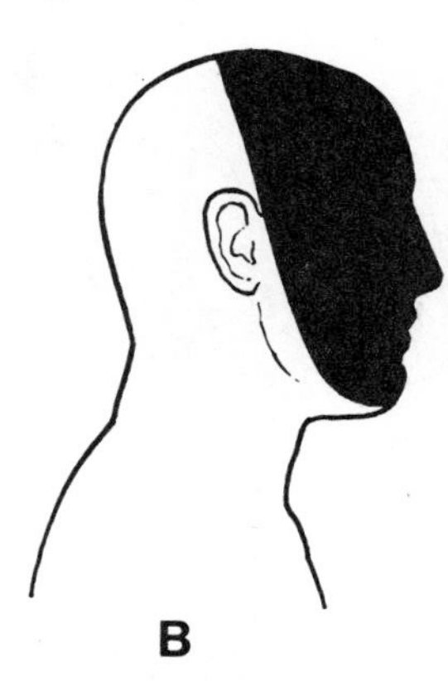

B. Organic facial anesthesia from a Vth nerve lesion spares the angle of the mandible (innervated by C_2). The border follows the distribution of the entire Vth nerve or one of its three branches. See also Fig. 9-13.

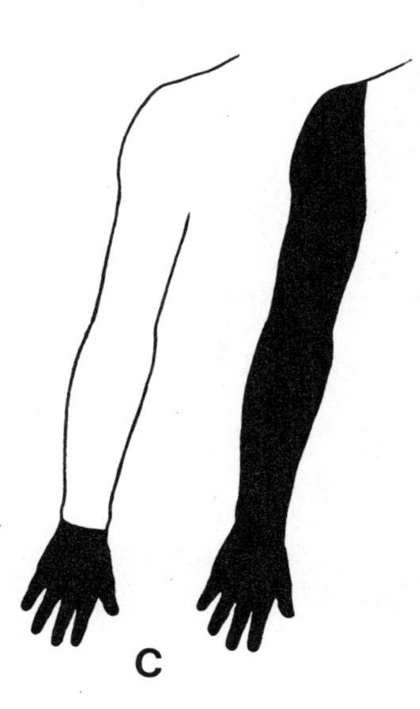

C. Functional loss of upper limb sensation usually cuts off at a joint, the wrist, elbow, or shoulder.

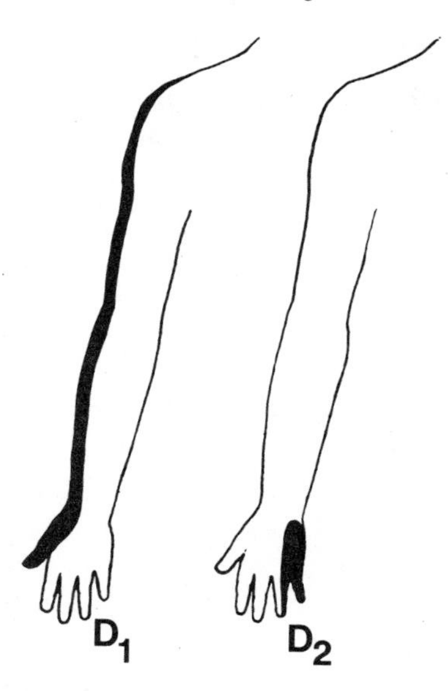

D. Organic sensory loss when limited to a region of an upper extremity follows an anatomic distribution, either dermatomal (D_1, C_6 dermatome) or peripheral nerve (D_2, ulnar nerve). See also Fig. 3-7, A and B.

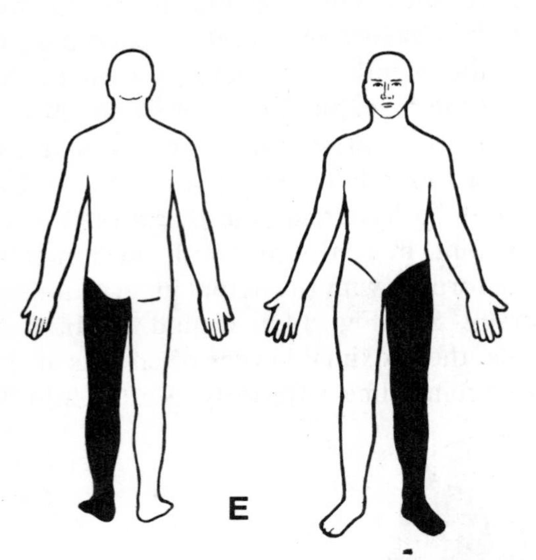

E. Functional loss of lower extremity sensation usually cuts off at a joint or the gluteal fold dorsally, or the inguinal line ventrally.

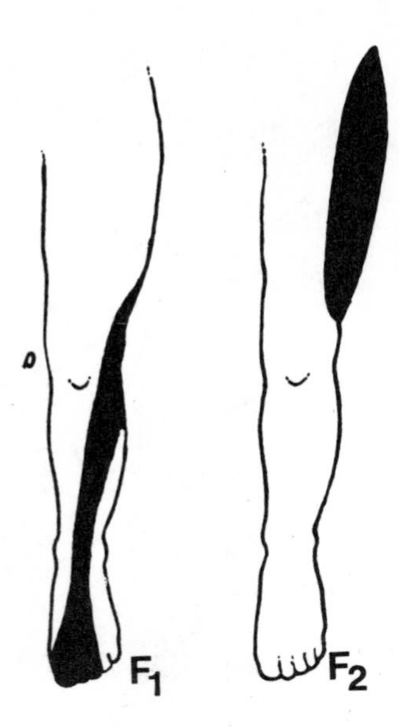

F. Organic sensory loss, when limited to a region of a lower extremity, follows an anatomic distribution, either dermatomal (F_1, L_5 dermatome) or peripheral nerve (F_2, ulnar nerve). See also Fig. 3-7, A and B.

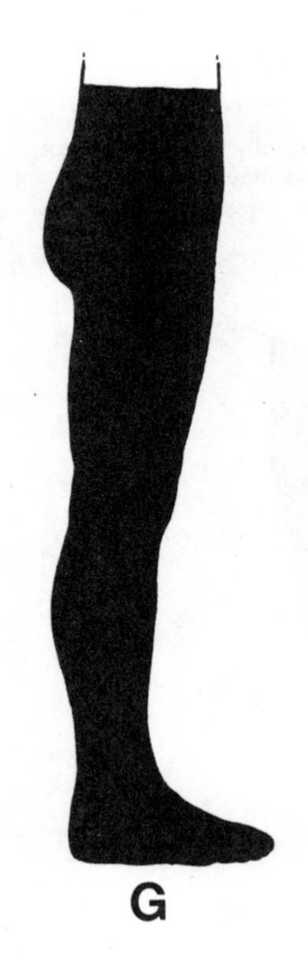

G. Functional sensory levels on the trunk run *horizontally*, in keeping with the patient's "body image."

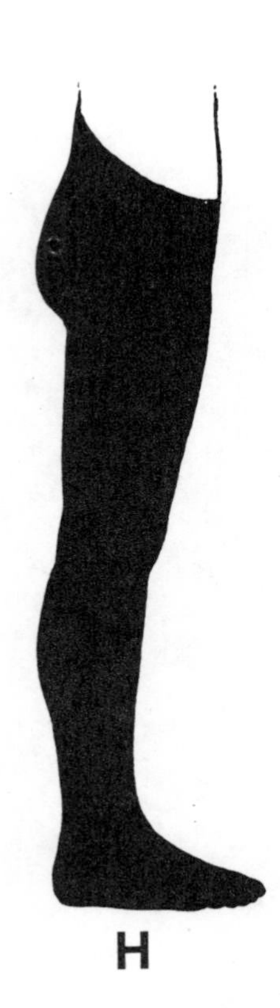

H. Organic sensory levels on the trunk from spinal cord lesions run *obliquely*, in keeping with the downward slant of the dermatomes.

FIG. 14-9. Contrast between functional and organic sensory losses.

paraplegia with a sensory level, the line circles the body horizontally, instead of having a dermatomal slant. See Fig. 14-9, G and H. A striking example of body image loss of sensation occurs in hysterical hemianesthesia. The patient not only loses all somatic sensation from one-half of the body but also may lose sight, hearing, taste, and smell on the affected side, an obvious anatomic impossibility.

The border between the anesthetic and normal zone, although usually sharp, may change from time to time. In hysterical hemianesthesia, the sensory loss occurs sharply at the midline and may run up the entire body and head as in the mental image of one-half of the body. Patients with organic hemisensory loss usually have an indistinct midline loss, whereas hysterics often have a sharp sensory boundary. The hysteric, for example, will report complete absence of vibratory sensation when the tuning fork applied to sternum or forehead falls just short of the midline on the anesthetic side. In fact, the vibration travels some distance through the bone. The intact side registers the vibration even with the fork some little distance away from the midline. Figs. 14-10 and 14-11 show the differences in the borders of organic and hysterical sensory losses.

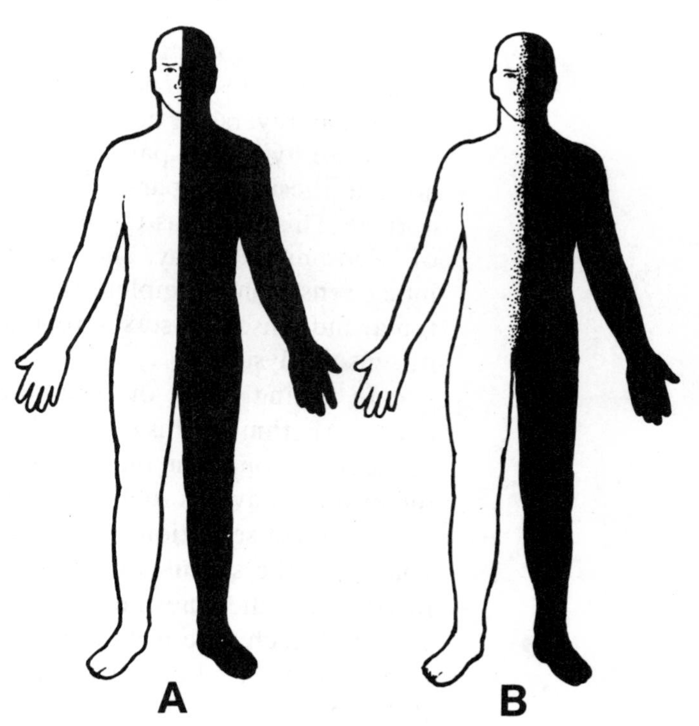

FIG. 14-10. Some characteristic differences in the borders of functional and organic sensory losses. (A) In functional hemianesthesia the sensory loss usually stops abruptly at the midline for all modalities. (B) In organic hemianesthesia, the sensory loss usually fades gradually at the midline, particularly for vibration.

Some inversions of the body parts can provide a quick answer to an hysterical hemisensory loss. In males with hemianesthesia, the penis can be twisted to reverse right and left. Then touching the previously anesthetic half, now reversed, will produce a sensory response, whereas

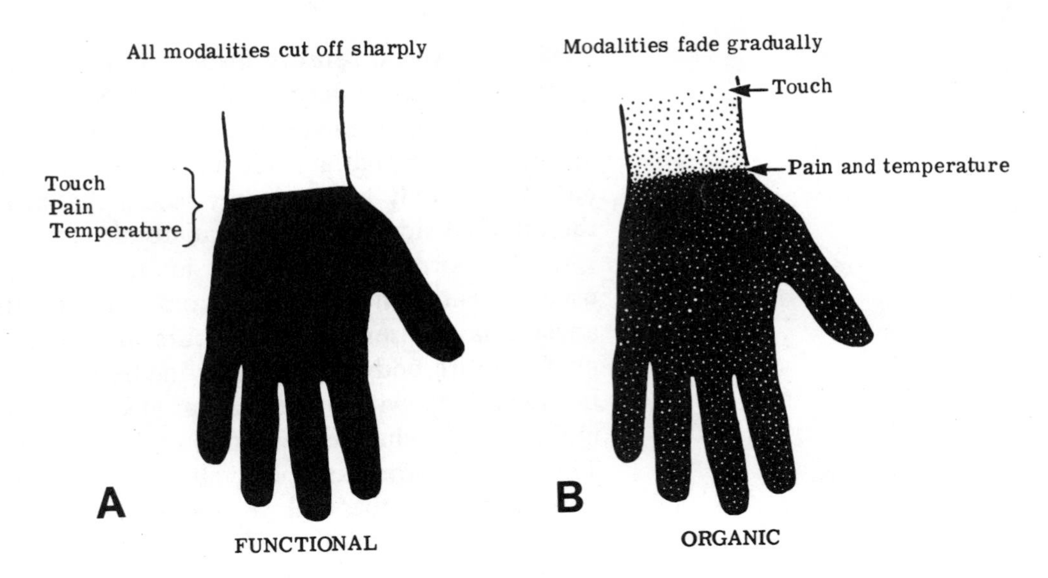

FIG. 14-11. Contrast between functional and organic stocking-glove sensory loss. (A) In functional stocking-glove sensory loss the proximal border usually stops sharply at a joint line or skin crevice for all modalities. (B) In organic stocking-glove sensory loss, the proximal border usually fades gradually and differs for the various modalities.

the previously normal side becomes anesthetic, a striking proof of the "body" image loss of sensation in hysteria. Similarly, reversal of the hands may reverse or confuse the sensory responses. See Fig. 14-12.

If the hysterical patient complains of anesthesia for all modalities, not anesthesia plus paralysis, the patient may use the part completely normal. This fact plus the *preservation* of stretch reflexes and *absence* of hypotonia, atrophy, and dystaxia, mean that the patient must have intact sensation. Complete sensory loss must produce areflexia, hypotonia, and sensory dystaxia (review Table 10-1, page 315, for the features of sensory dystaxia).

In testing touch or pain responses the examiner may be able to elicit a rhythm of answering that inadvertently discloses the integrity of the sensation in the putatively anesthetic or analgesic area. Ordinarily the examiner avoids such a rhythm in organic patients. Starting with an area of intact sensation, get the patient to respond by saying "yes" when you apply the stimulus or "no" when you withhold it. Then gradually incorporate the anesthetic region in the testing. Often the hysteric says "no" each time just after you touch the anesthetic zone, indicating that at some level of consciousness the patient has actually perceived the stimulus.

In responding to position sense testing the functional patient may display a pattern of exactly opposite answers, saying, for example, "down" each time for "up". The fact that the patient gives exactly the reverse response each time means that position sense has to be intact. Even with total absence of position sense the patient should guess the right answer about one-half of the time.

The astute clinician will frequently observe that hysterics respond very slowly and deliberately to sensory stimuli during the examination.

The patient gives the impression of trying very hard to feel the stimulus and report it correctly, a pseudocooperation. Other patients give a studied response of feeling it "just a little bit," even though the stimulus is strong. In hysterical analgesia, the physician should not continue to make increasingly strong pain stimuli to try to prove a point (or express frustration with a puzzling sensory examination). In contrast to these underreacting patients, others manifestly overreact to sensory stimuli. The physician soon learns to recognize the histrionic overreaction or studied underreaction of the patient as part of the diagnostic pattern.

Caveats: In deciding whether a sensory loss is organic or functional, review the *Steps in the Analysis of a Sensory Complaint* on page 327. Recall also that organic pain may be referred to or radiate beyond the confines of an anatomic territory. On some occasions patients with thalamic or parietal lesions will show hemisensory losses that suggest hysteria (Yarnell et al., 1978). Recall also that the patient may have an organic process with a functional overlay. Some patients with organic disease have true hyperesthesia, sometimes of excruciating type as in causalgia, or trigger zones where the slightest stimulus elicits unbearable pain, as in trigeminal neuralgia.

E. *Hysterical disorders of motor function*

Hysteria may cause paralysis or hyperkinesias. The hyperkinesias usually take the form of tremors or spasms. The paralysis may affect cranial nerve muscles causing aphonia or dysphagia, often with *globus hystericus,* a sensation of a lump in the throat, or the paralysis may affect the rest of the body in monoplegic, hemiplegic, or paraplegic distributions. Perhaps the commonest form of psychogenic or functional paralysis, impotence, generally is not regarded as a form of hysteria because it represents failure of automatic rather than willfully directed muscular activity.

1. *Oculomotor manifestations of hysteria*

Common oculo*motor* manifestations of hysteria include tics, blepharospasm, convergence spasm, and pseudo VIth-nerve palsy. In blepharospasm, the eyelids remain tonically closed and strongly resist any attempt of the patient or examiner to open them. Yet no other muscle may be involved, and no progression to recruit other muscles occurs as in a Jacksonian epileptic march. In convergence spasm, the pupils constrict along with the forceful adduction of the eyes, indicating an overactive accommodation mechanism. (Review accommodation in Table 2-3, page 63). Both blepharospasm and convergence spasm can have organic causes, but usually neighborhood signs of midbrain-pretectal region lesions accompany them.

In the pseudo VIth-nerve palsy syndrome of hysteria or malingering, the patient, on attempting to look to one side, say the right, will move the eyes conjugately to, or a little past, the midline, then as the *ad*ducting eye continues to progress to the right, the *ab*ducting eye deviates inward, as if the lateral rectus muscle had failed to act. Careful inspection will show that the patient has learned to utilize convergence. As the errant eye breaks off of conjugate movement to adduct, the pupil simultaneously constricts. Thus, a convergence stimulus has arrested the abduction of the eye, not failure of action of the lateral rectus muscle. In organic VIth-nerve palsy, the eye which fails to abduct does not show any change in pupillary size.

2. *Hysterical aphonia-dysphagia*
   Hysterical patients may become completely speechless. Often the patient, although aphonic, has normal vocal cord action during laryngoscopy, or shows pure adductor palsy. Yet a normally strong cough proves that the adductor muscles of the vocal cords can, in fact, act forcefully. The patient has no palatal palsy, and no difficulty with breathing, or swallowing, and whispers with perfect articulation. The patient may talk or phonate during sleep, establishing the integrity of the vocal apparatus.
3. *Hysterical disturbances of station and gait (astasia-abasia)*
   Some hysterical patients show an inability to stand (astasia) or an inability to walk (abasia), or both (astasia-abasia). The patient typically shows wild gyrations when standing or walking, but rarely falls, or falls into the examiner's arms or a chair, without suffering bodily injury. The wildness of the gyrations without falling leaves no doubt that the patient has competent balance. In bed, or sitting, the patient may show no disability or only minor disturbances of movement.

   In doing the Romberg swaying test, the patient with astasia-abasia may show a great increase in swaying upon eyelid closure. To analyze this problem, ask the patient to repeatedly perform the finger-to-nose test, or count slowly to 25. After the patient begins the test, ask the patient to close the eyes. Usually, with attention diverted to the primary task, the patient continues to maintain a normal upright posture upon eyelid closure, establishing the integrity of the dorsal columns of the cord. Of course, the hysterical patient will still retain muscle stretch reflexes and sensation.

   Caveats: Recall that the patient with the rostral or caudal vermis syndromes may show little dysfunction when reclining, but may show severe dystaxia in walking, particularly tandem walking. The patient with gait apraxia or the elderly patient with the *marche à petit pas* (tiny shuffling steps), or the swaying from dorsal column loss, as in the Romberg test, has to be distinguished from hysteria. Patients with involuntary movement syndromes, particularly chorea or dystonia musculorum deformans, frequently get diagnosed as having an hysteric gait in the early stages of their illness.
4. *Hysterical paresis or paralysis of trunk and limbs*
   The patient's demeanor during testing often provides a clue to hysteria. Usually the patient with hysterical paralysis makes a great show of effort to move the afflicted part. Thus the patient may grimace, grunt, or squirm, and show obvious strain. It is a dramatic performance meant to communicate sincerity of effort, rather than a simple attempt to make a movement, as in organic paralysis. The hysteric with an incompletely paralyzed part usually moves it very slowly. Often the examiner can see and feel that the putatively paralyzed muscles in such a movement in fact contract very strongly. Thus, in making a grip the patient contracts

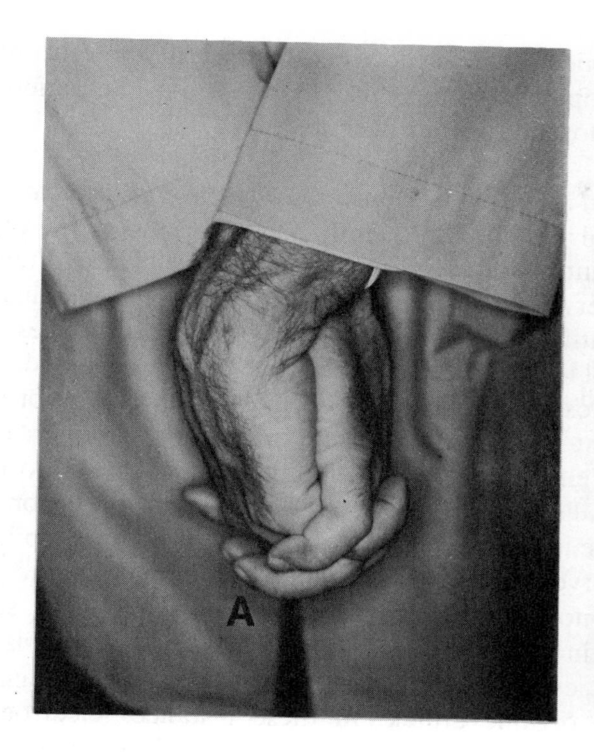

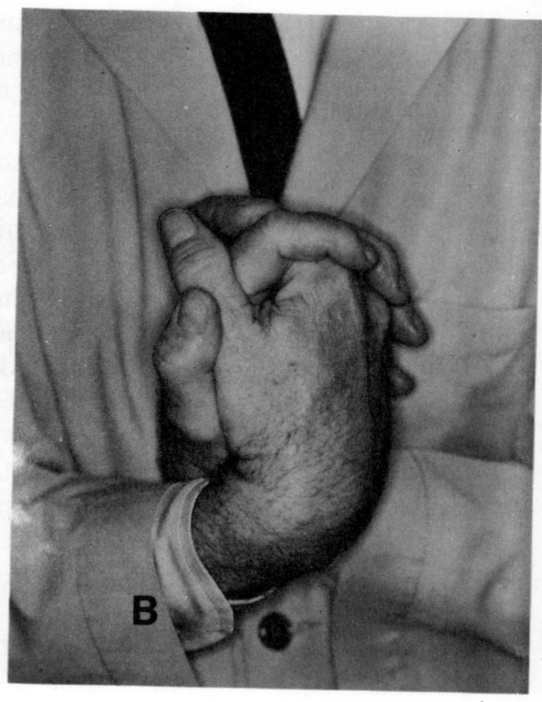

FIG. 14-12. Method of inverting hands to test for hysterical loss of sensation or motor function. The final posture in B reverses right for left. (A) Clasp fingers as shown. (B) Invert the hands.

the flexors and extensors very strongly, proving that their innervation is intact, although the patient grips the examiner's fingers with only slight power.

Several observations or maneuvers establish the integrity of the putatively paralyzed part by inadvertent or automatic mechanisms. The patient will move the part during sleep. When dressing, the patient may inadvertently reach out with the affected part or use it automatically for postural support. To test for a functional wrist drop, watch for action of the wrist extensors when you ask the patient to grip your fingers strongly. If intact, the putatively paralyzed wrist extensors automatically cock the hand up into the "anatomical position" when the patient makes a fist. Make a strong fist to notice this action on yourself.

The inverted hands test of Fig. 14-12 helps to identify hysterical hand paralysis. With the patient's hands in the inverted position, point to, but do not touch, a finger and ask the patient to move the finger. Usually the patient moves the finger of the opposite hand. Try this test on a partner. Notice that after a few trials the subject learns to respond accurately. Thus, it serves best the first few times you try it.

While hysterics may show paralysis in monoplegic, hemiplegic, or paraplegic distributions, they do not show paralysis in individual muscles or groups of muscles innervated by a single peripheral nerve or root, nor do their limbs assume organic postures. Of course, the muscle stretch reflexes and plantar responses remain normal. The hysterical patient with paraplegia, rarely loses bladder and bowel control. The organic paraplegic does lose bladder and bowel control. In any hysterical monoplegia, hemiplegia, or paraplegia, the patient moves the parts in the normal manner during sleep.

F. Hysterical seizures, syncope, and loss of consciousness

Hysterical patients frequently have various types of dizziness, blackout spells, fainting, or pseudoepileptic seizures. These often occur in association with hyperventilation. As part of the neurologic examination, have the patient hyperventilate for 3 min to see whether it reproduces the episodes. Usually hysterical lapses of consciousness occur after some identifiable precipitating event. Most commonly they occur in the presence of someone emotionally significant to the patient, such as a parent or lover, or to avoid some unpleasant circumstance. Usually hysterical patients do not injure themselves if they fall, nor do they bite their tongue, or become incontinent, all of which frequently occur with organic syncope or epileptic seizures. If you can observe an episode, you generally will find that the patient does not show the autonomic phenomena of organic syncope or seizures, with distinct changes in blood pressure, pulse rate, or pupillary size. In some instances, however, even an experienced observer cannot distinguish an hysteric attack from an organic attack. In these instances electroencephalographic and electrocardiographic monitoring may exclude epilepsy or organic syncope by showing normal records during an hysterical attack. Whenever you observe a patient with any undiagnosed type of attack which alters or obtunds consciousness, or results in a frank seizure, always draw a sample of blood to measure glucose.

G. Fevers of unknown origin

The physician always has to consider doing a lumbar puncture in patients with fever of unknown origin. Malingerers may produce false temperature elevations. In every patient with a puzzling fever of unknown origin, obtain a freshly passed sample of urine and measure its temperature yourself. The urine specimen will record the true body temperature rather than some manipulation the patient manages with the thermometer (Murray et al., 1977).

H. Vomiting

Some hysterical or malingering patients have functional vomiting. Usually the patient can, on some occasions, be observed to induce the vomiting by gagging, or the vomiting occurs in the presence of emotionally significant people.

I. Some final caveats in the diagnosis of hysteria

Some patients with puzzling organic disorders, in making the rounds from doctor to doctor, elaborate on or exaggerate their organic disorders in desparation as they try to convince the doctor of their illness. Thus the patient may display both organic and functional disease. This violates the parsimony principle of seeking a single diagnosis, but by keeping the issue open you may avoid a serious diagnostic error.

Don't let functional patients perceive you as trying to unmask or expose them. Once you have convinced yourself of the functional nature of the patient's complaint do not triumphantly confront the patient with the evidence and say, "Quit faking. It's all in your mind." Let the patient retain the dignity of patienthood. The symptom serves some need for the patient. The patient will relinquish it after resolution of the problem which has caused it. Don't rush things. You can suggest that your findings indicate a disorder from which the patient may ultimately make a complete recovery, but beyond that, avoid confrontation and parlor tricks such as hypnosis or electric shocks to "speed up" recovery. In other words, treat causes, not effects. Similar remarks hold for the patients with chronic pain syndromes which represent complicated mixtures of organic disease, functionally overlay, depression, and hostility. Physicians often assume a pejorative attitude to these puzzling and troublesome patients, calling them by such offensive and truly obscene names as, "crocks," "gomers," or "turkeys." Remember yet another aphorism: A patient who gets a pejorative label is a patient whom the physician has failed to understand.

Lastly, never diagnose a functional illness by exclusion because you cannot think of anything else. Call in a consultant who just may recognize the porphyria, smoldering collagen disease, occult carcinoma, parasitic infestation, chronic liver abscess, or multiple sclerosis that you didn't even think about. Remember this:

There are more things in heaven and earth, Horatio,
than are dreamt of in your philosophy.

William Shakespeare

V. And lastly remember this ancient adage, giving the goals of the physician:

A painless examination
A complete cure
Leaving no blemish behind

Bibliography

Abse, D. W.: *Hysteria and Related Mental Disorders,* Baltimore, Williams and Wilkins, 1966.

Aminoff, M. J., Dedo, H. H., Izdebski, K.: Clinical aspects of spasmodic dysphonia, *J. Neurol. Neurosurg. Psych.,* 41:361-365, 1978.

Benson, D. F., and Blumer, D.: *Psychiatric Aspects of Neurological Disease,* New York, Grune and Stratton, 1975.

Cavenar, J. O., Jr., Brantley, I. J., Braasch, E.: Blepharospasm: Organic or functional? *Psychosomatics,* 19:623-628, 1978.

DePaulo, J. R., and Folstein, M. F.: Psychiatric disturbances in neurological patients: Detection, recognition, and hospital course, *Annals of Neurol.,* 4: 225-228, 1978.

Ellis, J. M., and Lee, S. I.: Acute prolonged confusion in later life as an ictal state, *Epilepsia,* 19:119-128, 1978.

Finlayson, R. E., and Lucas, A. R.: Psuedo-epileptic seizures in children and adolescents, *Mayo Clin. Proc.,* 54:83-87, 1979.

Griffin, J. F., Wray, S. H., Anderson, D. P.: Misdiagnosis of spasm of the near reflex, *Neurology (Minneap),* 26:1018-1020, 1976.

Hill, O. W.: Psychogenic vomiting, *Gut,* 9:348-352, 1968.

Livingston, S.: Breathholding spells in children, *JAMA,* 212:2231-2235, 1970.

Markand, O. N., Wheeler, G. L., Pollack, S. L.: Complex partial status epilepticus, *Neurology,* 28:189-196, 1978.

Murray, H. W., Tuazon, C. U., Guerrero, I. C. et al.: Urinary temperature: A clue to early diagnosis of factitious fever, *New Eng. J. Med.,* 296:23, 1977.

Perley, M. J., and Guze, S. B.: Hysteria—the stability and usefulness of clinical criteria, *New Eng. J. Med.,* 266:421-426, 1962.

Woolsey, R. M.: Hysteria: 1875–1975, *Dis. Nerv. Syst.,* 37:379-386, 1976.

Yarnell, P., Melamed, E., Silverberg, R.: Global hemianesthesia: A parietal perceptual distortion suggesting non-organic illness, *J. Neurol. Neurosurg.* Psych., 9:843-846, 1978.

Neurologic examination

Brock, S., and Krieger, H.: *The Basis of Clinical Neurology,* 4th ed., Baltimore, The Williams and Wilkins Co., 1963.

Chusid, J., and McDonald, J.: *Correlative Neuroanatomy and Functional Neurology,* Los Altos, Lange Medical Publications, 14th ed., 1970.

DeJong, R.: *The Neurologic Examination,* 3rd ed., New York, Hoeber Medical Division, Harper & Row, 1967.

Haymaker, W.: *Bing's Local Diagnosis in Neurological Diseases,* 15th ed., St. Louis, The C. V. Mosby Co., 1969.

Mayo Clinic: *Clinical Examinations in Neurology,* 4th ed., Philadelphia, W. B. Saunders Co., 1976.

Monrad-Krohn, G.: *The Clinical Examination of the Nervous System,* 12th ed., New York, Hoeber Medical Division, Harper & Row, Publishers, 1964.

Paine, R., and Oppe, T.: *Neurological Examination of Children,* New York, William Heinemann Medical Books Ltd., 1966.

Van Allen, M.: *Pictorial Manual of Neurologic Tests,* Chicago, Year Book Medical Publishers, 1969.

Wartenberg, R.: *The Examination of Reflexes. A Simplification,* Chicago, Year Book Medical Publishers, 1945.

General neurology

Adams, R. D., and Victor, M.: *Principles of Neurology,* New York, McGraw-Hill, 1977.

Aita, J.: *Neurologic Manifestations of General Diseases,* Springfield, Charles C Thomas, Publisher, 1964.

Alpers, B., and Mancall, E.: *Clinical Neurology,* 6th ed., Philadelphia, F. A. Davis, 1971.

Baker, A., and Baker, L. (eds.): *Clinical Neurology,* vols. I–III, 3rd ed., New York, Hoeber Medical Division, Harper & Row, Publishers, 1973.

Bodechtel, G.: *Differentialdiagnose Neurologischer Krankheitsbilder,* 2nd ed., Stuttgart, Georg Thieme Verlag, 1963.

Bray, P.: *Neurology in Pediatrics,* Chicago, Year Book Medical Publishers, 1969.

Elliott, F.: *Clinical Neurology,* 2nd ed., Philadelphia, W. B. Saunders, 1971.

Farmer, T. (ed.): *Pediatric Neurology,* 2nd ed., New York, Hoeber Medical Division, Harper & Row, Publishers, 1975.

Ford, F.: *Diseases of the Nervous System in Infancy, Childhood and Adolescence,* 6th ed., Springfield, Charles C Thomas, Publisher, 1973.

Gamstorp, I.: *Pediatric Neurology,* New York, Appleton-Century-Crofts, 1970.

Gilroy, J., and Meyer, J.: *Medical Neurology,* London, The Macmillan Company, 1969.

Jabbour, J., Duenas, D., Gilmartin, R., and Gottlieb, M.: *Pediatric Neurology Handbook,* New York, Medical Examination Publishing Co., 1973.

Merritt, H. H.: *A Textbook of Neurology,* 6th ed., Philadelphia, Lea and Febiger, 1979.

O'Doherty, D. S., and Fermaglich, J. L.: *Handbook of Neurologic Emergencies,* Flushing, N. Y., Medical Examination Publishing Co., Inc., 1977.

Pryse-Phillips, W., and Murray, T. J.: *Essential Neurology,* Garden City, N. Y., Medical Examination Publishing Co., Inc., 1978.

Scheinberg, L., Taylor, J., and Schaumburg, H.: *Neurology Handbook,* Flushing, Medical Examination Publishing Co., 1972.

Wilson, S.: *Neurology,* vols I–III, 2nd ed., Baltimore, The Williams & Wilkins Co., 1955.

Index

Index